DVD Contents

*From Canale ST, Beaty JH. Campbell's Operative Orthopaedics, 11th Ed. Philadelphia: Mosby-Elsevier, 2008.

pediatric orthopaedic
surgery

OPERATIVE TECHNIQUES

pediatric orthopaedic
surgery

Mininder S. Kocher, MD, MPH
Associate Director, Division of Sports Medicine
Director, Clinical Effectiveness Research Unit
Children's Hospital Boston
Associate Professor of Orthopaedic Surgery
Harvard Medical School
Boston, Massachusetts

Michael B. Millis, MD
Director, Adolescent and Young Adult Hip Unit
Children's Hospital Boston
Professor of Orthopaedic Surgery
Harvard Medical School
Boston, Massachusetts

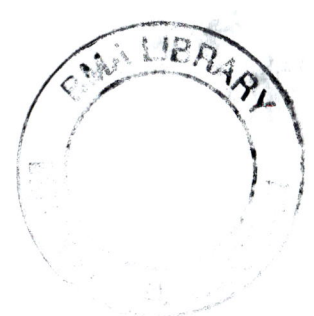

ELSEVIER
SAUNDERS

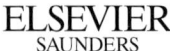

ELSEVIER
SAUNDERS

1600 John F. Kennedy Blvd.
Ste 1800
Philadelphia, PA 19103-2899

OPERATIVE TECHNIQUES: PEDIATRIC ORTHOPAEDIC SURGERY   ISBN: 978-1-4160-4915-9

Notices

Knowledge and best practice in this field are constantly changing. As new research and experience broaden our understanding, changes in research methods, professional practices, or medical treatment may become necessary.

Practitioners and researchers must always rely on their own experience and knowledge in evaluating and using any information, methods, compounds, or experiments described herein. In using such information or methods they should be mindful of their own safety and the safety of others, including parties for whom they have a professional responsibility.

With respect to any drug or pharmaceutical products identified, readers are advised to check the most current information provided (i) on procedures featured or (ii) by the manufacturer of each product to be administered, to verify the recommended dose or formula, the method and duration of administration, and contraindications. It is the responsibility of practitioners, relying on their own experience and knowledge of their patients, to make diagnoses, to determine dosages and the best treatment for each individual patient, and to take all appropriate safety precautions.

To the fullest extent of the law, neither the Publisher nor the authors, contributors, or editors, assume any liability for any injury and/or damage to persons or property as a matter of products liability, negligence or otherwise, or from any use or operation of any methods, products, instructions, or ideas contained in the material herein.

Library of Congress Cataloging-in-Publication Data

Pediatric orthopaedic surgery / [edited by] Mininder S. Kocher, Michael B. Millis.
    p. ; cm. — (Operative techniques)
  Includes bibliographical references and index.
  ISBN 978-1-4160-4915-9 (hardcover : alk. paper)
 1. Pediatric orthopedics. I. Kocher, Mininder S. II. Millis, Michael B. III. Series: Operative techniques.
  [DNLM: 1. Orthopedic Procedures—Atlases. 2. Adolescent. 3. Child. 4. Infant. WS 17]
  RD732.3.C48P4313 2011
  618.92'7—dc22   2010041114

Acquisitions Editor: Dolores Meloni
Developmental Editor: Taylor E. Ball
Publishing Services Manager: Pat Joiner-Myers
Senior Project Manager: Joy Moore
Design Direction: Steven Stave

Printed in the United States of America

Last digit is the print number: 9 8 7 6 5 4 3 2 1

We dedicate this book to Dr. John E. Hall, world-renowned healer of countless injured and deformed children, peerless surgeon and sensitive physician. He has mentored generations of orthopaedic surgeons around the globe. His standards of clinical excellence transcended technical skill. He has imbued in his pupils and colleagues a commitment to the highest possible level of execution in every step of the therapeutic process, particularly including operative care.

Dr. Hall, revered role model, mentor, senior colleague, and dear friend, we salute you and thank you.

CONTRIBUTORS

Jay C. Albright, MD
Director of Pediatric Sports Medicine, Arnold Palmer
Hospital for Children, Orlando, Florida
Proximal Humerus Fracture: Reduction and Fixation
with Elastic Nail; Osteochondritis Dissecans:
Arthroscopic Evaluation and Extra-articular
Drilling with or without Fixation

Sameer Badarudeen, MD, MPH
Resident, Department of Orthopaedic Surgery,
Boston Medical Center, Boston University, Boston,
Massachusetts
Radial Head/Neck Fracture: Closed Reduction,
Percutaneous Reduction, and Open Reduction

Robert M. Bernstein, MD
Director, Pediatric Orthopaedics, Cedars-Sinai
Medical Center, Los Angeles, California
Radial Head/Neck Fracture: Closed Reduction,
Percutaneous Reduction, and Open Reduction

Saul M. Bernstein, MD*
Clinical Professor of Orthopaedics, Keck School of
Medicine at the University of Southern California,
Los Angeles, California
Radial Head/Neck Fracture: Closed Reduction,
Percutaneous Reduction, and Open Reduction

Brian K. Brighton, MD, MPH
Pediatric Orthopaedic Surgeon, Department of
Orthopaedic Surgery, Carolinas Medical Center,
Charlotte, North Carolina
Open Reduction and Internal Fixation of Tibial
Tubercle Fractures

Michael Busch, MD
Surgical Director of Sports Medicine and Fellowship
Director, Children's Healthcare of Atlanta at
Scottish Rite, Atlanta, Georgia
Arthroscopic Management for Juvenile
Osteochondritis Dissecans of the Talus

Robert M. Campbell, Jr., MD
Attending Physician, Division of Orthopaedics, and
Director, The Center for Thoracic Insufficiency
Syndrome, The Children's Hospital of Philadelphia,
Philadelphia, Pennsylvania
Vertical Expandable Prosthetic Titanium Rib (VEPTR)
Expansion Thoracoplasty

Henry G. Chambers, MD
Pediatric Orthopedic Surgeon, Rady Children's
Hospital, San Diego; David Sutherland Director of
Cerebral Palsy Research, Director of CHAMPS
Sports Medicine, and Medical Affairs Officer, Rady
Children's Hospital and Health Center—
San Diego; Clinical Professor, Department of
Orthopedic Surgery, University of California, San
Diego, San Diego, California
Forearm Fractures: Intramedullary Rodding

Constantine A. Demetracopoulos, MD
Resident, Department of Orthopaedic Surgery,
Hospital for Special Surgery, New York, New York
Ponseti Method for Idiopathic Clubfoot Deformity;
Resection of Talocalcaneal Tarsal Coalition and Fat
Autograft Interposition; Resection of
Calcaneonavicular Coalition and Fat Autograft
Interposition

Mohammad Diab, MD
Associate Professor of Orthopaedic Surgery,
University of California, San Francisco, San
Francisco, California
Hip Pyarthritis

Matthew Diltz, MD
Eisenhower Medical Center, Rancho Mirage,
California
Repair of Proximal Hamstring Avulsion; Femur
Fracture: Closed Reduction and Spica Cast;
Osteochondritis Dissecans Fixation

Craig J. Finlayson, MD
Attending Physician, Children's Memorial Hospital,
Chicago, Illinois
Transphyseal ACL Reconstruction in Skeletally
Immature Patients Using Autogenous Hamstring
Tendon

John M. Flynn, MD
Associate Professor of Orthopaedic Surgery,
University of Pennsylvania School of Medicine;
Associate Chief of Orthopaedic Surgery, The
Children's Hospital of Philadelphia, Philadelphia,
Pennsylvania
Femur Fracture: Flexible Intramedullary Nailing

*Deceased.

Jeremy S. Frank, MD
Department of Orthopaedic Surgery, Children's
Hospital Boston, Boston, Massachusetts
Chevron Osteotomy for Adolescent Hallux Valgus

Theodore J. Ganley, MD
Sports Medicine Director and Attending Physician,
The Children's Hospital of Philadelphia; Assistant
Professor of Orthopaedic Surgery, University of
Pennsylvania School of Medicine, Philadelphia,
Pennsylvania
Discoid Lateral Meniscus

Purushottam Arjun Gholve, MD
Assistant Professor of Orthopaedic Surgery, Tufts
University School of Medicine; Pediatric
Orthopaedist, Floating Hospital for Children at
Tufts Medical Center, Boston, Massachusetts
Femur Fracture: Flexible Intramedullary Nailing

Michael Glotzbecker, MD
Department of Orthopaedic Surgery, Children's
Hospital Boston, Boston, Massachusetts
Tibialis Posterior Tendon Transfer

Charles A. Goldfarb, MD
Associate Professor of Orthopaedic Surgery,
Washington University School of Medicine;
Associate Professor of Orthopaedic Surgery,
Barnes-Jewish Hospital, St. Louis, Missouri
Modified Woodward Procedure for Sprengel's
Deformity

J. Eric Gordon, MD
Associate Professor, Washington University School of
Medicine; Associate Professor, St. Louis Children's
Hospital, St. Louis, Missouri
Femur Fracture: Lateral Trochanteric Entry Rigid
Nailing

Daniel J. Hedequist, MD
Assistant Professor of Orthopaedic Surgery, Harvard
Medical School, Boston, Massachusetts
Hemivertebra Resection; Posterior Surgical
Treatment for Scheuermann's Kyphosis; Scoliosis
Correction

William Hennrikus, MD
Professor of Orthopaedics and Pediatrics and
Associate Dean of Education, Penn State Medical
School, Hershey, Pennsylvania
Open Reduction and Internal Fixation of Displaced
Medial Epicondyle Fracture Using a Screw and
Washer

John E. Herzenberg, MD, FRCSC
Director of the Rubin Institute for Advanced
Orthopaedics, International Center for Limb
Lengthening, Sinai Hospital of Baltimore,
Baltimore, Maryland
Femoral Lengthening with External Fixation; Tibial
Lengthening with Circular External Fixation

Douglas T. Hutchinson, MD
Associate Professor, Department of Orthopaedics,
University of Utah, Salt Lake City, Utah
Digital Syndactyly Release

Michelle A. James, MD
Chief, Division of Pediatric Orthopaedics, and
Professor of Clinical Orthopaedic Surgery,
University of California, Davis, School of Medicine,
Sacramento; Clinical Professor of Orthopaedic
Surgery, University of California, San Francisco,
San Francisco; Chief of Orthopaedic Surgery,
Shriners Hospital for Children Northern California,
Sacramento, California
Shoulder External Rotation Tendon Transfers for
Brachial Plexus Birth Palsy

Lawrence I. Karlin, MD
Department of Orthopaedic Surgery, Children's
Hospital Boston, Boston, Massachusetts
Anterior Spinal Instrumentation and Fusion for
Lumbar and Thoracolumbar Idiopathic Scoliosis

Kathryn A. Keeler, MD
Assistant Professor, Department of Orthopaedic
Surgery, Washington University School of
Medicine; St. Louis Children's Hospital; Shriners
Hospital, St. Louis, Missouri
Femur Fracture: Lateral Trochanteric Entry Rigid
Nailing; Triplane Fractures

Young-Jo Kim, MD, PhD
Associate Professor of Orthopaedic Surgery, Harvard
Medical School; Department of Orthopaedic
Surgery, Children's Hospital Boston, Boston,
Massachusetts
Triple Pelvic Osteotomy

Mininder S. Kocher, MD, MPH
Associate Director, Division of Sports Medicine, and
Director, Clinical Effectiveness Research Unit,
Children's Hospital Boston; Associate Professor of
Orthopaedic Surgery, Harvard Medical School,
Boston, Massachusetts
Repair of Proximal Hamstring Avulsion; Femur
Fracture: Closed Reduction and Spica Cast;
Osteochondritis Dissecans Fixation; Transphyseal
ACL Reconstruction in Skeletally Immature
Patients Using Autogenous Hamstring Tendon;
Physeal-Sparing ACL Reconstruction in Skeletally
Immature Patients Using Iliotibial Band Technique

Dennis E. Kramer, MD
Instructor, Department of Orthopaedic Surgery,
Children's Hospital Boston, Boston, Massachusetts
Closed Reduction and Pinning of Distal Radius
Fractures; Patellar Instability: Lateral Release and
Medial Plication; Tibial Spine Fracture:
Arthroscopic and Open Reduction and Internal
Fixation

James A. Krcik, MD
South Suburban Hospital, Hazel Crest; Ingalls
Memorial Hospital, Harvey, Illinois
Physeal-Sparing ACL Reconstruction in Skeletally
Immature Patients Using Iliotibial Band Technique;
Chevron Osteotomy for Adolescent Hallux Valgus

Paul R.T. Kuzyk, MASc, MD, FRCS(C)
Clinical Fellow, Harvard University, Boston,
Massachusetts
Flexion Osteotomy for Slipped Capital Femoral
Epiphysis

Jennifer C. Laine, MD
Resident, Department of Orthopaedic Surgery,
University of California, San Francisco, San
Francisco, California
Hip Pyarthritis

Jakub S. Langer, MD
Clinical Instructor of Orthopaedics, and Hand and
Upper Extremity Fellow, University of Utah, Salt
Lake City, Utah
Modified Woodward Procedure for Sprengel's
Deformity

Justin M. LaReau, MD
Hinsdale Orthopaedic Associates, Hinsdale, Illinois
Bernese Periacetabular Osteotomy

Scott J. Luhmann, MD
Associate Professor, Department of Orthopaedic
Surgery, Washington University School of
Medicine; Associate Professor, St. Louis Children's
Hospital, St. Louis, Missouri
Triplane Fractures

Susan T. Mahan, MD, MPH
Instructor in Orthopaedic Surgery, Harvard Medical
School; Orthopaedic Staff Surgeon, Children's
Hospital Boston, Boston, Massachusetts
Lateral Humeral Condyle Fracture: Closed Reduction
and Percutaneous Pinning and Open Reduction
and Internal Fixation; Flexor Tenotomy for
Congenital Curly Toe

Lisa D. Maskill, MD
Clinical Fellow, Shriners Hospital for Children
Northern California, Sacramento, California
Shoulder External Rotation Tendon Transfers for
Brachial Plexus Birth Palsy

Travis Matheney, MD
Instructor, Department of Orthopaedic Surgery,
Harvard Medical School; Staff Surgeon,
Department of Orthopaedic Surgery, Children's
Hospital Boston, Boston, Massachusetts
Bernese Periacetabular Osteotomy; Tibialis Posterior
Tendon Transfer; Split Transfer of the Tibialis
Anterior Tendon

Lyle J. Micheli, MD
Clinical Professor of Orthopaedic Surgery and Sports
Medicine, Harvard Medical School; O'Donnell
Family Professor of Sports Medicine, Children's
Hospital Boston, Boston, Massachusetts
Chevron Osteotomy for Adolescent Hallux Valgus

Michael B. Millis, MD
Director, Adolescent and Young Adult Hip Unit,
Children's Hospital Boston; Professor of
Orthopaedic Surgery, Harvard Medical School,
Boston, Massachusetts
Surgical Dislocation of the Hip; Percutaneous in situ
Cannulated Screw Fixation of Slipped Capital
Femoral Epiphysis; Bernese Periacetabular
Osteotomy; Greater Trochanteric Transfer/Relative
Femoral Neck Lengthening

Scott J. Mubarak, MD
Clinical Professor, Department of Orthopedics,
University of California, San Diego; Director of
Orthopedic Program, Children's Hospital, San
Diego, California
Osteotomies of the Foot for Cavus Deformities;
Calcaneal-Cuboid-Cuneiform Osteotomy for the
Correction of Valgus Foot Deformities

Adam Nasreddine, MA
Clinical Research Coordinator, Department of
Orthopaedic Surgery, Children's Hospital Boston,
Boston, Massachusetts
Transphyseal ACL Reconstruction in Skeletally
Immature Patients Using Autogenous Hamstring
Tendon

Peter O. Newton, MD
Associate Clinical Professor, Department of
Orthopedic Surgery, University of California, San
Diego; Chief, Scoliosis Service, Rady Children's
Hospital, San Diego, California
Thoracoscopic Release and Instrumentation for
Scoliosis

J. Megan M. Patterson, MD
Assistant Professor, Department of Orthopaedics, University of North Carolina, Chapel Hill, North Carolina
Digital Syndactyly Release

Charles T. Price, MD
Professor of Orthopedic Surgery, University of Central Florida College of Medicine; Director of Pediatric Orthopedic Education, Arnold Palmer Hospital for Children, Orlando, Florida
Forearm Fractures: Closed Treatment

Maya E. Pring, MD
Pediatric Orthopedic Surgeon, and Vice Chair, Department of Orthopedic Surgery, Rady Children's Hospital; Assistant Clinical Professor, University of California, San Diego, San Diego, California
Forearm Fractures: Intramedullary Rodding

Gleeson Rebello, MD
Instructor in Orthopaedic Surgery, Harvard Medical School; Attending Orthopedic Surgeon, Massachusetts General Hospital for Children, Boston, Massachusetts
Triple Pelvic Osteotomy

Wudbhav N. Sankar, MD
Assistant Professor of Orthopaedic Surgery, Division of Orthopaedic Surgery, The Children's Hospital of Philadelphia, Philadelphia, Pennsylvania
Surgical Dislocation of the Hip

David M. Scher, MD
Associate Professor of Clinical Orthopaedic Surgery, Weill Cornell Medical College; Associate Attending Orthopaedic Surgeon, Hospital for Special Surgery, New York, New York
Ponseti Method for Idiopathic Clubfoot Deformity; Resection of Talocalcaneal Tarsal Coalition and Fat Autograft Interposition; Resection of Calcaneonavicular Coalition and Fat Autograft Interposition

Benjamin J. Shore, MD, FRCSC
Instructor, Orthopaedic Surgery, Harvard Medical School; Attending Orthopaedic Surgeon, Children's Hospital Boston, Boston, Massachusetts
Chiari Pelvic Osteotomy; Percutaneous in situ Cannulated Screw Fixation of Slipped Capital Femoral Epiphysis; Greater Trochanteric Transfer/Relative Femoral Neck Lengthening; Knee Surgery for Children with Cerebral Palsy I: Hamstring Lengthening; Knee Surgery for Children with Cerebral Palsy II: Distal Rectus Femoris Transfer

Ernest L. Sink, MD
Associate Professor, University of Colorado Health Sciences Center, Aurora; Pediatric Orthopaedic Surgeon and Director of the Hip Program, The Children's Hospital, Denver, Colorado
Submuscular Plating for Pediatric Femur Fractures

Hua Ming Siow, MBChB (Glasgow), MMed (Orth), FRCSEd (Orth), FAMS
Clinical Tutor, Yong Loo Lin School of Medicine, National University of Singapore; Consultant and Director of Sports Medicine, Alexandra Hospital; Visiting Consultant, Department of Orthopaedic Surgery, KK Women's and Children's Hospital, Singapore
Discoid Lateral Meniscus

Brian G. Smith, MD
Associate Professor and Director of Pediatric Orthopaedics, Department of Orthopaedics, Yale University School of Medicine; Director of Pediatric Orthopaedics, Yale New Haven Children's Hospital, New Haven, Connecticut
Operative Treatment of Tillaux Fractures of the Ankle

Brian Snyder, MD, PhD
Director of Cerebral Palsy, Department of Orthopedics, Children's Hospital Boston, Boston, Massachusetts
Chiari Pelvic Osteotomy; Knee Surgery for Children with Cerebral Palsy I: Hamstring Lengthening; Knee Surgery for Children with Cerebral Palsy II: Distal Rectus Femoris Transfer

Samantha A. Spencer, MD
Clinical Instructor, Harvard Medical School; Staff Orthopaedic Surgeon, Children's Hospital Boston, Boston, Massachusetts
Epiphysiodesis of the Distal Femur/Proximal Tibia-Fibula; Sofield Osteotomy with Intramedullary Rod Fixation of the Long Bones of the Femur/Tibia

Paul D. Sponseller, MD, MBA
Lee H. Riley, Jr., Professor and Head, Division of Pediatric Orthopaedics, Johns Hopkins Medical Institutions, Baltimore, Maryland
Posterior Instrumented Reduction and Fusion for Spondylolisthesis

Craig J. Spurdle, MD
Voluntary Assistant Professor, University of Miami Miller School of Medicine; Attending Pediatric Orthopaedic Surgeon, Miami Children's Hospital; United States Ski Team Physician, Miami, Florida
Arthroscopic Management for Juvenile Osteochondritis Dissecans of the Talus

Shawn C. Standard, MD
Head of Pediatric Orthopaedics, Rubin Institute for
Advanced Orthopaedics, International Center for
Limb Lengthening, Sinai Hospital of Baltimore,
Baltimore, Maryland
Femoral Lengthening with External Fixation; Tibial
Lengthening with Circular External Fixation

Deborah F. Stanitski, MD, FRCS(C)
Emeritus Professor of Orthopaedic Surgery, Medical
University of South Carolina, Charleston, South
Carolina
Proximal Tibial Osteotomy for Blount's Disease

Peter M. Stevens, MD
Professor of Orthopaedics, University of Utah, Salt
Lake City, Utah
Guided Growth—Hemiepiphysiodesis

Eric W. Tan, BA
Medical Student, Johns Hopkins Medical Institutions,
Baltimore, Maryland
Posterior Instrumented Reduction and Fusion for
Spondylolisthesis

John E. Tis, MD
Assistant Professor, Department of Orthopaedic
Surgery, Johns Hopkins Medical Institutions,
Baltimore, Maryland
Thoracoscopic Release and Instrumentation for
Scoliosis

John Hunt Udall, MD
Fellow, Department of Orthopaedic Surgery,
Children's Hospital Boston, Boston, Massachusetts
Patellar Instability: Lateral Release and Medial
Plication

John H. Wedge, OC, MD, FRCSC
Professor of Surgery, University of Toronto; Staff
Surgeon, The Hospital for Sick Children, Toronto,
Ontario, Canada
Innominate Osteotomy

Stuart L. Weinstein, MD
Ignacio V. Ponseti Chair and Professor of
Orthopaedic Surgery, Department of Orthopaedic
Surgery, University of Iowa, Iowa City, Iowa
Anteromedial Approach to a Developmentally
Dislocated Hip

Yi-Meng Yen, MD, PhD
Instructor in Orthopaedic Surgery, Harvard Medical
School; Department of Orthopaedic Surgery,
Children's Hospital Boston, Boston, Massachusetts
Open Reduction and Internal Fixation of Tibial
Tubercle Fractures

Ira Zaltz, MD
Section Chief, Pediatric Orthopaedics, Department
of Orthopaedic Surgery, William Beaumont
Hospital, Royal Oak; Senior Staff Surgeon, Section
of Pediatric Orthopaedics, Henry Ford Health
System, Detroit, Michigan
Single-Incision Supraperiosteal Triple Innominate
Osteotomy

PREFACE

We editors are fortunate to have been taught many of our most important surgical techniques directly, in hands-on fashion, by some of the surgical giants of orthopaedic surgery. This text is envisioned as an important part of the next-best-thing to learning pediatric orthopaedic surgical techniques directly from a master.

We have selected 60 important and frequently done procedures that a pediatric orthopaedist should have in his or her armamentarium for optimal patient care. The contributors work in many different centers and clinical environments, but all contributions uniformly reflect deep experience with techniques of recognized clinical utility.

The format is clear, easy to use, and it has been very effective in previous titles in this series. While no text can completely replace either personal experience or direct, face-to-face learning from an expert, we offer this focused text as a useful handbook of contemporary pediatric orthopaedic surgical practice.

Mininder S. Kocher, MD, MPH
Michael B. Millis, MD

FOREWORD

The history of orthopaedics as a medical discipline is based in pediatric orthopaedics. In 1741, Nicholas Andry published a small monograph entitled "L'Orthopedie," deriving the term from the Greek words meaning "straight child." In addition, Andry provided an illustration of a crooked tree tied to a straight stake, which has become the emblem of orthopaedics.

In fact, many of the oldest and seminal procedures in orthopaedics are derived from pediatric orthopaedics, such as bracing and manipulation for deformity, osteotomy for deformity, amputation for congenital abnormalities, and spinal fusion for scoliosis. Although many surgical techniques in pediatric orthopaedics have remained the same over the years, there has also been much innovation. In general, procedures in pediatric orthopaedics must take into consideration the growth of the child and the long-term outcome and sequelae in adulthood. In addition, the biology of the child differs from the adult, allowing for more rapid healing, remodeling with growth, more robust periosteum, and more biologic fixation.

This volume of *Operative Techniques: Pediatric Orthopaedic Surgery* provides an excellent overview of modern procedures in pediatric orthopaedics. The range of topics is broad from the hand and upper extremity, to the spine, to the foot and lower extremity. Both "classic" pediatric orthopaedic procedures, such as innominate osteotomy and Woodward

procedure, and "contemporary" pediatric orthopaedic procedures, such as submuscular plating of femur fractures and surgical dislocation of the hip, are included. Some procedures, such as spica casting for femur fracture and Ponseti correction of clubfoot deformity are both "classic" and "contemporary."

This volume provides concise surgical techniques and excellent illustrations. However, pearls of wisdom, indications, and pitfalls are not skipped. This volume will serve as an excellent resource for resident, pediatric orthopaedic fellow, general orthopaedist, and pediatric orthopaedic surgeon. The chapter authors are eminent in their field and are to be commended for their excellent contributions.

The tradition of pediatric orthopaedics is strong at Children's Hospital Boston. The teaching of surgical mastery is a fundamental part of this tradition, emphasized from Frank Ober, to W.T. Green, to John Hall. Doctors Kocher and Millis continue this tradition and are to be congratulated on this important resource.

James R. Kasser, MD
Surgeon-in-Chief, Children's Hospital Boston
Orthopaedic Surgeon-in-Chief
Children's Hospital Boston
Catherine Ormandy Professor of
Orthopaedic Surgery, Harvard Medical School
Boston, Massachusetts

Contents

xx

Contents

SHOULDER

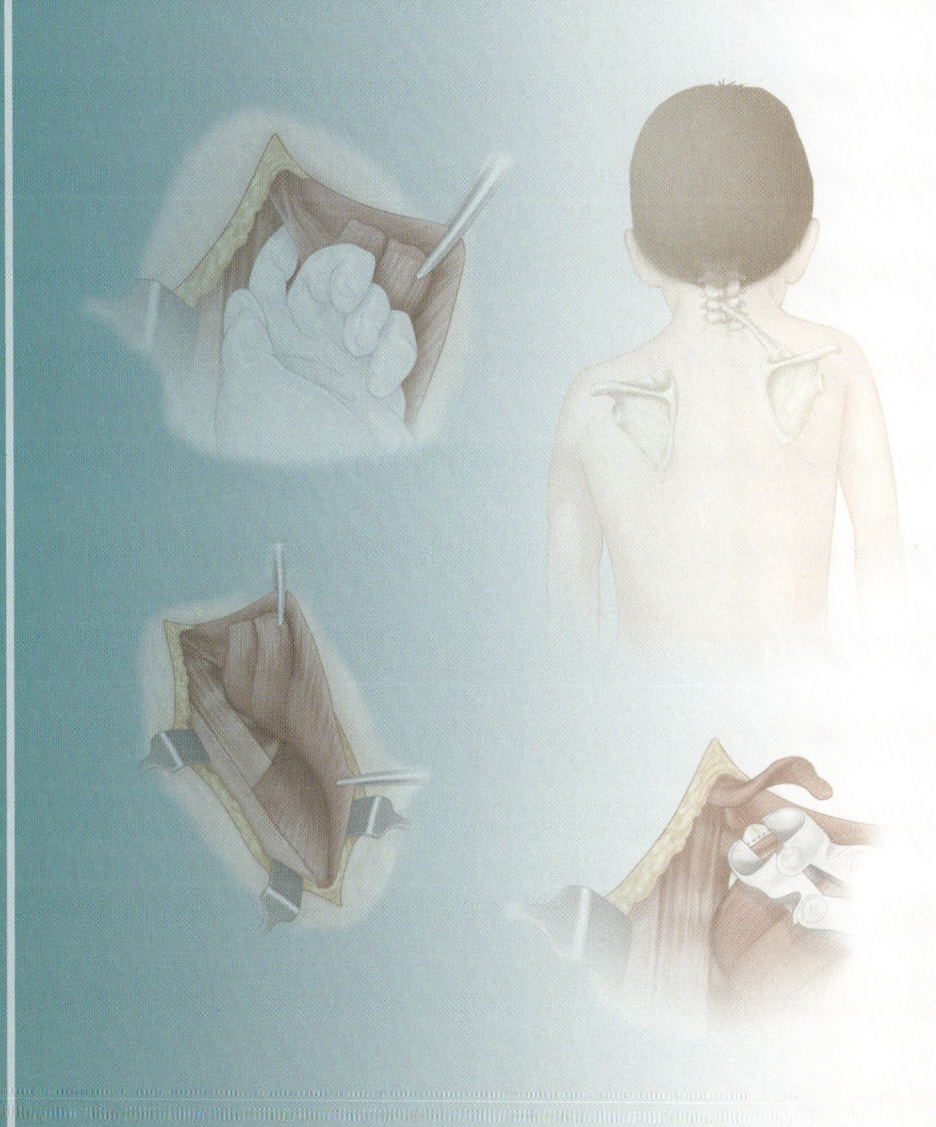

Modified Woodward Procedure for Sprengel's Deformity

Charles A. Goldfarb and Jakub S. Langer

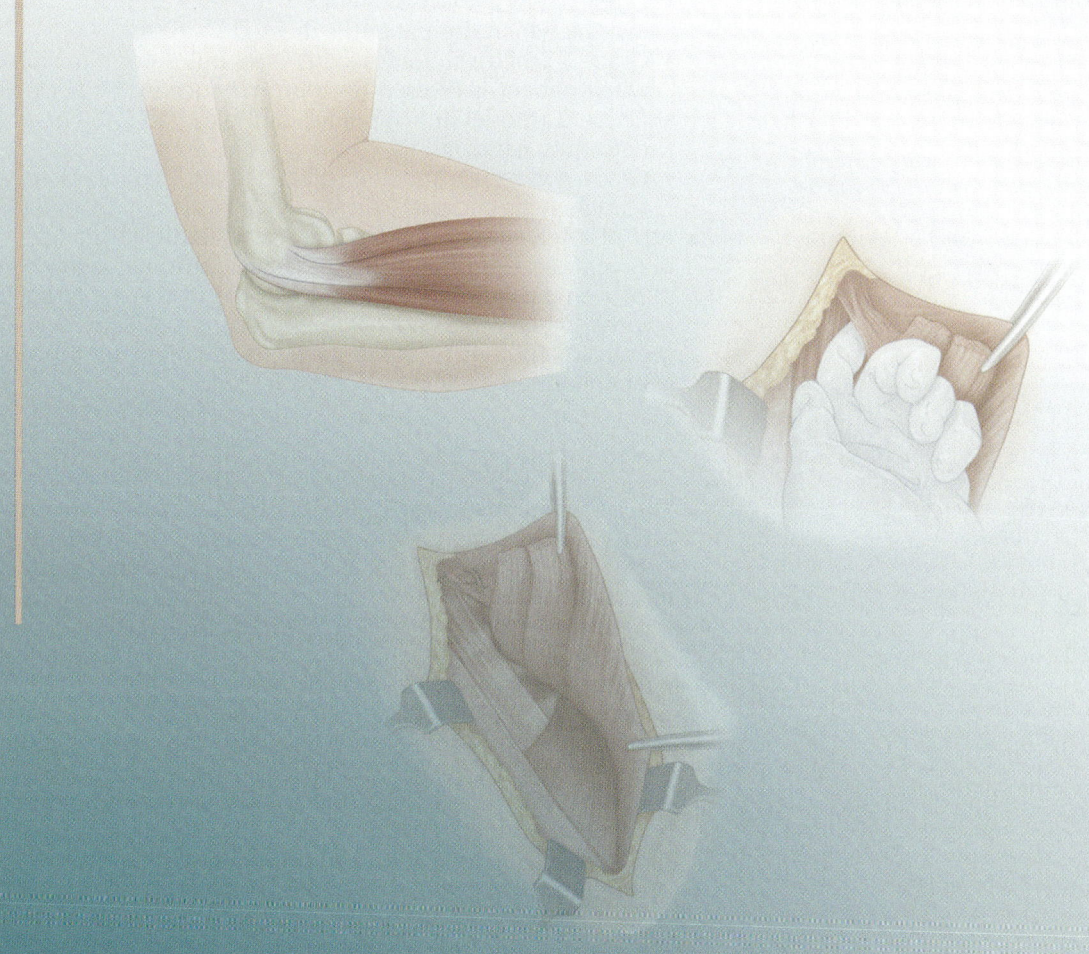

INDICATIONS

- Operative intervention is considered in children with functional limitations, including those with decreased shoulder forward flexion and/or abduction. Children with a range of motion of less than 120° in either plane have the greatest potential for improvement after surgery.

- Operative intervention is also considered for aesthetic reasons due to the fact that the undescended scapula is quite noticeable.

- The Cavendish classification of Sprengel's deformity (Cavendish, 1972) may be helpful in assessing the need for operative intervention based on appearance. A limited intervention such as excision of superomedial scapular prominence may be utilized for grades 1 and 2 whereas a more significant procedure to relocate the scapula, such as the Woodward procedure, may be more appropriate for grades 3 and 4.
  - Grade 1 (very mild): shoulder joints level and deformity invisible when the patient is dressed
  - Grade 2 (mild): shoulder joints level but deformity visible even when patient is dressed (as a prominence in the neck web)
  - Grade 3 (moderate): shoulder joint elevated 2–5 cm with deformity easily visible
  - Grade 4 (severe): shoulder greater than 5 cm elevated with scapula near occiput

- Age of intervention: The trend in treatment is for earlier intervention as it offers a better chance at functional improvement. Intervention between 3 and 6 years of age is favored, while others advocate intervention as early as 6–9 months. Nonetheless, some surgeons still offer the procedure in later childhood (5–9 years) or adolescence.

EXAMINATION/IMAGING

- The general appearance of the patient is assessed, with specific attention to the symmetry of the shoulders. The patient is evaluated with the arms at the sides and in various positions of function. When both scapulae are undescended, there is less asymmetry but still a noticeable abnormality. Figure 1 demonstrates the typical appearance of a right-sided unilateral deformity as seen in the anterior clinical view of a 3-year-old patient.

- Shoulder range of motion is measured, with particular attention to active forward flexion and abduction. Figure 2 shows posterior clinical views of a 4-year-old patient with deficient right-sided abduction secondary to Sprengel's deformity preoperatively (Fig. 2A) and postoperatively (Fig. 2B). Passive glenohumeral abduction and rotation are typically normal, whereas scapulothoracic motion is most severely affected. Additionally, upper extremity strength may be decreased.

- An anteroposterior radiograph to include both shoulders and centered on the clavicles is recommended to allow side-to-side comparison of the bony anatomy. The bilateral shoulder radiograph in Figure 3 demonstrates a typical hypoplastic, undescended, and rotated right scapula in the 3-year-old patient with right-sided deformity seen in Figure 1.

- Computed tomography of both shoulders, including a three dimensional assessment, may be considered as it will provide a more detailed understanding of the anatomy.

- The physician should clinically evaluate for an accessory omovertebral bone connecting the superomedial aspect of the scapula to the mid- to lower cervical spinous process (Fig. 4); oblique shoulder radiographs and/or computed tomography scan may also be obtained.

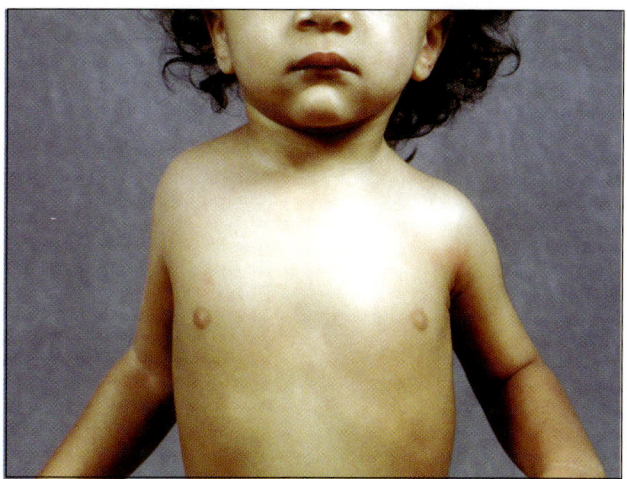

FIGURE 1

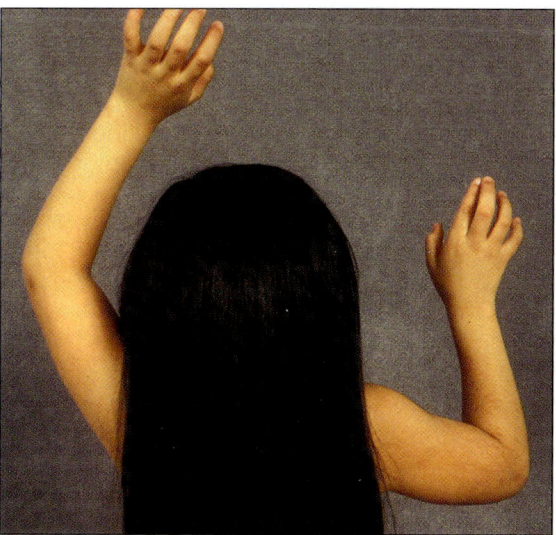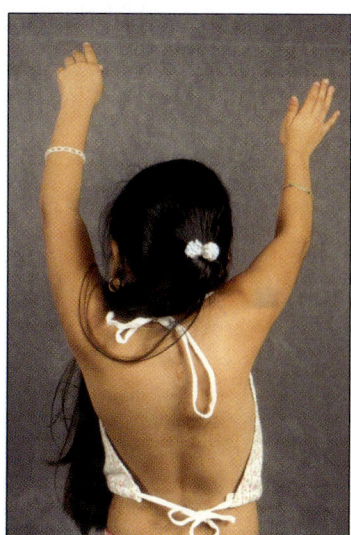

FIGURE 2 A

B

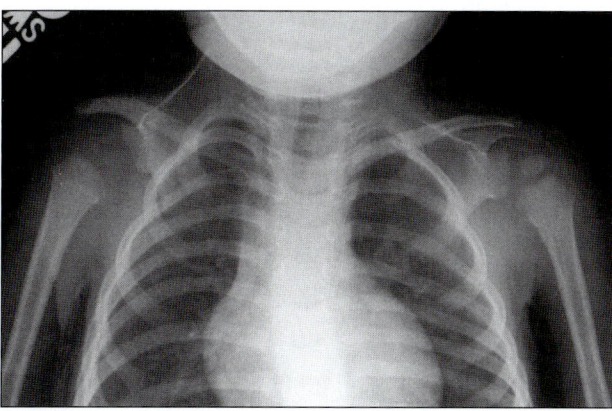

FIGURE 3

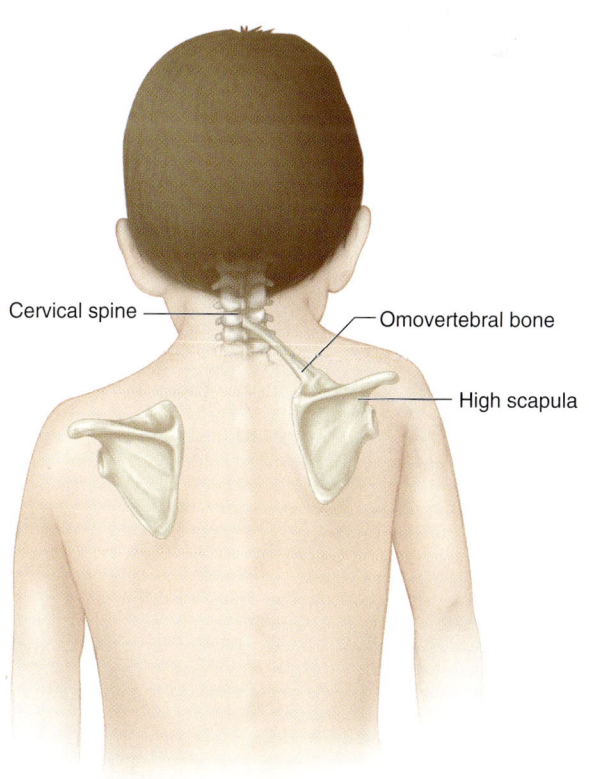

Cervical spine — — Omovertebral bone

— High scapula

FIGURE 4

Treatment Options

- Minimal deformity (Cavendish grade 1) may be treated with conservative measures, including therapy focusing on range of motion, stretching, and strengthening.
- Patients with a lesser degree of deformity (Cavendish grade 2) may be treated with resection of the prominent superior-medial scapular angle without muscle detachment and without scapular relocation.
- The modified Green procedure involves detachment of all scapular stabilizers at their insertion on the scapula and creation of an inferior pocket in the latissimus to place the scapula in a more inferior, anatomic position.
- An alternative option is a vertical scapular osteotomy with resection of the superior-medial angle and distal translation of the lateral scapula (modified Konig procedure).

PEARLS

- *Include the contralateral side in the anterior and, especially, the posterior operative fields, for ease of comparison and palpation.*
- *A radiolucent operating table will allow, if necessary, intraoperative fluoroscopy to assure satisfactory mobilization of the scapula.*

Controversies

- Some authors advocate semilateral or "floppy lateral" positioning to allow for access to the clavicle and posterior structures in one operative field, eliminating the need for redraping. We find this makes the posterior procedure awkward and prefer to simply redrape.

- The patient is evaluated for the most common associated abnormalities, including cervical vertebral deformities, such as Klippel-Feil syndrome (30%), congenital scoliosis (25%), chest wall defects/hypoplasia (25%), and renal/genitourinary disorders (10%). Other associated anomalies include diastematomyelia, long bone deficits, and ray abnormalities of the hand or foot. Renal ultrasound and cervical spine computed tomography or magnetic resonance imaging should be considered (Ross and Cruess, 1977).
- Consultations from spine and/or plastic surgeons are obtained prior to intervention to allow treatment of associated spine or chest wall deformities as needed.

SURGICAL ANATOMY

- The trapezius, one of the primary muscles released during the Woodward procedure, has a very broad origin from the occiput to the T12 spinous processes (Fig. 5).
- Thirty percent of patients will have an osseous or cartilaginous omovertebral bone linking the superior-medial angle of the scapula to the cervical spine (see Fig. 4). This is resected to allow for correction.
- Neurovascular structures to be protected:
  - The spinal accessory nerve provides innervation to the trapezius muscle and courses longitudinally along its anterior surface with the descending branch of the superficial cervical artery (deep surface when approached from posterior).
  - Branches of the dorsal scapular nerve innervate the rhomboid muscles.
  - The transverse cervical artery lies just anterior to the insertion of the levator scapulae and is at risk while releasing this muscle from the superomedial aspect of the scapula (Fig. 6).
  - Lateral dissection at the proximal scapula should be limited to avoid injury to the suprascapular neurovascular structures, located at the suprascapular notch.
  - The subclavian vessels are at risk during the clavicular osteotomy; curved Hohmann retractors placed subperiosteally will provide protection.

POSITIONING

- Initially, for the clavicular osteotomy, the patient is placed in the supine or beach chair position with a bump in the midline between the scapulae. A wide sterile field is created to include the entire upper extremity (to allow control of the clavicle) and the contralateral medial clavicle and sternum (Fig. 7).
- Following clavicular osteotomy and closure of the wound, a sterile dressing is applied and the patient is placed prone.
  - The head and neck are carefully supported with the head in a neutral to slightly flexed position. Longitudinal bolsters avoid undue pressure on the abdomen.
  - Again, the entire arm and shoulder girdle past the midline, including the opposite scapula, are prepped into the field to allow for adequate mobilization of the scapula and easy visualization and palpation of contralateral structures (Fig. 8).

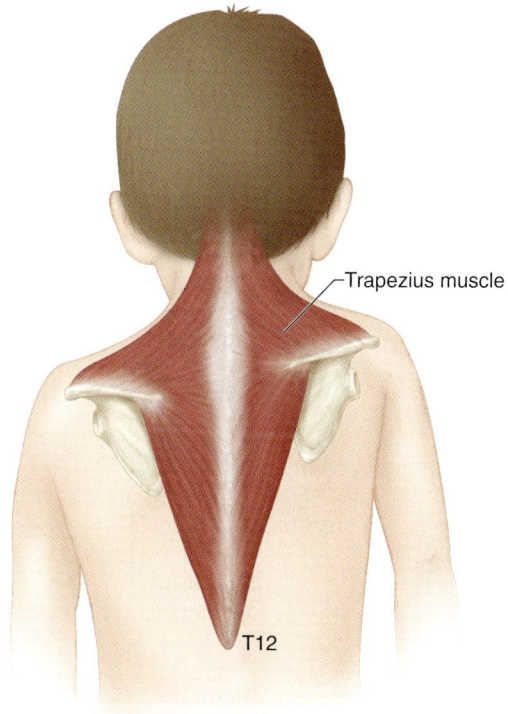

FIGURE 5

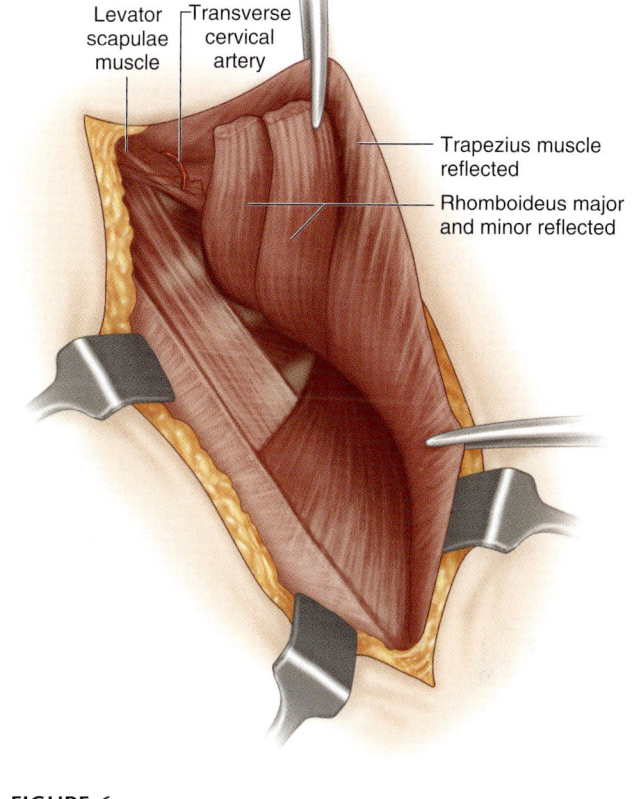

Levator scapulae muscle

Transverse cervical artery

Trapezius muscle reflected

Rhomboideus major and minor reflected

FIGURE 6

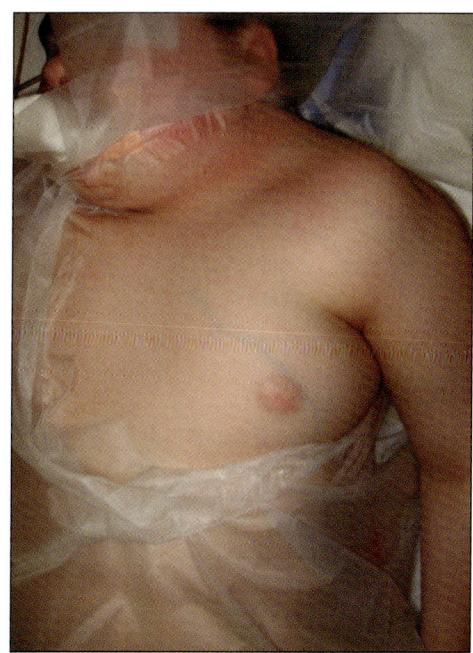

FIGURE 7

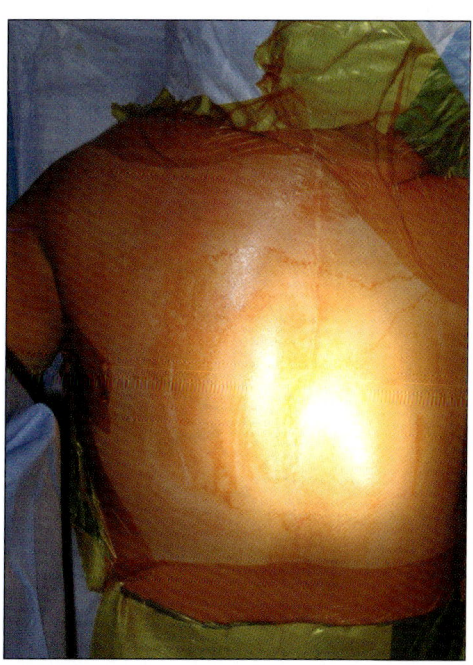

FIGURE 8

Controversies

- Some authors do not routinely perform a clavicular osteotomy, citing good results without this step especially in younger patients and those with a lesser degree of deformity. This is further discussed below.

PORTALS/EXPOSURES

- Anterior approach
  - A minimal, 2-cm incision is made over the midportion of the clavicle, with dissection carried to the periosteum (Fig. 9A). The superficial sensory nerves are protected and the platysma is detached as necessary.
  - The periosteum is incised in line with the clavicle and blunt, circumferential subperiosteal elevation is performed.
  - Subperiosteal mini-Hohmann retractors protect the subclavian vein and artery beneath the clavicle (Fig. 9B).
- Posterior approach
  - A 10- to 15-cm incision slightly lateral to midline is used from the level of the C5 spinous process to the T8 spinous process (Fig. 10).
  - Sharp dissection is carried out through the skin and subcutaneous tissue to the level of the dorsal fascia. The overlying tissues are elevated laterally to create a flap allowing visualization of the scapula and supporting musculature (see Fig. 10).

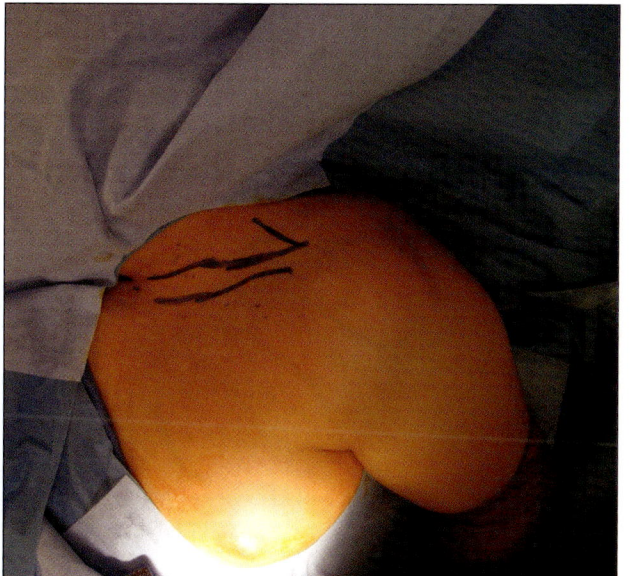 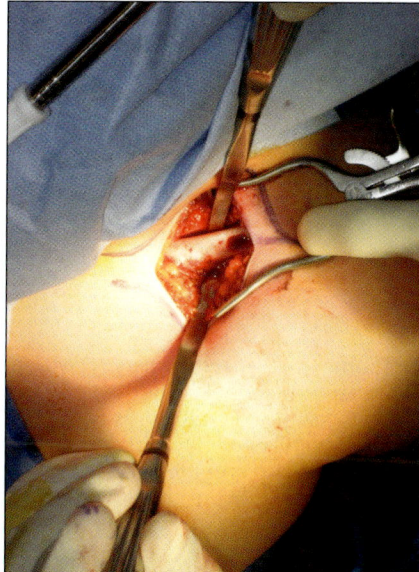

A

B

FIGURE 9

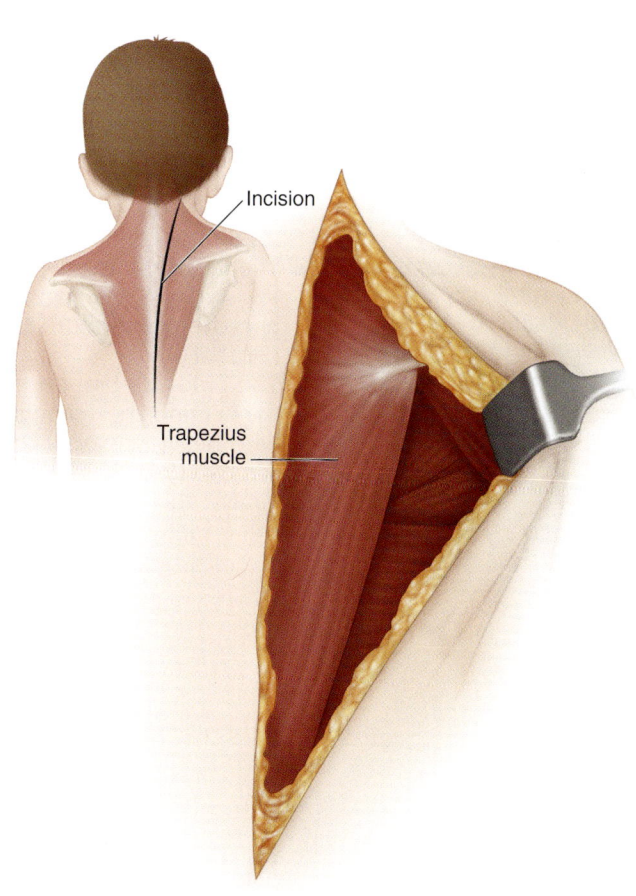

Incision

Trapezius
muscle

FIGURE 10

Controversies

- Some authors recommend clavicular osteotomy only in older patients (>6 years) or in cases of severe deformity, citing low risk of brachial plexus palsy and adequate correction without this osteotomy.
- In adolescents, it has been described that the coracoid should also be osteotomized to prevent compression of neurovascular structures against a rib.

PROCEDURE

STEP 1

- We routinely perform a clavicular osteotomy to minimize the risk of a brachial plexus traction injury that may result from mobilization of the scapula.
- A bone biter or rongeur is used to create an osteotomy through the midaspect of the clavicle (Fig. 11).
- A simple osteotomy or morcellization of a small segment of the clavicle is performed.
- The wound is irrigated and the skin is closed with subcutaneous 4-0 or 5-0 absorbable sutures and a 5-0 running, absorbable subcuticular stitch.
- The wound is dressed, and patient is turned prone for posterior exposure.

STEP 2

- The lateral aspect of the distal trapezius is identified and dissected free from the underlying latissimus dorsi and paraspinal musculature (Fig. 12). This step helps identify the key surgical plane. Adhesions or hypoplastic musculature can make identification of this surgical plane difficult.
- The trapezius is sharply dissected from the thoracic and cervical spinous processes from caudad to cephalad. As the dissection progresses proximally, the origins of the rhomboid major and minor are reflected as well. Figure 13 shows the trapezius and rhomboids detached at their origins and elevated, with the levator scapulae exposed at the superomedial aspect of the scapula. The tendinous insertion of these muscles is preserved to allow later, more caudal, reattachment. At the level of the C4 spinous process, the trapezius muscle is divided transversely to allow adequate release.
- In the proximal aspect of the incision, the levator scapulae and, in 30% of cases, the omovertebral bone are evident. The spinal accessory nerve innervating the trapezius and branches of the dorsal scapular nerve innervating the rhomboids are carefully preserved.
- The surgeon must avoid injuring the descending branch of the superficial cervical artery or the transverse cervical artery.
- The levator scapulae is released at its superomedial insertion on the scapula. The transverse cervical artery travels directly beneath the levator scapulae and is protected during the release (Fig. 14).
- The omovertebral bone or fibrous bands in its location connecting the scapula to the cervical spine must be released with heavy scissors or bone biters. The omovertebral bone is removed extraperiosteally.
- Finally, the undersurface of the scapula is swept bluntly free of the underlying chest wall and any remaining fibrous adhesions are released.

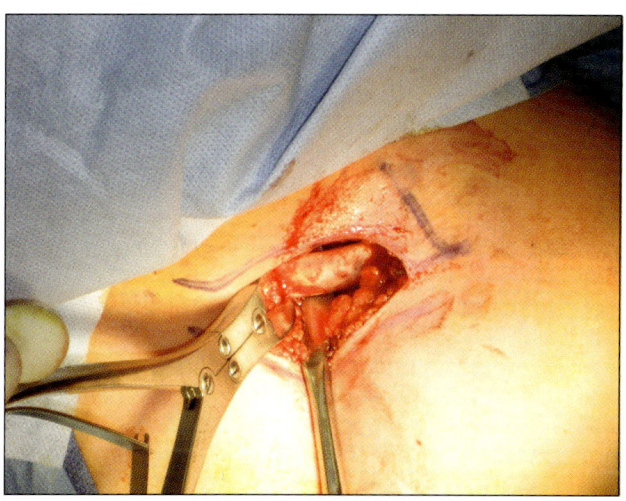

FIGURE 11

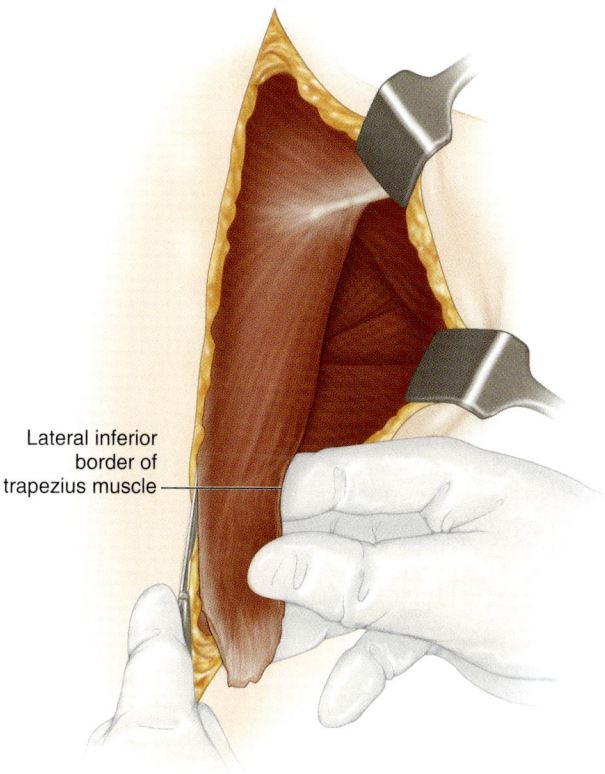

Lateral inferior border of trapezius muscle

FIGURE 12

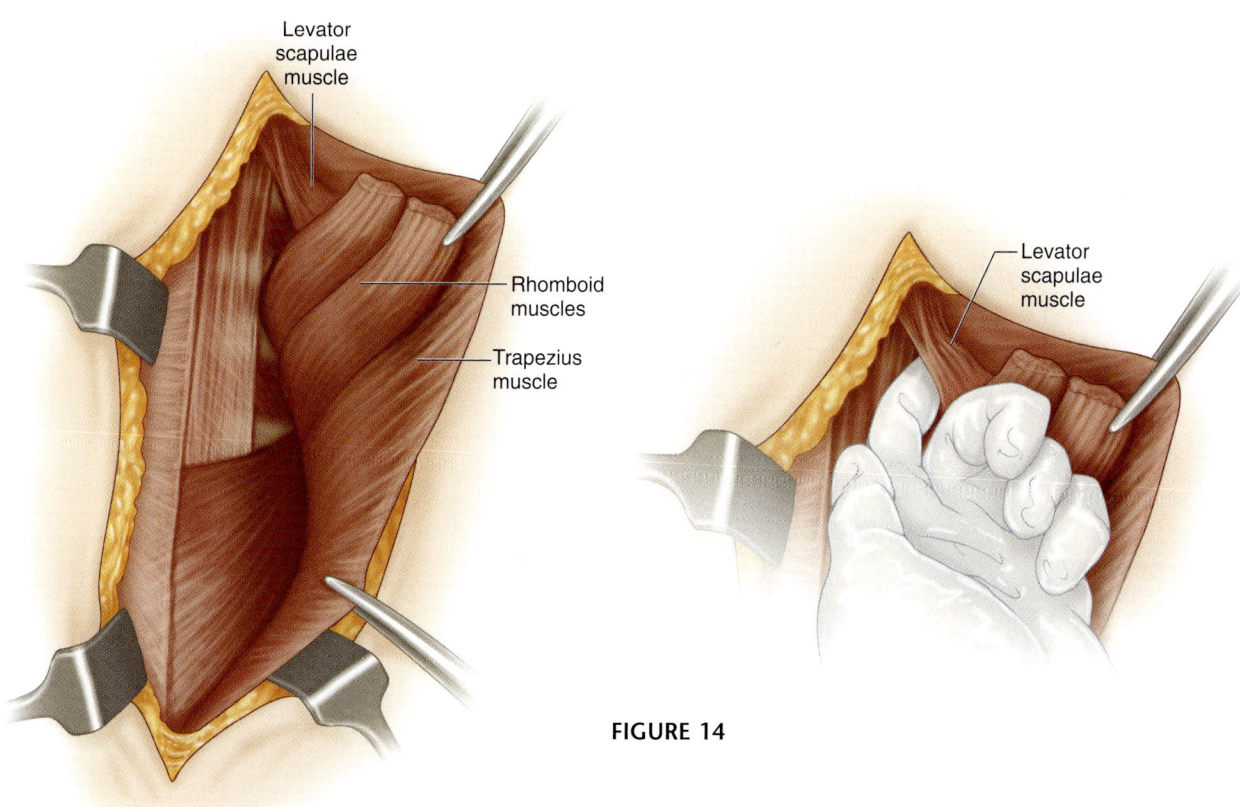

Levator scapulae muscle

Rhomboid muscles

Trapezius muscle

FIGURE 13

Levator scapulae muscle

FIGURE 14

Controversies

• Some authors advocate greenstick fracture transversely through the superomedial portion of the scapula rather than excision for correction of its prominent curvature.

Controversies

• Some authors recommend release of the subscapularis and serratus anterior to allow mobilization of the scapula caudally. If released, those muscles may be repaired after the scapula is stabilized in the inferior position. We have not found this step to be necessary.

STEP 3

■ The prominent superomedial aspect of the scapula is resected using bone biters in a medial to lateral direction (Fig. 15). The suprascapular neurovascular structures are protected.

■ This resection is performed extraperiosteally to minimize bone regrowth.

STEP 4

■ The scapula should be fully mobile and is reduced to a more caudal position.

   • The spine of the scapula is placed at the level of the contralateral scapular spine.

   • The previously elevated aponeurosis of trapezius and rhomboid muscles is sutured in place with multiple heavy nonabsorbable sutures in a more caudal position (Fig. 16). The redundant distal trapezius may be folded over or trimmed.

■ A pocket may be created in the latisimuss dorsi muscle to accommodate the lowered inferior angle of the scapula.

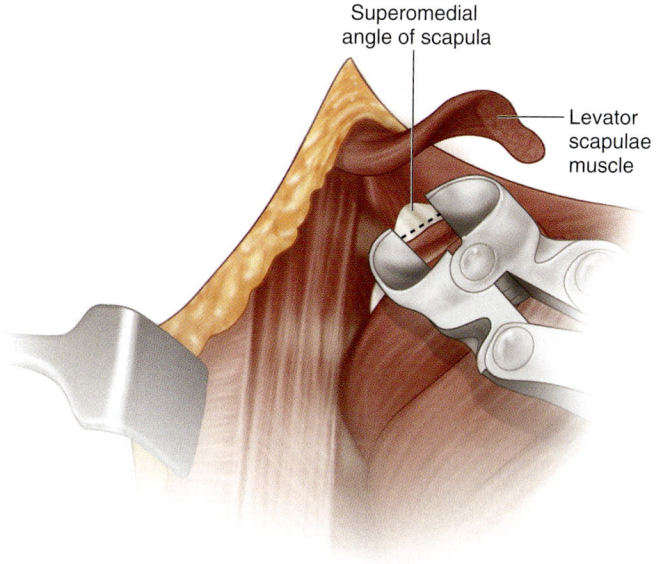

Superomedial angle of scapula

Levator scapulae muscle

FIGURE 15

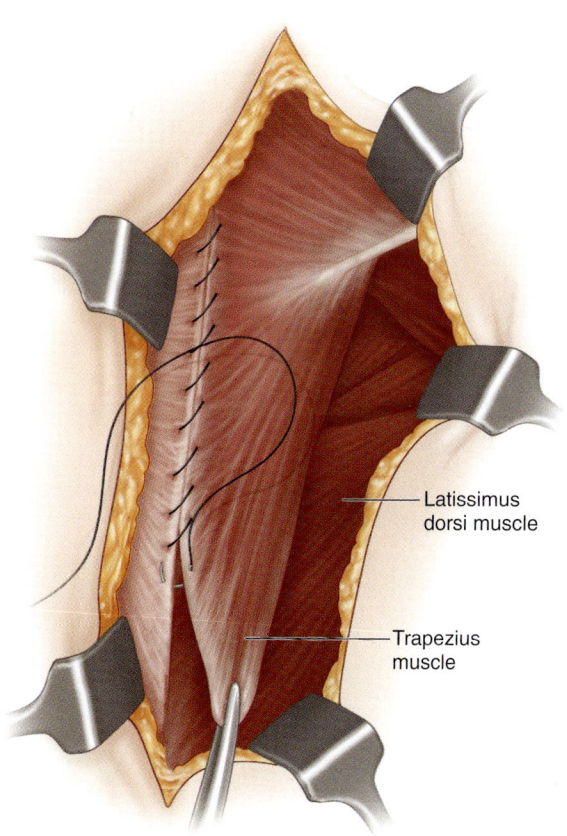

Latissimus dorsi muscle

Trapezius muscle

FIGURE 16

STEP 5: CLOSURE

■ The wound is closed with a 4-0 absorbable subcutaneous and a 5-0 absorbable subcuticular suture.
■ Bleeding is typically minimal, and a drain is rarely required.
■ Figure 17 shows the aesthetic (Fig. 17A) and functional (Fig. 17B) outcome from the modified Woodward procedure.

POSTOPERATIVE CARE AND EXPECTED OUTCOMES

■ Postoperatively, the patient is placed in a prefitted sling and swath. The patient remains in the hospital for 1–2 days for pain control. Immediate gentle neck motion, symmetric posture training, isometric scapular depression, and elbow, wrist, and hand motion exercises are initiated as indicated based on patient age.
■ At 3 weeks postoperatively, a home therapy program is advanced to include Codman exercises and passive and active-assistive shoulder motion to 90° while stabilizing the clavicle.
■ At 5 weeks postoperatively, radiographs are taken and the patient is weaned of the sling and swath. Active and passive range of motion beyond 90° is begun and scapular depression exercises are emphasized.
■ At 3 months postoperatively, a more rigorous strengthening protocol is initiated.
■ Complications include disfiguring scar, transient brachial plexus palsy, recurrence of deformity secondary to bone regeneration or cephalad migration of the scapula, and inability to improve deformity because of other factors (scoliosis, cervical spine abnormality).

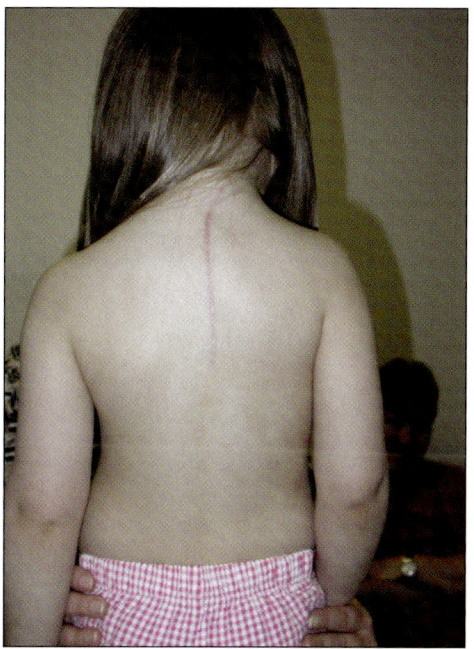 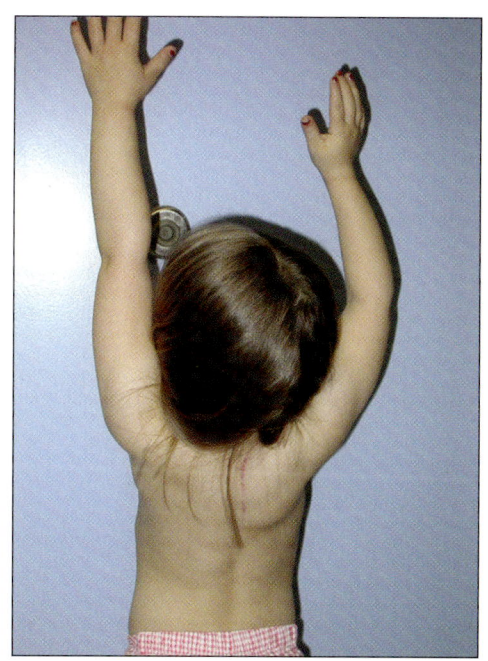

A

B

FIGURE 17

EVIDENCE

Borges JLP, Shah A, Torres BC, Bowen JR. Modified Woodward procedure for Sprengel deformity of the shoulder: long-term results. J Pediatr Orthop. 1996;16:508–13.

In this retrospective review over 3 to 15 years of follow-up, 15 patients had an 86% satisfaction rate and 14 of 15 had markedly improved appearance as per the Cavendish grading system. Average abduction improved by 35° and scapular lowering by 2.7 cm. The authors advocated removal of the medial border of the scapular, hypothesizing that it may prevent postoperative winging. One case of brachial plexus palsy was reported, which resolved after clavicular osteotomy. (Level IV evidence)

Carson WG, Lovell WW, Hitesides TE. Congenital elevation of the scapula: surgical correction by the Woodward procedure. J Bone Joint Surg [Am]. 1981;63:1199–1207.

This 11-patient case series of the Woodward procedure with clavicular osteotomy demonstrated 9 of 11 patients were satisfied with their outcome, with one of the unsatisfied patients having an unsightly scar and the other scapular winging. Better outcomes were achieved in patients with more severe limitations in preoperative range of motion. (Level IV evidence)

Cavendish ME. Congenital elevation of the scapula. J Bone Joint Surg [Br]. 1972;54:395–408.

This comprehensive review of 100 cases of Sprengel's deformity focused on description of surgical techniques and a classification system aimed at tailoring an appropriate surgical approach based on degree of deformity. (Level IV evidence)

Greitemann B, Rondhuis J, Karbowski A. Treatment of congenital elevation of the scapula: 10 (2–18) year follow-up of 37 cases of Sprengel's deformity. Acta Orthop Scand. 1993;64:365–8.

In this retrospective analysis of 23 operative procedures, including 6 Woodward procedures without clavicular osteotomy, the latter yielded the best results and satisfaction rates secondary to improved scar appearance and larger scapular mobilization. There was one transient brachial plexus palsy. (Level IV evidence)

Grogan DP, Stanley EA, Bobechko WP. The congenital undescended scapula: surgical correction by the Woodward procedure. J Bone Joint Surg [Br]. 1983;65:598–605.

This retrospective review of 21 Woodward procedures without clavicular osteotomy yielded 80% good to excellent results with average follow-up of nearly 9 years. One patient had transient brachial plexus palsy and one had worsening of preoperative scapular winging. One patient had recurrence of resected superomedial scapula. The authors indicated a trend toward improved scar appearance with a subcuticular stitch. (Level IV evidence)

Ross DM, Cruess RL. The surgical correction of congenital elevation of the scapula: a review of seventy-seven cases. Clin Orthop Relat Res. 1977;(125):17–23.

The authors presented a comprehensive review of all operatively treated Sprengel's deformity cases at U.S. Shriners Hospitals between 1935 and 1970. The review included 17 Woodward procedures, 3 of which led to recurrence or scapular winging, and 1 case with transient brachial plexus palsy. (Level IV evidence)

Woodward JW. Congenital elevation of the scapula: correction by release and transplantation of muscle origins, a preliminary report. J Bone Joint Surg [Am]. 1961;43:219–28.

In his original paper, Woodward described his technique, which did not include clavicular osteotomy, and his experience with nine patients. One patient experienced transient brachial plexus palsy and three patients had unsightly scars. (Level IV evidence)

Shoulder External Rotation Tendon Transfers for Brachial Plexus Birth Palsy

Lisa D. Maskill and Michelle A. James

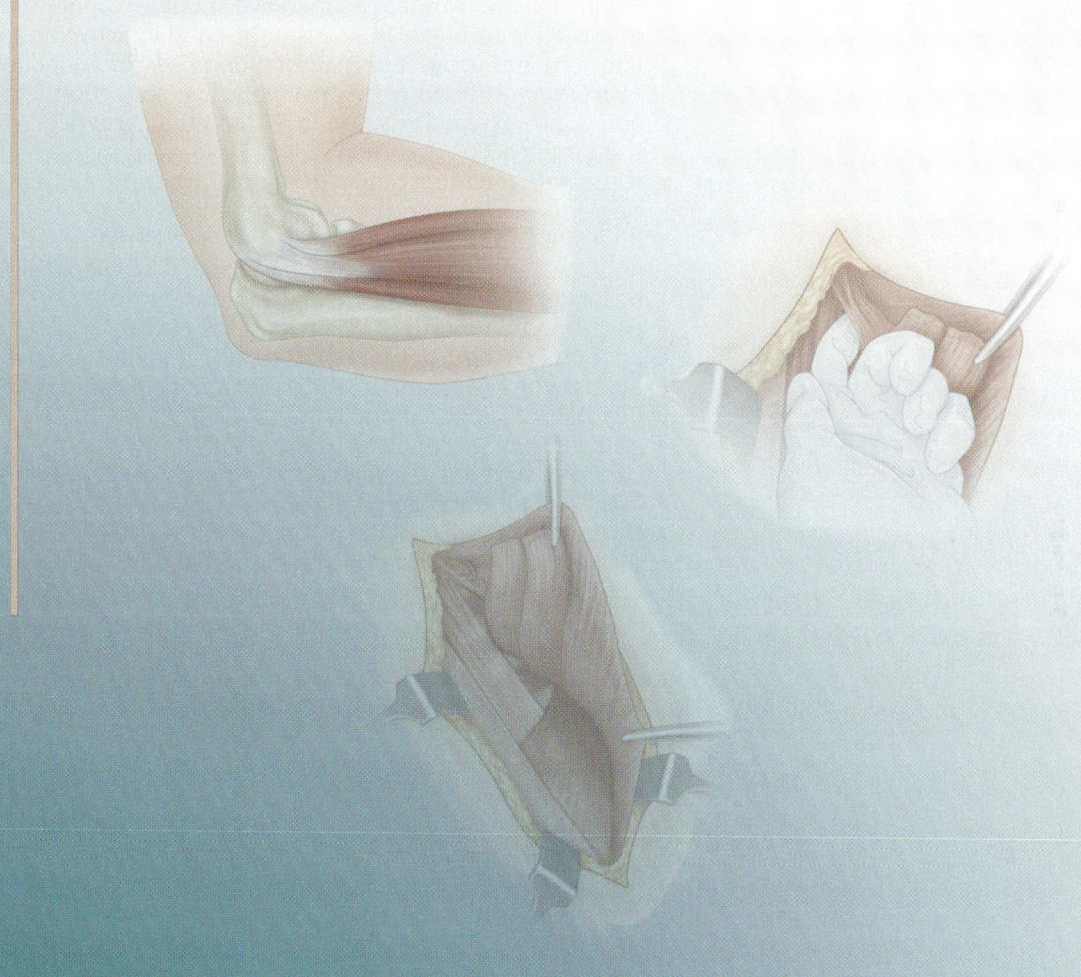

Controversies

- Timing of external rotation tendon transfer (ERTT)
  - ERTT should be performed before contracture (diminished PROM) occurs; this can be seen in infancy.
  - Compliance with postoperative therapy (which is limited in infants and toddlers) may improve outcomes.
  - ERTT may halt progression of glenohumeral dysplasia; early dysplasia is a possible indication.
- Poor hand function limits functional improvement from ERTT.

Treatment Options

- Botulinum toxin injections to the supraspinatus and pectoralis major, followed by shoulder spica casting
- Subscapularis release (arthroscopic, open, or origin "slide")
- Humerus external rotation osteotomy

INDICATIONS

- Weak shoulder external rotation associated with C5-6 palsy and:
  - Strong donor muscles (latissimus dorsi and teres major) on Active Movement Scale (AMS) for infant assessment
  - Active shoulder abduction ≥ 60° on AMS
  - Well-maintained passive range of motion (PROM) of the shoulder
  - Impairment of bimanual overhead activities
  - Good hand function on AMS

EXAMINATION/IMAGING

- Physical examination should document PROM and active range of motion (AROM) and strength of the shoulder and elbow, in addition to hand function.
  - Figure 1 demonstrates preoperative shoulder range of motion in a child with brachial plexus birth palsy in active abduction (Fig. 1A) and active external rotation in 90° of abduction (Fig. 1B). Figure 2 shows postoperative active abduction (Fig. 2A) and active external rotation in 90° of abduction (Fig. 2B) in the same child.
  - If supination contracture is developing, biceps rerouting may be performed during the same surgery as ERTT.
  - If wrist extension is weak, active finger extension is adequate, and a suitable donor muscle is available (brachioradialis or flexor carpi ulnaris), wrist extension transfer may be performed during the same surgery as ERTT.
- Glenohumeral joint status should be documented with serial examinations and imaging studies. Magnetic resonance imaging (MRI) will reveal glenohumeral dysplasia (Fig. 3).
  - All ages: passive shoulder external rotation with scapula stabilized and arm at side and in 90° of shoulder abduction
  - Infants: ultrasonography or MRI
  - Under age 3 years: MRI
  - Over age 3 years: anteroposterior and axillary radiographs or computed tomography
- Preoperative physical and/or occupational therapy should be scheduled to accustom the child to therapy, optimize range of motion and function, and strengthen donor muscles.

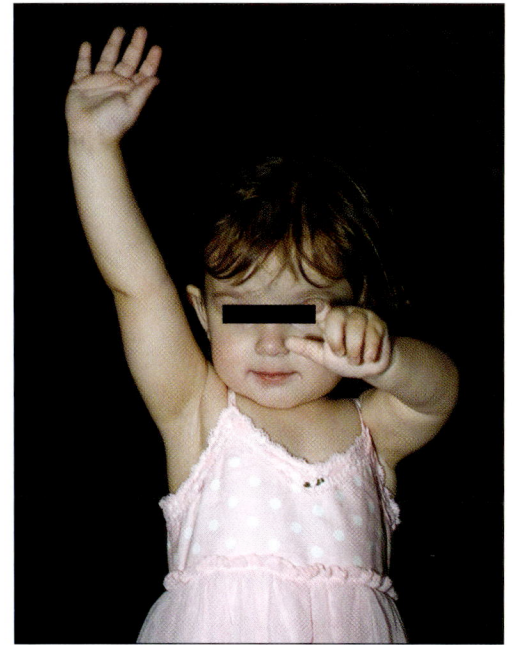 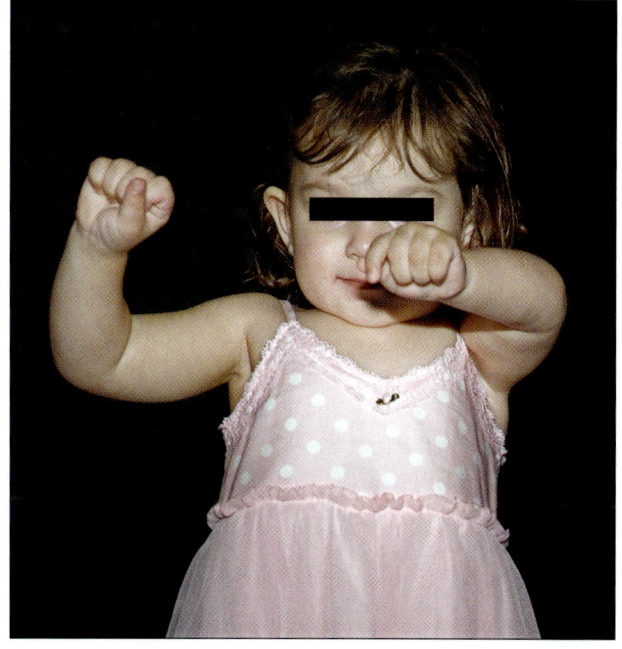

FIGURE 1 A   B

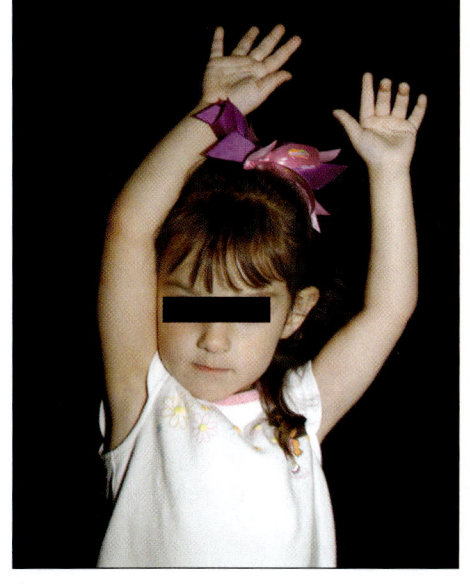 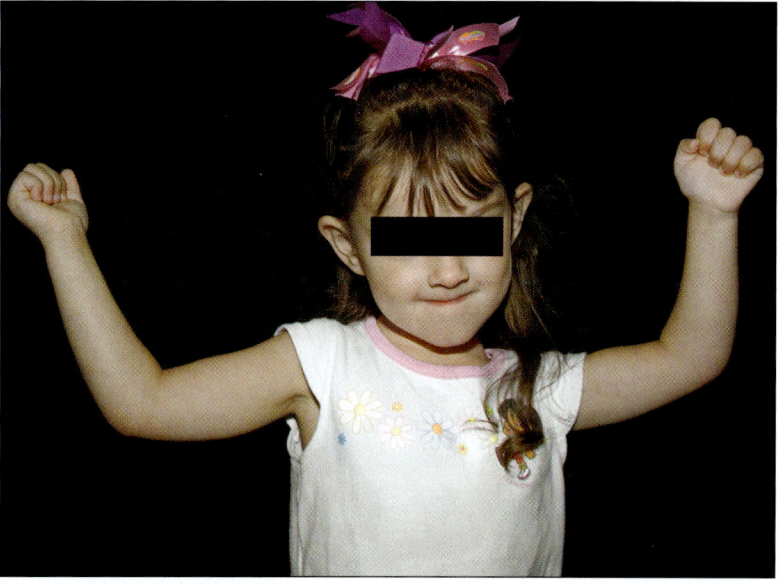

A   B

FIGURE 2

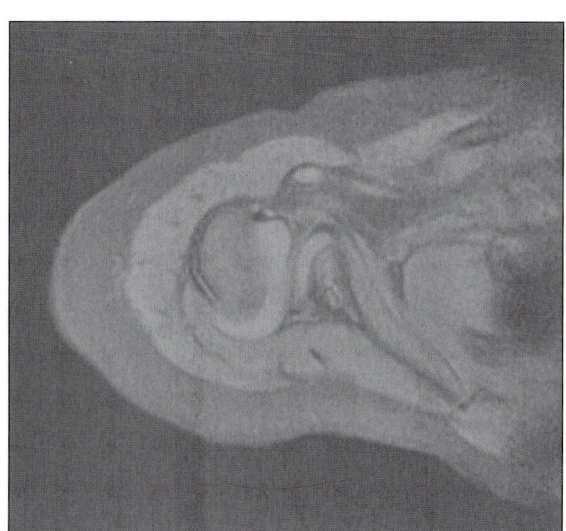

FIGURE 3

SURGICAL ANATOMY

- The axillary nerve is at risk in two locations during this operation.
  - The nerve and the posterior humeral circumflex artery are exposed in the quadrangular space when the latissimus dorsi and teres major are detached.
  - In addition, the tendon transfer passes through the deltoid-triceps interval, and care should be taken to develop the opening in this interval proximal to where the axillary nerve enters the posterior deltoid.
- The teres major and latissimus dorsi tendons are usually conjoined.
- Posterior subluxation of the humeral head attenuates the capsule and displaces the supraspinatus tendon superiorly and the infraspinatus tendon inferiorly, making attachment of the transfer more difficult.

POSITIONING

- The patient is positioned in the lateral decubitus position with the affected extremity superior, stabilized with a beanbag.
- Range of motion is assessed prior to draping, in order to determine if subscapularis release is necessary.
- The affected extremity is draped free, and if release of the subscapularis origin is planned, the scapula is in the surgical field.

PORTALS/EXPOSURES

- A transverse skin incision extends across the axillary fold from the pectoralis major to the interval between the deltoid and triceps (Fig. 4).

PROCEDURE

STEP 1

- If the shoulder cannot reach 90° of external rotation while abducted, fractional lengthening of the pectoralis major is performed. The posterior, tendinous portion of the muscle is released near its insertion on the humerus.
- If the shoulder does not reach 30° of external rotation in adduction, the subscapularis origin is released ("subscapularis slide") through a separate incision over the inferolateral scapula.

STEP 2

- With the shoulder placed in maximum internal rotation, the teres major and latissimus dorsi muscles are detached from their insertion on the humerus and tagged with nonabsorbable suture. Care must be taken to avoid damaging the axillary nerve and posterior humeral circumflex vessels (Fig. 5A and 5B).

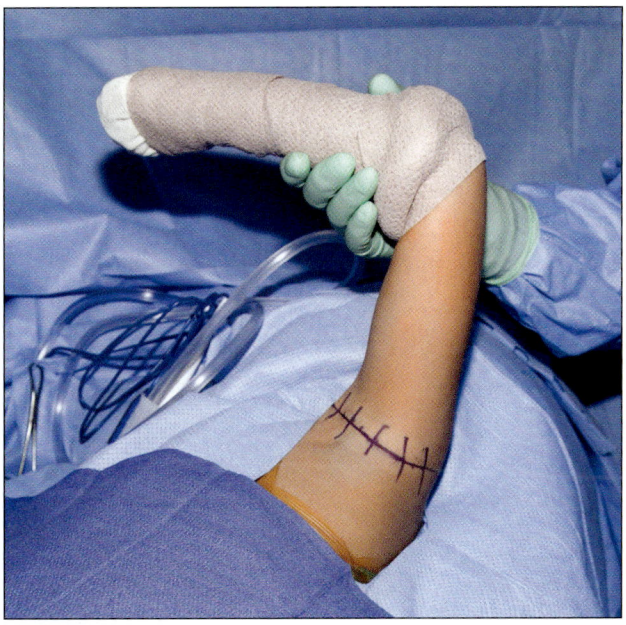

FIGURE 4

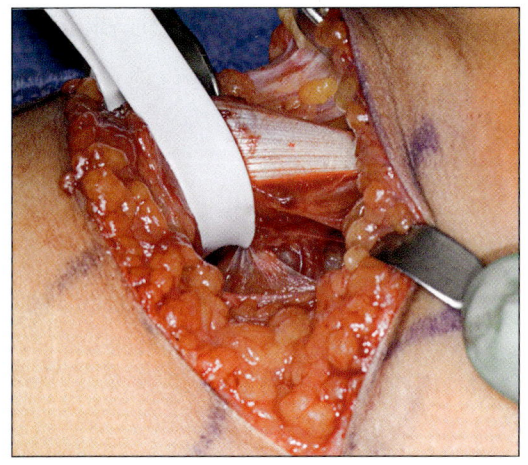

A
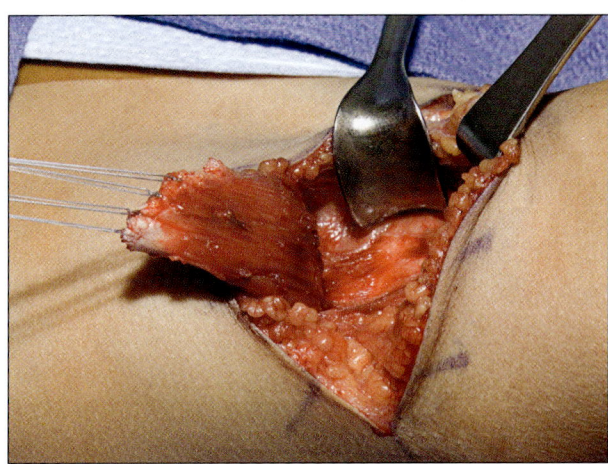

B

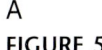
FIGURE 5

Controversies

- Anterior capsular release and subscapularis release help reduce a subluxated glenohumeral joint, but risk the development of anterior subluxation and/or an external rotation contracture, which is more debilitating than an internal rotation contracture because it makes performance of bimanual midline activities difficult.

STEP 3

- With the shoulder in 90° of abduction and 60–80° of external rotation, the latissimus dorsi and teres major tendons are passed posterior to the triceps muscle (Fig. 6) and then sutured into the tendons of the supraspinatus and infraspinatus tendons, taking care not to damage the axillary nerve where it enters the deltoid.
- Tension on the transfer is tested by placement of the surgeon's finger on the repair as the shoulder is gently ranged. This helps the surgeon decide the optimal position of abduction and external rotation for postoperative immobilization.

POSTOPERATIVE CARE AND EXPECTED OUTCOMES

- The waist portion of a shoulder spica cast is fabricated preoperatively with the child standing, then univalved and removed for reapplication immediately postoperatively. While the child is still under general anesthesia, the waist portion is applied and attached to a long-arm cast with wooden dowels, in optimal abduction and external rotation.
- The shoulder spica cast is left in place for 4–5 weeks.
- After the cast is removed, the child is placed in an airplane splint for nighttime wear for 1–3 months, depending on how well the transfer is working.
- Intensive therapy is begun when the cast is removed and continued for 3–6 months, focusing on bimanual overhead activities.

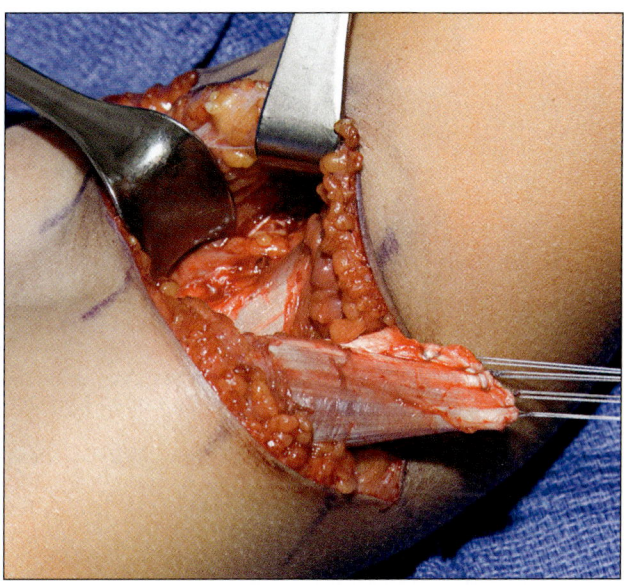

FIGURE 6

EVIDENCE

Al-Zahrani S. Combined Sever's release of the shoulder and osteotomy of the humerus for Erb's palsy. J Hand Surg [Br]. 1997;22:591–3.

The author presented a case series of a technique to improve shoulder external rotation and abduction. (Level IV evidence [therapeutic])

Anderson KA, O'Dell MA, James MA. Shoulder external rotation tendon transfers for brachial plexus birth palsy. Tech Hand Up Extrem Surg. 2006;10:60–7.

This paper presented a description of the technique of shoulder external rotation tendon transfer and postoperative rehabilitation.

Bae DS, Waters PM. External rotation humeral osteotomy for brachial plexus birth palsy. Tech Hand Up Extrem Surg. 2007;11:8–14.

The authors described the technique of humeral external rotation osteotomy.

Bennett JB, Allan CH. Tendon transfers about the shoulder and elbow in obstetrical brachial plexus palsy. J Bone Joint Surg. 1999;81(A):1612–27.

This paper presented a review of tendon transfers.

Carlioz H. La place de la disinsertion interne du sous-scapulaire dans le traitement de la paralysie obstetricale du membre superieur chez l'enfant. Ann Chir Infant. 1971;12:159–68.

The author described release of the origin of the subscapularis muscle in order to reduce the shoulder internal rotation contracture associated with external rotation weakness, while lowering the risk of anterior instability caused by releasing the subscapularis at its insertion.

Chen L, Gu YD, Hu SN. Applying transfer of trapezius and/or latissimus dorsi with teres major for reconstruction of abduction and external rotation of the shoulder in obstetrical brachial plexus palsy. J Reconstr Microsurg. 2002;18:275–80.

Based on the results of this case series, the authors advocated the addition of trapezius transfer when preoperative active abduction is less than 90°. (Level IV evidence [therapeutic])

Covey DC, Riordan DC, Milstead ME, Albright JA. Modification of the L'Episcopo procedure for brachial plexus birth palsies. J Bone Joint Surg [Br]. 1992;74:897–901.

This paper described a modification of the technique for shoulder external rotation transfers, involving rerouting the latissimus and teres. (Level IV evidence [therapeutic])

Curtis C, Stephens D, Clarke HM, Andrews D. The Active Movement Scale: an evaluative tool for infants with obstetric brachial plexus palsy. J Hand Surg [Am]. 2002;27:470–8.

The authors presented a validation of a method of evaluating progress in infants with birth palsy by examination. (Level IV evidence [diagnostic, case-control])

Desiato MT, Risina B. The role of botulinum toxin in the neuro-rehabilitation of young patients with brachial plexus birth palsy. Pediatr Rehabil. 2001;4:29–36.

Results of this case series indicated that botulinum toxin injections may have a role in improving global movements in children with brachial plexus birth palsy. (Level IV evidence [therapeutic])

El-Gammal TA, Saleh WR, El-Sayed A, Kotb MM, Iman HM, Fathi NA. Tendon transfer around the shoulder in obstetric brachial plexus paralysis: clinical and computed tomographic study. J Pediatr Orthop. 2006;26:641–46.

Results of this case series indicated that shoulder tendon transfers were associated with improved range of motion and glenohumeral deformity when performed before age 2; between ages 2 and 4, motion was improved but not deformity, and after age 4 neither was significantly impacted. (Level IV evidence [therapeutic])

Hoffer MM, Wickenden R, Roper B. Brachial plexus birth palsies: results of tendon transfers to the rotator cuff. J Bone Joint Surg [Am]. 1978;60:691–5.

This paper provided a description of the technique of attaching the donor tendons to the rotator cuff and results of a case series. (Level IV evidence [therapeutic])

Javid M, Shahcheraghi GH. Shoulder reconstruction in obstetric brachial plexus palsy in older children via a one-stage release and tendon transfers. J Shoulder Elbow Surg. 2009;18:107–13.

The authors reported improvement in range of motion with shoulder release and transfers in older children. (Level IV evidence [therapeutic])

L'Episcopo JB. Tendon transplantation in obstetrical paralysis. Am J Surg. 1934; 25:122–5.

The author presented the original description of tendon transfer technique to restore external rotation.

Pagnotta A, Haerle M, Gilbert A. Long-term results on abduction and external rotation of the shoulder after latissimus dorsi transfer for sequelae of obstetric palsy. Clin Orthop Relat Res. 2004;(426):199–205.

Results of this case series indicated that external rotation gains following shoulder external rotation tendon transfer may diminish with time. (Level IV evidence [therapeutic])

Pearl ML, Edgerton BW, Kazimiroff PA, Burchette RJ, Wong K. Arthroscopic release and latissimus dorsi transfer for shoulder internal rotation contractures and glenohumeral deformity secondary to brachial plexus birth palsy. J Bone Joint Surg [Am]. 2006;88:564–74.

In this study, arthroscopic release of the capsule and subscapularis was found to diminish posterior subluxation and possibly improve range of motion, but was also associated with decreased internal rotation. (Level IV evidence [therapeutic])

Phipps GJ, Hoffer MM. Latissimus dorsi and teres major transfer to rotator cuff for Erb's palsy. J Shoulder Elbow Surg. 1995;4:124–9.

Results of this case series indicated that this tendon transfer is associated with improved shoulder abduction and external rotation. (Level IV evidence [therapeutic])

Waters PM. Comparison of the natural history, the outcome of microsurgical repair, and the outcome of operative reconstruction in brachial plexus birth palsy. J Bone Joint Surg [Am]. 1999;81:649–59.

This case series examined outcomes for infants with brachial plexus birth palsy who do not recover biceps function by age 6 months. Some benefited from nerve exploration and grafting. (Level IV evidence [therapeutic])

Waters PM. Update on management of pediatric brachial plexus palsy. J Pediatr Orthop. 2005;25:116–26.

The author reviewed the treatment of brachial plexus birth palsy in infants and children.

Waters PM, Bae DS. Effect of tendon transfers and extra-articular soft-tissue balancing on glenohumeral development in brachial plexus birth palsy. J Bone Joint Surg [Am]. 2005;87:320–5.

Results of this case series indicated that shoulder tendon transfers improve global shoulder motion but have little effect on glenohumeral dysplasia. (Level IV evidence [therapeutic])

Waters PM, Peljovich AE. Shoulder reconstruction in patients with chronic brachial plexus birth palsy: a case control study. Clin Orthop Relat Res. 1999;(364):144–52.

A comparison of outcomes of tendon transfers and osteotomy indicated that both are associated with improved motion. (Level III evidence [therapeutic])

HUMERUS AND ELBOW

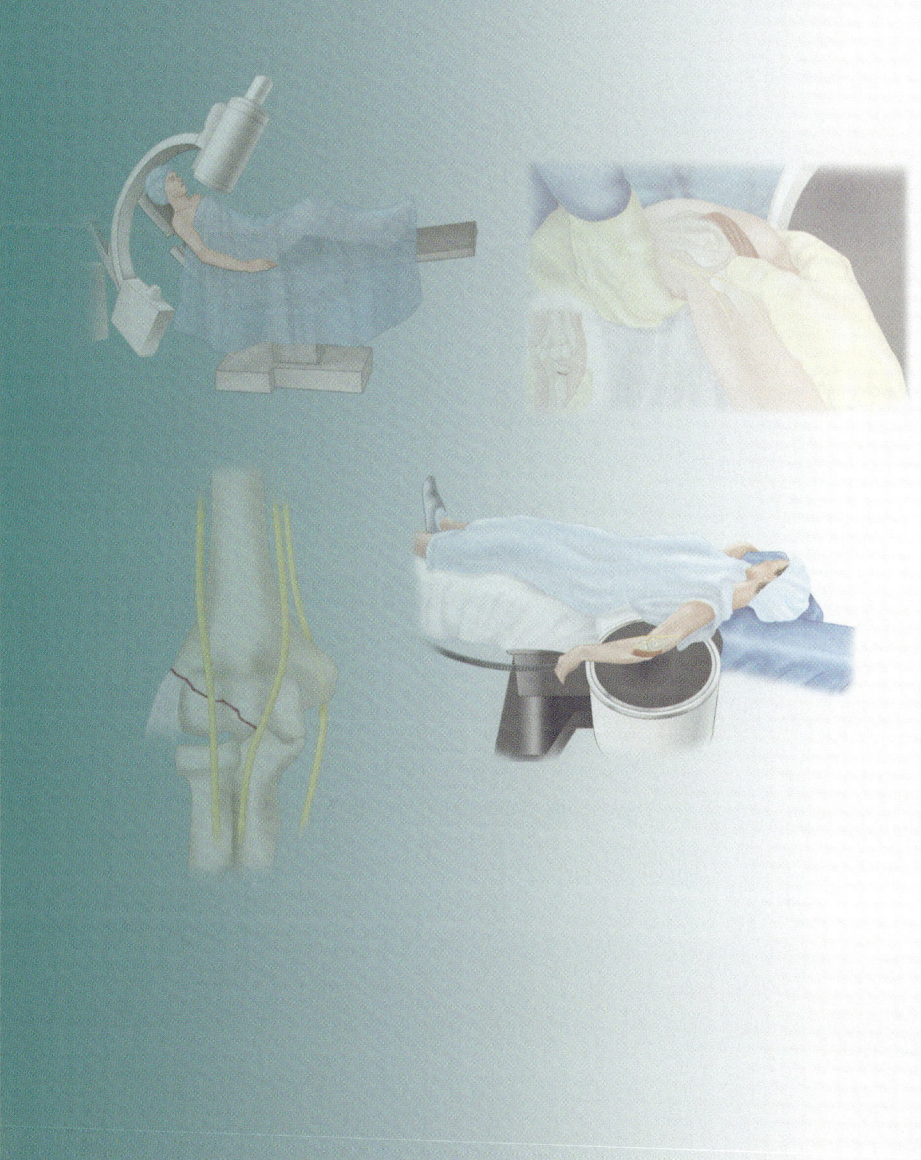

Proximal Humerus Fracture: Reduction and Fixation with Elastic Nail

Jay C. Albright

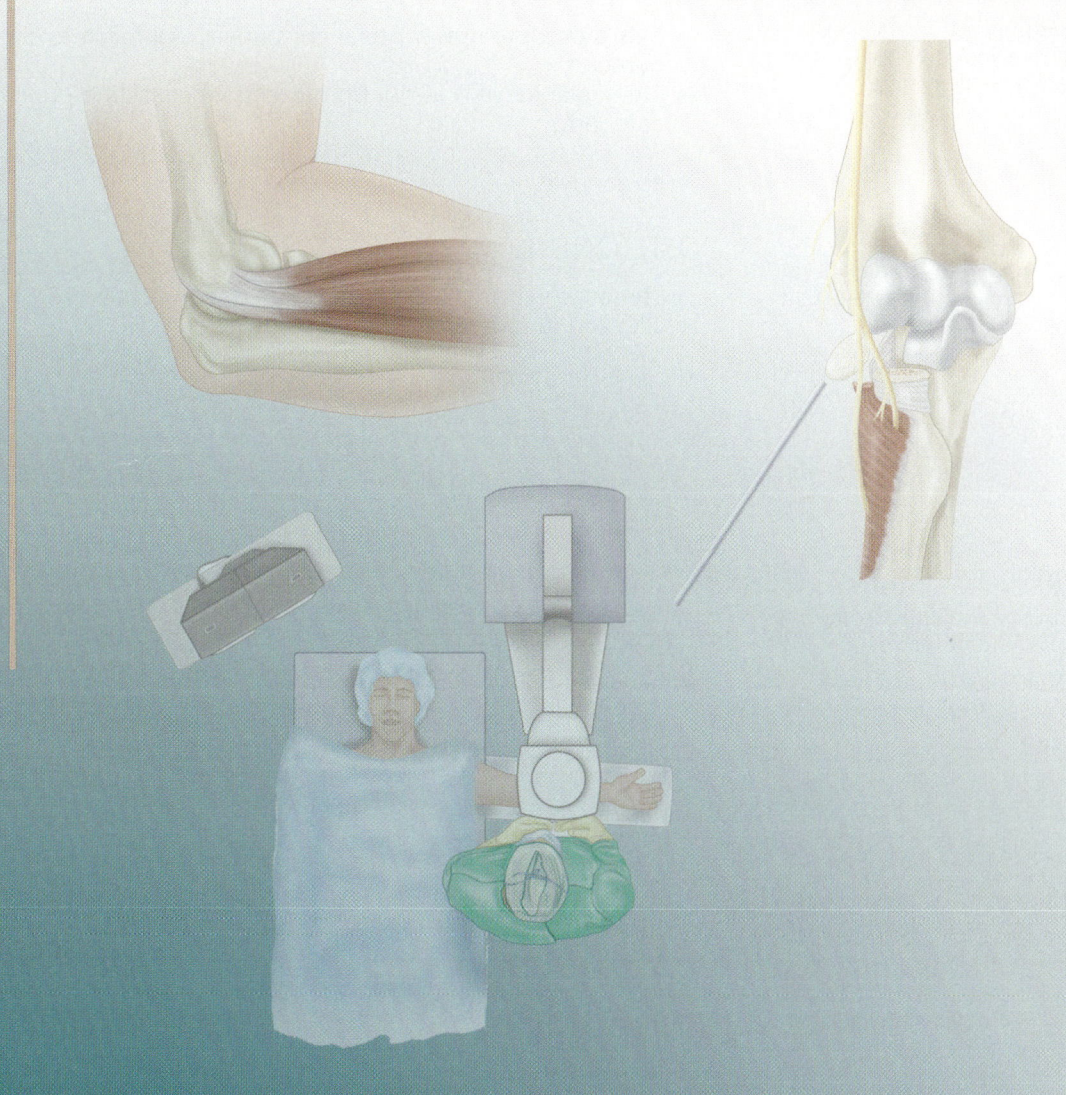

Controversies

• Patients with more than 2–3 years of growth remaining will likely remodel adequately even in displaced fractures, provided no growth arrest occurs.

Treatment Options

• Closed reduction with percutaneous pin fixation

• Closed reduction with percutaneous screw fixation

• Open reduction and internal fixation

Equipment

• The fluoroscope should enter from the cephalad end of the room.

• The operating table should be turned to accommodate this position.

Controversies

• Supine or beach chair position can be used for this procedure.

INDICATIONS

■ Significantly displaced proximal humeral physeal fracture in an older adolescent (2 or less years of growth remaining)

■ Closed injury

■ No distal trauma (ipsilateral elbow fractures)

EXAMINATION/IMAGING

■ Adequate anteroposterior (AP) (Fig. 1A) and orthogonal radiographs, either an axillary lateral or a scapular Y view (Fig. 1B), are needed to visualize the position of the fracture.

SURGICAL ANATOMY

■ This procedure uses a lateral epicondylar approach to the distal humerus.

■ The radial nerve is at risk from excessive dissection proximally or anteriorly.

■ The extensor origins are at risk distally, inserting onto the epicondyle.

POSITIONING

■ The beach chair position can be used with relative ease, allowing for adequate fluoroscopic imaging (Fig. 2).

PEARLS

• *Ensure that adequate radiographic images can be obtained in both a true AP and an axillary lateral view.*

• *Rotate the image intensifier to obtain the orthogonal views.*

• *Use standard padding for all extremities.*

• *Beach chair positioning can facilitate reduction with the help of gravity.*

PITFALLS

• *Neutral head position is absolutely necessary.*

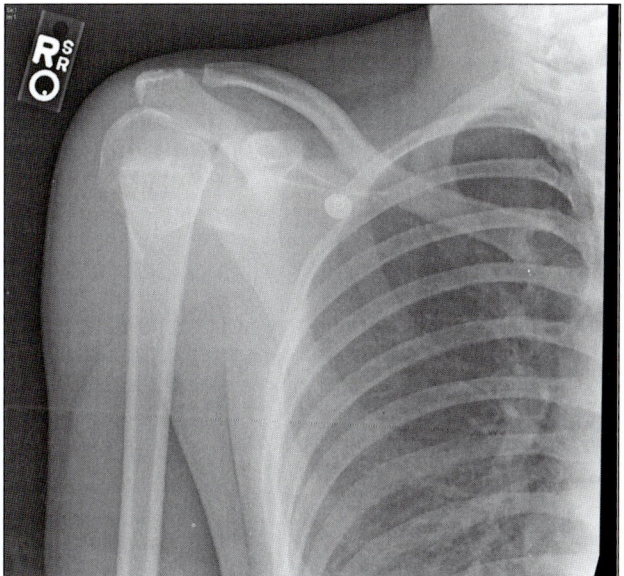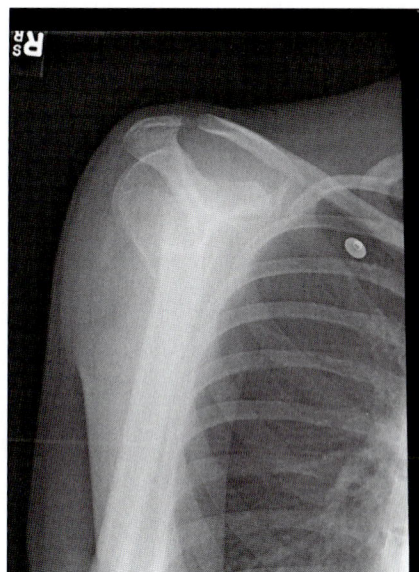

A

B

FIGURE 1

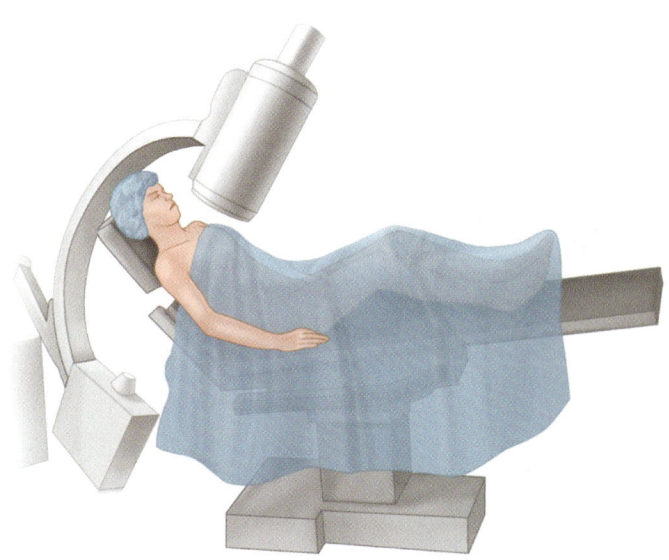

FIGURE 2

PITFALLS

• *Too low an entry site into the lateral column will result in prominence of the implant.*

PEARLS

• *Overdrill the lateral cortex by 0.5 mm obliquely to ease passage of the implant.*

PITFALLS

• *Drilling less obliquely will make passing the nail more challenging.*

• *Choosing an implant too large or small will make control more difficult, and the implant may have less strength or ability to help in reduction.*

Instrumentation/ Implantation

• Passing the implant upward may be initially accomplished by hand.

• Use of a chuck or other inserter may be necessary to control the direction of the implant.

PORTALS/EXPOSURES

■ A 2-cm incision is utilized with its distal end over the lateral epicondyle (Fig. 3).
■ Dissection is carried down to the superior aspect of the epicondyle, where subperiosteal dissection is carried a few centimeters proximally.

PROCEDURE

STEP 1

■ The size of elastic implant to be used is determined.
■ An appropriate-size hole is drilled obliquely into the cortex of the lateral column, a centimeter or two above the lateral epicondyle.
■ The implant is prebent into a gentle C or S configuration.
■ An elastic nail is passed up to the fracture site under fluoroscopic guidance (Fig. 4).

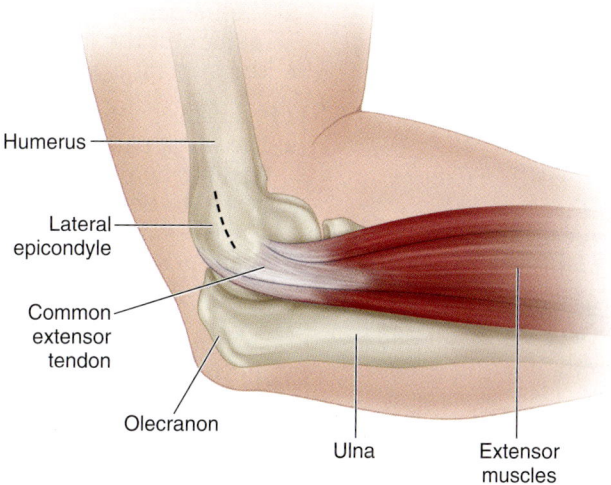

Humerus

Lateral epicondyle

Common extensor tendon

Olecranon

Ulna

Extensor muscles

FIGURE 3

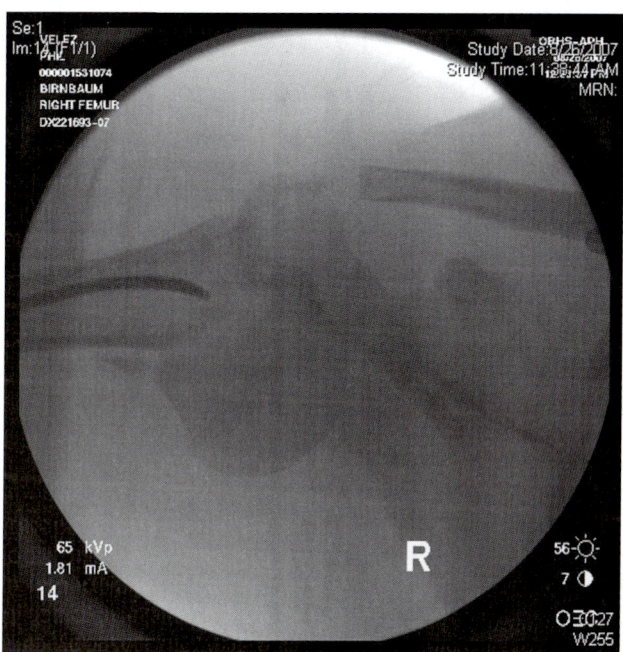

FIGURE 4

Instrumentation/Implantation

- Use an implant insertion device to rotate the implant and aid reduction.

- A mallet insertion device can be used to seat the implant across the physis into the epiphysis.

STEP 2

- The fracture is reduced with closed reduction techniques and rotation of the implant.
- The implant is seated across into the epiphysis (Fig. 5).

STEP 3

- The distal end of the implant as is cut flush with the skin as possible by placing torque on the implant with the insertion device to bend it in the cephalad direction.
- The wounds are closed in a standard fashion.
- Figure 6 shows radiographs of an elastic nail postoperatively on the AP (Fig. 6A) and internal rotation lateral (Fig. 6B).

POSTOPERATIVE CARE AND EXPECTED OUTCOMES

- A sling or shoulder immobilizer is used for 3–4 weeks.
- Elbow range-of-motion and shoulder pendulum exercises are begun immediately.
- Physical therapy starts at week 3–4 for range of motion and gentle strengthening.
- Restriction of activities continues for 12 weeks.
- Removal of the implant may be done anytime after complete healing.

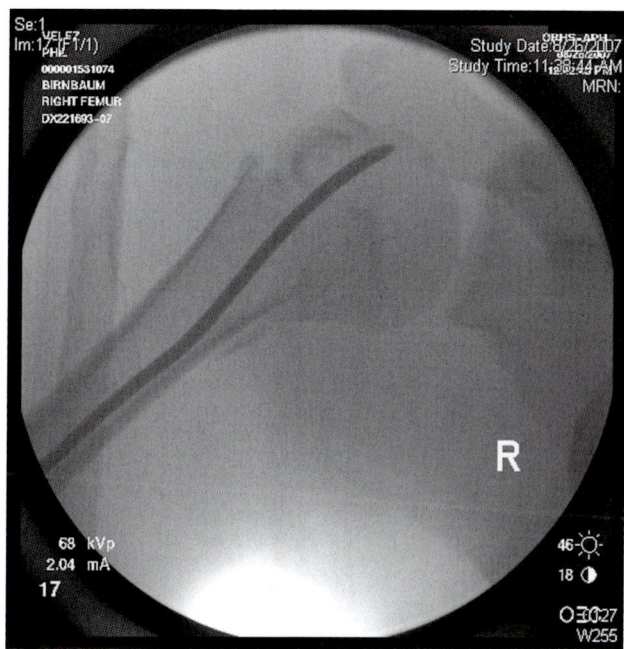

FIGURE 5

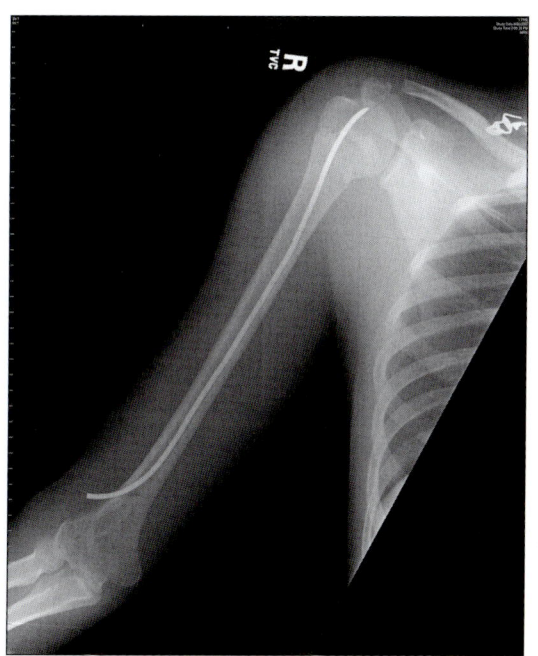

A

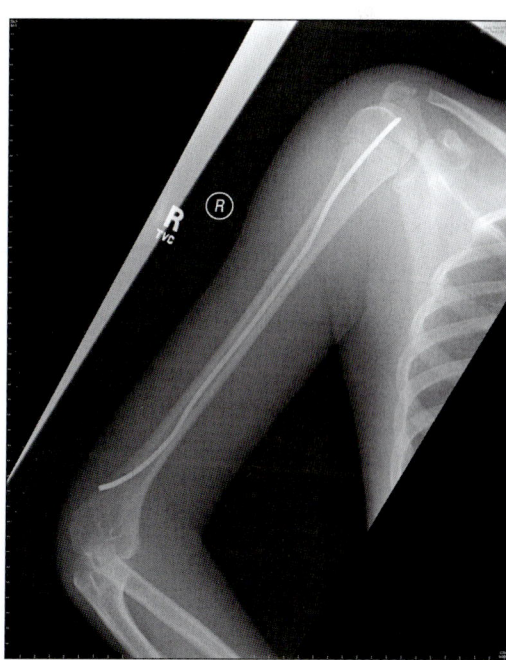

B

FIGURE 6

EVIDENCE

Metaizeau JP, Lascombes P, Lemelle JL, Finlayson D, Prevot J. Reduction and fixation of displaced radial neck fractures by closed intramedullary pinning. J Pediatr Orthop. 1993;13:355–60.

Radial neck fractures in children are serious injuries with frequent sequelae when the tilt exceeds 60°. Conservative treatment is often inadequate in such cases and open reduction may produce iatrogenic complications. The authors report their experience with an original technique. An intramedullary wire introduced from below and projected upward allows reduction of the displacement and maintenance of the correction without infringing the joint. The operative technique is described. This method was used in 31 fractures with between 30° and 80° of tilt and in 16 fractures with >80° of tilt. Excellent and good functional results were obtained in 30 cases in the first group and in 11 cases in the second group.

Rajan RA, Hawkins KJ, Metcalfe J, Konstantoulakis C, Jones S, Fernandes J. Elastic stable intramedullary nailing for displaced proximal humeral fractures in older children. J Child Orthop. 2008;2:15–9.

This paper demonstrates the effectiveness of intramedullary fixation of severely displaced proximal humeral physeal fractures in skeletally immature children using the elastic stable intramedullary nail (ESIN). There was retrospective recruitment of 14 patients aged 10–15 years old with severely displaced proximal humeral physeal fractures between 1999 and 2004 in a single regional specialist pediatric orthopaedic hospital. The fractures were graded using the Neer classification; severe displacement constituted Neer II–IV or displacement >1 cm and angulation >45°. The authors recommend stabilization using ESIN in the management of the displaced proximal humeral physeal fracture in older children, once reduction of the fracture has been achieved by either closed or open means. ESIN is safe and allows early return to pre-injury function.

Open Reduction and Internal Fixation of Displaced Medial Epicondyle Fracture Using a Screw and Washer

William Hennrikus

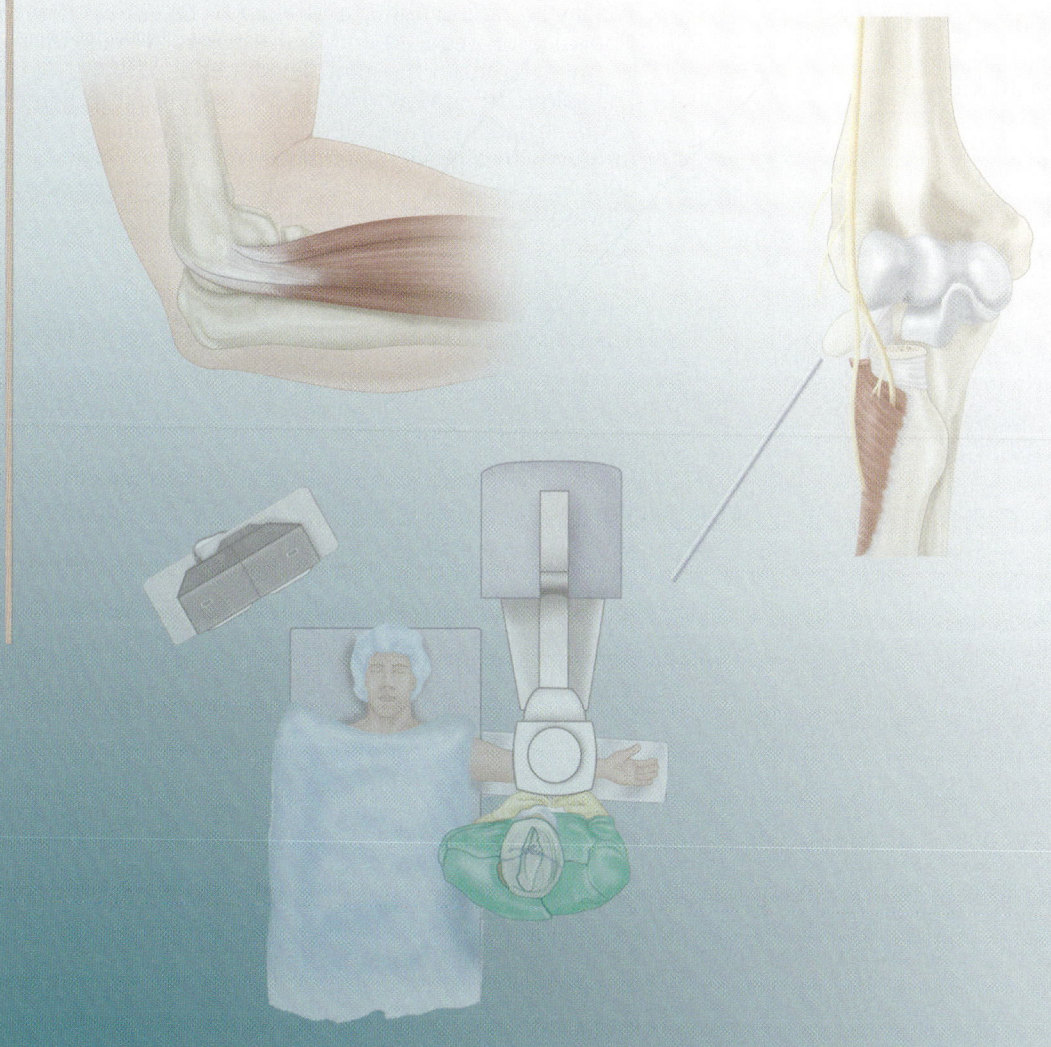

Controversies

- Some authors advocate nonoperative treatment for all medial epicondyle fractures (Farsetti et al., 2001; Josefsson and Danielsson, 1986). Nonoperative treatment usually leads to a nonunion. In the nonathlete, the nonunion is rarely symptomatic. However, in athletes who are involved in overhead activities, the nonunion can result in valgus instability of the elbow and limit the athlete's performance (Gilchrist and McKee, 2002; Sugita et al., 1994; Takeishi et al., 2001; Woods and Tullos, 1977).

Controversies

- Some authors suggest that opening of the medial joint by the valgus stress test is an indication for open reduction and internal fixation. Other authors discount this test and state that all patients with significant displacement of the epicondyle will demonstrate a positive valgus stress test. Instead, the decision to operate should be based on the patient's need to have a stable elbow for his or her sport or work (Wilkins, 1991).

INDICATIONS

- An acute, displaced medial epicondyle fracture associated with an elbow dislocation or subluxation in an adolescent athlete

EXAMINATION/IMAGING

- The skin is examined for abrasions or open injuries.
- The sensory and motor function of the ulnar nerve, the radial pulse, and capillary refill of the hand are evaluated.
- The wrist and shoulder are also examined for possible additional injuries.
- Plain radiographs should be obtained in anteroposterior (AP), lateral, and valgus stress views.
  - The AP radiograph is best for determining the amount of displacement of the medial epicondyle fracture (Fig. 2).
  - The lateral radiograph is examined to be certain that the elbow joint is reduced and that the medial epicondyle fragment is not in the joint (Fowles et al., 1984) (Fig. 3).
  - The valgus stress view (Fig. 4) can be utilized to demonstrate valgus instability of the elbow. This can be done prior to surgery with a gravity valgus stress test, or under anesthesia prior to making the skin incision (Case and Hennrikus, 1997; Schwab et al., 1980; Woods and Tullos, 1977).

Treatment Options

- Nonoperative treatment is acceptable for some nonathletes. For these patients, treatment can include a brief period of splinting followed by range-of-motion exercises. Prolonged casting is not recommended. Many medial epicondyle fractures occur with an elbow dislocation or subluxation. Casting may lead to permanent elbow stiffness (Linscheid and Wheeler, 1965; Ross et al., 1999).

- Other techniques for fixation exist for operative treatment, such as a Kirshner wire (K-wire) rather than a screw and washer (Hines et al., 1987). However, the K-wire does not produce compression of the fracture. In addition, the less rigid and often prominent K-wire can inhibit the ability of the athlete to perform early motion. Early motion is necessary to prevent permanent elbow stiffness.

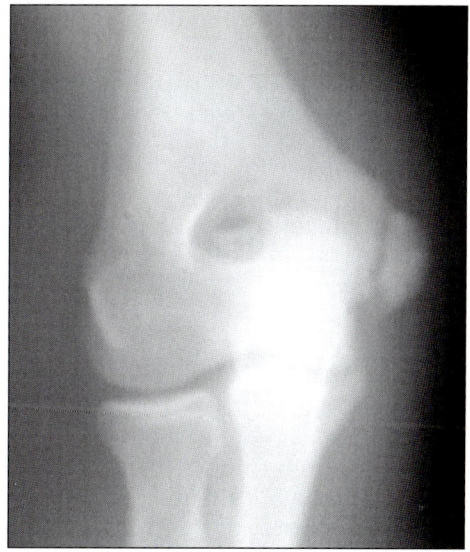

FIGURE 1

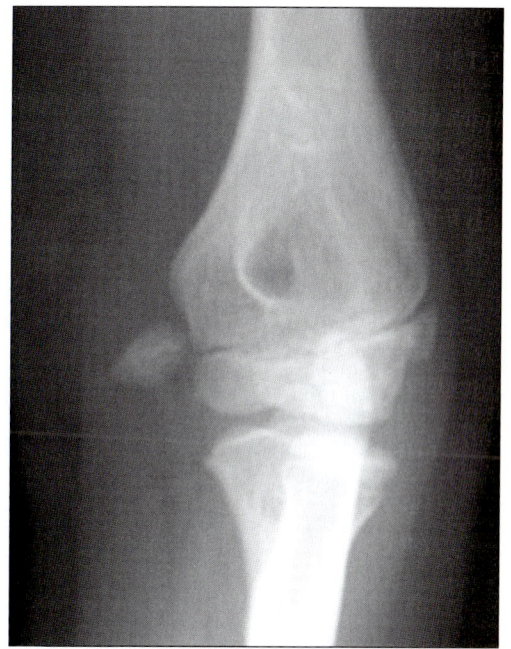

FIGURE 2

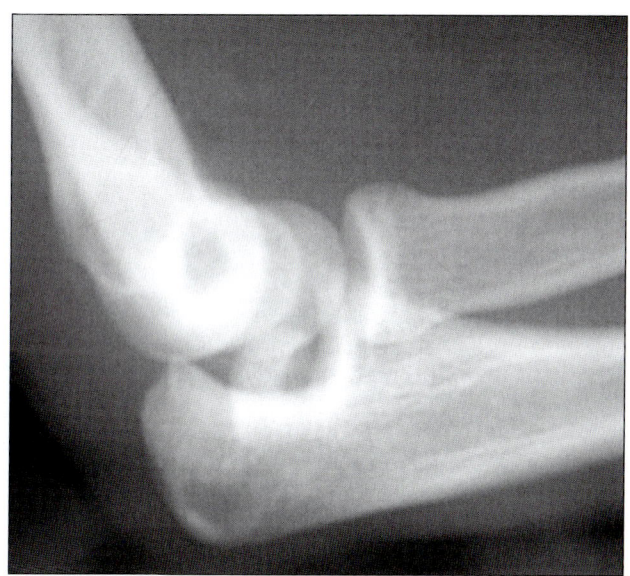

FIGURE 3

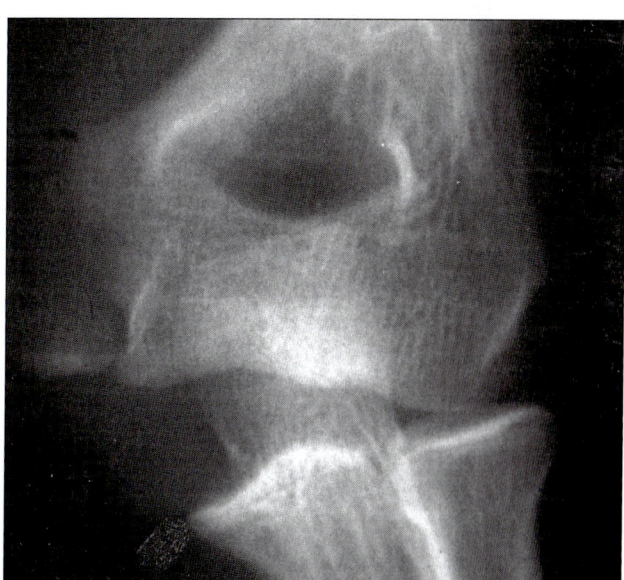

FIGURE 4

Equipment

• C-arm fluoroscope.

• Plexiglass radiolucent upper extremity table. This can be as simple as a 3 foot × 5 foot × ½-inch piece of plexiglass placed under the patient's shoulders and trunk and extending out about 3 feet on the side of injury.

• Sterile tourniquet.

Instrumentation

• A small self-retaining retractor can be utilized to spread the skin.

• A skin hook is used to retract the medial epicondyle distally to expose the bed in which the fragment originated.

Instrumentation/ Implantation

• Small-fragment screw set

• 2.5-mm drill bit

• Power drill

• Soft tissue guide

SURGICAL ANATOMY

■ The medial epicondyle is the last growth plate to fuse in the elbow (Fig. 5). Fusion occurs between the ages of 14 and 18. Fusion occurs later in males.

■ The ulnar collateral ligament originates on the inferior surface of the medial epicondyle.

■ Muscles in the flexor-pronator mass, including the pronator teres, flexor carpi radialis, palmaris longus, flexor digitorum superficialis, and flexor carpi ulnaris, originate from the medial epicondyle.

POSITIONING

■ Supine positioning is used, with a plexiglass radiolucent upper extremity table for the injured elbow (Fig. 6).
  • The C-arm is brought in under the radiolucent table perpendicular to the patient.
  • The surgeon sits on the ulna side of the upper extremity table.

■ A sterile tourniquet is utilized on the operative arm.

PORTALS/EXPOSURES

■ A longitudinal skin incision about 4 cm long is made in the skin centered on the medial epicondyle. In the swollen injured elbow, fluoroscopy can be utilized to mark the site of the medial epicondyle and place the skin incision.

■ The displaced medial epicondyle is identified and reflected distally with a skin hook to expose the origin of the epicondyle fragment and to identify and protect the ulnar nerve inferiorly.

PROCEDURE

STEP 1

■ Following exposure, a 2.5-mm drill bit with soft tissue guide is placed into the center of the site of origin of the medial epicondyle fragment from the medial condyle of the distal humerus.
  • The soft tissue guide is used to prevent inadvertent injury to the adjacent ulnar nerve. Fluoroscopy is used to guide the direction of the drill.

■ The drill bit is passed up the medial column of the distal humerus (Fig. 7). Care is taken to avoid drilling into the olecranon fossa.

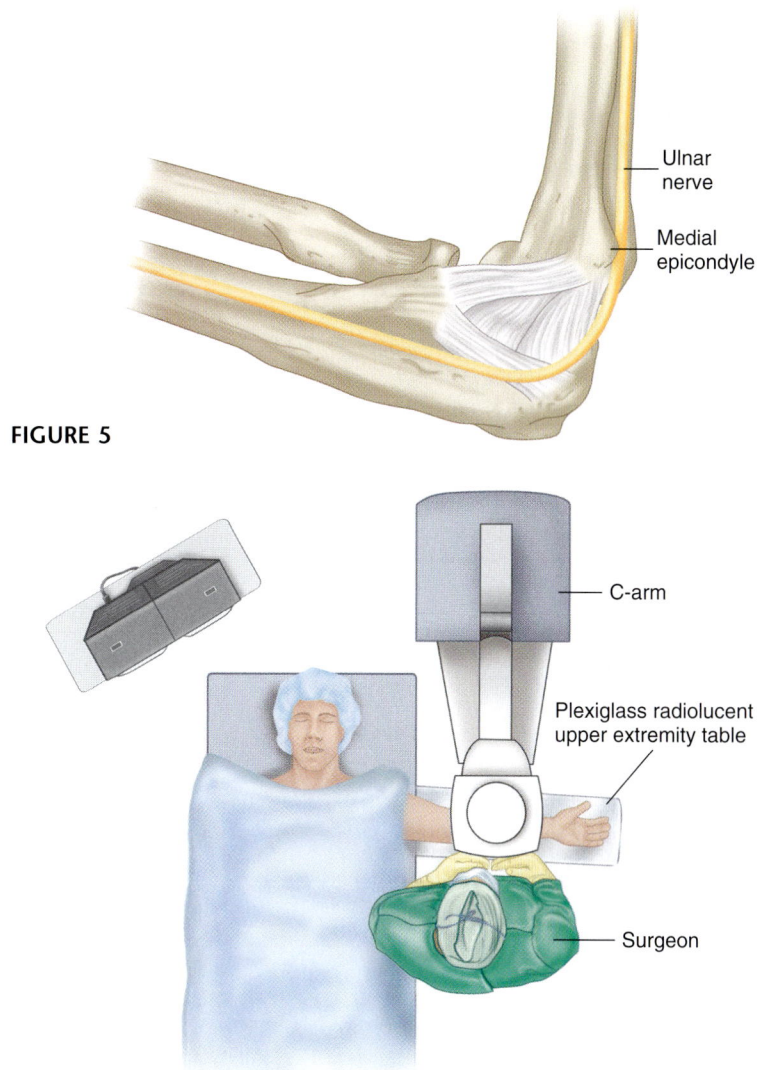

Ulnar nerve

Medial epicondyle

FIGURE 5

C-arm

Plexiglass radiolucent upper extremity table

Surgeon

FIGURE 6

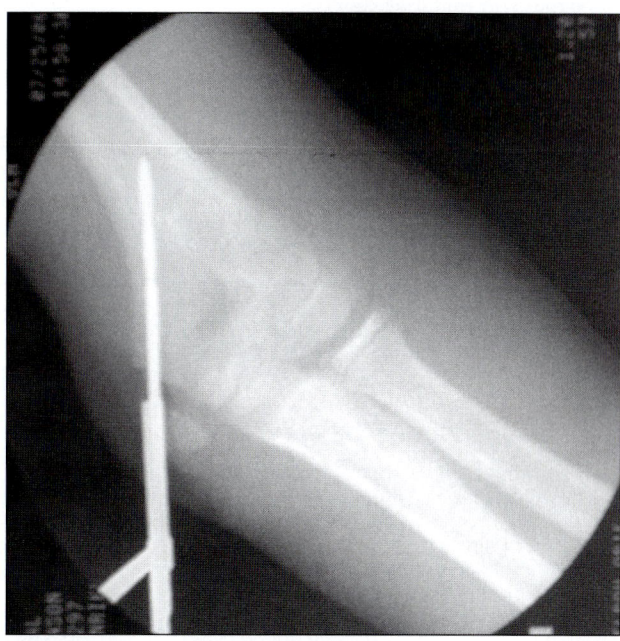

FIGURE 7

Instrumentation/ Implantation

• A 40-mm-long small-fragment screw and metal washer.

STEP 2

■ The 2.5-mm drill bit with soft tissue guide is used to drill a hole in the center of the medial epicondyle fragment. This can be done simply by flipping the medial epicondyle over, identifying the center of the epicondyle, and drilling from inside out.

STEP 3

■ A small-fragment screw and metal washer are selected for fixation.
  • The screw is typically about 40 mm long. The screw does not need to reach the far cortex. Tapping is not necessary.
  • The metal washer is utilized to increase the surface area for compression and to prevent the screw head from penetrating or fragmenting the apophyseal epicondylar fragment.
■ The screw and washer are hand screwed through the medial epicondylar fragment from outside in until the screw tip is protruding about 10 cm through the epicondyle.
■ The tip of the screw is then placed into the predrilled hole in the medial condyle. With the elbow flexed to about 90° and the forearm in supination, the screw is slowly hand screwed up the medial column of the distal humerus.
■ The epicondylar fragment is gradually compressed back to its origin. Anteroposterior (Fig. 8A) and lateral (Fig. 8B) fluoroscopic images are obtained to document repair of the medial epicondyle and appropriate screw and washer position.

Controversies

• For the typical teenager patient with a large epicondyle fragment, a screw and washer provides rigid fixation that allows for early motion (Case and Hennrikus, 1997). Prolonged postfixation casting is not recommended because elbow stiffness may result. However, for the less common case of a small epicondyle fragment in young children, a smaller buried K-wire can be utilized for fixation. In these cases, casting may be needed for 2 weeks to prevent displacement. Elbow motion should be started after cast removal.

• A cannulated small-fragment screw can also be used for fixation. However, hardware breakage complications may occur when using small cannulated systems (Schwend et al., 1997).

STEP 4

■ The wound is irrigated and the tourniquet is released and removed. All bleeding should be controlled.
■ The subcutaneous tissues are closed using interrupted Vicryl suture. The skin is closed with interrupted Monocryl or nylon suture.
■ The arm is placed into a well-padded splint with the elbow at about 80° of flexion and the forearm in supination.

POSTOPERATIVE CARE AND EXPECTED OUTCOMES

■ The splint is removed on postoperative day 3 or 4 and elbow motion is started. Instruction and monitoring of motion, strengthening, and home exercises by a physical therapist is recommended.
■ Athletes should anticipate returning to their preinjury sport by about 12 weeks postsurgery with near-full range of motion and no valgus instability.

Displaced Medial Epicondyle Fracture

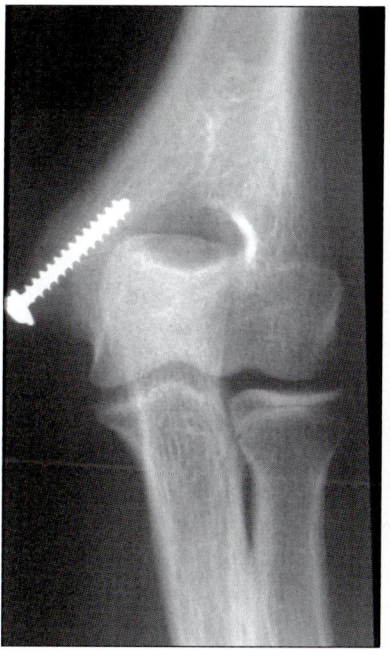 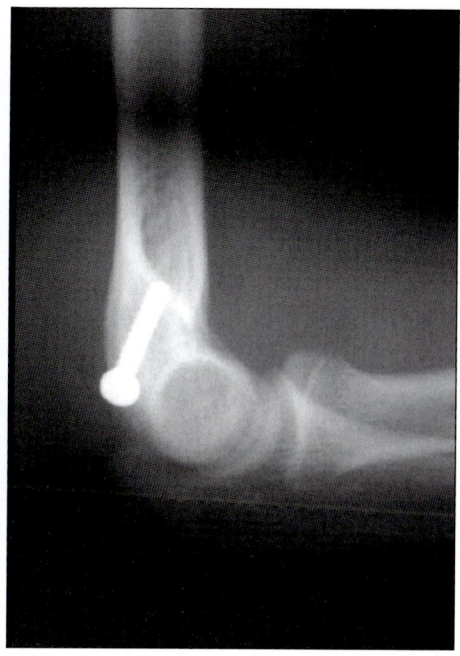

A   B

FIGURE 8

EVIDENCE

Bede WB, Lefebvre AR, Rosman MA. Fractures of the medial humeral epicondyle in children. Can J Surg. 1975;18:137–142.

(Level IV evidence)

Case S, Hennrikus W. Surgical treatment of displaced medial epicondyle fractures in adolescent athletes. Am J Sports Med. 1997;25:682–686.

(Level IV evidence)

Farsetti P, Potenza V, Caterini R, et al. Long term results of treatment of fractures of the medial epicondyle in children. J Bone Joint Surg [Am]. 2001;83:1299–1305.

(Level IV evidence)

Fowles JV, Kassab MT, Moula T. Untreated intra articular entrapment of the medial epicondyle. J Bone Joint Surg [Br]. 1984;66:562–565.

(Level IV evidence)

Gilchrist AD, McKee MD. Valgus instability of the elbow due to medial epicondyle non-union: a report of 5 cases. J Shoulder Elbow Surg. 2002;11:493–497.

(Level IV evidence)

Hines RF, Herndon WA, Evans JP. Operative treatment of medial epicondyle fractures in children. Clin Orthop Relat Res. 1987;(223):170–174.

(Level IV evidence)

Josefsson PO, Danielsson LG. Epicondylar fractures in children. Acta Orthop Scand. 1986;57:313–315.

(Level IV evidence)

Linscheid RL, Wheeler DK. Elbow dislocations. JAMA. 1965;194:1171–1173.

(Level IV evidence)

Ross G, McDevitt ER, Chronister R, et al. Treatment of elbow dislocation with an immediate motion protocol. Am J Sports Med. 1999;27:308–311.

(Level IV evidence)

Schwab G, Bennett JB, Woods GW, et al. Biomechanics of elbow instability: the role of the medial collateral ligament. Clin Orthop Relat Res. 1980;(146):42–52.

(Level V evidence)

Schwend R, Hennrikus W, Millis M, et al. Complications when using the cannulated 3.5 mm screw set. Orthopedics. 1997;20:221–223.

(Level IV evidence)

Smith FM. Medial epicondyle injuries. JAMA. 1950;142:396–402.

(Level V evidence)

Speed JS, Boyd HB. Fractures about the elbow. Am J Surg. 1937;38:727–730.

(Level V evidence)

Sugita A, Konani H, Ueo T, et al. Recurrent dislocation of the elbow. Nippon Geka Hokan. 1994;63:181–185.

(Level IV evidence)

Takeishi H, Oka Y, Ikeda M. Reconstructing an unstable medial elbow complicated by medial epicondyle nonunion. Tokai J Exp Clin Med. 2001;2:77–80.

(Level IV evidence)

Woods GW, Tullos HG. Elbow instability and medial epicondyle fractures. Am J Sports Med. 1977;5:23–30.

(Level V evidence)

Wilkins KE. Fractures of the medial epicondyle in children. Instr Course Lect. 1991;40:3–10

(Level V evidence)

Radial Head/Neck Fracture: Closed Reduction, Percutaneous Reduction, and Open Reduction

Sameer Badarudeen, Robert M. Bernstein, and Saul M. Bernstein

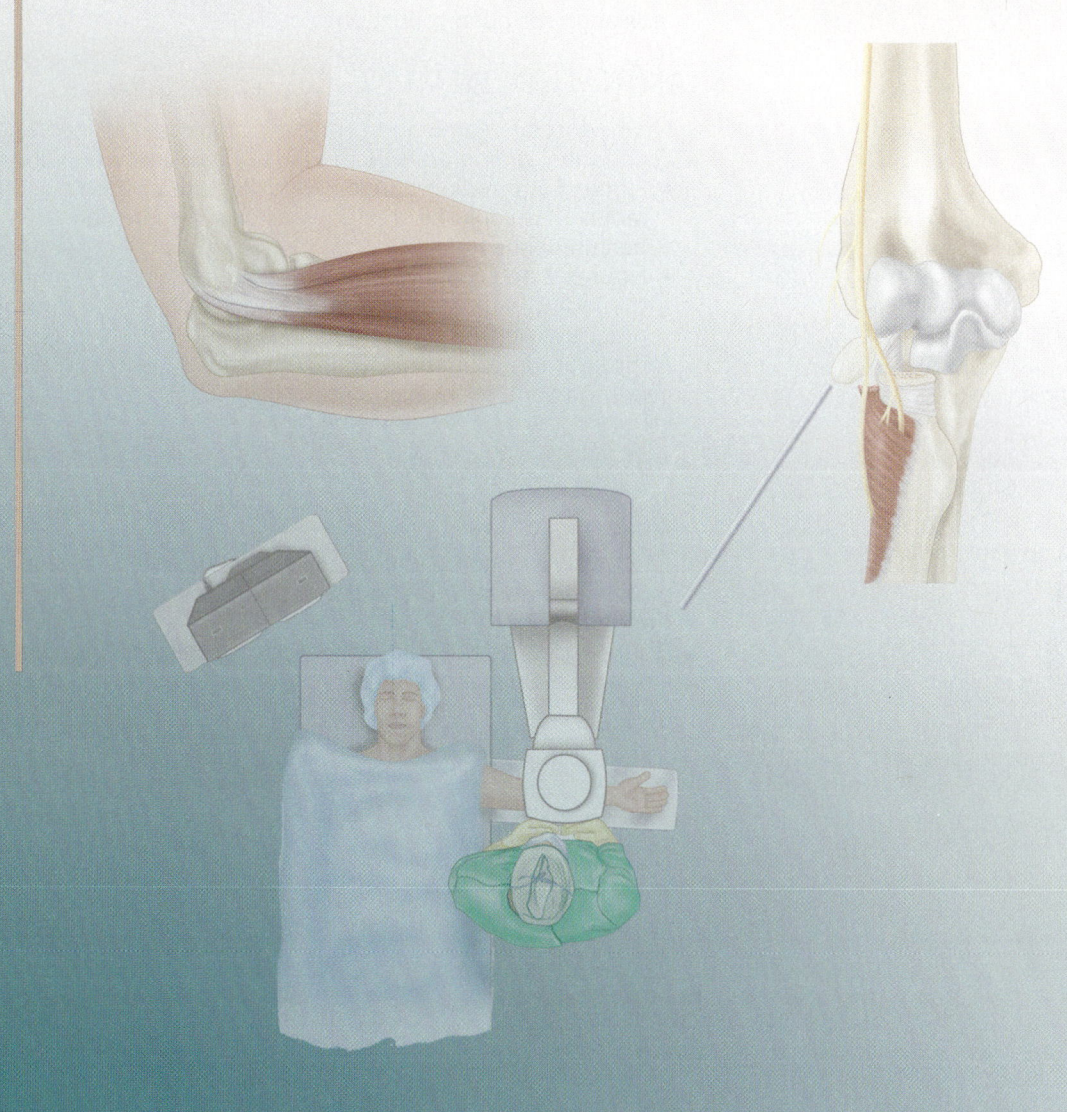

Controversies

- Radial neck angulation greater than 65° and completely displaced fractures may be difficult or impossible to reduce closed.
- Localized infection (cellulitis, abscess) over the radial head may complicate percutaneous reduction using Steinmann pin.
- Open reduction is only rarely needed since almost all radial head/neck fractures can be reduced by closed or percutaneous means.

Treatment Options

- Acceptance of position
- Closed reduction
- Percutaneous reduction with a Steinmann pin
- Open reduction

INDICATIONS

- Depending upon the extend of fracture displacement and angulation, there might be better indications for each of the three different techniques: closed reduction, percutaneous reduction, and open reduction.
- Closed reduction indications: Fractures with displacement greater than 2 mm or lateral angulation greater than 20–30°.
- Percutaneous reduction indications: Fractures with displacement greater than 2 mm or fractures with lateral angulation greater than 20–30° that are not reducible by closed method.
- Open reduction indications: Fractures with displacement greater than 2 mm or fractures with lateral angulation greater than 20–30° that are not reducible by closed or percutaneous methods. Also, reversal of the radial head (180° rotation) is an indication for open reduction.

EXAMINATION/IMAGING

- Neurovascular examination (posterior interosseous nerve)
- Orthogonal radiographs of the radial head and elbow joint
  - Figure 1 is a radiograph showing fracture of the neck of the radius that could be treated with closed reduction or percutaneous reduction.
  - Figures 2 and 3 are radiographs of a fracture of the neck of the radius with complete dislocation that may be difficult to reduce closed.
- Arthrogram in children in whom the radial head secondary center has not yet ossified

SURGICAL ANATOMY

- The radial head and neck are subcutaneous on the lateral side of the elbow, just distal to the lateral epicondyle.
- The posterior interosseous nerve penetrates the supinator muscle just distal to the radial neck and may lie directly upon the bone (Fig. 4).
- Figure 5 depicts the surface anatomy of the posterior interosseous nerve in relation to the radial neck.

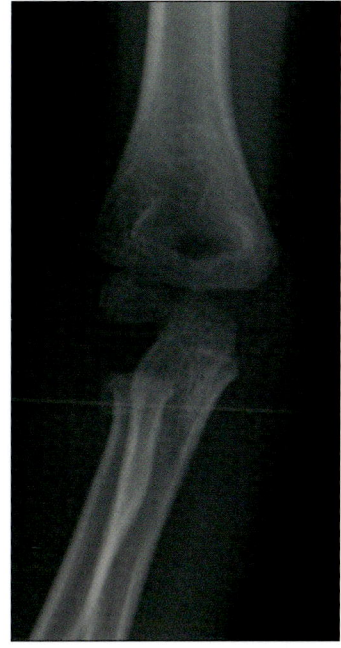

FIGURE 1

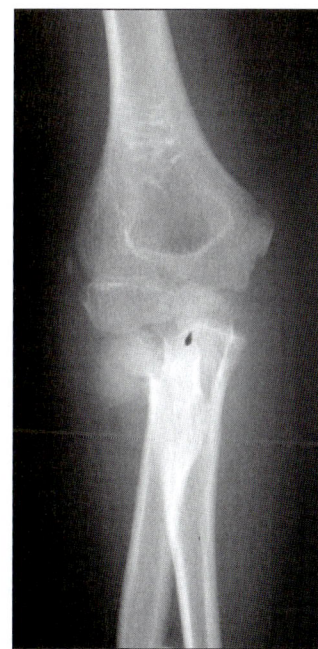

FIGURE 2

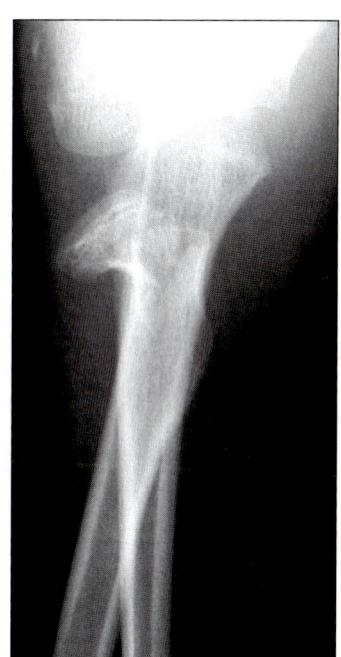

FIGURE 3

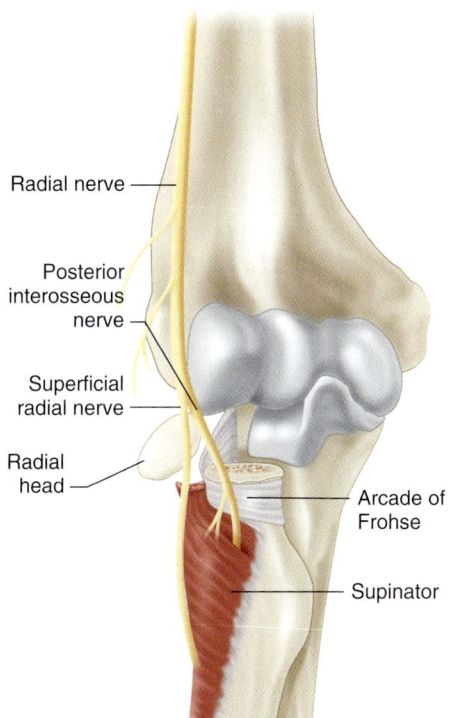

Radial nerve

Posterior
interosseous
nerve

Superficial
radial nerve

Radial
head

Arcade of
Frohse

Supinator

FIGURE 4

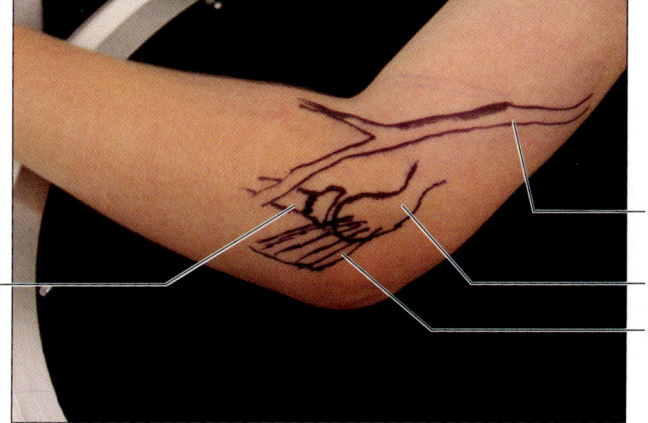

Proximal end
of radius

Posterior
interosseous nerve

Distal end
of humerus
Anconeus muscle

FIGURE 5

Equipment

- Armboard

Equipment

- Armboard

CLOSED REDUCTION

POSITIONING

- The patient is placed in the supine position on the table with the armboard at the ipsilateral head, folded in, to act as a headboard extension.
- The elbow is positioned over the fluoroscopic receiver (C-arm) (Fig. 6).
- The surgical assistant should stand at the ipsilateral head of the table, stabilizing the distal humerus.
- Figure 7 depicts the authors' preferred set up of the operating room for a "left" radial neck fracture, with the armboard and C-arm on the same side and the monitor on the opposite side of the table.

PROCEDURE

- The forearm is supinated and the surgeon places his or her thumb over the radial head (Fig. 8).
- Varus stress is applied to the elbow while the assistant stabilizes the distal humerus (Fig. 9).
- Direct pressure is placed over the radial head while the forearm is gradually rotated into full pronation.
- Radiographic views (Figs. 10 and 11) are taken in two planes to confirm reduction.

PERCUTANEOUS REDUCTION WITH A STEINMANN PIN

POSITIONING

- The patient is placed in the supine position on the table with the armboard at the ipsilateral head, folded in, to act as a headboard extension.
- The forearm and hand are prepped, and the elbow is then positioned over the fluoroscopic receiver (C-arm) (see Fig. 6).
- The surgical assistant should stand at the ipsilateral head of the table, stabilizing the distal humerus.

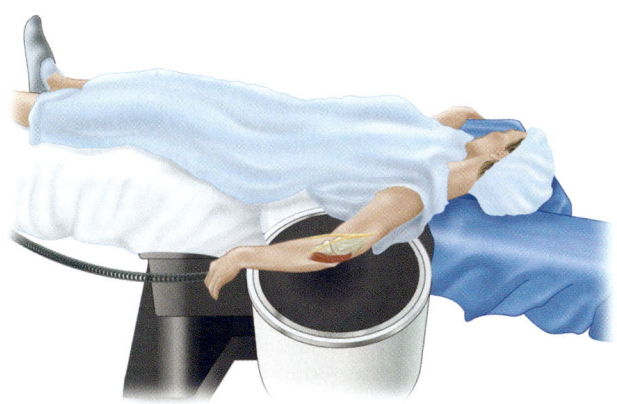

FIGURE 6

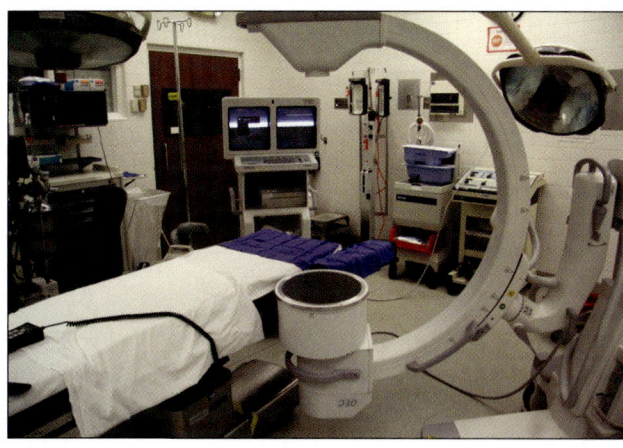

FIGURE 7

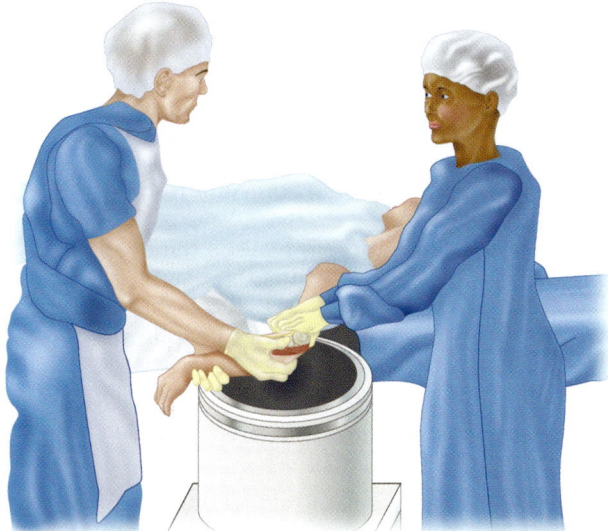

FIGURE 8

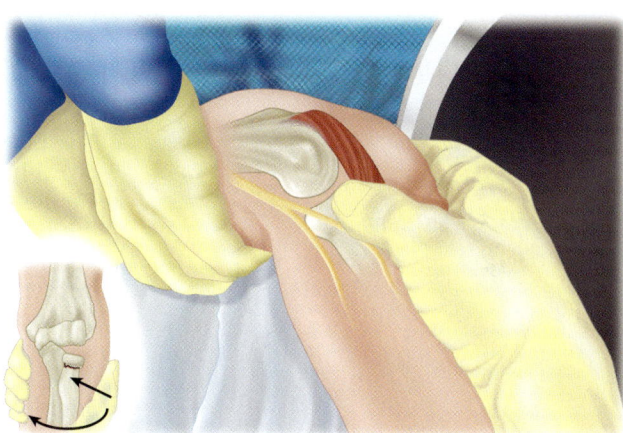

FIGURE 9

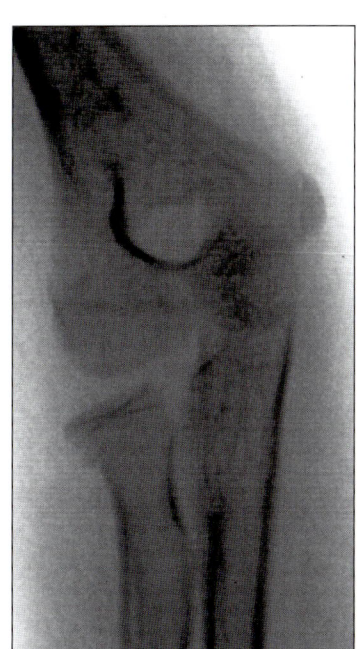

FIGURE 10

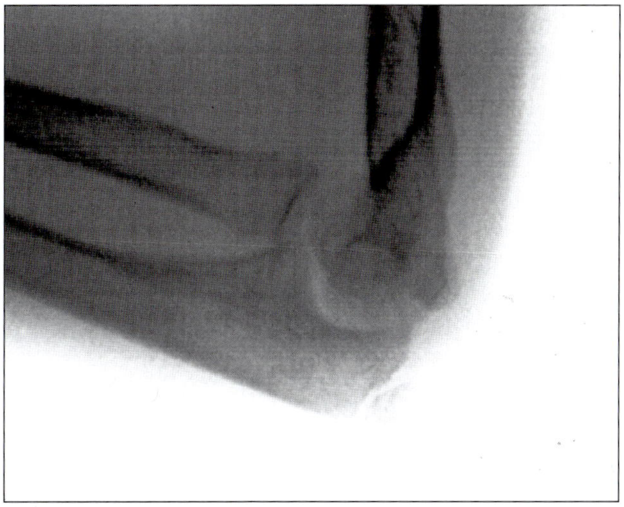

FIGURE 11

PORTALS/EXPOSURES

- The portal is through a stab incision made just distal to the radial head/neck on the lateral side of the forearm.
- A fluoroscopic view is taken with the knife blade or metallic marker over the distal radial neck to accurately identify the site of puncture (Fig. 12), which is then marked on the skin (Fig. 13).

PROCEDURE

STEP 1

- The forearm is slightly supinated and the stab incision is made with a knife blade just distal to the radial head.
- A hemostat is used to spread down to bone, angling in a slightly proximal direction to the fracture site.
- A large (3-mm), blunt-ended Steinmann pin is advanced manually up to the radial head.

STEP 2

- Varus stress is applied to the elbow while the assistant stabilizes the distal humerus.
- The blunt end of the Steinmann pin is used to manipulate the radial head fragment into place (Figs. 14 and 15).
- Gentle pronation may be performed as pressure is applied to the fragment.
- If partial reduction is obtained, the pin may be removed and further manipulation by the closed technique may be attempted.
- Radiographic views are taken in two planes to confirm reduction (Fig. 16).
- Simple 4.0 chromium suture is used to repair the incision.

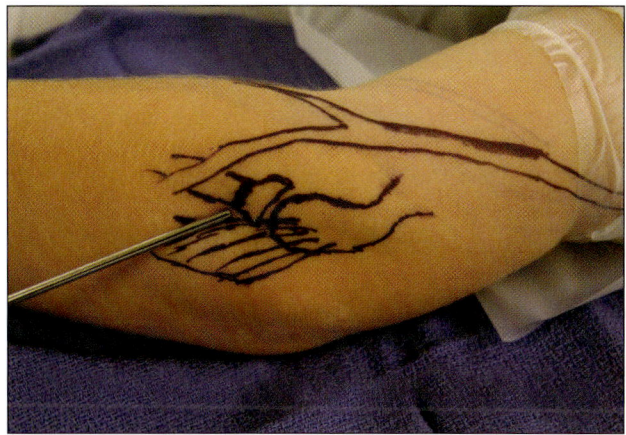

FIGURE 12

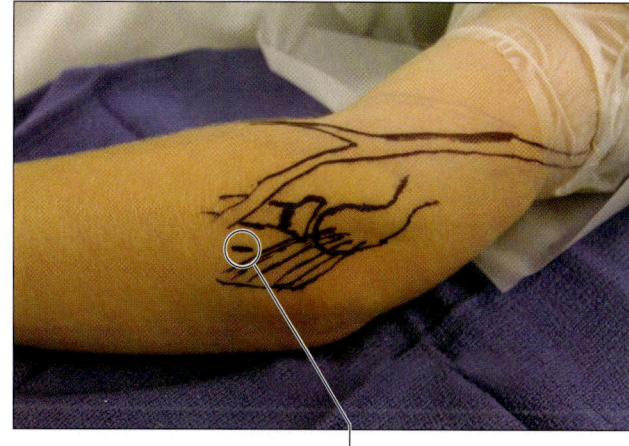

Mark the site of puncture

FIGURE 13

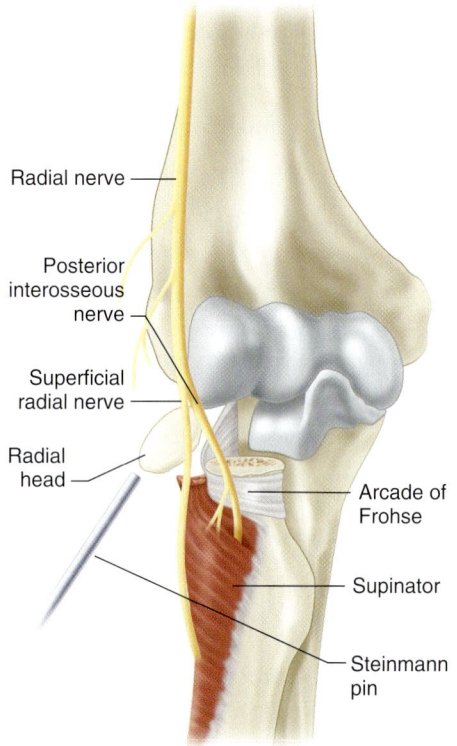

Radial nerve

Posterior interosseous nerve

Superficial radial nerve

Radial head

Arcade of Frohse

Supinator

Steinmann pin

FIGURE 14

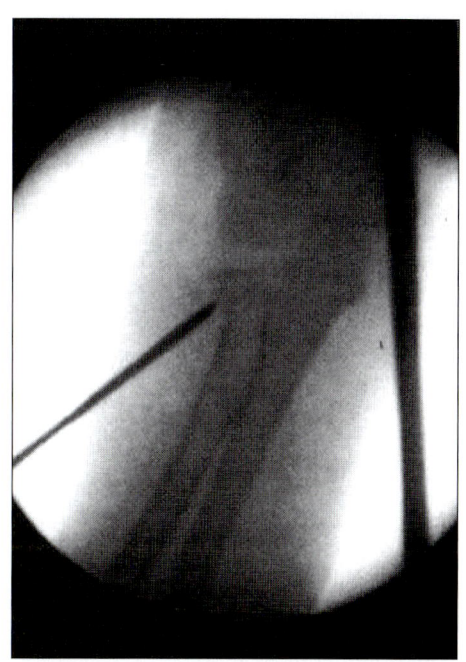

FIGURE 15

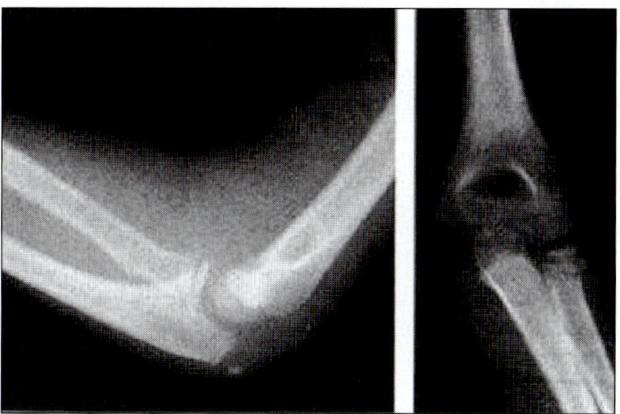

FIGURE 16

Equipment
- Armboard

OPEN REDUCTION

POSITIONING
- The patient is placed in the supine position on the table with the forearm and elbow lying on the armboard or hand table.
- A tourniquet is applied to the upper arm.
- The elbow, forearm, and hand are prepped and draped.

PORTALS/EXPOSURES
- A standard Kocher incision is made over the lateral side of the elbow.
- The anconeus is reflected anteriorly off the ulna and the joint capsule is exposed and entered.

PROCEDURE

STEP 1
- After giving preoperative antibiotics, the tourniquet is inflated and the hand and arm are exsanguinated.
- A curvilinear incision is made over the lateral side of the elbow, extending distally from the tip of the lateral epicondyle to just distal to the radial neck.

STEP 2
- The anconeus is reflected off the proximal ulna, exposing the capsule of the radiocapitellar joint.
- The joint is opened if the capsule has not already been disrupted.

STEP 3
- The joint is irrigated, removing any clot.
- The radial head fragment is gently manipulated and reduced onto the distal fragment, with care not to disrupt any residual soft tissue attachments if they exist.
- The capsule is repaired if possible.
- Radiographic views are taken in two planes to confirm reduction (Figs. 17 and 18).
- The skin is repaired in a standard fashion.

POSTOPERATIVE CARE AND EXPECTED OUTCOMES
- Postoperative care is similar for all three procedures described; after adequate reduction, a sterile dressing is applied to any surgical wound.
- A long-arm cast is applied at 90° of flexion with the forearm in neutral or slight supination.
  - The cast should be bivalved or a large window should be removed anteriorly over the cubital fossa to allow for swelling.
- Cast immobilization is continued for 3–4 weeks.

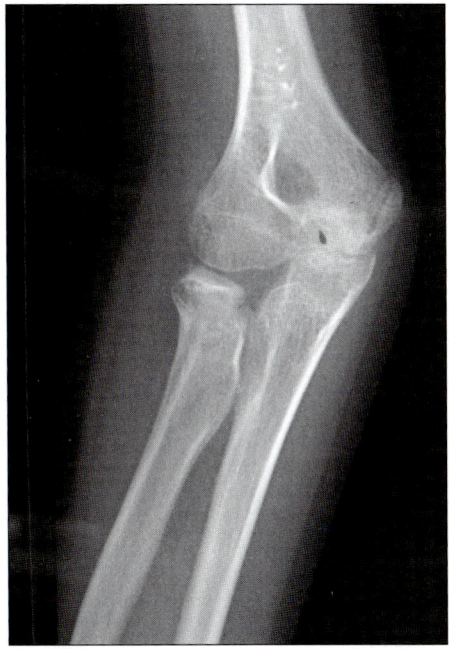

FIGURE 17

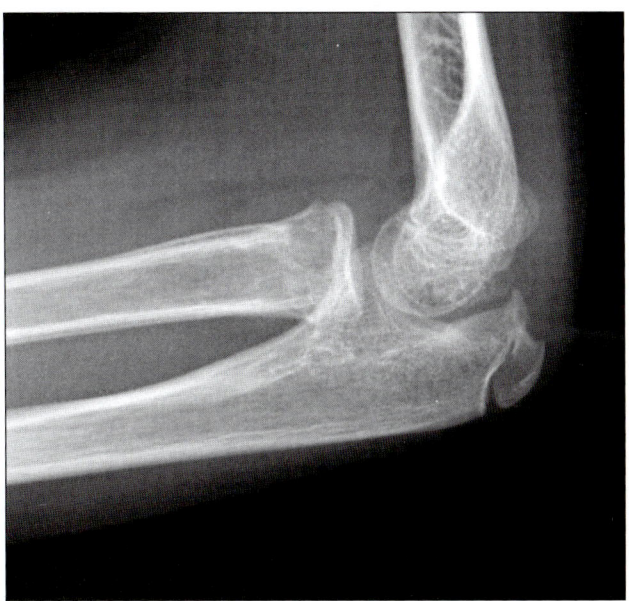

FIGURE 18

EVIDENCE

Bernstein SM, McKeever P, Bernstein L. Percutaneous reduction of displaced radial neck fractures in children. J Pediatr Orthop. 1993;13(1):85–8.

Eighteen patients who failed closed reduction treated by percutaneous reduction using Steinmann pin. Successful reduction in fifteen patients. (Level IV evidence)

D'souza S, Vaishya R, Klenerman L. Management of radial neck fractures in children: a retrospective analysis of one hundred patients. J Pediatr Orthop. 1993;13:232–8.

This is a retrospective review of 100 children with radial neck fractures. Closed reduction had better results than open reduction. Most common complications were avascular necrosis, radial head enlargement and radial neck notching. (Level III evidence)

Steele JA, Graham HK. Angulated radial neck fractures in children. A prospective study of percutaneous reduction. J Bone Joint Surg [Br]. 1992;74(5):760–4. Erratum in: J Bone Joint Surg [Br]. 1993;75:169.

Prospective study of angulated radial neck fractures treated by percutaneous reduction. Successful reduction in 33 of the 36 patients and over 90% good to excellent results (Level II evidence)

Steinberg EL, Golomb D, Salama R, Wientroub S. Radial head and neck fractures in children. J Pediatr Orthop. 1988;8:35–40.

This is long-term followup report of 42 consecutive radial neck fractures. The most important factor affecting results was primary angulation. (Level IV evidence)

Lateral Humeral Condyle Fracture: Closed Reduction and Percutaneous Pinning and Open Reduction and Internal Fixation

Susan T. Mahan

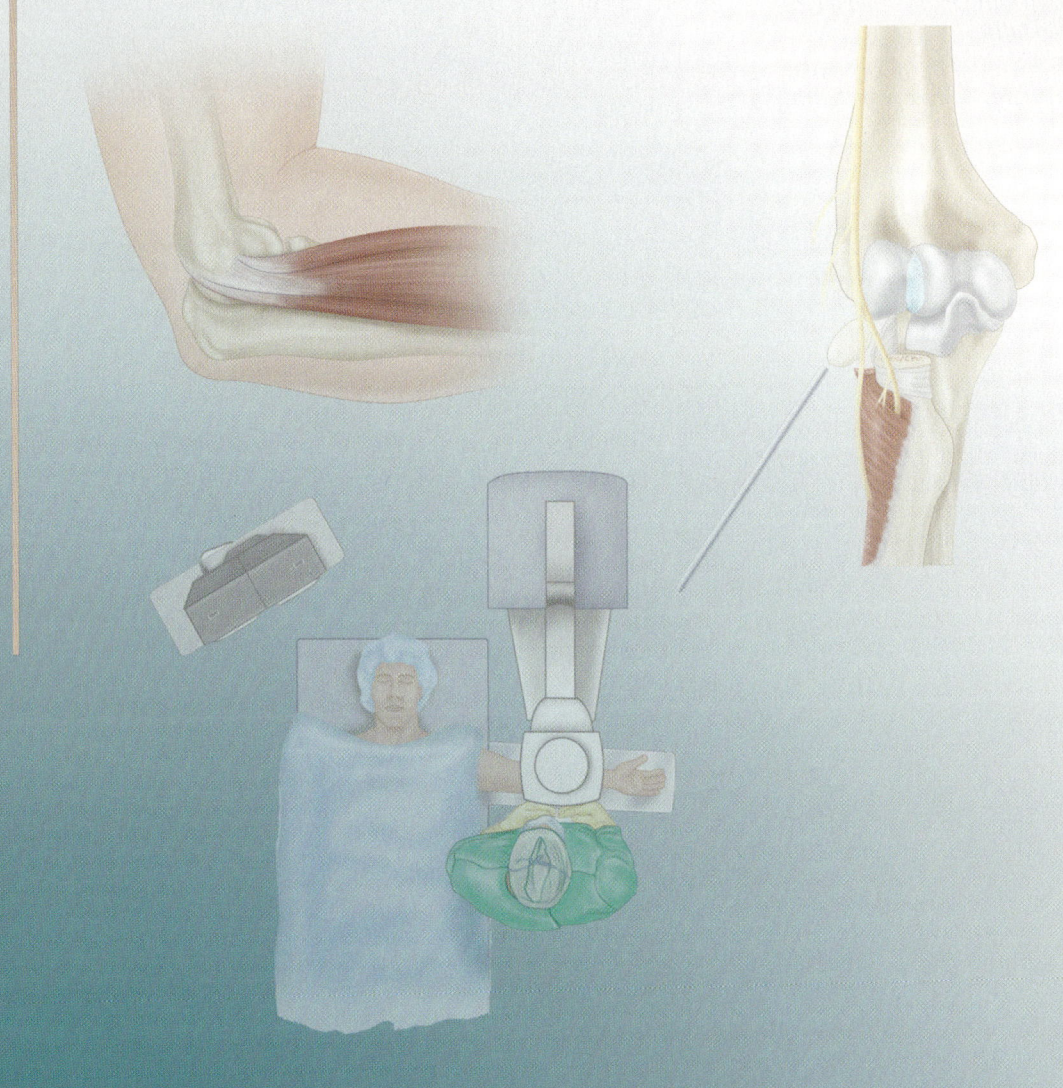

Treatment Options

- Closed reduction with percutaneous pinning (with or without arthrogram) or open reduction and internal fixation

INDICATIONS

- For closed reduction and percutaneous pinning (CRPP)
  - Greater than 2 mm but less than 4 mm of displacement with the appearance of articular congruity
  - Nondisplaced fractures (<2 mm) in cases in which the social environment is concerning and/or close follow-up is not possible
- For open reduction and internal fixation (ORIF)
  - Greater than 4 mm of displacement and possibly rotated
  - Articular incongruity

Controversies

- Treatment of nondisplaced and minimally displaced lateral condyle fractures remains controversial. Many support use of cast immobilization and close follow-up, while other advocate for internal fixation. Nonunion of even minimally displaced fractures has been reported.

- Some advocate for arthrography to determine joint congruity after CRPP in all fractures displaced less than 2 mm; however, some feel these can be treated with only a cast.

- Some advocate for ORIF for any displacement of the fracture (Badelon et al., 1988), noting the instability of the fragments even in minimally displaced fractures.

EXAMINATION/IMAGING

- The injured elbow should be assessed with anteroposterior (AP), lateral, and (often) internal oblique radiographs to determine displacement and optimal treatment.
- Figure 1 shows preoperative AP (Fig. 1A) and lateral (Fig. 1B) radiographs in a 2-year-old girl with a minimally displaced lateral condyle fracture.
- Figure 2 shows preoperative AP (Fig. 2A) and lateral (Fig. 2B) radiographs in a 6-year-old girl with a fully displaced lateral condyle fracture.

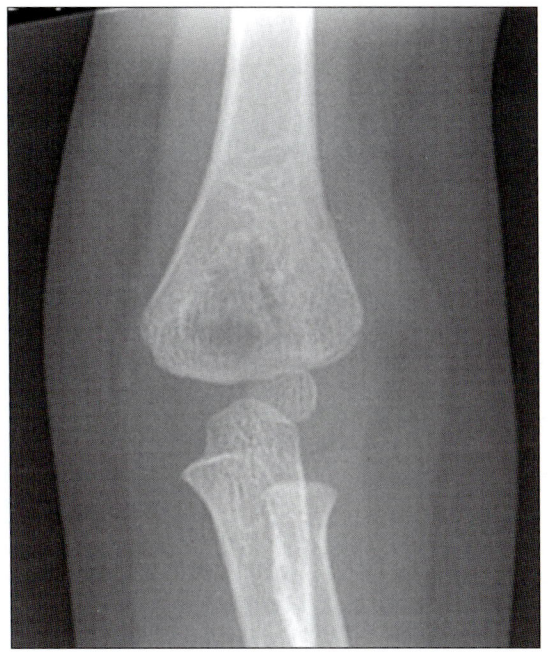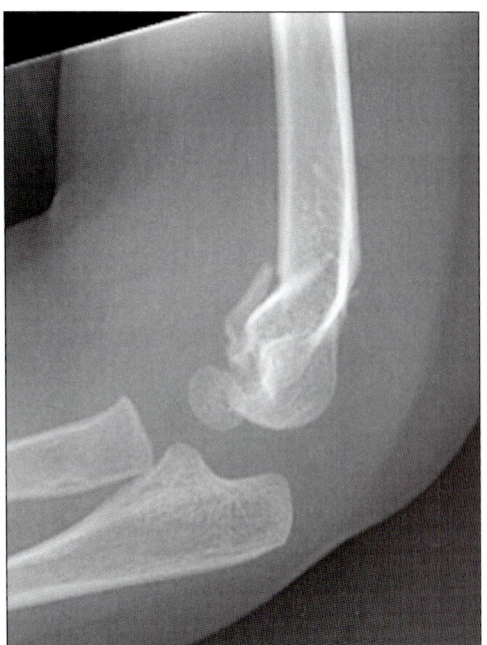

A

FIGURE 1

B

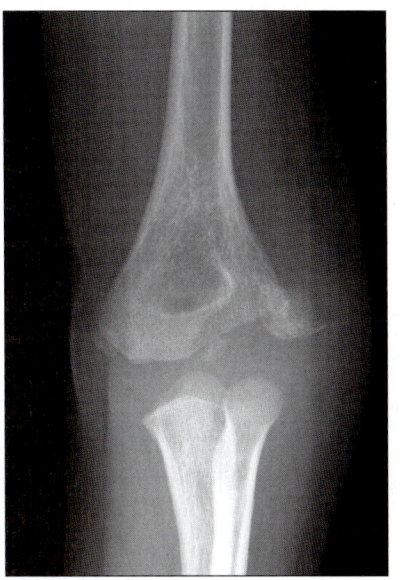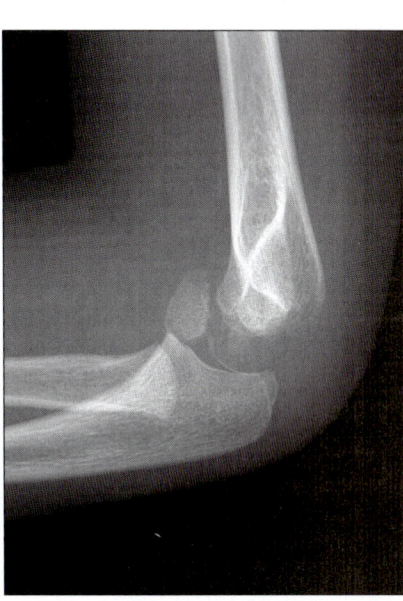

A

FIGURE 2

B

SURGICAL ANATOMY

- Lateral wrist extensors and forearm supinators (brachioradialis, extensor carpi radialis longus, and extensor carpi radialis brevis), originating from the lateral epicondyle, serve as deforming forces for the fracture.
- Be aware of the ulnar nerve and its course around the medial epicondyle (Fig. 3) when using any penetrating pins. Avoid placing a Hohmann-type retractor anteriorly around the medial side.
- The radial nerve crosses the elbow joint anterior to this approach, between the brachialis and brachioradialis muscles.
- Avoid dissection along the posterior part of the capitellum as this may lead to avascular necrosis.

POSITIONING

- The patient is placed in the supine position with the arm on a translucent armboard.
  - Figure 4 shows positioning of the arm. The patient's head is to the right and the arm is resting on a stack of towels. Note the placement of a sterile tourniquet.
  - The fluoroscopic image intensifier may be used as a table, particularly when an arthrogram and CRPP are likely.
- Patient positioning must plan for adequate fluoroscopic visualization.

PORTALS/EXPOSURES

- For open reduction and internal fixation, a direct longitudinal lateral incision is made slightly anterior to the lateral humeral condyle.
- Figure 5 shows the incision marked on a swollen elbow. The circle corresponds to the expected location of the lateral epicondyle in the reduced elbow.
- The skin and subcutaneous tissue are divided, as is any remaining thin fascia covering the fracture hematoma.
  - The interval is between the brachioradialis and the triceps. The dissection is carried down to the lateral humeral condyle.
  - Often the brachioradialis muscle is torn, leading the surgeon directly to the fracture site.

PEARLS

- *Some have advocated use of the prone position to allow positioning of the elbow that relaxes the distracting muscles during reduction.*

- *Drape out the entire humerus to the armpit to facilitate exposure and sterile tourniquet placement.*

- *A stack of towels can be placed under the elbow to elevate it slightly.*

- *If the surgeon is certain that the fracture can be adequately fixed with closed reduction and percutaneous pinning, the arm can be draped directly on the base of the fluoroscope.*

PITFALLS

- *Do not place a nonsterile tourniquet as this may regretfully interfere with the operative exposure. especially in small children with short humeri.*

Equipment

- A headlight or lighted sucker tip can be useful for visualization during ORIF.

PEARLS

- *Place the incision slightly anterior to facilitate exposure across the front of the joint and leave skin directly over the lateral condyle for pin placement (see Fig. 5).*

- *Avoid dissecting any remaining muscle from the fractured fragment.*

PITFALLS

- *The arm is often quite swollen (and the fractured lateral condyle may be flipped or rotated), making the appropriate landmarks difficult to find. Flexing the elbow to 90° and locating the radial head in addition to utilizing skin landmarks proximally and distally can give the best approximation.*

- *Avoid distal and posterior dissection!*

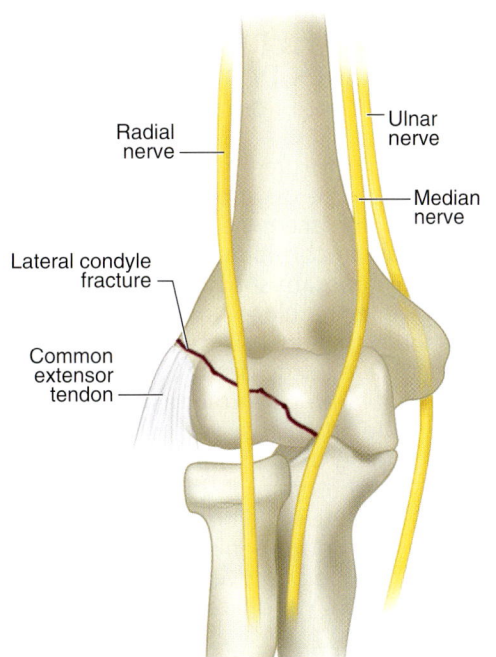

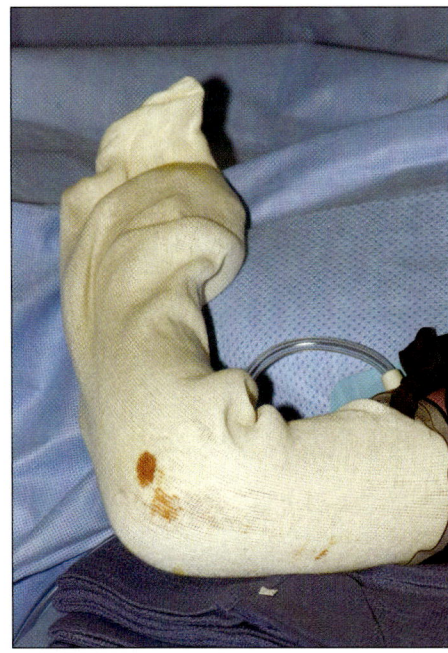

Radial
nerve

Ulnar
nerve

Median
nerve

Lateral condyle
fracture

Common
extensor
tendon

FIGURE 4

FIGURE 3

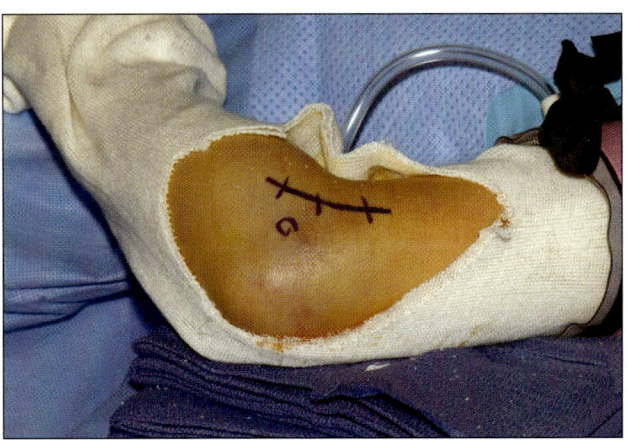

FIGURE 5

PROCEDURE

STEP 1: CLOSED REDUCTION AND PERCUTANEOUS PINNING

- The amount of displacement of the fracture fragment is assessed.
  - If the fractured fragment is more than 4 mm displaced, ORIF should be performed (see Step 2).
  - For displacement of less than 4 mm, percutaneous pinning may be considered.
- An arthrogram should be performed by injecting 0.5–1 ml of dye into the elbow joint. The congruity of the articular surface should then be assessed.
  - If there is any disruption in the articular surface, then ORIF should be performed (see Step 2).
  - If the articular surface is congruent, then percutaneous pinning of the fragment can be performed.
- After arthrogram and CRPP of the patient in Figure 1, intraoperative radiographs show reduction of the fracture, pinning, and the joint congruity from AP (Fig. 6A) and lateral (Fig. 6B) perspectives. Follow-up radiographs 6 months later in AP (Fig. 6C) and lateral (Fig. 6D) views show a healed fracture.

STEP 2: FRACTURE EXPOSURE

- After incision, dissection is carried down to the brachioradialis. In Figure 7, the muscle is torn, revealing the edge of the fracture fragment that is flipped and rotated.
- The fracture is entered and the hematoma and fracture sites are copiously irrigated.
- The periosteum is gently elevated at the fracture edges in order to assess alignment and reduction.
- If the fracture fragment is rotated or flipped (see Fig. 7), it can be grasped with a towel clip or forceps and gently rotated back into place.
- The muscle should be bluntly elevated off the anterior aspect of the distal humerus to allow visualization across the anterior articular surface.

PITFALLS

- *Excessive stripping of the periosteum and its accompanying blood supply must be avoided.*

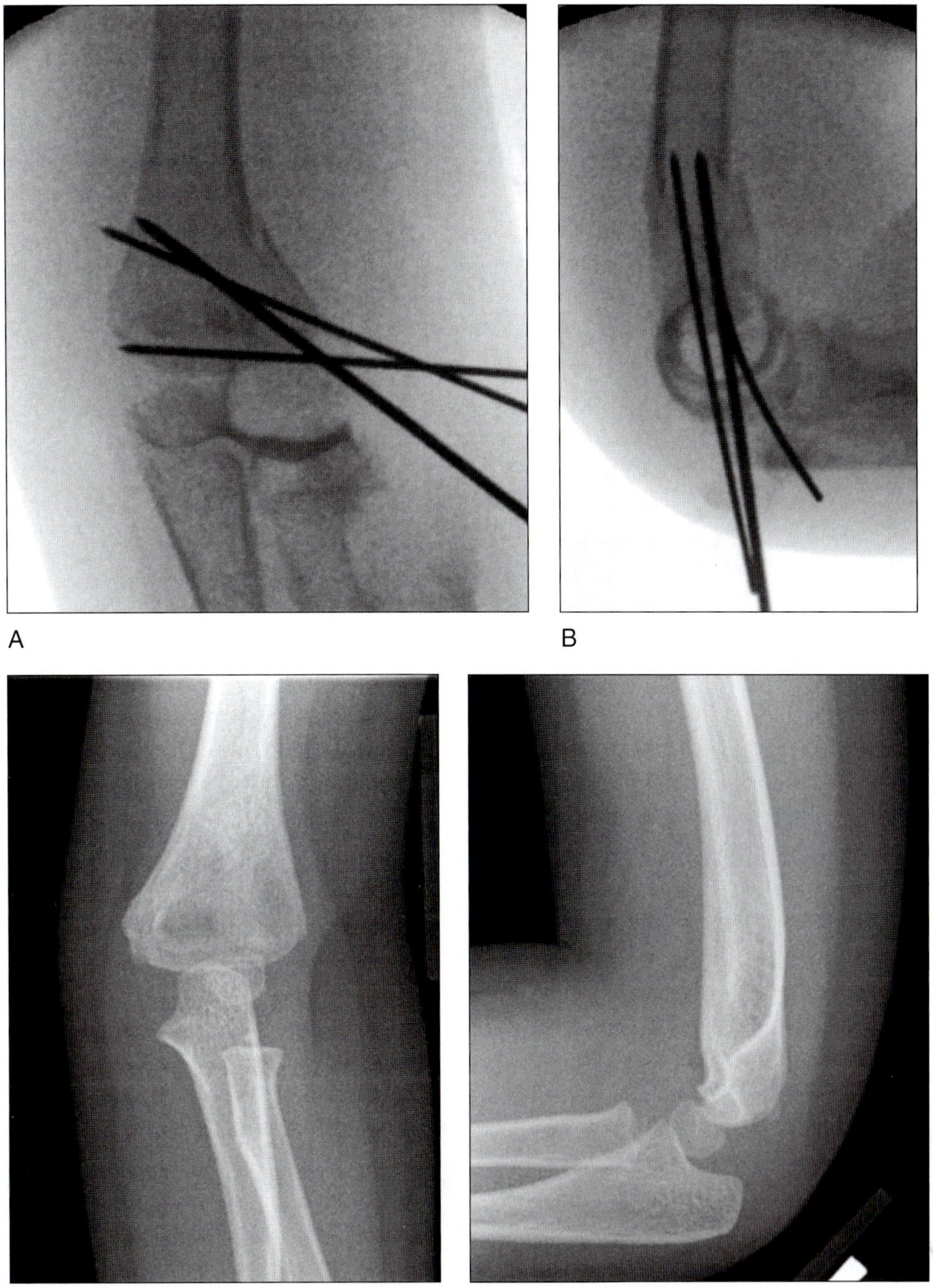

A

B

FIGURE 6 C

D

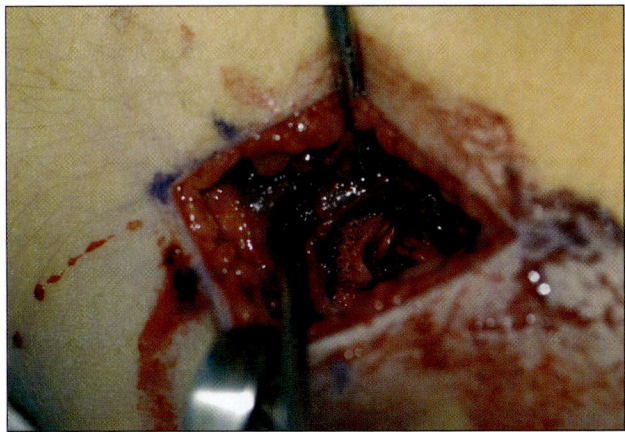

FIGURE 7

- *Be sure both the articular surface and metaphyseal fragments are accurately reduced.*

Instrumentation/ Implantation

- Ideal place for pins is in the metaphyseal fragment. Diverging pins are necessary for the stability of the construct.

- Be sure not to cross the pins at the fracture!

- Pins that are to be left outside the skin should go through a separate stab incision posterior to the main incision.

PEARLS

- *Delayed union and nonunion are possible in this fracture. Some fractures take longer to heal and require more than 4 weeks in a cast.*

- *Watch the trochlea and capitellum for signs of avascular necrosis.*

- *Because this is a Salter-Harris IV fracture, long-term follow-up is necessary to assess for possible growth arrest.*

PITFALLS

- *Malunions may result in valgus deformity of the elbow.*

STEP 3: OPEN REDUCTION

- Reduction is achieved by manually placing the fracture fragment back into its donor site. This can be done with a Freer elevator, using a Kirschner wire (K-wire) as a joystick, and/or using a towel clip to carefully place the fractured piece back in place.
  - In Figure 8, the fracture fragment has been mostly reduced and the first K-wire is introduced in the fragment. This wire can also be used as joystick to facilitate final reduction.
  - Note the retractor anteriorly allowing visualization across the anterior aspect of the distal humerus and articular surface.
- The reduction is assessed both visually and by digital palpation across the anterior aspect of the articular surface.
- At least two smooth K-wires are placed through the fractured condyle, across the physis, and into the humeral metaphysis.
- The position of the reduction and the wires is checked both directly and fluoroscopically.
  - After ORIF of the patient in Figure 2, intraoperative radiographs show the reduction from the AP (Fig. 9A) and lateral (Fig. 9B) perspectives.
  - Postoperative AP (Fig. 9C) and lateral (Fig. 9D) films show the healing injury.
- Bend and cut the ends of the wires and leave them beneath the skin. In Figure 10, the fracture has been reduced and pinned with three K-wires. These wires have been cut and bent to allow the skin to be closed over them. Note the suture closing the rent in the periosteum at the right of the field.

Controversies

- Some advocate using screw osteosynthesis instead of K-wires for fixation. This is thought to be more stable, leading to more reliable union and a decrease in the lateral condyle hypertrophy seen commonly after K-wire fixation. Others have concern with possible growth disturbance from the screw. In the older adolescent, screw fixation may be best.

POSTOPERATIVE CARE AND EXPECTED OUTCOMES

- A long-arm, well-padded, bivalve cast or split is applied with the elbow flexed 60–90° and the forearm in neutral rotation.
- The patient returns in 7–10 days for radiographs and wound check. Anteroposterior, lateral, and oblique radiographs of the distal humerus out of the cast may be obtained to assess maintenance of reduction and hardware fixation. A snugger non-bivalve cast should be placed.
- Follow-up is scheduled at 4 weeks postsurgery with radiographs to assess healing. Pending satisfactory radiographic evidence of healing, the cast may be removed and range of motion initiated.
- Outpatient removal of pins may be scheduled once solid healing has occurred, typically 8 weeks after surgery.
- Hypertrophy of the lateral humeral condyle often occurs.

Controversies

- Due to the risk of delayed union, leaving the pins buried allows fixation to remain after the cast is removed, although it requires surgical removal of the pins at a later date. Some choose to leave the pins outside the skin, necessitating earlier removal.

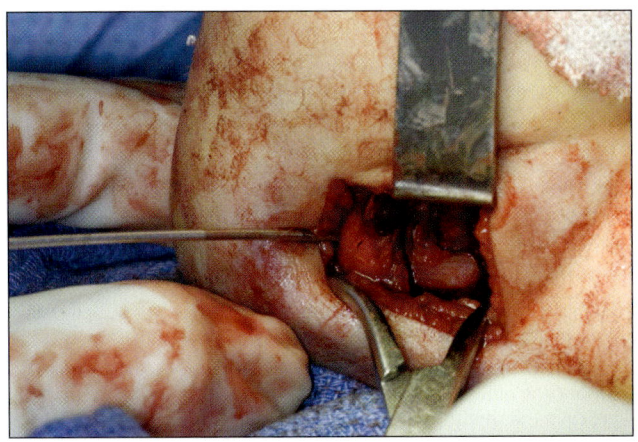

FIGURE 8

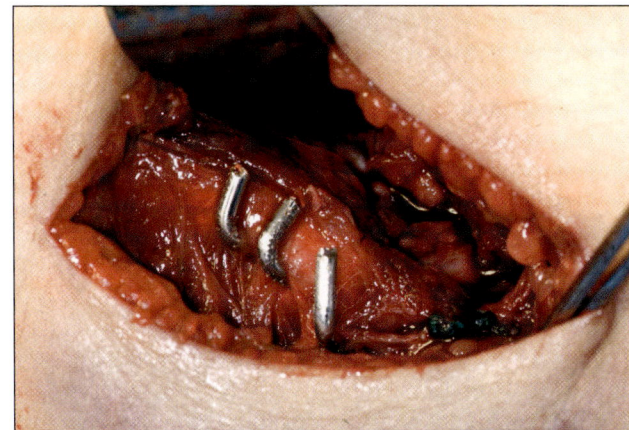

FIGURE 10

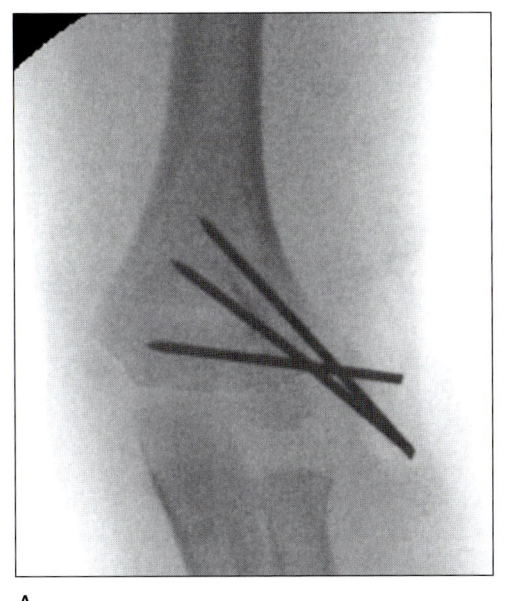

A

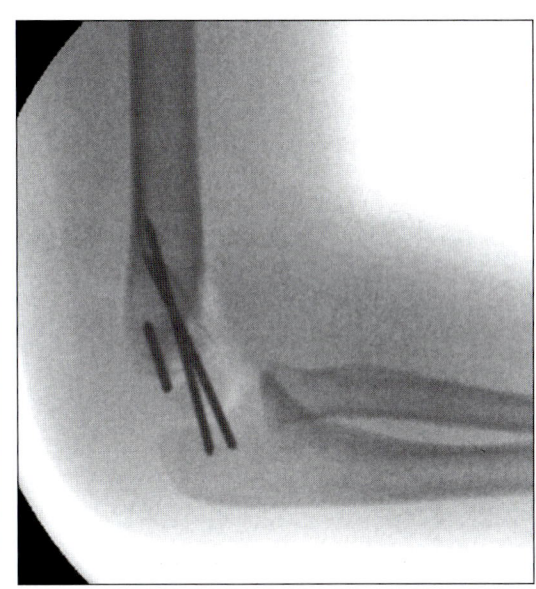

B

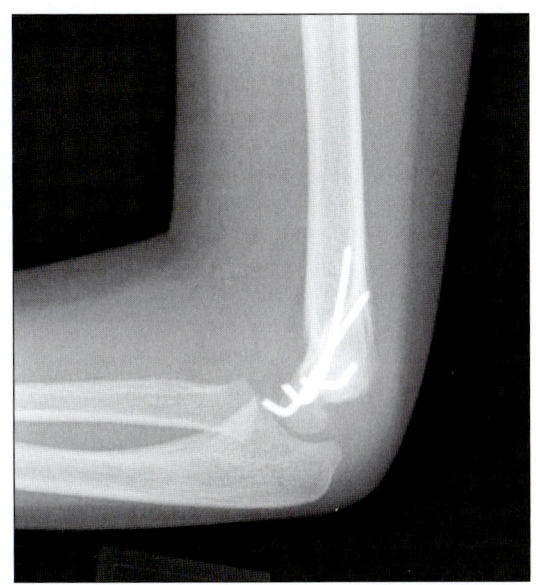

FIGURE 9 C

D

EVIDENCE

Bast SC, Hoffer MM, Aval S. Nonoperative treatment for minimally and nondisplaced lateral humeral condyle fractures in children. J Pediatr Orthop. 1998;18:448–450.

This retrospective review of 95 children who sustained a nondisplaced or minimally displaced lateral condyle fracture was conducted to determine which type of fracture, when treated closed, displaced and required further treatment. Two fractures displaced requiring ORIF; the other 98% healed in 3–7 weeks. The authors noted that minimally displaced and nondisplaced fractures may be treated closed with close follow-up. (Level IV evidence)

Badelon O, Bensahel H, Mazda K, Vie P. Lateral humeral condyle fractures in children: a report of 47 cases. J Pediatr Orthop. 1988;8:31–34.

The authors made a distinction between fractures that are undisplaced and those that are displaced and the implication of treatment. (Level IV evidence)

Jakob R, Fowles JV, Rang M, Kassab MT. Observations concerning fractures of the lateral humeral condyle in children. J Bone Joint Surg [Br]. 1975;57:430–436.

This classic article described open reduction and internal fixation of lateral condyle fractures. (Level V evidence)

Mintzer CM, Waters PM, Brown DJ, Kasser JR. Percutaneous pinning in the treatment of displaced lateral condyle fractures. J Pediatr Orthop. 1994;14:462–465.

In this retrospective review of 12 patients who sustained a lateral condyle fracture with greater than 2 mm of displacement and congruent articular surface as seen by intraoperative arthrogram, all patients did well. Percutaneous pinning may be an effective treatment in this group. (Level IV evidence)

Sullivan JA. Fractures of the lateral condyle of the humerus. J Am Acad Orthop Surg. 2006;14:58–62.

The author presented a well-written review article on lateral condyle fractures.

FOREARM AND WRIST

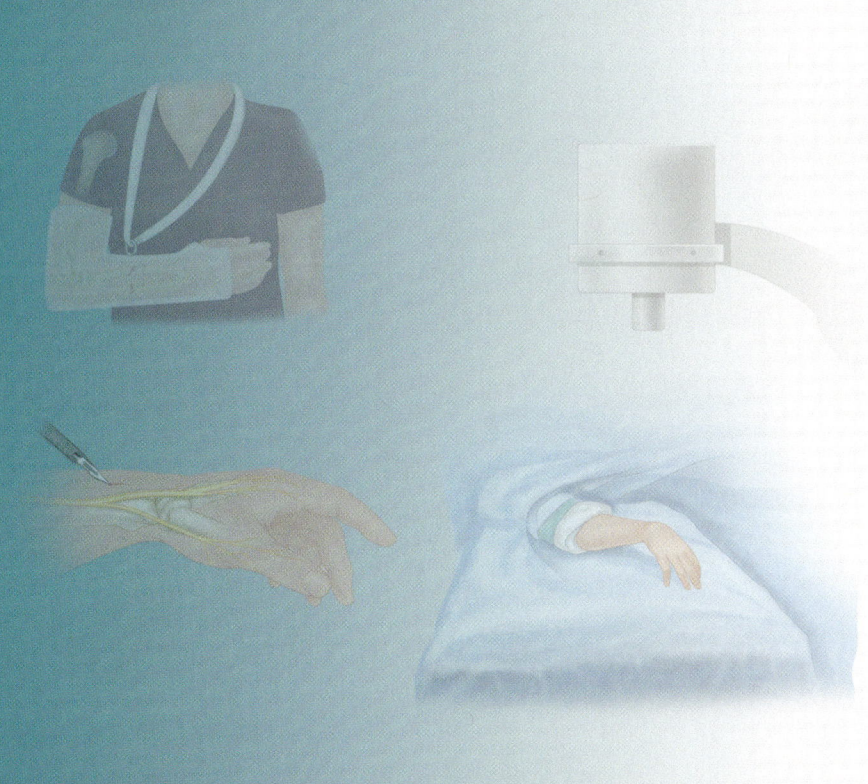

Forearm Fractures: Closed Treatment

Charles T. Price

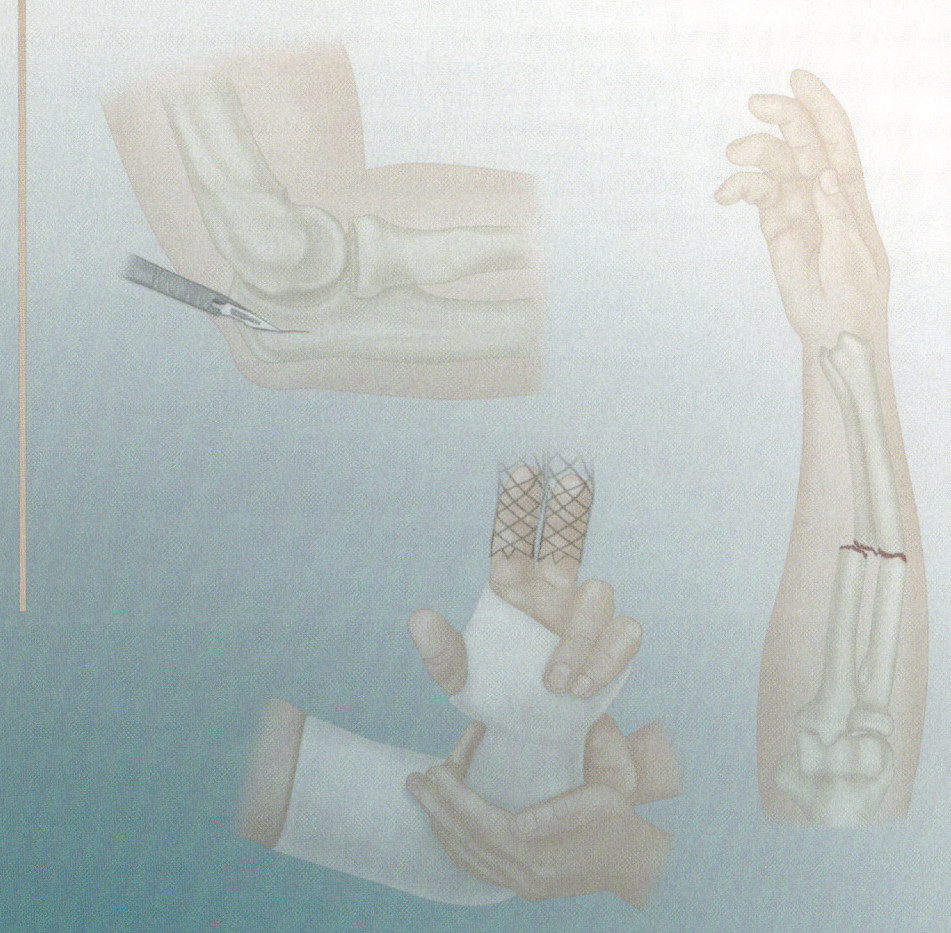

Figure 7 redrawn from Evans E. Fractures of the radius and ulna. J Bone Joint Surg [Br]. 1951;33:548–61.

Controversies

- Some surgeons prefer internal fixation for all displaced fractures after 8 years of age instead of attempting closed treatment.

INDICATIONS

- All angulated greenstick and nondisplaced fractures with angulation more than
  - 20° age < 6 years.
  - 15° age 6–10 years.
  - 10° age 10 years to maturity.
- Displaced fractures in the distal two thirds of the radius and ulna with greater than 2 years of growth remaining
  - Consider closed treatment for proximal-third fractures in children less than 6 years of age.
- Plastic deformation injuries

EXAMINATION/IMAGING

- Anteroposterior (AP) and lateral radiographs of the forearm should be made perpendicular to the distal humerus regardless of forearm pronation or supination.
  - Figure 1 shows AP (Fig. 1A) and lateral (Fig. 1B) radiographs of a volar-angulated forearm fracture (Case 1). Note the volar apex of the deformity with a nondisplaced fracture of the radius and ulna. The proximal radius crosses the ulna on the AP radiograph, suggesting pronation of the proximal fragment, although there is no true malrotation of the radius.
  - Figure 2 shows the initial radiograph of a displaced and angulated midshaft fracture of the radius and ulna in a 9-year-old girl (Case 2).
- Comparison radiographs may be obtained with the contralateral forearm in the same position of pronation or supination as the injured forearm.

Treatment Options

- Surgical stabilization is generally recommended for
  - Displaced proximal fractures
  - Refractures with displacement
  - Fractures within 2 years of skeletal maturity
  - Open fractures
  - Polytrauma
  - Fractures that lose their initial closed reduction position

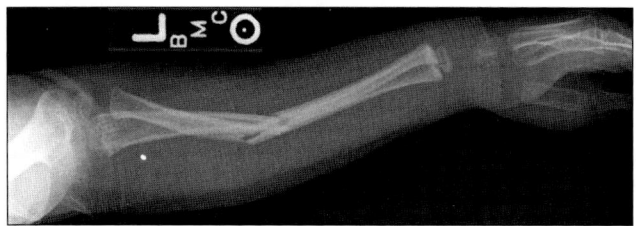
A

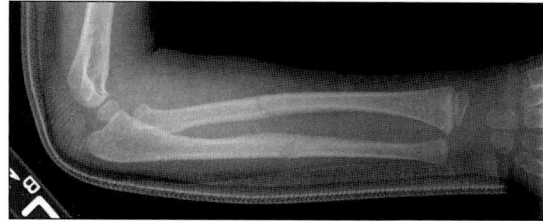
B

FIGURE 1

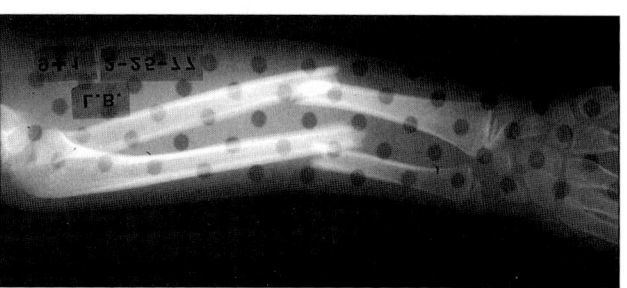

FIGURE 2

SURGICAL ANATOMY

- Figure 3A shows the normal shape of the radius. Note that the apex of the radial bow is lateral in supination. The radial tuberosity and the styloid are seen approximately on opposite sides of the radius.
- Figure 3B shows the normal shape of the ulna. Note the varus bow of the proximal ulna. A line down the shaft passes through the lateral aspect of the olecranon. The coronoid and styloid can be used to judge rotation in older children and adults.
- Figure 4 illustrates the position of the proximal and distal forearm in various degrees of pronation or supination. Note that the radial tuberosity is approximately opposite the radial styloid and therefore opposite the position of the thumb. Also note that the proximal radius does not cross the proximal ulna when resting in a supinated position.
- Greenstick and nondisplaced fractures have rotational deformity that is influenced by mechanism of injury.
  - When both bones are fractured at the same level, there may be angular deformity without malrotation.
  - There may be pronation or supination deformity when the fractures are at different levels in the diaphysis.
  - Volar bowing is associated with supination of the distal fragment relative to the proximal fragment (Fig. 5A). Note that the proximal forearm is in a pronated position, but the distal forearm is in a neutral position. This indicates 90° torsional deformity in addition to the volar angulation.
  - Dorsal bowing is associated with pronation deformity of the distal fragment relative to the proximal fragment (Fig. 5B). Note that the proximal forearm is in a supinated position, but the distal forearm is in neutral. This indicates 90° torsional deformity in addition to the dorsal angulation.
- Completely displaced fractures have rotational deformity that is influenced by muscular forces acting on the proximal fragment rather than by the mechanism of injury. Angulation and rotation of the proximal fragment of the radius depends on level of injury.
  - Figure 6 shows the anatomy of the principal muscles affecting proximal fragment position for displaced fractures of the radius.
  - Proximal fractures of the radius rest in supination due to the unopposed action of the biceps and supinator muscles.
  - Midshaft fractures of the radius rest in neutral rotation because the pronator teres opposes the supinator and biceps while moving the radius toward the ulna as expected in the neutral pronation-supination position.
- Plastic deformation is due to microfractures or slip lines that require constant pressure applied for several minutes to achieve reduction without osteoclysis.

POSITIONING

- Greenstick and nondisplaced fractures are reduced without any special positioning.
- Completely displaced fractures often benefit from finger traps to facilitate positioning, manipulation, and molding of the cast during reduction.
  - Countertraction is applied through a sling around the arm.
  - The image intensifier is positioned in a transverse position so the reduction can be visualized for alignment during immobilization.

PEARLS

- *Greenstick and nondisplaced fractures are reduced without any special positioning. Pronation or supination of distal fragment is the key to successful reduction.*
- *Completely displaced fractures may benefit from finger traps with countertraction applied through a sling around the arm. The image intensifier is positioned horizontally.*

PITFALLS

- *When the thumb is also placed in a finger trap, the thumb and index finger must not be spread too far apart.*

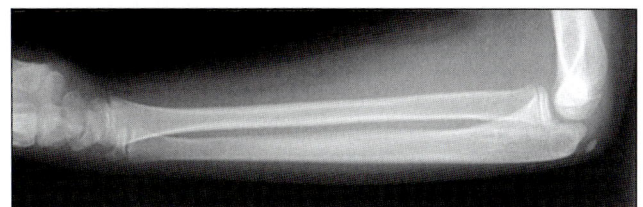

A

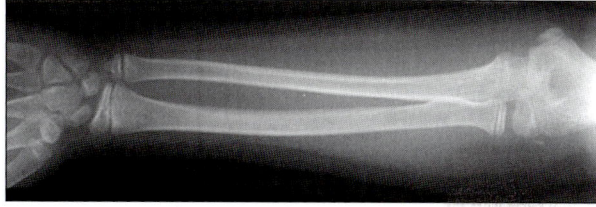

B

FIGURE 3

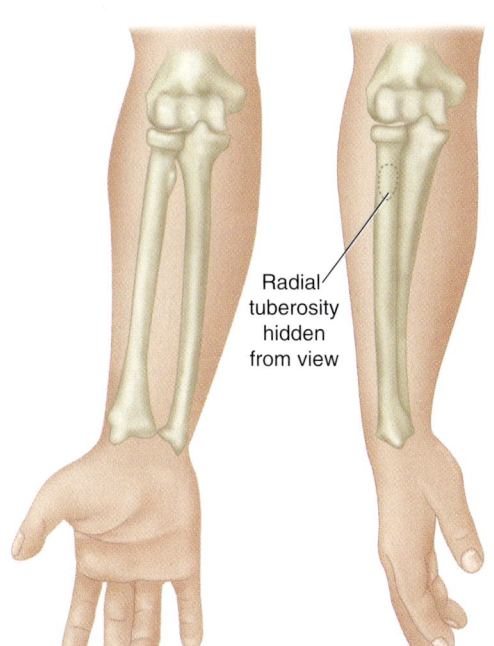

Radial tuberosity hidden from view

FIGURE 4

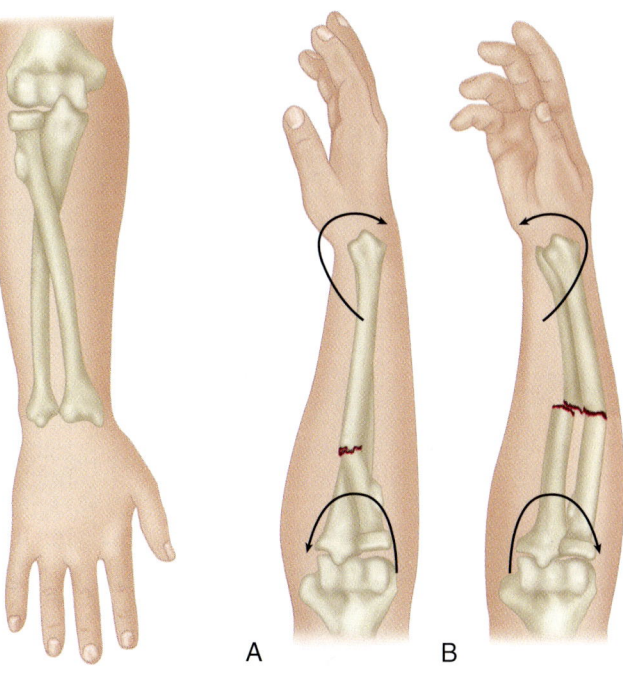

A

B

FIGURE 5

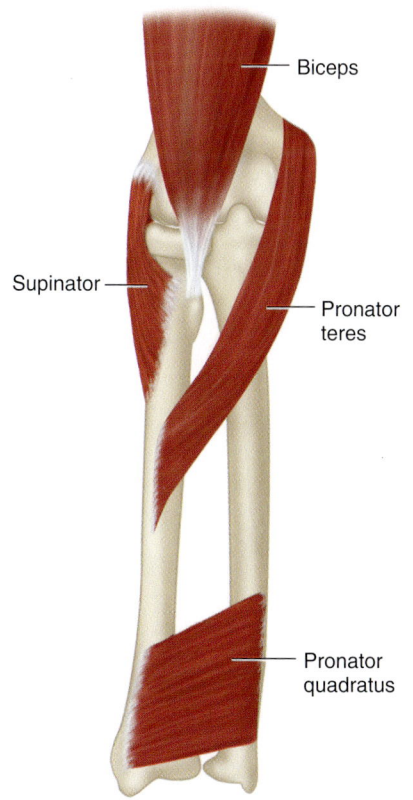

Biceps

Supinator

Pronator teres

Pronator quadratus

FIGURE 6

Controversies

- The need to maintain interosseous space is controversial. Some loss of interosseous distance is well tolerated in children, but the acceptable amount is unknown. End-to-end reduction with straightening of the radial bow may create more tension on the interosseous membrane and greater loss of motion than overlapped fractures that allow relaxation of the interosseous membrane.

PROCEDURE

STEP 1

- Greenstick or nondisplaced fractures are fully pronated or supinated to obtain reduction. Pronation is required when the bow is volar, and supination is required when the bow is dorsal.
  - For simplicity, the thumb is rotated toward the apex of angulation while pressure is applied to the apex of deformity. This maneuver often fractures the intact cortex of a greenstick fracture. Fracturing the opposite cortex is not necessary but does facilitate maintenance of reduction and also decreases the risk of refracture.
  - Following reduction, the forearm may be immobilized in a position slightly less than full pronation or full supination if radiographs demonstrate maintenance of alignment.
  - Deformity in the proximal forearm should be corrected to less than 10° degrees of angulation.
- Completely displaced fractures are aligned manually by matching the position of the distal fragments to the position of the proximal fragments.
  - Neutral rotation of the distal forearm is generally the best position for fractures of the middle and distal diaphysis. Figure 7 illustrates the position of the forearm relative to the location of a completely displaced diaphyseal fracture. Note that proximal fractures require more supination than midshaft fractures, but none of the completely displaced diaphyseal fractures in this study required pronation (Evans, 1951).
  - Figure 10 shows reduction of the volar-angulated forearm fracture in Case 1. Anteroposterior (Fig. 8A) and lateral (Fig. 8B) radiographs demonstrate inadequate reduction following attempted reduction at another facility without pronating the distal forearm. Subsequent AP (Fig. 8C) and lateral (Fig. 8D) radiographs demonstrate satisfactory final reduction after the distal fragment was pronated with pressure on the volar apex.
  - Complete displacement can be accepted, but angulation less than 10° is the objective of initial reduction. Figure 9 shows lateral and AP radiographs of the displaced midshaft fracture in Case 2 following closed reduction. Note complete displacement, but excellent angular and rotational alignment.
  - Proximal fractures often require some supination of the distal fragments, but the author recommends surgical stabilization for the majority of displaced proximal-third fractures due to frequent loss of motion from fractures in this location.
  - Attempts to obtain end-to-end reduction are unnecessary as long as alignment is maintained within acceptable guidelines.

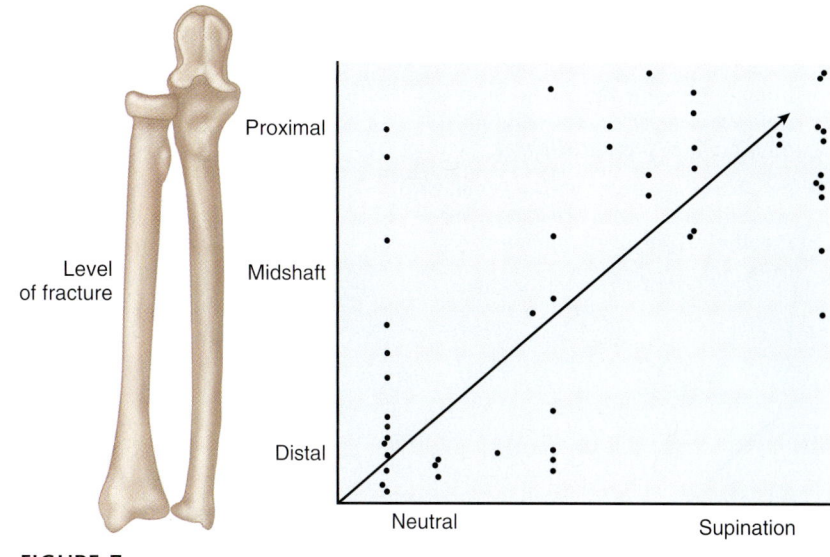

Proximal

Level
of fracture

Midshaft

Distal

Neutral

Supination

FIGURE 7

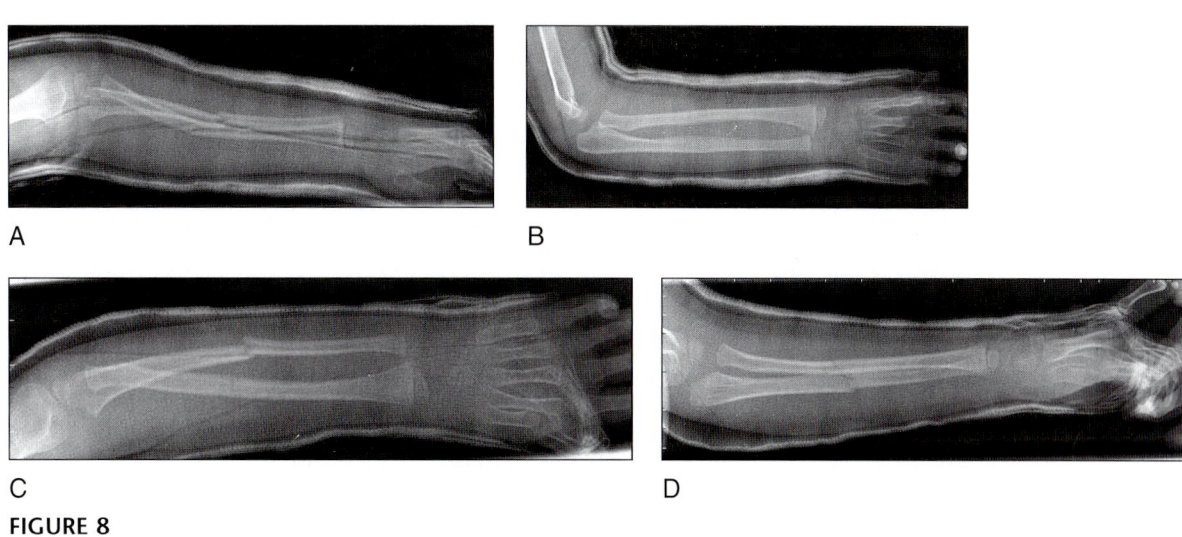

A

B

C

D

FIGURE 8

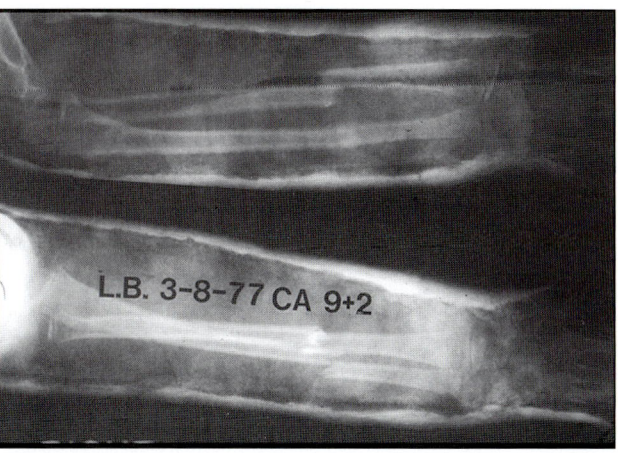

L.B. 3-8-77 CA 9+2

FIGURE 9

PEARLS

- *Immobilize with the elbow in extension for younger children and include the thumb to prevent slippage.*

- *An oval-shaped cast with appropriate molding and limited cast padding is essential for maintenance of reduction.*

STEP 2

- Immobilization following reduction is usually maintained in a double sugar tong splint.
  - One U-shaped splint is wrapped around the elbow with dorsal and volar support of the forearm and wrist. This may sufficiently immobilize the elbow, but a second U-shaped splint can be applied around the upper arm for additional stability and comfort.
  - The sugar tong splint is overwrapped with an elastic bandage and carefully molded with three-point pressure during hardening.
- Alternatively, a long-arm cast can be applied when the reduction is stable, or when minimal three-point molding is required as the cast hardens. When a cast is used, it is bivalved and loosely overwrapped with an elastic bandage to allow for swelling.
- Molding without excessive padding is essential for maintenance of the reduction.
  - An oval-shaped cast is preferred to preserve the interosseous distance and alignment (Fig. 10). However, some loss of interosseous space is acceptable in the distal and middle forearm. It is more critical to maintain angular and rotational alignment within acceptable guidelines.
  - Three-point pressure with appropriate rotation may be more important than molding for greenstick or nondisplaced fractures.
- Approximately 80–90° elbow flexion is the position of immobilization for most fractures of the forearm.
- A sling or cast loop should be positioned to support the elbow.
  - The ulnar border of the cast needs to be well molded so that the forearm does not slip proximally into the cast as the swelling subsides.
  - Figure 11A shows proper cast fitting and location of support if a neck sling is used. Figure 11B shows a poorly molded ulnar border and improper support.
- Extension of the elbow is preferred for small children because the contour of the proximal forearm makes it difficult to mold the cast adequately with the elbow in a flexed position (Fig. 12A). The thumb is included in an extended position to prevent slippage of the cast. Anteroposterior (Fig. 12B) and lateral (Fig. 12C) radiographs of the same forearm demonstrate acceptable alignment in the extended position.

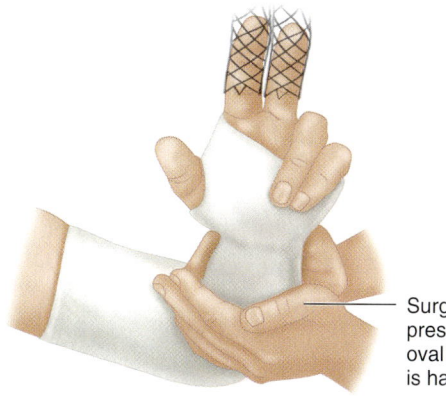

Surgeon applying pressure to maintain oval shape as splint is hardening

FIGURE 10

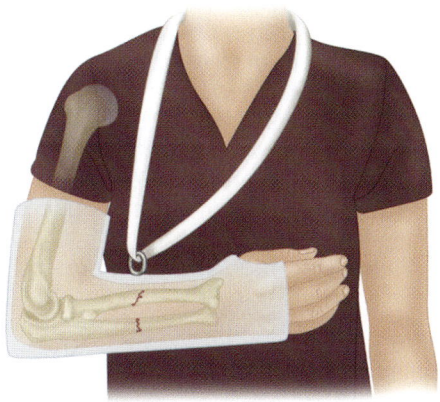

A

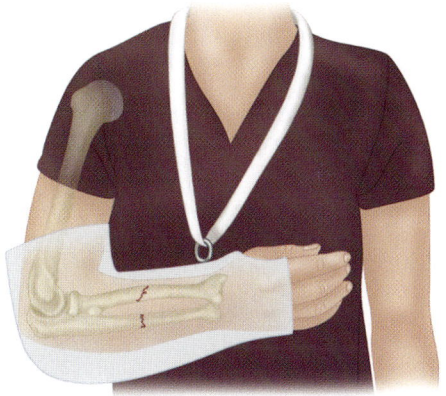

B

FIGURE 11

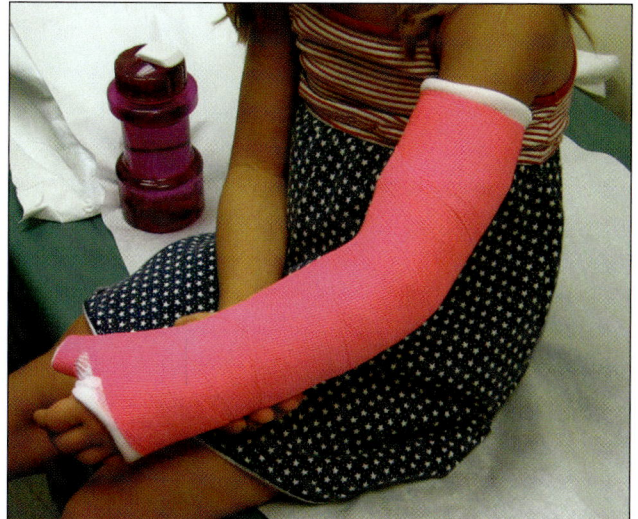

A

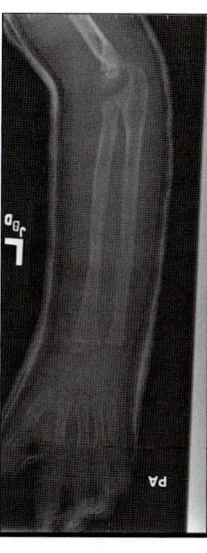

B

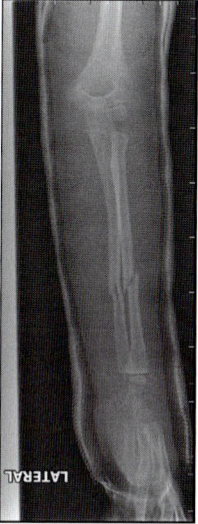

C

FIGURE 12

POSTOPERATIVE CARE AND EXPECTED OUTCOMES

■ Follow-up radiographs in the splint or cast are obtained 7–10 days after initial reduction.
  • As swelling subsides, some loss of reduction is common, but reduction should remain within the guidelines for acceptable alignment. Adjustments in angular alignment are made by applying a new cast and gently molding the forearm as the cast is hardening. Molding in a new cast is well tolerated by patients with or without oral analgesics, although the latter provide parental reassurance.
  • Forceful remanipulation in the clinic is not recommended. When major malalignment is identified at follow-up, the surgeon should consider remanipulation with internal fixation under general anesthesia.
■ Regardless of alignment, follow-up radiographs are recommended after another 7–10 days so that the patient is seen in follow-up twice during the first 3 weeks for cast change and gentle realignment if necessary.
■ Immobilization is continued until union is complete. Six to 8 weeks of immobilization are sufficient for complete fractures. Splinting of greenstick fractures is recommended for an additional 6 weeks following cast removal unless the opposite cortex was fractured at the time of reduction.
■ Malunion of ≤ 20° should be observed for 6 months prior to consideration for osteotomy.
  • Functional limitation is uncommon with alignment in ≤ 20° of angulation.
  • Ulnar angulation is more cosmetically objectionable than angulation of the radius, but angulation of the radius is more likely to limit forearm rotation.
  • Note that ≤ 15° of angulation is the guideline for acceptable alignment during the early stages of management because some loss of alignment may occur in the final stages of healing in the cast.
■ Remodeling is expected as long as there are 2 or more years of growth remaining. Anteroposterior (Fig. 13A) and lateral (Fig. 13B) radiographs taken 7 years postfracture in Case 2 demonstrate complete remodeling of displacement. Photographs taken 7 years postfracture demonstrate normal pronation (Fig. 14A) and supination (Fig. 14B) motion.

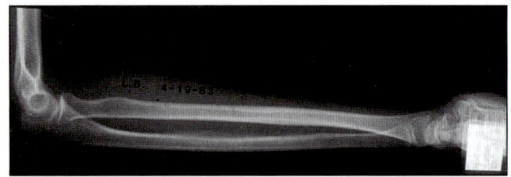

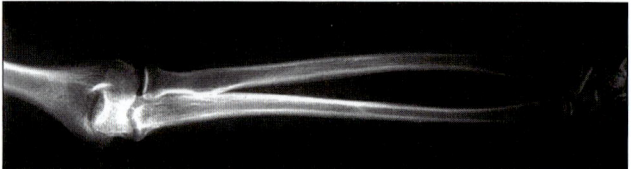

A

B

FIGURE 13

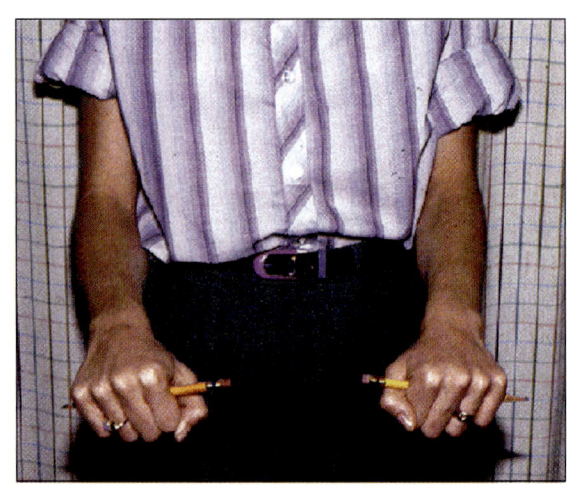

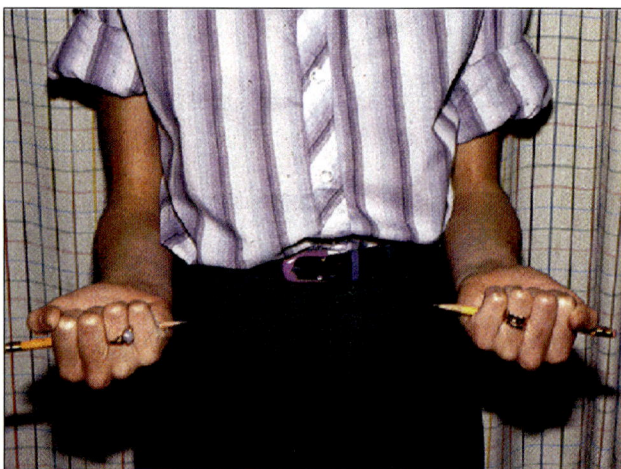

A

B

FIGURE 14

EVIDENCE

Bhatia M, Housden PH. Re-displacement of paediatric forearm fractures: role of plaster moulding and padding. Injury. 2006;37:259–68.

The authors found that redisplacement is significantly related to excessive cast padding and poor molding of the cast. Improvement in plaster application skills reduced the redis-placement rate by 50%. (Level II evidence [diagnostic study])

Bochang C, Jie Y, Zhigang W, Weigl D, Bar-On E, Katz K. Immobilisation of forearm fractures in children: extended versus flexed elbow. J. Bone Joint Surg [Br]. 2005;87:994–6.

In this study, redisplacement did not occur in any of 60 fractures immobilized with the elbow in extension. Nine of 51 children (17.6%) treated with the elbow in flexion failed to maintain acceptable reduction. (Level II evidence [therapeutic study])

Carey PJ, Alburger PD, Betz RR, Clancy M, Steel HH. Both-bone forearm fractures in children. Orthopedics. 1992;15:1015–9.

In this study, 33 both-bone forearm fractures were reduced in finger-trap traction and immobilized in neutral rotation. Twenty-seven patients recovered full range of forearm rotation. Six patients lost 20–35(of forearm rotation, but none had functional limitations. Neutral rotation position was recommended to avoid extremes of position that may lead to functional loss of forearm rotation. (Level II evidence [case series])

Evans E. Fractures of the radius and ulna. J Bone Joint Surg [Br]. 1951;33:548–61.

Classic paper identifying the rotational deformities associated with complete or greenstick fractures of the forearm. Methods are identified for assessment and treatment to avoid rotational malunion of these two types of fractures. (Level IV evidence [case series])

Fuller DJ, McCullough CJ. Malunited fractures of the forearm in children. J Bone Joint Surg [Br]. 1982;64:364–7.

Twenty-six patients with diaphyseal malunion greater than 20° were reviewed in this study. Nine patients remodeled completely and 17 had incomplete remodeling. At long-term follow-up, only two patients noted functional or cosmetic deformity. These two patients had severe rotational malalignment at time of union and both lost 90° of pronation. (Level IV evidence [case series])

Matthews LS, Kaufer H, Garver DF, Sonstegard DA. The effect on supination-pronation of angular malalignment of fractures of both bones of the forearm: an experimental study. J Bone Joint Surg [Am]. 1982;64:14–7.
Tarr RR, Garfinkel AI, Sarmiento A. The effects of angular and rotational deformities of both bones of the forearm. J Bone Joint Surg [Am]. 1984;66:65–70.

These two human cadaver studies confirmed that 10° of midshaft angulation does not limit forearm rotation. Angulation of 15° restricted forearm rotation by an average of 30–40%. Angulation of 20° resulted in functionally important loss of forearm rotation. It should be noted that cadaver studies do not allow for remodeling or physiologic recovery, but these studies do provide evidence that 10–15° of angulation corresponds with published guidelines for acceptable alignment.

Price CT, Scott DS, Kurzner ME, Flynn JC. Malunited forearm fractures in children. J Pediatr Orthop. 1990;10:705–12.

In this long-term follow-up study of 39 patients with greater than 10° angulation at time of union, there were 32 excellent, 4 good (30° loss of rotation), and 3 fair results (30–90° loss of rotation); none was poor. Proximal-third fractures have a worse prognosis for recovery of motion than more distal fractures. Angulation of up to 10° can be accepted with complete displacement and mild malrotation. (Level IV evidence [case series])

Zionts LE, Zalavras CG, Gerhardt MB. Closed treatment of displaced diaphyseal both-bone forearm fractures in older children and adolescents. J Pediatr Orthop. 2005;25:507–12.

In this study, 25 patients with an average age of 13 years were managed with closed reduction and cast immobilization. Three patients (12%) lost 35–40° of forearm rotation, while 22 (88%) had full motion or minor degrees of motion loss. The authors concluded that complete displacement and up to 15° of angulation can be accepted in children and adolescents rather than resorting to open reduction and internal fixation. (Level IV evidence [case series])

Closed Reduction and Pinning of Distal Radius Fractures

Dennis E. Kramer

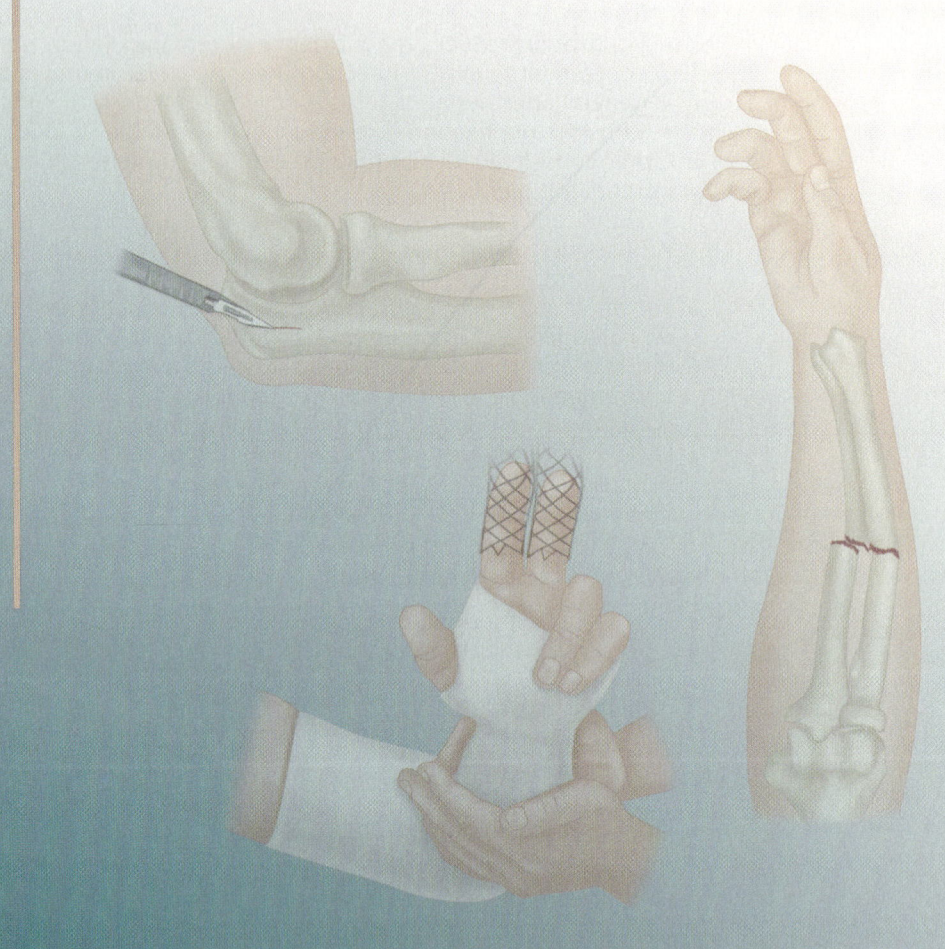

Controversies

- Late displacement following initial fracture reduction occurs in approximately one third of cases and is most related to initial fracture displacement, degree of fracture obliquity, and inadequate initial closed reduction.

Treatment Options

- Repeat closed reduction and casting in the clinic or emergency department
- Repeat closed reduction and casting in the operating room
- Closed reduction and pinning in the operating room

INDICATIONS

- Unstable distal radius fracture unable to be controlled by cast alone
- Displaced distal radius fracture that is in unacceptable alignment following a reduction and casting maneuver
  - If greater than 2 years of growth remaining, acceptable alignment includes:
    - 20–25° of dorsal or volar angulation
    - 10° of radial-ulnar deviation
    - 50% translational displacement
- Redisplacement following a previous reduction and casting maneuver
  - Completely displaced fractures have 60–80% rate of redisplacement after incomplete reduction.
  - Following redisplacement, outcomes and complications are similar with re-reduction and casting vs. re-reduction and pin fixation.
  - Pin fixation reduces the incidence of remanipulation but caries concomitant risks for infection, neurovascular injury, and general anesthesia.
  - Consider pin fixation if re-reduction is unstable or incomplete.
- Other consideration that may preclude circumferential cast immobilization:
  - Significant soft tissue swelling
  - Neurovascular compromise
  - Open fractures or skin issues
- For distal radial physeal fractures, multiple reduction attempts or repeated late reduction attempts should be avoided. If reduction remains unacceptable, consider allowing the fracture to heal and observing the deformity over time, proceeding with late corrective osteotomy if remodeling does not occur.
- Distal ulnar fractures often accompany distal radial fractures. Acceptable alignment for distal ulnar fractures includes up to 50% translation and 20° of angulation.

EXAMINATION/IMAGING

- Posteroanterior and lateral wrist films are obtained.
- Dorsal/volar angulation and radial tilt are evaluated. The lateral radiographic wrist view in Figure 1 shows a displaced distal radial fracture with over 30 degrees of dorsal angulation.

SURGICAL ANATOMY

- Dorsal sensory branch of the radial nerve (DSBRN)
  - The DSBRN pierces the brachioradialis (BR) and emerges between the extensor carpi radialis longus and brevis 8 cm proximal to the radial styloid.
  - It then crosses over the extensor retinaculum before dividing into medial and lateral branches.
  - It lies dorsal to proper pin position (Fig. 2).
- Radial artery
  - The radial artery runs with the DSBRN between the BR and flexor pollicis longus.
  - It runs radial to the flexor carpi radialis at the wrist.
  - It lies palmar to proper pin position (see Fig. 2).

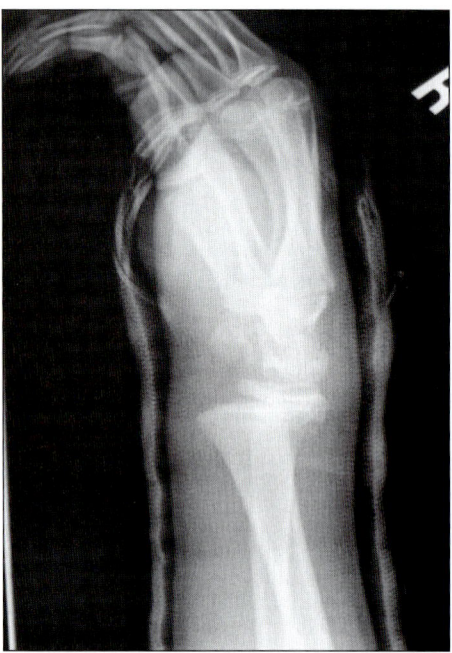

FIGURE 1

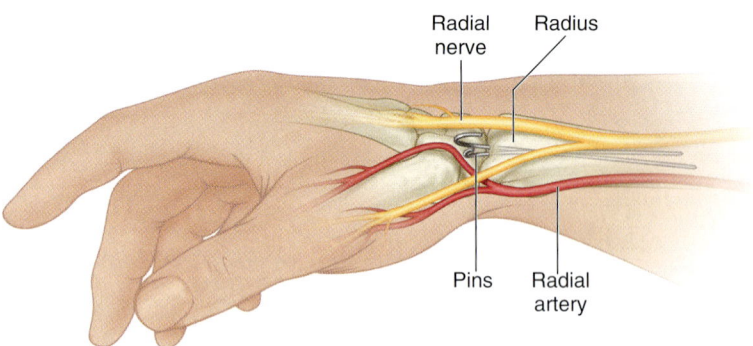

Radial nerve   Radius

Pins   Radial artery

FIGURE 2

POSITIONING

■ The patient is placed in the supine position with a nonsterile high-arm tourniquet.
■ The arm is positioned on a hand table (Fig. 3).

PORTALS/EXPOSURES

■ Pins are placed using a "nick-and-spread" technique.
■ For physeal fractures or fractures near the physis, the pin entry site is through the radial styloid (Fig. 4A).
■ For more proximal metaphyseal fractures, the pin entry site is started just proximal to the distal radial physis to avoid placing pins across the physis.
■ Fluoroscopy is used to plan the incision site (Fig. 4B).

PROCEDURE

STEP 1: CLOSED REDUCTION

■ Multiple reduction maneuvers are described. Our preferred reduction technique for dorsally angulated displaced distal radius fractures follows these steps:
   • The deforming force is reproduced by dorsiflexing the wrist (this relaxes the intact periosteum).
   • Traction is applied.
   • The surgeon uses the thumb to apply volar pressure to the dorsal aspect of the distal radius (Fig. 5).
   • Volar translation is then applied to the carpus to complete the reduction maneuver.
   • The wrist is ulnar deviated as needed to restore the radial tilt.

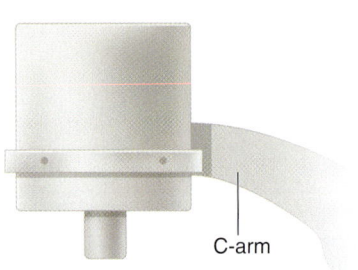

C-arm

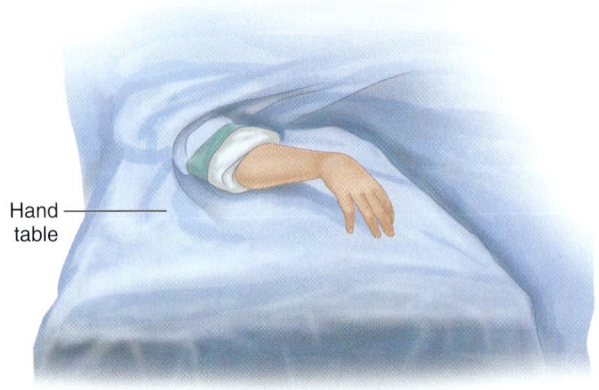

Hand table

FIGURE 3

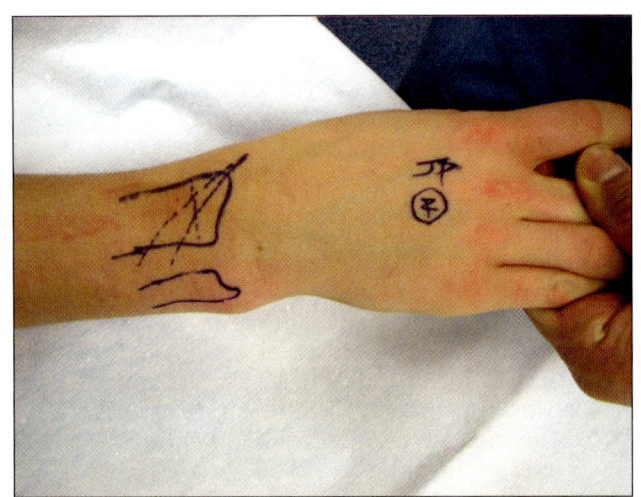

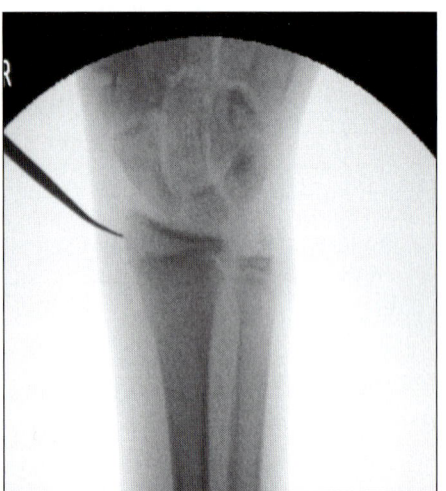

FIGURE 4 A

B

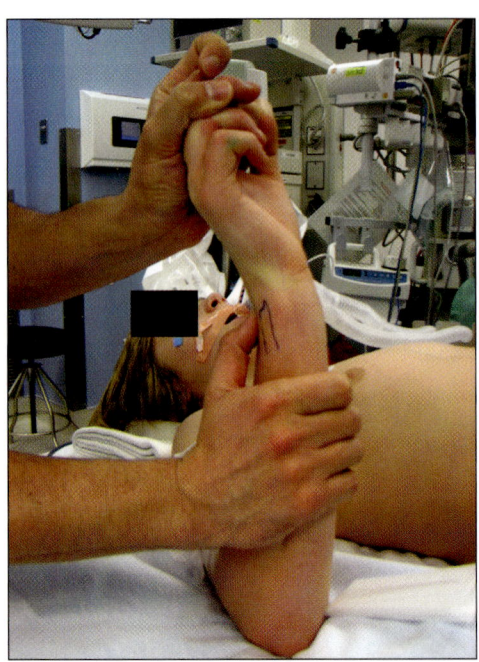

FIGURE 5

PEARLS

- *A stack of towels placed at the distal forearm can help with palmar flexion and ulnar deviation to hold reduction during pin fixation.*

PITFALLS

- *Feel the cortical bone during pin placement and check AP and lateral fluoroscopic views to ensure that the pin has crossed the fracture site and achieved solid bicortical purchase.*

Instrumentation/ Implantation

- For older adolescents, use 0.0062-inch K-wires. For younger patients, smaller wires are acceptable.

Controversies

- Pins can be buried underneath the skin for later removal in the operating room if concerns for pin site infection exist or it is felt that the fracture may take a longer time to heal.

PEARLS

- *Ulnar styloid fractures have a high rate of nonunion (most are asymptomatic) and may be associated with triangular fibrocartilage complex injuries.*

PITFALLS

- *Avoid multiple reduction attempts and multiple pin passes across the physis to minimize risk of physeal injury.*

Controversies

- Smooth pin fixation across the distal radial physis has been reported to be a successful treatment option with low risk of iatrogenic disruption to the distal radial physis.

STEP 2: PERCUTANEOUS PIN FIXATION

- Pins are placed through a nick-and-spread technique to avoid injury to a branch of the DSBRN.
  - A small nick is made in the skin (Fig. 6A).
  - A blunt instrument is used to spread down to the radial styloid (Fig. 6B).
- The fracture is held reduced during pin placement (Fig. 7).
- One or two Kirschner wires (K-wires) should be used to stabilize the fracture site. Two divergent K-wires provide the most stability but may be difficult to place (Fig. 8).
  - For physeal fractures, the starting point is the dorsal distal radial styloid, aiming distal-to-proximal and radial-to-ulnar. In Figure 9, pre- and postfixation radiographic views showing acceptable reduction and pin placement of a distal radius physeal fracture.
  - For more proximal metaphyseal fractures, the starting point is just proximal to the distal radial physis on the radial aspect of the radial metaphysis. Figure 10 shows fixation of a metaphyseal distal radius fracture with pins placed proximal to the physis.
- Fluoroscopic images in AP and lateral views are checked during pin placement to ensure that the pin is remaining in bone.
- The surgeon should feel for cortical bone at the proximal aspect of the fracture site to be sure bicortical purchase is achieved.
- A K-wire can also be placed in the distal fragment and used to lever the distal fragment into place, correcting dorsal angulation and radial inclination to achieve an acceptable reduction before driving the pin across the fracture site.
- Single K-wire fixation of the distal radial fracture is acceptable if the fracture site is deemed to be stable following pin placement and a well-molded cast is applied.
- Cross-pinning (one K-wire retrograde, one antegrade) across the distal radial or ulnar fracture site is acceptable in cases in which parallel or divergent retrograde pins cannot be accomplished due to fracture position or pattern.
- Stability of the fracture is checked under fluoroscopy by taking the wrist through a gentle range of motion.
- The pins are bent and cut and left out of the skin for removal later in the clinic (Fig. 11).

STEP 3: OTHER FRACTURE CONSIDERATIONS

- Open reduction through a volar approach may be necessary in irreducible fractures in which soft tissue interposition precludes closed reduction. The volar periosteum and pronator quadratus are most commonly trapped in the fracture site.
- For more proximal metaphyseal-diaphyseal distal radial fractures, flexible intramedullary nail fixation or open reduction with volar plating are acceptable options. If plate fixation is chosen, the goal is to obtain four to six cortices of fixation in the distal fragment.
- Fractures through the ulna styloid or distal ulnar physis are usually stable following reduction and pinning of the distal radius fracture. If instability exists, the surgeon may consider retrograde pinning through the ulnar styloid and across the distal ulnar fracture site.
- Fractures through the ulnar styloid base that are associated with distal radioulnar joint instability may benefit from open reduction and internal fixation with a tension band construct.

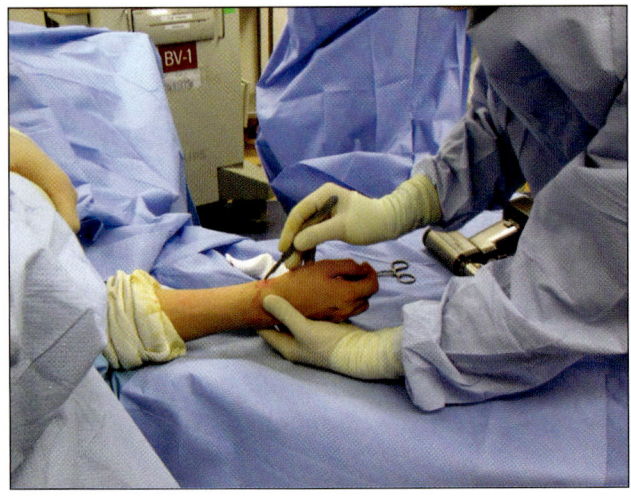

A

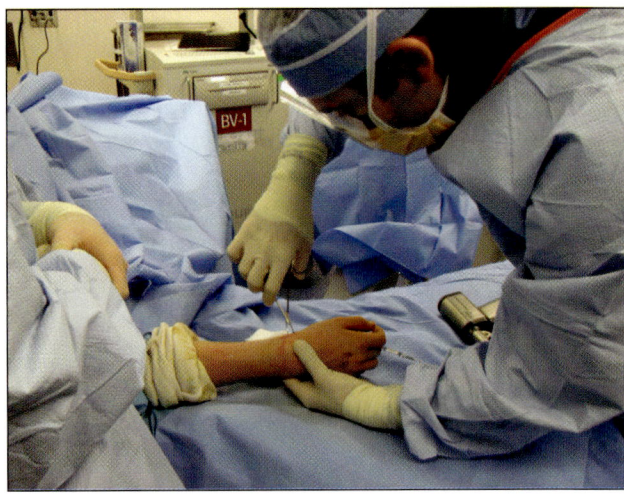

B

FIGURE 6

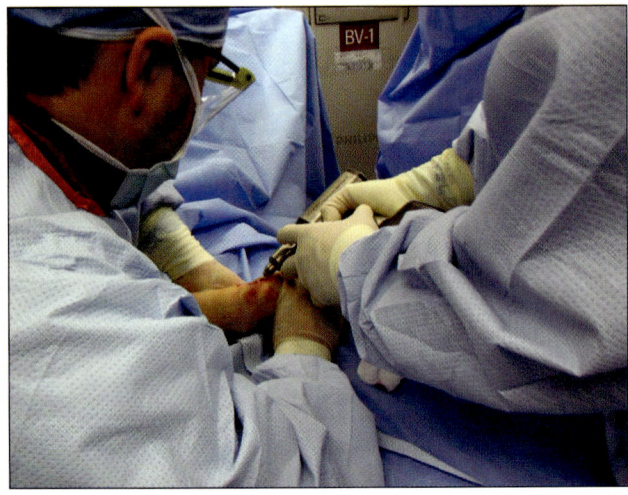

FIGURE 7

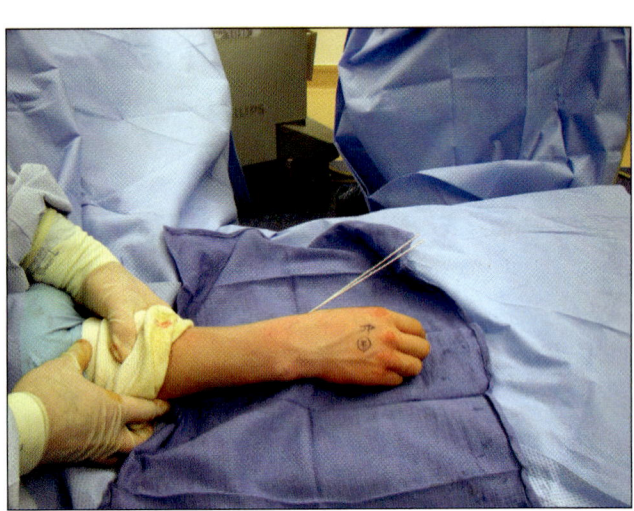

FIGURE 8

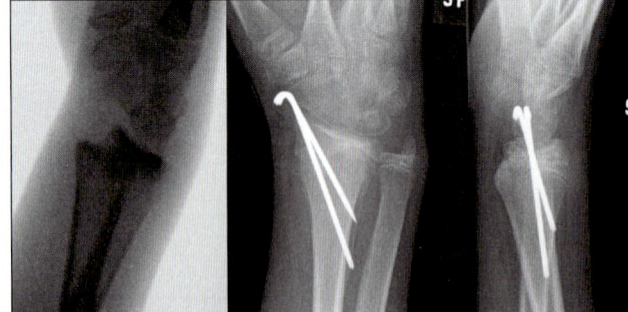

FIGURE 9

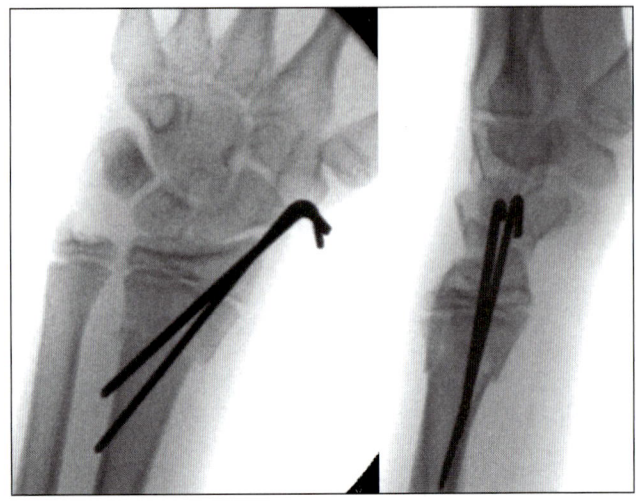

FIGURE 10

PEARLS

- *Maintain a low threshold for removing the cast and inspecting the K-wires to rule out pin tract infection if there are any complaints of fever, drainage, or pain.*

PITFALLS

- *Distal radial physeal growth arrest occurs in 1–4% of cases, while distal ulnar physeal arrest may occur in up to 50% of ulnar physeal injuries.*

Controversies

- Given the enormous remodeling potential of the distal radius, distal radial malunions are typically observed in skeletally immature patients. If deformity persists, corrective osteotomy is considered.

POSTOPERATIVE CARE AND EXPECTED OUTCOMES

- Protocols vary; our preference follows:
  - A well-molded short-arm cast over pins is put on in the operating room.
    - A bivalve cast may be used if there is concern for compartment syndrome or postoperative swelling.
  - A follow-up radiograph is obtained in 1 week in the cast to confirm stability of the fracture.
  - K-wire removal is done in the clinic at 3 or 4 weeks after fixation.
    - K-wires that are buried underneath the skin can be removed in the operating room anytime after the fracture has healed.
  - The arm is placed back into a cast after K-wire removal for a total casting time of 6 weeks.
  - Transition to a volar-based wrist splint is done at 6 weeks postoperatively.
  - The patient is followed with radiographs for 1–2 years after injury to ensure that there is no physeal growth arrest.

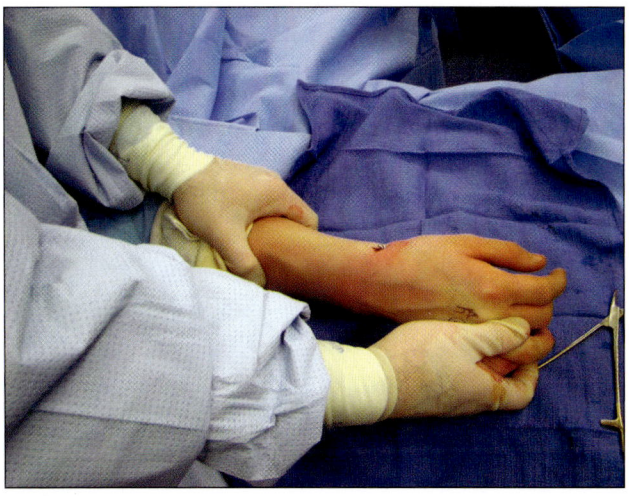

FIGURE 11

EVIDENCE

Abraham A, Handoll HH, Khan T. Interventions for treating wrist fractures in children. Cochrane Database Syst Rev. 2008;(2):CD004576.

The authors perform a systemic review of randomized controlled trials to evaluate types and position of casts and the use of surgical fixation for distal radius fractures in children. Ten trials involving 827 children were identified. The authors found limited evidence to support the use of above elbow casts after reduction of displaced fractures. Percutaneous wire fixation was found to prevent redisplacement although long term outcome improvement was not demonstrated. Further research is warranted. (Level II evidence)

Alemdaroğlu KB, Iltar S, Cimen O, Uysal M, Alagöz E, Atlihan D. Risk factors in redisplacement of distal radial fractures in children. J Bone Joint Surg [Am]. 2008;90:1224–30.

The authors performed a prospective study to evaluate the causes of redisplacement following closed treatment of distal metaphyseal radial fractures in children. Initial complete displacement and the degree of obliquity of the fracture were the most important risk factors for displacement. A radiographic "three-point index" was described and predicted redisplacement better than previously described measures. (Level I evidence)

Bae DS. Pediatric distal radius and forearm fractures. J Hand Surg [Am]. 2008;33:1911–23.

The author presents a "current concepts" style review of treatment and results of pediatric distal radius and forearm fractures.

Bae DS, Waters PM. Pediatric distal radius fractures and triangular fibrocartilage complex injuries. Hand Clin. 2006;22:43–53.

The authors describe the management of distal radius fractures, indications for surgical treatment, complications and treatment of growth arrest of the distal radius. Triangular fibrocartilage complex (TFCC) injuries are discussed as a source of ulnar sided wrist pain in children and adolescents. Pertinent subtle physical exam findings are described. Management includes conservative treatment (activity modification and therapy) and surgery (for repair of peripheral tears) in cases of persistent pain.

Cannata G, De Maio F, Mancini F, Ippolito E. Physeal fractures of the distal radius and ulna: long-term prognosis. J Orthop Trauma. 2003;17:172–9; discussion 179–80.

The authors present a retrospective case series analyzing the long term results of injuries to the distal physis of the forearm bones. One hundred sixty-three physeal fractures treated non-operatively were identified. Physeal arrest causing shortening > 1 cm was observed in 7 out of 157 (4.4%) distal radial lesions (2 were cases of open fractures and infection) and 3 out of 6 (50%) distal ulnar lesions. At long term follow-up all patients who had <1 cm of shortening were asymptomatic (including 53 cases of ulnar styloid non-union). Of the 10 patients with shortening >1 cm, only 2 had significant functional problems. (Level IV evidence)

Hove LM, Brudvik C. Displaced paediatric fractures of the distal radius. Arch Orthop Trauma Surg. 2008;128:55–60.

The authors present a prospective review of closed manipulation of distal radial fractures. Eighty-eight patients were identified and followed over time. Mean angulation pre-reduction was 19 degrees, post-reduction 5 degrees and at union 4 degrees. All fractures with more than 15 degrees of malangulation at union completely remodeled over seven years. The authors concluded that the remodeling capacity of the distal radial physis is excellent and conservative treatment remains the gold standard for this injury. (Level II evidence)

Price CT. Surgical management of forearm and distal radius fractures in children and adolescents. Instr Course Lect. 2008;57:509–14.

The author presents a comprehensive review of the management of forearm and distal radius fractures in children and adolescents. Closed manipulation and surgical techniques for management of these injuries are described.

Forearm Fractures: Intramedullary Rodding

Maya E. Pring and Henry G. Chambers

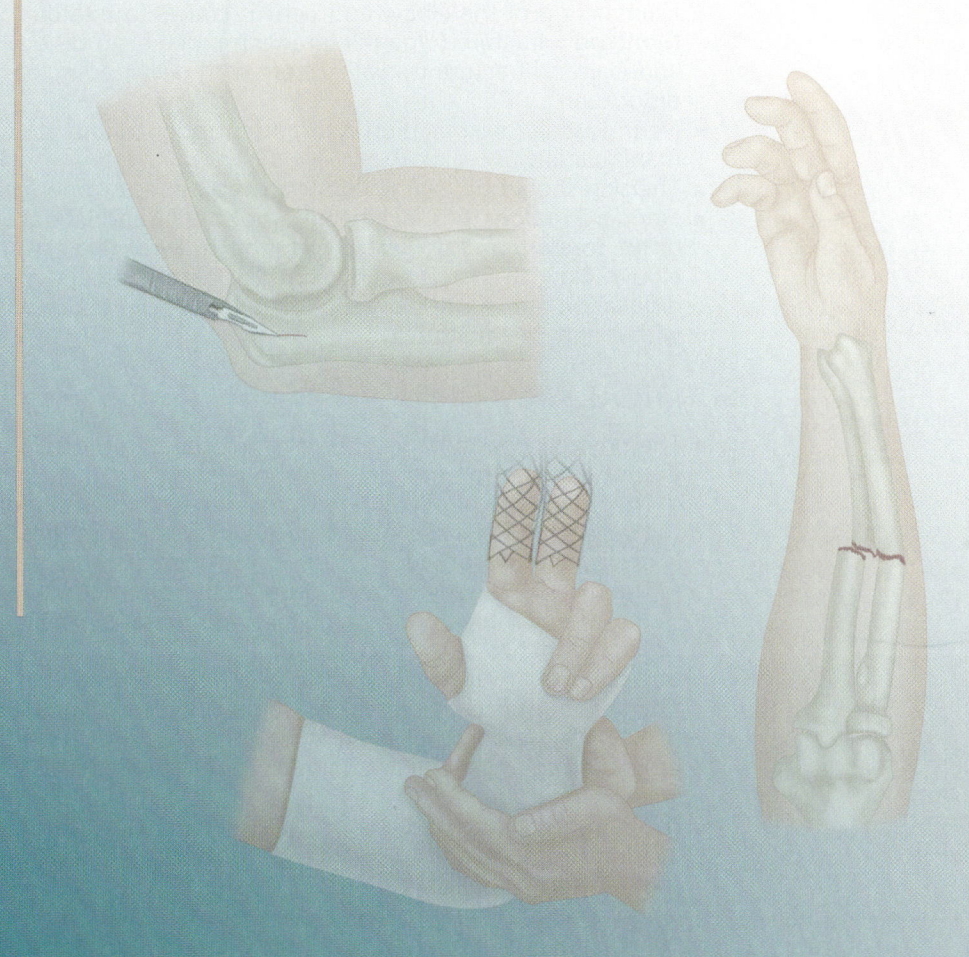

Controversies

- What constitutes a failed reduction can be controversial. A casting expert may be able to stabilize what many would consider too unstable for conservative management. Cast wedging can also be used to help realign a fracture that is angulating in the cast. This may be dangerous as there can be skin breakdown.
- Acceptable alignment varies with age. The younger the child, the more remodeling potential he or she will have.

Treatment Options

- Closed reduction and casting (can be used for the majority of children's forearm fractures)
- Closed reduction and percutaneous Kirschner wire (K-wire) fixation for distal metaphyseal fractures
- Closed (and possibly open) reduction with placement of intramedullary pins/rods
- Open reduction and internal fixation with plates and screws
- External fixation

INDICATIONS

- Intramedullary nails are designed for long-bone shaft (diaphyseal) fractures:
  - Fractures that fail closed reduction
  - Fractures that are associated with proximal or distal radioulnar joint dislocation when the joint reduction is unstable
  - Open radius and ulna shaft fractures
  - Fractures with associated compartment syndrome requiring fasciotomies
  - Refractures
  - Ipsilateral humerus fractures ("floating elbow")

EXAMINATION/IMAGING

- Deformity and swelling of the forearm typically indicate fracture location.
- Examination of the elbow and wrist is critical to rule out Monteggia fracture (ulna fracture with radial head dislocation) and Galeazzi fracture (radial fracture with distal radioulnar joint dislocation).
- Neurovascular examination is important prior to and after any manipulation.
- The skin should be examined for any abrasions or open areas.
- Standard radiographs include anteroposterior and lateral views of the forearm and dedicated views of the wrist (Fig. 1A) and/or elbow (Fig. 1B) to rule out proximal or distal radioulnar joint dislocation above or below the fracture that can be associated with diaphyseal fractures.

SURGICAL ANATOMY

- The physes need to be localized so that the intramedullary nails do not damage the growth cartilage.
  - The radius is typically entered proximal to the distal radial physis, and the nail should stop prior to touching the proximal radial physis.
  - The ulna is typically entered distal to the olecranon apophysis, and the nail stops prior to touching the distal ulnar physis.
- Several branches of the superficial branch of the radial nerve traverse the dorsal radial aspect of the distal forearm and are often encountered when making the incision for the radial nail (Fig. 2). These branches need to be protected during the procedure to avoid creating an area of numbness distal to the incision.
- The tendons on the radial aspect of the wrist at the level of incision (from radial to ulnar) are the abductor pollicis longus (APL), extensor pollicis brevis (EPB), extensor carpi radialis longus (ECRL), extensor carpi radialis brevis (ECRB), and extensor pollicis longus (EPL). Figure 3 shows the tendons and appropriate intervals for nail insertion at the distal radius.
- The ulnar nerve is medial to the olecranon, so nail entry should always be on the lateral side of the olecranon to avoid ulnar nerve injury (Fig. 4).

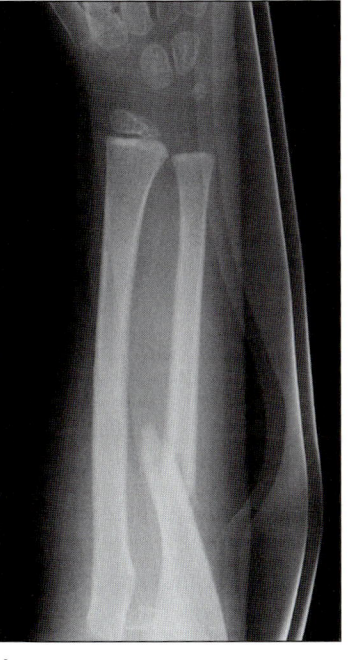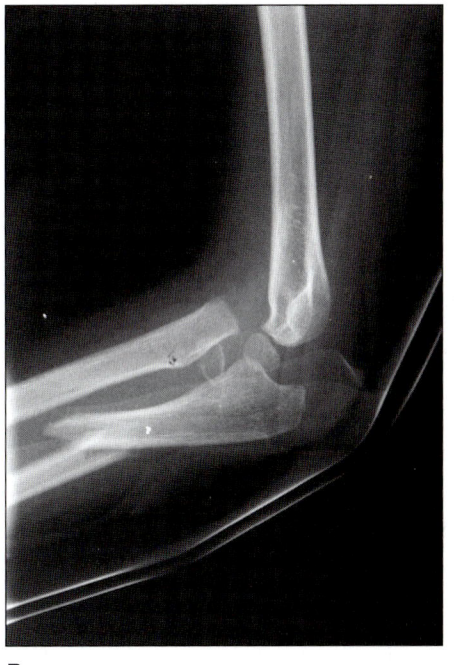

A   B

FIGURE 1

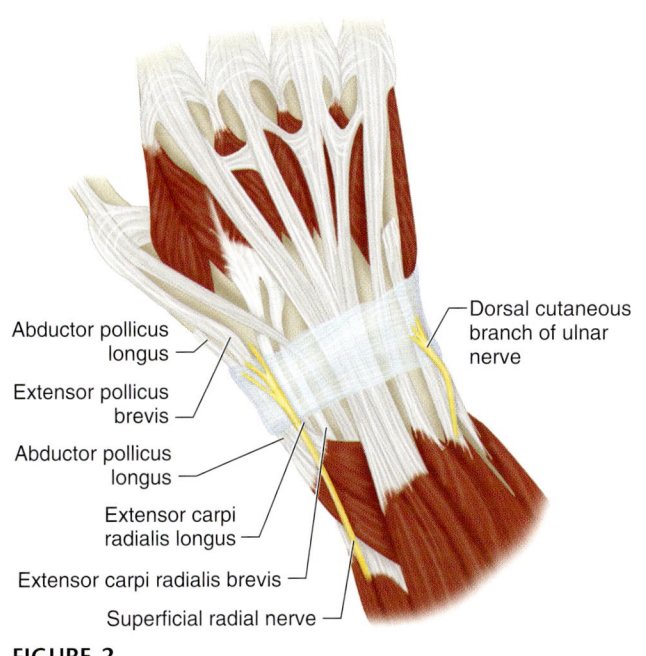

Abductor pollicus
longus

Extensor pollicus
brevis

Abductor pollicus
longus

Extensor carpi
radialis longus

Extensor carpi radialis brevis

Superficial radial nerve

Dorsal cutaneous
branch of ulnar
nerve

FIGURE 2

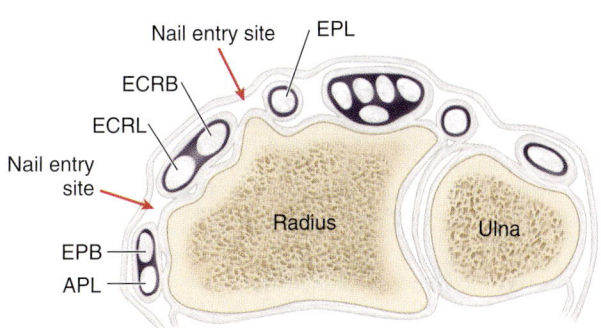

Nail entry site   EPL

ECRB

ECRL

Nail entry
site

EPB

APL

Radius   Ulna

FIGURE 3

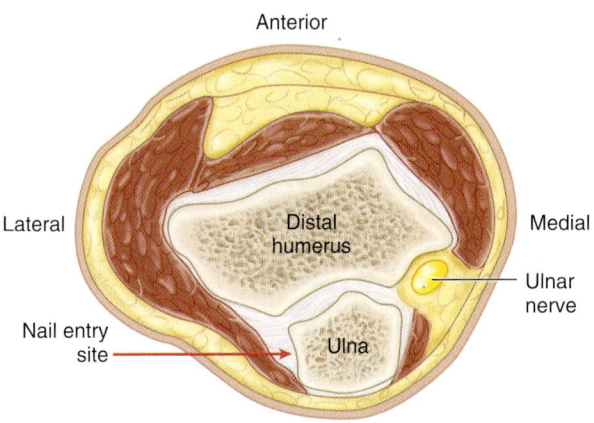

Anterior

Lateral   Distal
humerus   Medial

Ulnar
nerve

Nail entry
site   Ulna

FIGURE 4

Equipment

• Radiolucent armboard (a Lucite board can be placed between the patient and bed to support the operative forearm)

POSITIONING

■ The patient is positioned supine on the operating table with a radiolucent armboard.
■ A tourniquet is placed on the arm but may not need to be inflated.
■ C-arm fluoroscopy should be brought in parallel to the bed to minimize disruption to the surgical team (Fig. 5).

PORTALS/EXPOSURES

RADIUS

■ A small incision is made on the dorsal radial aspect of the wrist just proximal to the physis (Fig. 6). Care is taken to protect the superficial branches of the radial nerve.
■ The interval between the first and second compartments (extensor pollicis brevis and extensor carpi radialis longus tendons), or that between the second and third compartments (extensor carpi radialis brevis and extensor pollicis longus tendons), can be utilized.
■ A proximal starting point should not be used for the radius.

ULNA

■ A small incision is made on the lateral aspect of the olecranon midway between the ulnohumeral joint and the posterior aspect of the olecranon and approximately 2 cm from the tip of the olecranon (Fig. 7).
■ If the ulna fracture is proximal, an entry site through the distal ulna can be used, making the incision just proximal to the physis and along the subcutaneous border of the ulna. This starting location, however, is technically more difficult and leaves a prominent nail tip without much soft tissue coverage. The dorsal cutaneous branch of the ulnar nerve must be protected during the approach to the distal ulna.

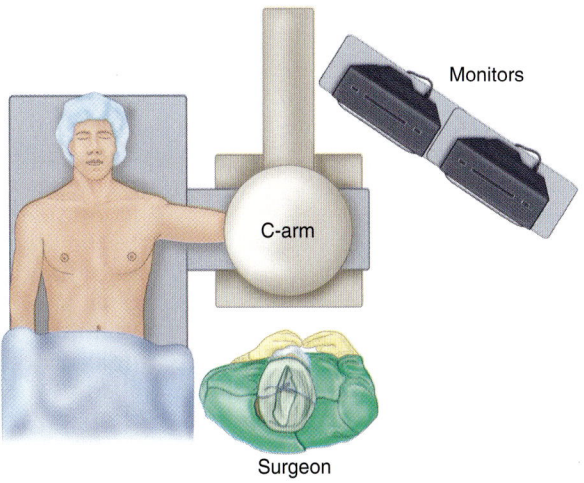

FIGURE 5

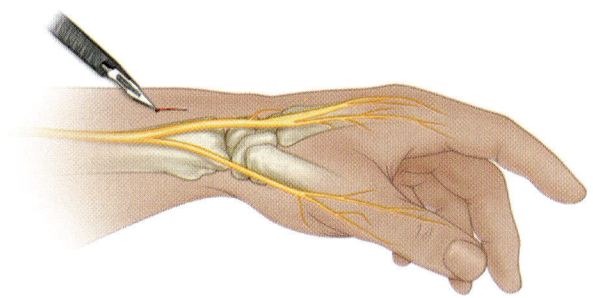

FIGURE 6

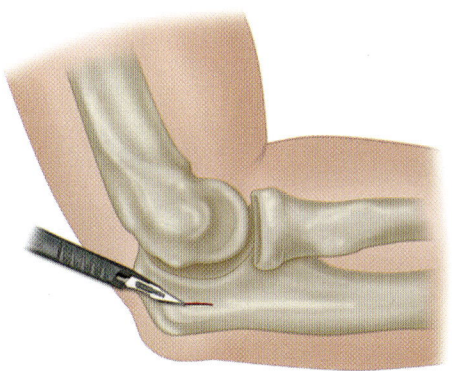

FIGURE 7

PROCEDURE

STEP 1: NAIL ENTRY SITES

■ Entry site for radial nail

• Once the surgeon has safely dissected down to the distal radius, a soft tissue protector that is 1–2 mm larger than the diameter of the planned nail should be used for the drill.

• Fluoroscopy is used to confirm that the entry site is proximal to the physis. A lateral view will ensure that the entry site is not too anterior on the radius.

• Only one cortex should be drilled through.

• With just the tip of the drill through the cortex (Fig. 8A), the drill is angled so the trajectory is approximately 30° to the shaft of the bone (angled distal to proximal) to facilitate passing the nail (Fig. 8B).

■ Entry site for ulnar nail

• Blunt dissection down to bone is done through the incision on the lateral side of the olecranon.

• The drill is inserted with a soft tissue protector.

• The drill is used to gently feel the joint and the posterior aspect of the olecranon. The drill hole is started midway between these two landmarks.

• Only one cortex is drilled through, with the drill bit perpendicular to the bone (Fig. 9A).

• Once the first cortex has been drilled through, the drill is kept running and is angled so that it is aiming down the canal (Fig. 9B).

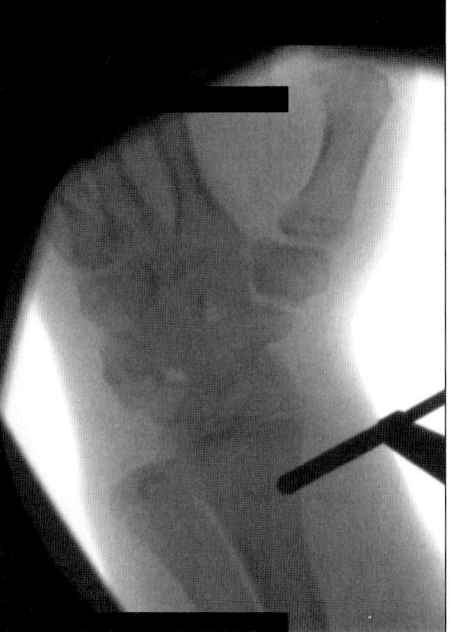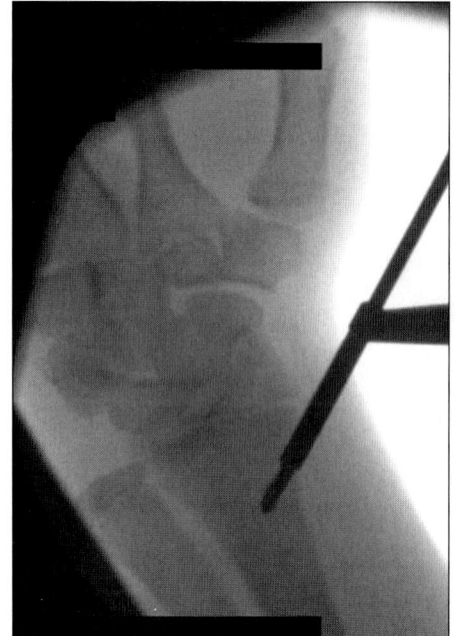

A

B

FIGURE 8

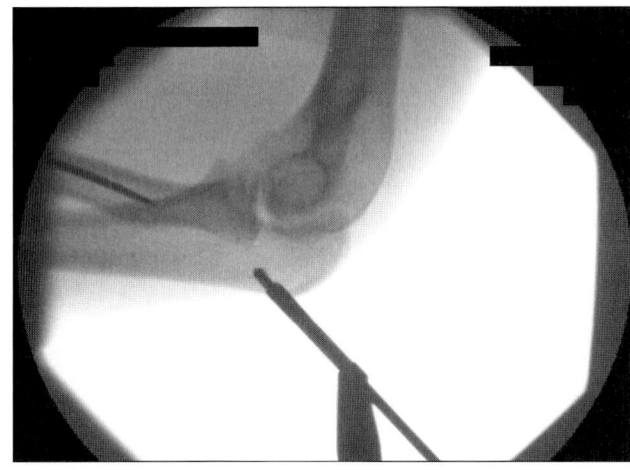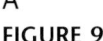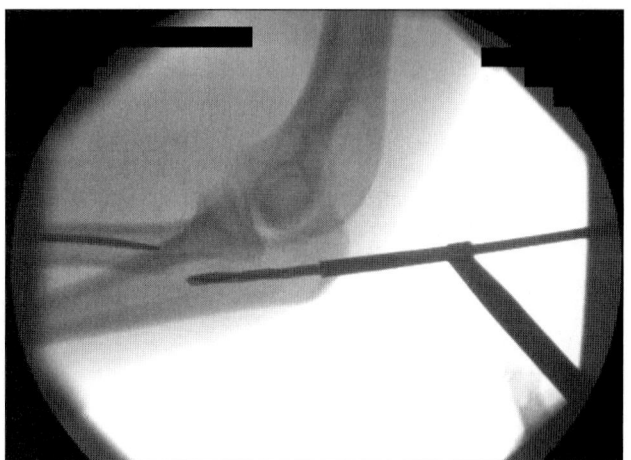

A

B

FIGURE 9

Instrumentation/Implantation

- Several brands of flexible nails can be used; both titanium and stainless steel nails are offered. They typically come in a set with the instrumentation for bending, passing, and cutting the nail.

- Flexible titanium nails already have a curve at the tip, but will still need some contouring to facilitate passage down the radial canal.

- For smaller children, we recommend simple K-wires. The technique is the same regardless of the type of implant, but the straight K-wires will require more contouring.

Controversies

- Titanium nails are more flexible, which facilitates passing the nail down the canal.

- Stainless steel nails are more rigid, which increases stability during healing.

Step 2: Nail Preparation and Insertion

- The appropriate-diameter nail for each bone is chosen (60–80% of the medullary canal diameter).
- Radial nail
  - The tip of the nail is curved so that it will bounce off the far cortex of the radius and pass easily down the IM canal, and then the nail is contoured to mimic the radial and dorsal bow of the radius (Fig. 10).
  - The tip of the nail is inserted into the previously drilled hole.
  - With a gentle rocking motion, the nail is passed down the canal to the fracture site. With the tip initially pointing radially, once the nail is traveling down the canal, it can be rotated to obtain the best path.
- Ulnar nail
  - This nail needs very little contour.
  - A slightly curved tip may help create the path and catch the distal fragment, but the ulna is very straight and the nail needs to maintain this alignment (Fig. 11). Often, we create the path with the curved tip but then remove the nail, cut the tip off or turn it over, and insert the straight tip, which will now follow the path that was previously created.
  - If the tip is too curved, the distal canal gets very narrow and the nail may distract the fracture site.

PEARLS

- *Radial nail*

  - *The contouring of the nail will determine how easy the nail is to pass. The nail needs to smoothly bounce off the ulnar cortex to pass into the canal.*

  - *While contouring the nail, think about the natural dorsal and radial bow of the radius.*

  - *If a K-wire is used, cut off the sharp tip or use the blunt end. The sharp tip will embed in the cortex and will not pass easily down the canal.*

- *Ulnar nail*

  - *Occasionally the curved tip of the Titanium Elastic Nail is too wide to pass into the distal ulna and may distract the fracture as it is pushed distally. If this is the case, we recommend inserting the curved tip first to create a path heading down the shaft; then the nail is removed and reinserted with the straight end first. It will follow the path created by the first insertion.*

PITFALLS

- *If the radial nail is overbent, the nail tip may embed in the radial cortex. If it is not curved enough, it will not bounce off the ulnar cortex.*

- *An ulnar nail with too much curve at the tip will be difficult to pass into the distal ulna and may distract the fracture site.*

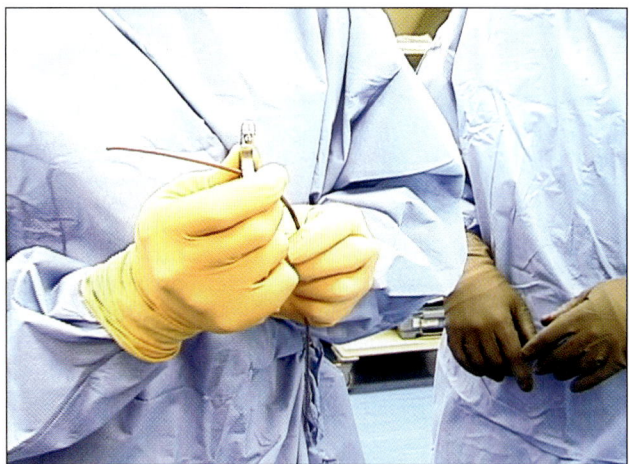

FIGURE 10

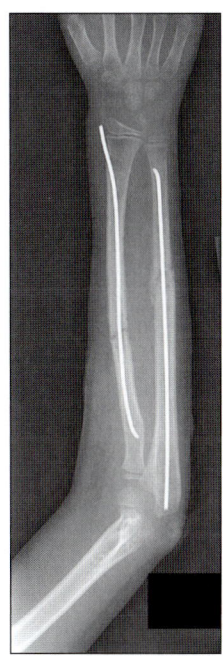

FIGURE 11

STEP 3: FRACTURE REDUCTION

- Once both nails are to the fracture site, the fractures must be reduced to pass the nails across the fractures. Fluoroscopy will help confirm reduction.

- Manual traction or finger-trap traction is usually necessary to get the fractured ends out to length.

- The bones can then be manipulated to align them. The nails can also be used as a joystick to maneuver one end to the other. The curved tip of the radial nail can be used to catch the proximal fragment (Fig. 12A–C) and help reduce the fracture.
  - After three passes across either fracture without getting into the second fragment, closed intramedullary nailing should be abandoned and the fracture site should be opened to directly visualize reduction and passing of the nail. This can usually be done through a small 2- to 3-cm incision, using an anterior approach for the radius or along the subcutaneous border for the ulna.

- Once the nail is across the radius fracture site, it is passed into the proximal radius and the tip is curved into the bicipital tuberosity. Once across the ulnar fracture, the nail is passed into the distal ulna, stopping 1 cm short of the physis.

- The radial nail should point toward the ulna and the ulnar nail should point toward the radius to help maintain the interosseous space. Angulation of one bone toward the other must be avoided as supination and pronation will be adversely affected by narrowing of the interosseous distance.

- The nails should then be pulled away from the bone, cut 6–8 mm from the entry site, and allowed to snap back against the bone. The radial pin should not rest on the physis.

- The nails can be tamped against the bone, but the surgeon must be careful not to tamp them significantly further into the bone as this will make later removal very difficult as well as potentially resulting in loss of three-point fixation.

- The cut end of the radial nail must not be under the tendons as rubbing over a sharp tip will rupture the tendons.

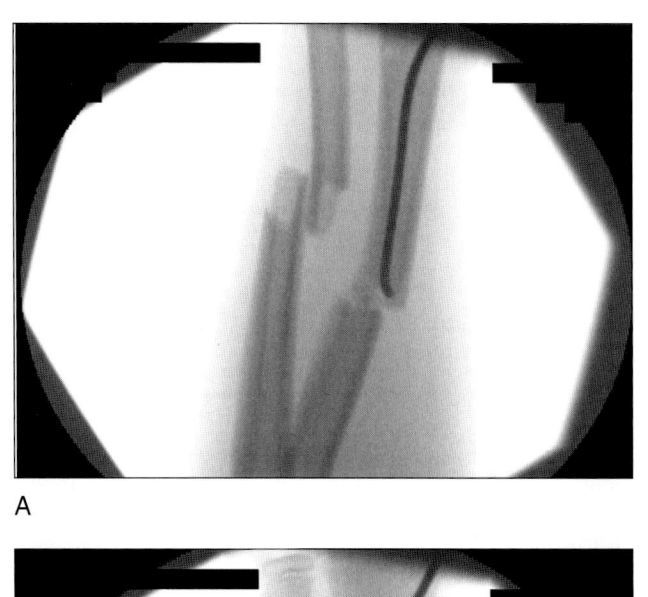

A

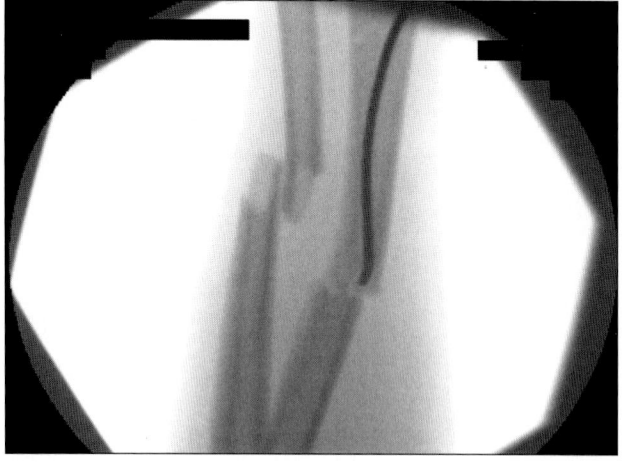

B

C

FIGURE 12

Controversies

• Nail removal: Nails can be left in place; however, in skeletally immature patients, we recommend nail removal 6–12 months postoperatively to prevent bony overgrowth and the long-term risk of infection with a foreign body. The literature is not clear on this point.

STEP 4: WOUND CLOSURE

■ Incisions can be closed with an absorbable suture.
■ A local anesthetic is injected at the insertion sites.
■ The forearm should be examined before applying any dressings to ensure there is not swelling that will cause compartment syndrome. If there is any concern, compartment pressures should be checked before the patient leaves the operating room.

POSTOPERATIVE CARE AND EXPECTED OUTCOMES

■ Although many surgeons use no postoperative immobilization, we recommend casting postoperatively to allow the soft tissues to heal and to stabilize the fractures until bony healing begins.
■ For fractures in the distal two thirds of the forearm, a short-arm cast is usually adequate. Proximal fractures are better stabilized with a long-arm cast.
■ All casts should be univalved for the first week to allow for swelling. The cast can be tightened and overwrapped with fiberglass once the swelling decreases.
■ Patients should be monitored at least overnight to watch for any signs or symptoms of compartment syndrome.
■ Nails should be removed 6–12 months postoperatively following complete healing of the fractures.

EVIDENCE

Flynn JM. Pediatric forearm fractures: decision making, surgical techniques, and complications. Instr Course Lect. 2002;51:355–60.

Flynn JM, Waters PM. Single-bone fixation of both-bone forearm fractures. J Pediatr Orthop. 1996;16:655–9.

Huber RI, Keller HW, Huber PM, Rehm KE. Flexible intramedullary nailing as fracture treatment in children. J Pediatr Orthop. 1996;16:602–5.

Kanellopoulos AD, Yiannakopoulos CK, Soucacos PN. Flexible intramedullary nailing of pediatric unstable forearm fractures. Am J Orthop. 2005;34:420–4.

Kapoor V, Theruvil B, Edwards SE, Taylor GR, Clarke NM, Uglow MG. Flexible intramedullary nailing of displaced diaphyseal forearm fractures in children. Injury. 2005;36:1221–5.

Lascombes P, Haumont T, Journeau P. Use and abuse of flexible intramedullary nailing in children and adolescents. J Pediatr Orthop. 2006;26:827–34.

Perry CR, Brueckmann FR, Pankovich AM, Sanders RW, Waddell JP. Flexible intramedullary nailing of long bone fractures. Instr Course Lect. 1993;42:57–66.

Simanovsky N, Tair MA, Simanovsky N, Porat S. Removal of flexible titanium nails in children. J Pediatr Orthop. 2006;26:188–92.

Shoemaker SD, Comstock CP, Mubarak SJ, Wenger DR, Chambers HG. Intramedullary Kirschner wire fixation of open or unstable forearm fractures in children. J Pediatr Orthop. 1999;19:329–37.

Yuan PS, Pring ME, Gaynor TP, Mubarak SJ, Newton PO. Compartment syndrome following intramedullary fixation of pediatric forearm fractures. J Pediatr Orthop. 2004;24:370–5.

SECTION IV

HAND

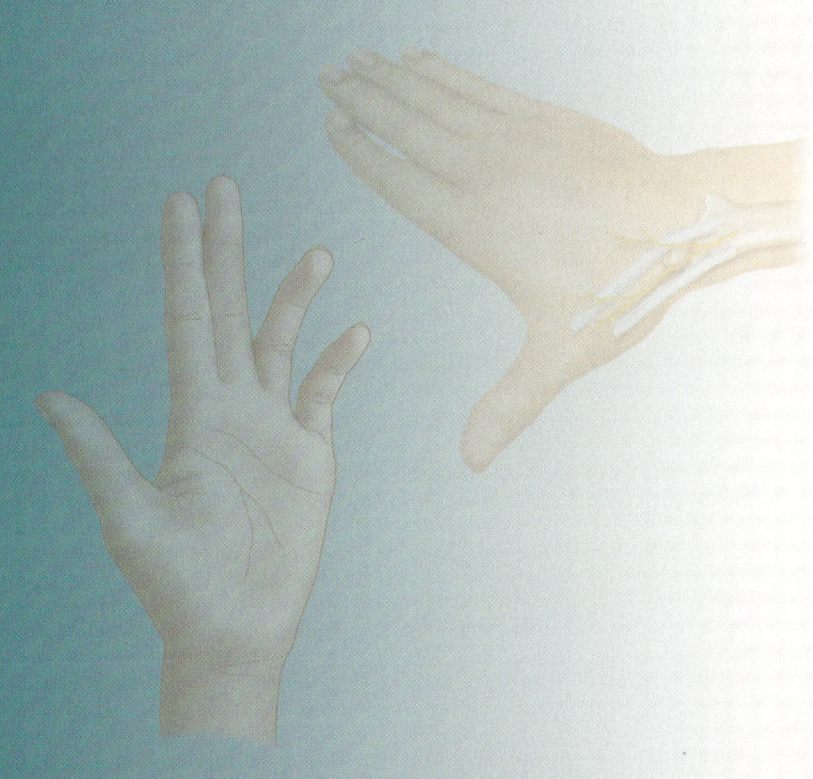

Digital Syndactyly Release

J. Megan M. Patterson and Douglas T. Hutchinson

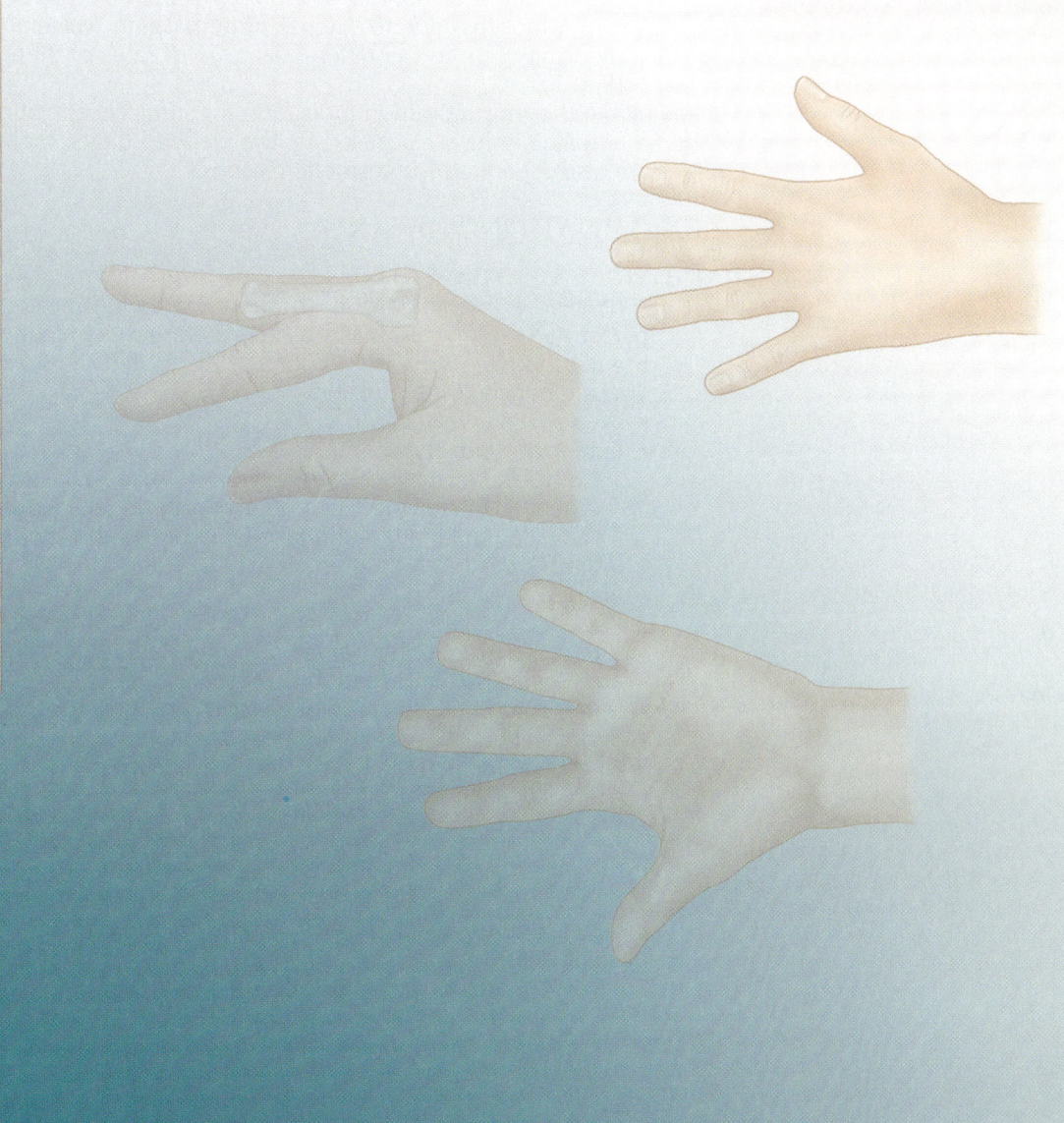

Controversies

• Multiple-digit syndactyly release is best performed as a staged procedure to decrease the risk of digital vascular compromise that is associated with release on both sides of one digit.

Treatment Options

• The most common controversy regarding syndactyly separation is whether to use skin grafts or local flaps only. Skin grafts allow for easy closure of all incisions; however, they are associated with complications including hyperpigmentation, hair growth, donor site morbidity, scar contracture, and web creep. Syndactyly release without skin grafts decreases surgical time, and may have improved cosmesis and fewer complications; however, a direct comparison of syndactyly release with skin grafting versus without skin grafting has not been done.

INDICATIONS

■ Surgical separation is indicated in almost all cases as syndactyly can have functional, cosmetic, and developmental implications that can worsen with growth of the child.

• Most surgeons recommend waiting until the child is at least 6 months old to allow tissues to grow and to reduce the anesthetic risk to the child, and some authors recommend waiting until the child is over the age of 2. All surgical releases should be completed before the child reaches school age.

• An exception to waiting until the child is 6 months of age is when the syndactyly involves the ring and small finger or the thumb and index finger. These are released earlier (between 3 and 6 months) due to the risk of developing worsening deformity due to the differential growth rates of these digits (Fig. 1).

■ While the most common indication for surgical separation is functional limitations caused by the webbed digits, many digits are also separated for cosmetic reasons.

EXAMINATION/IMAGING

PHYSICAL EXAMINATION

■ A detailed examination of both upper extremities needs to be performed and, occasionally, a more detailed examination of the child is necessary to rule out any associated syndromes.

■ Specific details to note include:

• Web space involvement.

• Extent of syndactyly.

◆ Complete versus incomplete. Figure 2A shows a complete syndactyly involving the long and ring fingers. Figure 2B shows an incomplete syndactyly involving the same fingers.

◆ Simple versus complex.

• Nail involvement (Fig. 3).

• Presence or absence of independent motion of the digits.

• The presence of joint creases can help determine if the joints are functioning and motion is present.

■ Features that may indicate associated syndromes include:

• Short webbed fingers (symbrachydactyly).

• Chest wall defects.

• Craniofacial abnormalities.

• Foot/toe abnormalities.

PLAIN RADIOGRAPHS

■ Plain radiographs are used to evaluate for bony fusions (which indicate a complex syndactyly), a concealed extra digit (Fig. 4), or joint deformities.

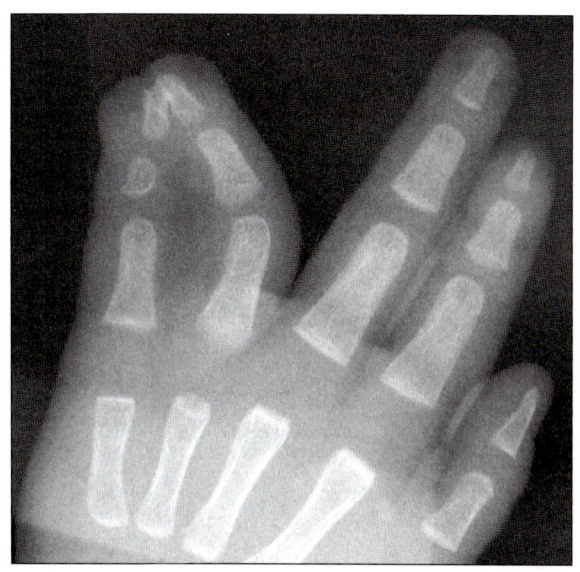

FIGURE 1

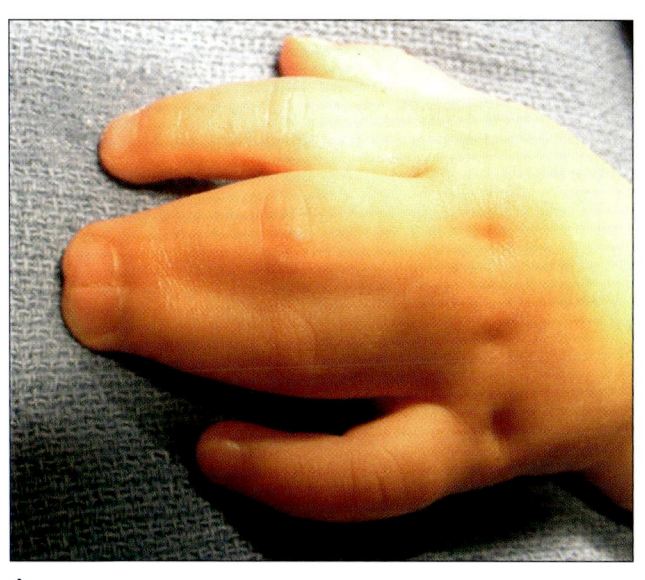

A
FIGURE 2

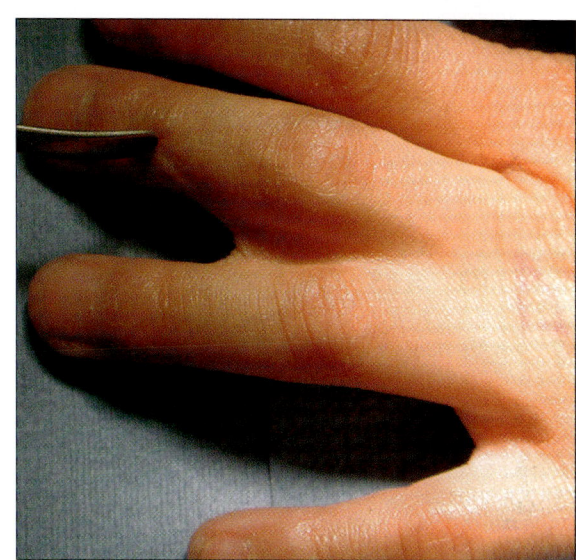

B

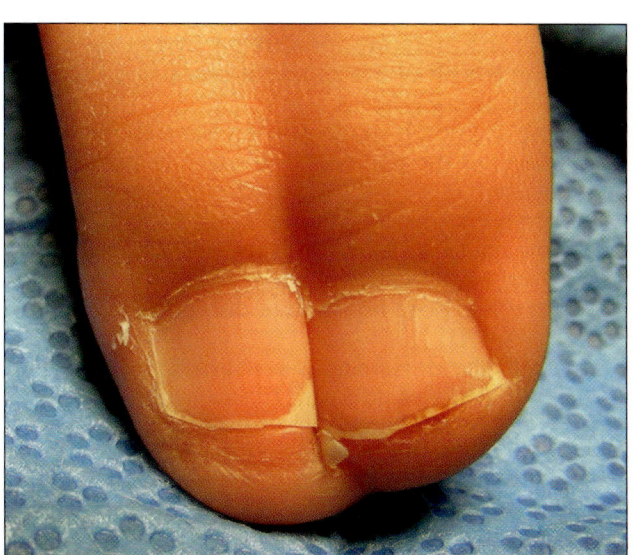

FIGURE 3

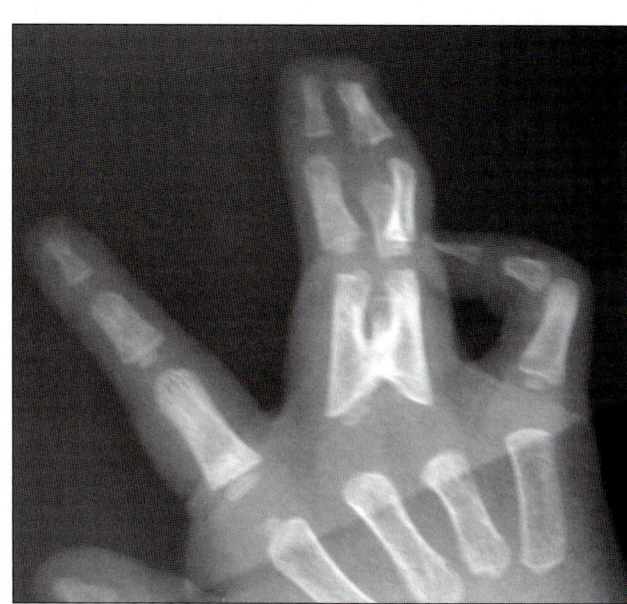

FIGURE 4

SURGICAL ANATOMY

- As the digits are separated, the neurovascular structures must be identified and protected.
  - The digital artery and nerve are often easiest to identify proximally. Proper digital arteries that bifurcate distal to the planned web space will need to be ligated. If this is necessary, the proper digital artery to the more midline digit is usually preserved.
  - Digital nerves that bifurcate distal to the planned web space can be separated by interfasicular microdissection.
- The lateral eponychial fold is often absent in complex or simple complete syndactyly. It can be reconstructed using tissue from the distal tip of the adjoined digit, and its careful reconstruction will improve the cosmetic outcome of the procedure.
- Re-creation of the web space
  - A normal web space is wider distally than proximally and begins its dorsal-to-palmar slope of about 35–45° at the level of the metacarpal head.
  - Many different local skin flaps have been described to re-create the web space.
    - Dorsal rectangular, trapezoidal, V-Y, and island pedicle flaps
    - A combination of dorsal and volar flaps
  - Care is taken at the beginning of the procedure to plan the location of the web space such that it will follow the normal cascade of the hand.

POSITIONING

- The child is positioned supine with the involved extremity extended on an armboard.
- A tourniquet is placed high on the upper arm.
- If a skin graft is going to be harvested, the donor site must also be prepped out.

PORTALS/EXPOSURES

COMMISSURE RECONSTRUCTION

- A dorsal flap is created for commissure reconstruction.
- Design of the flap is dependent on surgeon preference and whether skin grafting is planned for wound closure.
  - Syndactyly release with skin grafting
    - A proximally based rectangular dorsal flap that extends from the level of the metacarpophalangeal (MCP) joints to two thirds of the length of the proximal phalanx is used to re-create the web space (Fig. 5).
    - A corresponding incision is made at the volar base of the fingers at the level of the planned web space to accept the dorsal commissure flap.
  - Syndactyly release without skin grafting
    - A V-Y dorsal metacarpal island flap is used and is centered at the level of the MCP joint (Fig. 6).
    - The artery to the flap does not require dissection to allow for flap advancement.
    - The distal edge of the dorsal flap is concave, and the flap is slightly narrowed in the middle and triangular proximally. The triangular shape proximally allows for primary closure.
    - The dorsal flap is one-half the length of the proximal phalanx and extends from midsagittal line to midsagittal line.
    - A slightly convex volar incision is made to accept the dorsal commissure flap.

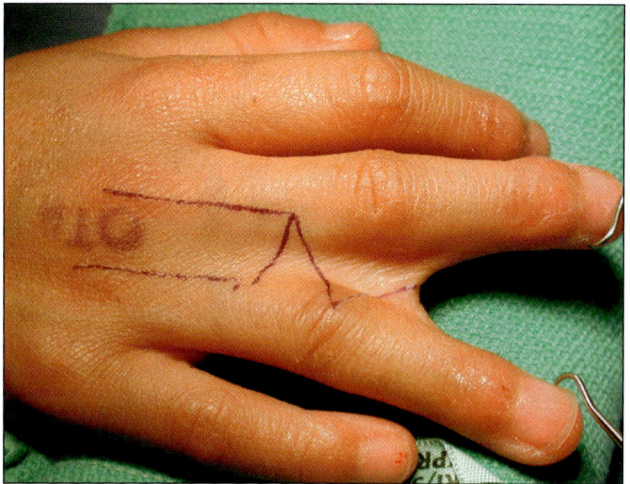

FIGURE 5

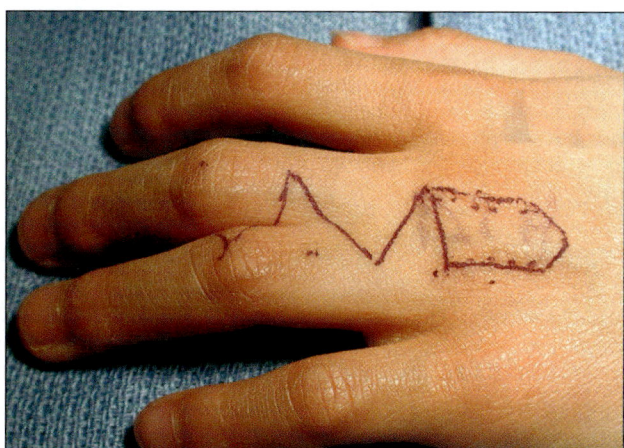

FIGURE 6

Controversies

- The design of the commissural flap is variable and determines the need for skin grafting during wound closure.

- We prefer using large triangle flaps both dorsally and volarly. Other methods have been described, including rectangular flaps and small triangles.

PEARLS

- *Both the dorsal and volar incision are made and then dissection is started from dorsal to volar, looking for the "light" of the volar incisions.*

- *Care must be taken to avoid crushing the tips of the flaps with forceps. This can be facilitated by using a microdouble skin hook to retract the flaps.*

DORSAL AND VOLAR EXPOSURE

- Dorsal exposure is created via multiple zigzag incisions extending from the midsagittal surface of each of the involved digits (Fig. 7).
- Corresponding palmar flaps are created opposite the dorsal zigzag flaps (Fig. 8).

PROCEDURE

STEP 1: ELEVATION OF SKIN FLAPS

- Using a combination of sharp and blunt dissection, the dorsal flaps are elevated first, followed by the volar flaps (Fig. 9).
- Blunt dissection is used to identify the neurovascular bundles, which is often easiest to do near their bifurcation.

STEP 2: SEPARATION OF THE DIGITS

- The digits are separated in a distal-to-proximal direction.
- Separation is facilitated by manual distraction of the two involved digits as this will put the tissues on tension.
- Interfascicular microdissection of digital nerves is required when the common digital nerves bifurcate distal to the level of the planned commissure.
- Ligation of a proper digital artery may be required to allow for proper commissure placement, though this is rare.
  - The smaller digital artery is sacrificed when both digits have two intact digital arteries.
  - In hands which require multiple syndactyly releases, the proper digital artery to the more midline digit is preserved.
  - If there is any question as to the vascular status of the digit, a vascular clamp can be placed on the digital arteries and the tourniquet deflated to ensure adequate blood flow to each of the digits prior to any planned arterial ligation.
- Small osteotomes or a scalpel is used to separate any bony component of the syndactyly.
- Any concealed polydactyly bone remnants should be removed.
- Separation of the nail
  - The nail is split longitudinally.
  - Laterally based triangular flaps (Buck-Gramcko flaps) are created on the pulp of the fingers that are rotated to form the lateral nail folds. The design of nail flaps is shown in Figure 10, while the elevation and placement of nail flaps is demonstrated in Figure 11.

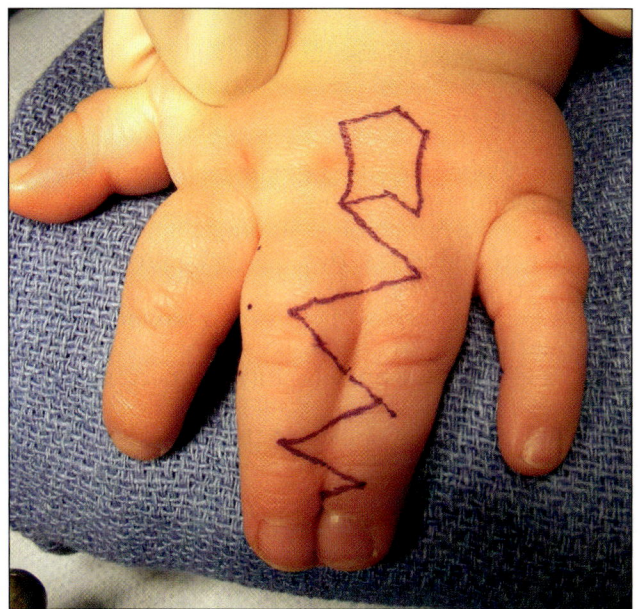

FIGURE 7

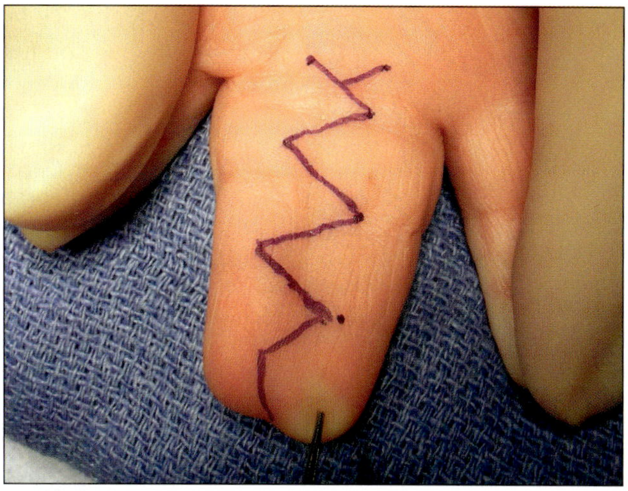

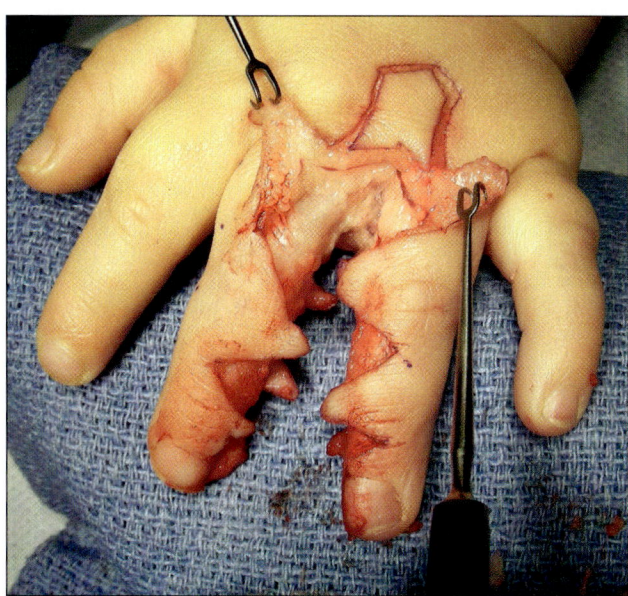

FIGURE 9

FIGURE 8

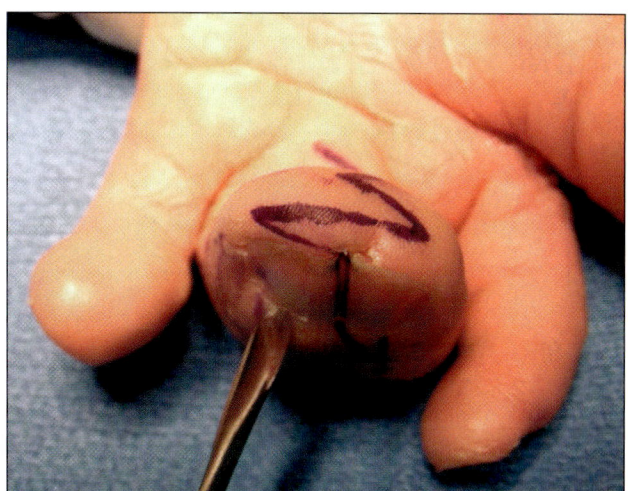

FIGURE 10

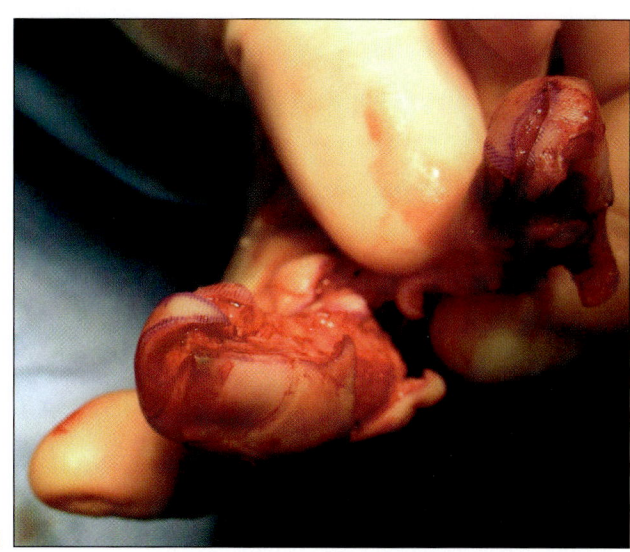

FIGURE 11

STEP 3: INSETTING OF THE FLAPS

- The fingers are defatted prior to insetting the flaps to decrease bulk (Fig. 12).
  - More extensive defatting is necessary if no skin grafting is planned.
  - Care must be taken when defatting the fingers near the commissure and neurovascular bundles.
- The flaps are inset using a 5-0 chromic suture.
  - The commissure flap is inset first (Fig. 13) to ensure proper position of the web space (Fig. 14).
  - The digital flaps are then inset without excess tension (Figs. 15 and 16).
  - Incisions may be left partially open (< 2 mm) if necessary to decrease tension.
- The tourniquet is released prior to placing the dressing to assess the vascular status of the digit.
  - Fingers that are not pink suggest that the flaps have been sutured too tight or there may be a problem with the vascular supply to the finger (spasm vs. vascular injury or insufficiency), and these must be addressed prior to placing the dressing. Stitches should be removed, and gaps of less than 2 mm may be left to decrease tension on the flaps.
  - The flaps may appear white, which is less of a concern.

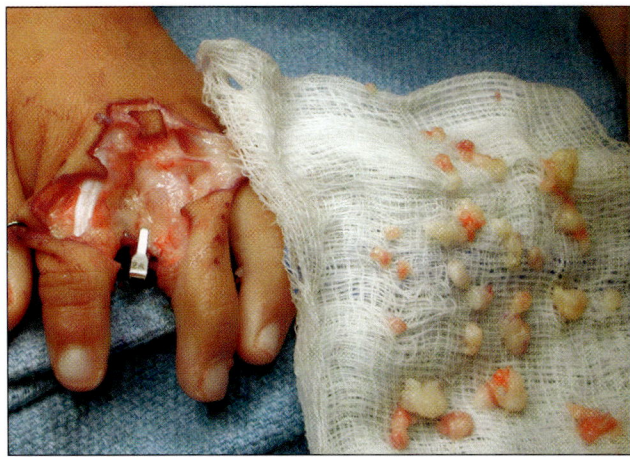

FIGURE 12

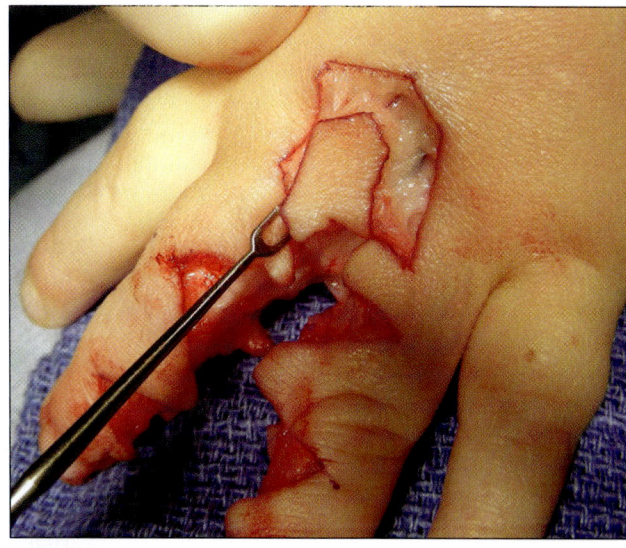

FIGURE 13

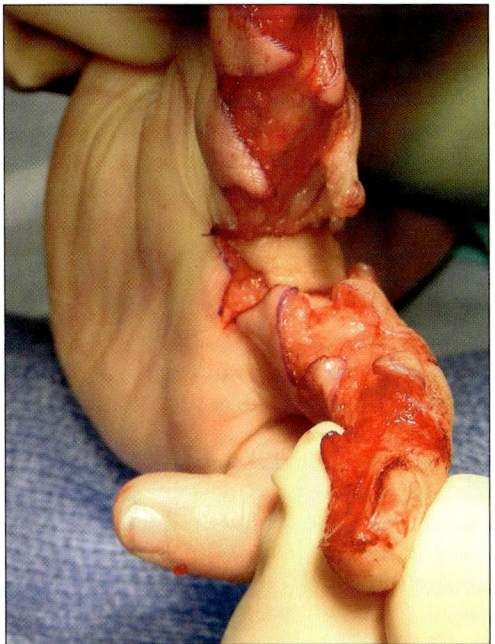

FIGURE 14

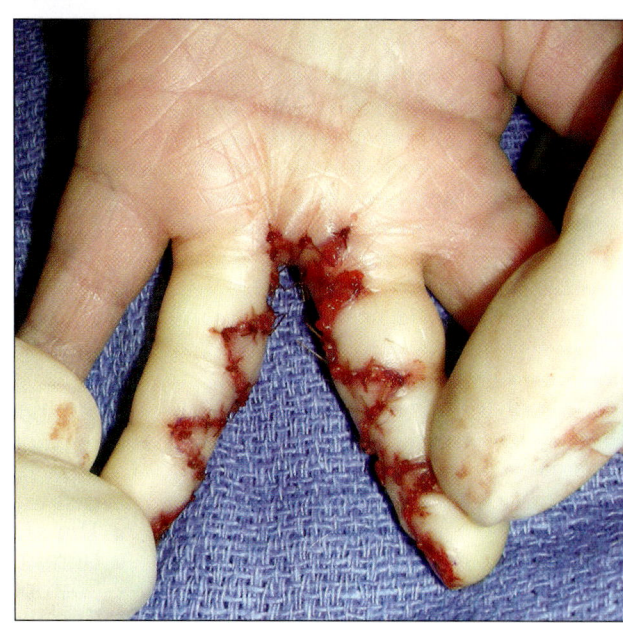

FIGURE 15

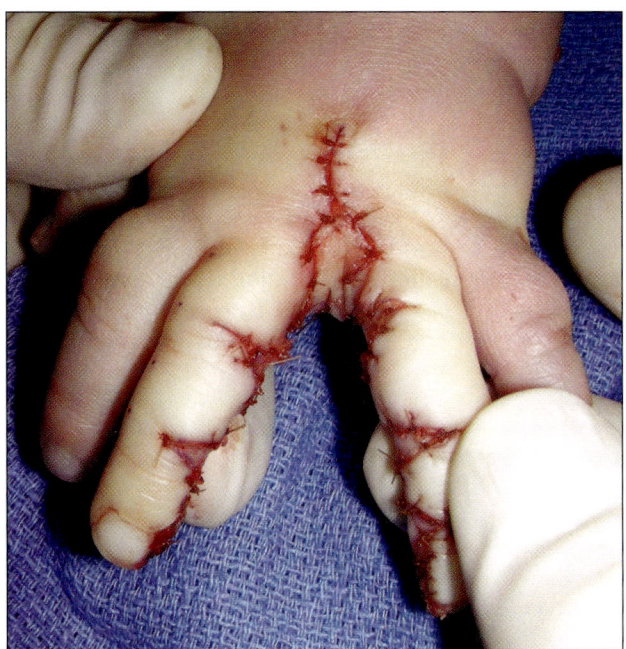

FIGURE 16

STEP 4: SKIN GRAFTING (IF NECESSARY)

- Full thickness skin grafts are preferred, and these should be defatted as they are harvested.
- Harvest sites include the hypothenar area, volar wrist, antecubital fossa, and groin. Our preferred site is the hypothenar area (Figs. 17 and 18), followed by the volar wrist and antecubital fossa.
  - Use of the antecubital fossa as a donor site will require a narrow, sterile tourniquet to be used.
  - Use of the groin as a donor site will require a separate sterile field. The groin donor site has fallen out of favor due to problems with cosmesis, including skin hyperpigmentation (Fig. 19) and hair growth. If groin grafts are to be used, they should be taken from the lateral aspect of the groin and within the inguinal crease to keep the scar concealed and help minimize hair growth. However, even with lateral harvest of the graft, the scar does tend to migrate as patients grow.
- An appropriate-size elliptical incision is made and the graft is elevated.
- The donor site is undermined and closed primarily.
  - We prefer to use temporary closing sutures to take tension off the wound as necessary, followed by subcuticular closure to prevent "train-track" scars at these locations.

POSTOPERATIVE CARE AND EXPECTED OUTCOMES

- Nonadherent dressings are placed between the fingers and in the web space. We prefer to place cotton balls soaked in mineral oil over the graft sites.
- An above-the-elbow splint or bulky soft dressing will help prevent removal of the dressing in the postoperative period, especially in the young child. We place an above-the-elbow tape cast as it eliminates the problem of cast/dressing slippage.
- The postoperative dressings are removed in 4 weeks.
- Unrestricted use of the hand is encouraged after the initial postoperative dressing is removed.
- Complications can occur both early and late and include:
  - Vascular compromise
  - Nerve injury
  - Infection
  - Wound dehiscence
  - Graft failure
  - Scar contracture (Fig. 20)
  - Web creep (Fig. 21)
    - This is worsened by longitudinal scars placed at the base of the finger, skin graft loss, and use of split-thickness skin grafts.
  - Digital deformities (angulation, malrotation, joint contracture) or instability

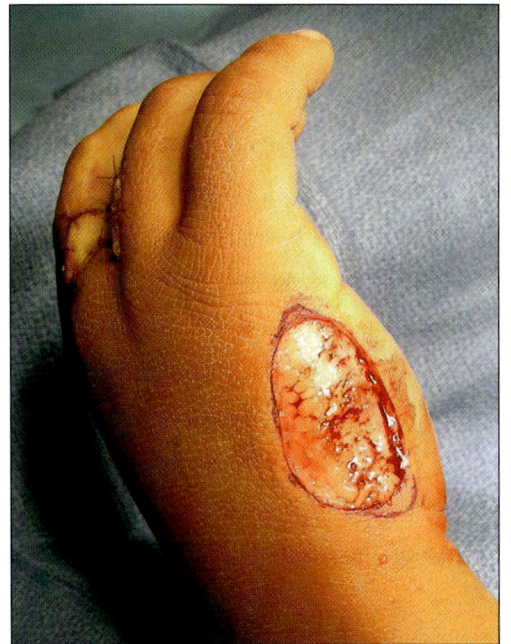

FIGURE 17

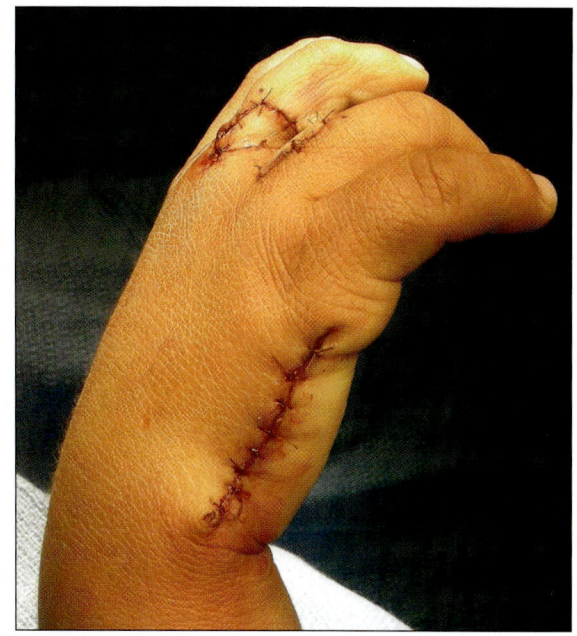

FIGURE 18

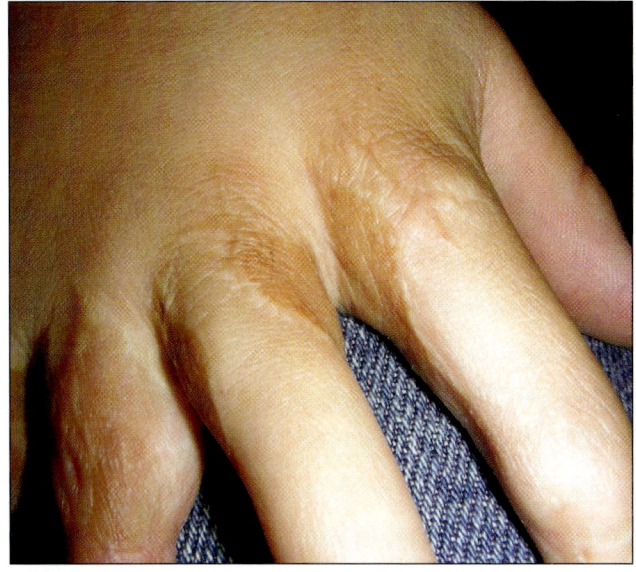

FIGURE 19

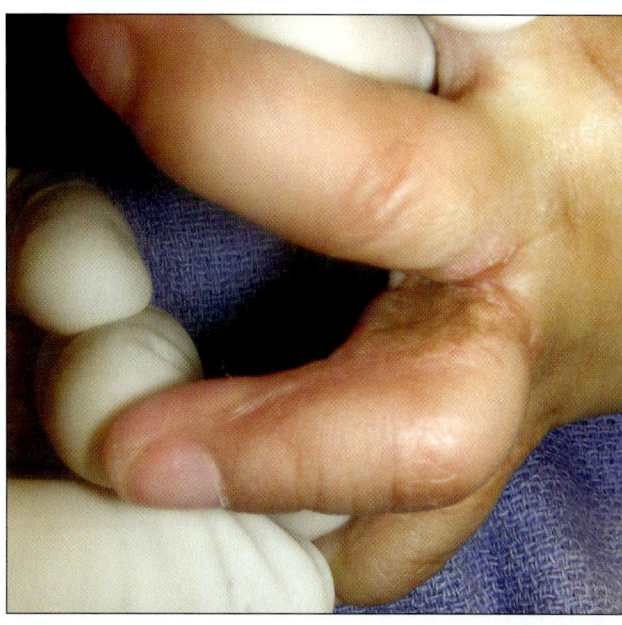

FIGURE 20

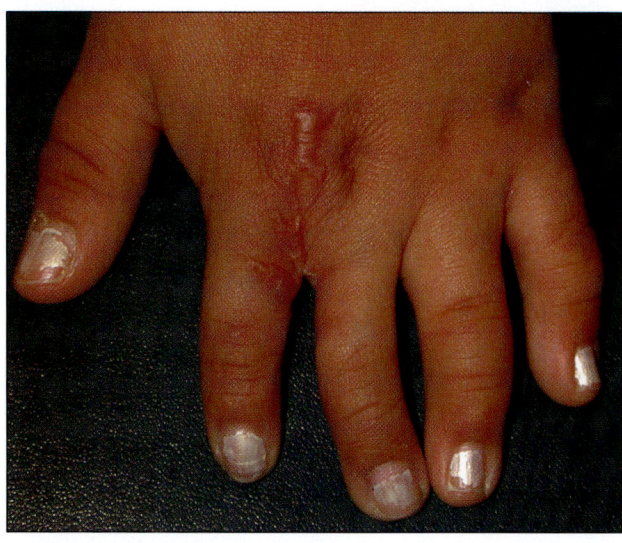

FIGURE 21

EVIDENCE

Dao KD, Shin AY, Billings A, Oberg KC, Wood VE. Surgical treatment of congenital syndactyly of the hand. J Am Acad Orthop Surg. 2004;12:39–48.

This paper gives an overview of congenital syndactyly, covering its embryology, epidemiology, treatment, and outcomes.

Deunk J, Nicolai JP, Hamburg SM. Long-term results of syndactyly correction: full-thickness versus split-thickness skin grafts. J Hand Surg [Br]. 2003;28:125–30.

This study evaluated 27 patients with an average follow-up of 21 years and found that those patients who had received split-thickness skin grafts had more flexion and extension lags and less interdigital separation when compared to the uninvolved fingers. The authors also found more web creep in patients who had received full-thickness grafts, and these patients also had more hyperpigmentation and hair growth. (Level IV evidence)

Eaton CJ, Lister GD. Syndactyly. Hand Clin. 1990;6:555–75.

The authors presented a review of syndactyly.

Greuse M, Bruno CC. Congenital syndactyly: defatting facilitates closure without skin graft. J Hand Surg [Am]. 2001;26:589–94.

In this study, 16 patients with 24 syndactylies were treated without the use of skin grafts. The authors found that defatting the full length of the finger and the interdigital space allowed for tension-free closure that was independent of flap configuration and that the defatted digits were of similar contour as the nonsyndactylized digits. (Level IV evidence)

Sherif MM. V-Y dorsal metacarpal flap: a new technique for the correction of syndactyly without skin graft. Plast Reconstr Surg. 1998;101:1861–6.

In this study, 12 patients with syndactyly were treated using a dorsal metacarpal artery island flap for web reconstruction, thereby avoiding skin grafting. No web creep was noted at follow-up ranging from 6 months to 2 years. (Level IV evidence)

Toledo LC, Ger E. Evaluation of the operative treatment of syndactyly. J Hand Surg [Am]. 1979;4:556–64.

The authors reviewed the records of 61 patients with 176 surgically treated syndactylies at an average follow-up of 14 years. They found that the use of split-thickness skin grafts was associated with a higher incidence of web creep and digital contractures. More secondary procedures were required in those patients who had been treated prior to 18 months of age and those who had a complex syndactyly. (Level IV evidence)

PELVIS AND HIP

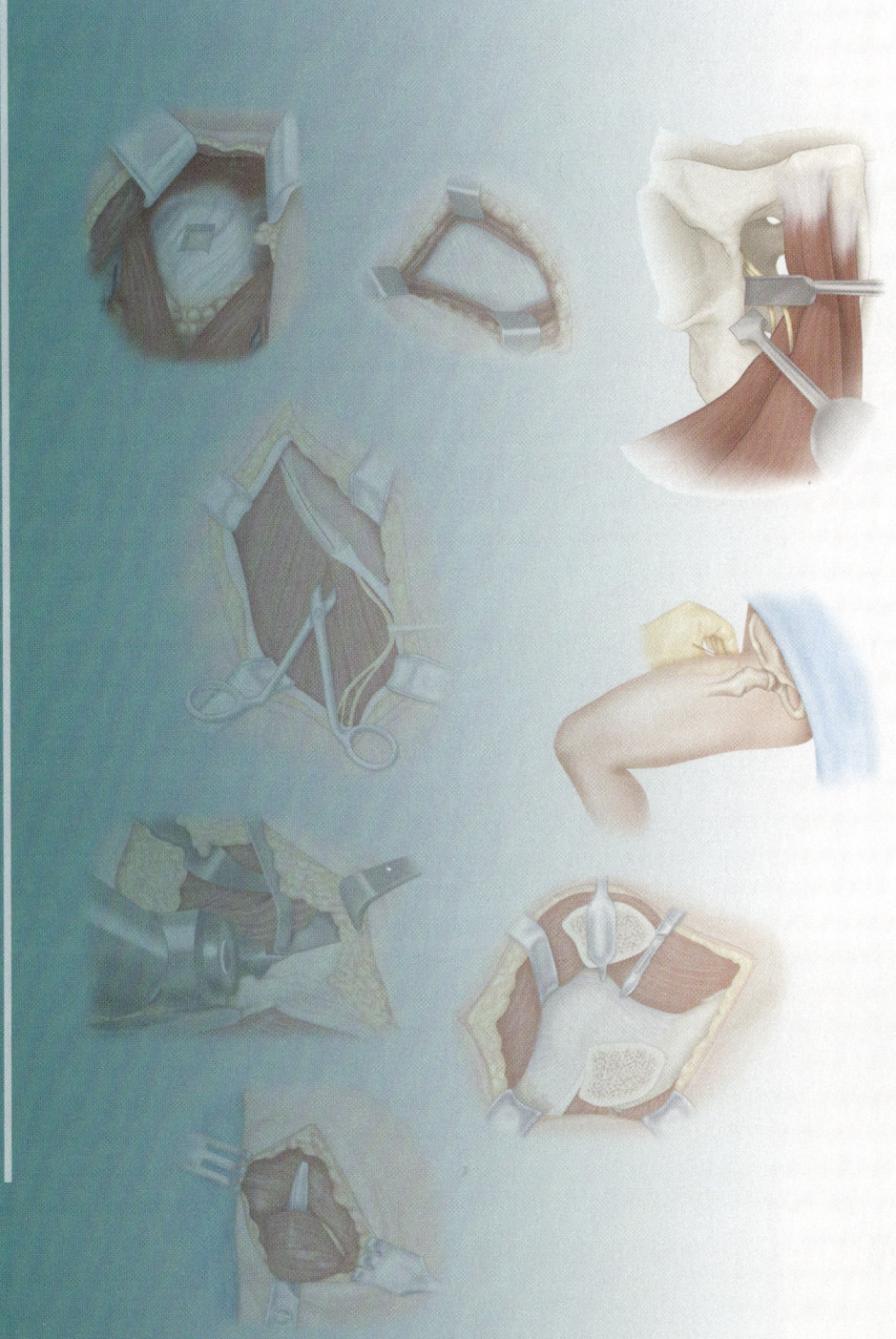

Innominate Osteotomy

John H. Wedge

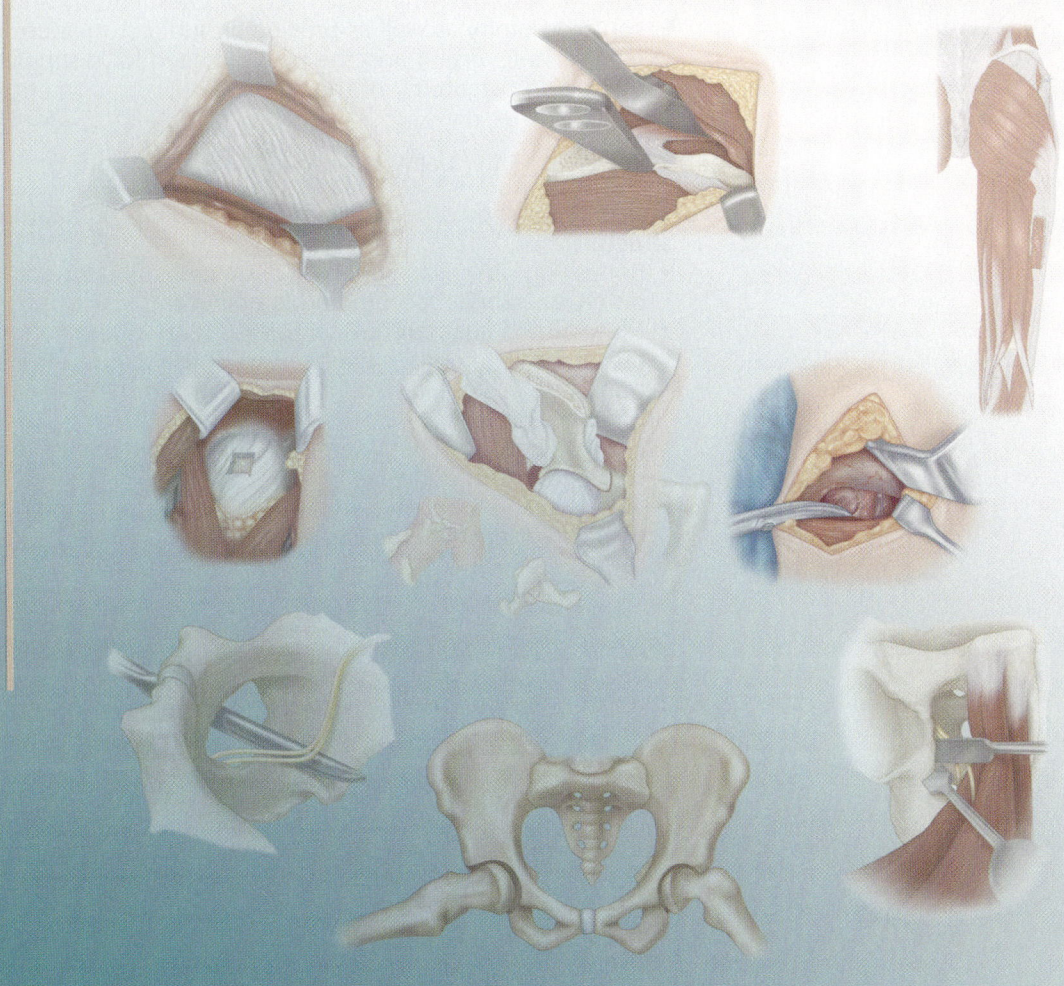

Controversies

• Experience with this procedure after closure of the acetabular triradiate growth plate has been mixed. Periacetabular or triple osteotomy should be considered instead of innominate osteotomy in the adolescent.

INDICATIONS

- Developmental dislocation of the hip (dislocated hip)
- Acetabular dysplasia and subluxation of the hip in the child and adolescent

EXAMINATION/IMAGING

- Anteroposterior (Fig. 1A) and frog-leg view radiographs are obtained.
- A supine anteroposterior radiograph with the thighs fully abducted and internally rotated is obtained to predict postoperative congruency of the hip when the hip is subluxated (Fig. 1B).
  - This will also determine the need for capsulotomy and capsulorrhaphy as well as provide an indirect measure of femoral anteversion and the possible need for a supplemental derotation osteotomy of the femur.

SURGICAL ANATOMY

- The surgeon should be familiar with the following anatomic structures:
  - Bones (Fig. 2A): iliac apophysis, iliac crest, greater sciatic notch, acetabular labrum and lateral acetabular epiphysis
  - Muscles and ligamentous complexes (Fig. 2B): sartorius and tensor fascia femoris, straight head of the rectus femoris, transverse acetabular ligament, ligamentum teres, iliopsoas muscle/tendon
  - Nerves (Fig. 2C): lateral femoral cutaneous nerve of the thigh, superior gluteal nerve
  - Vessels in the greater sciatic notch and the surrounding soft tissues of the ilium (see Fig. 2C)

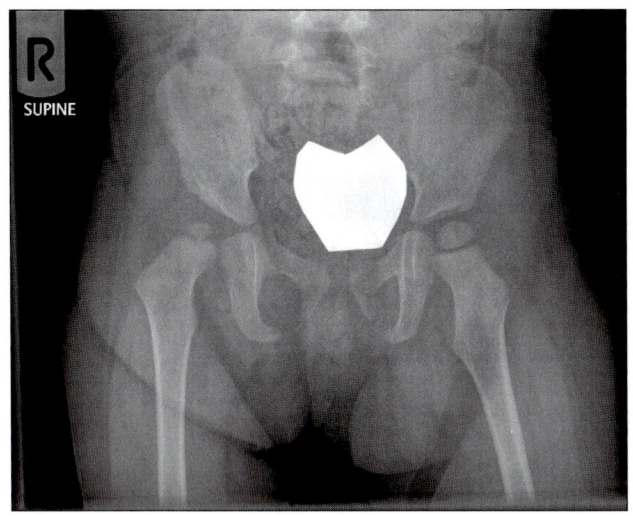

A

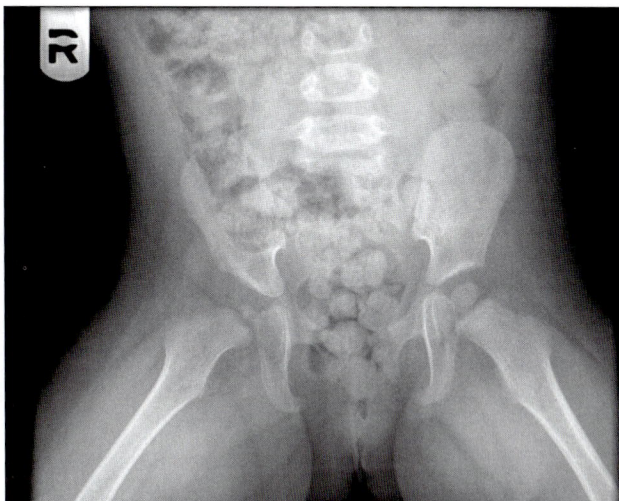

B

FIGURE 1

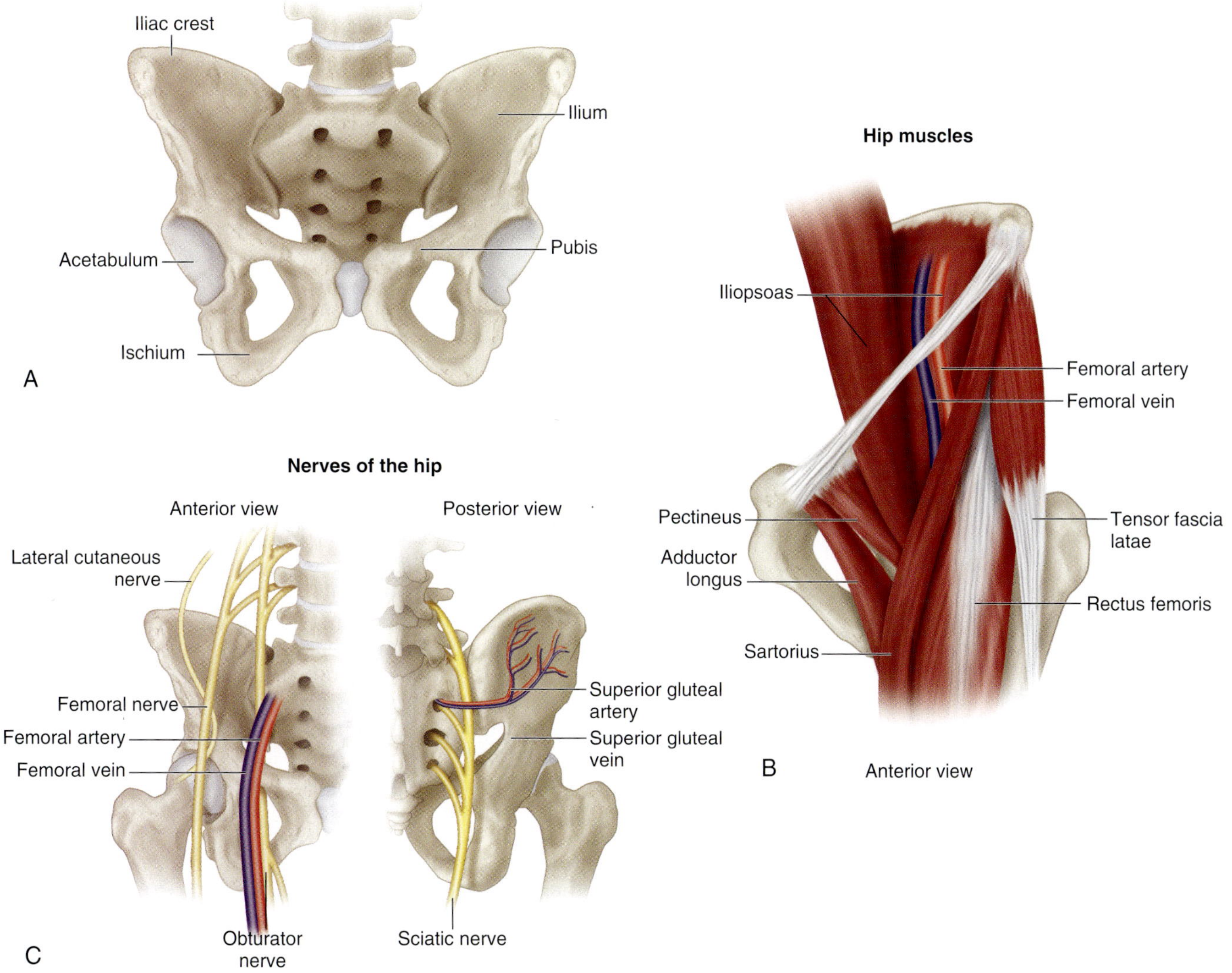

Iliac crest

Ilium

Acetabulum

Pubis

Ischium

A

Hip muscles

Iliopsoas

Femoral artery

Femoral vein

Pectineus

Adductor longus

Sartorius

Tensor fascia latae

Rectus femoris

B   Anterior view

Nerves of the hip

Anterior view   Posterior view

Lateral cutaneous nerve

Femoral nerve

Femoral artery

Femoral vein

Superior gluteal artery

Superior gluteal vein

Obturator nerve   Sciatic nerve

C

FIGURE 2

Instrumentation

- Rang Sciatic notch retractors (see Fig. 5)

POSITIONING

- The child is placed supine with a bolster beneath the ipsilateral thorax to achieve a 30° elevation of the ipsilateral pelvis (Fig. 3).

PORTALS/EXPOSURES

- A transverse "bikini line" incision is made centered on and just distal to the anterior superior iliac spine.
- The interval between the sartorius and tensor fascia femoris is separated, taking care to protect the lateral femoral cutaneous nerve of the thigh.
- If capsulorrhaphy is to be done for dislocation, the straight head of the rectus femoris is separated from the hip joint capsule, tagged with a suture, and divided just distal to the anterior inferior iliac spine.
- The iliac apophysis is split equally with a scalpel from the anterior inferior iliac spine to the junction of the anterior and middle thirds of the iliac crest.
- The iliac crest is stripped subperiosteally both medially and laterally to the greater sciatic notch (Fig. 4A and 4B). Rang sciatic notch retractors (Fig. 5) facilitate protection of the superior gluteal nerve and vessels in the notch and the surrounding soft tissues when cutting the ilium with the Gigli saw.

PROCEDURE

STEP 1

- Prior to making the skin incision, a percutaneous tenotomy of the adductor longus is done.
- An anterolateral approach via a transverse (bikini line) incision is used (see Portals/Exposures).
- The tendon of the rectus femoris is retracted from the hip joint capsule and the straight and reflected heads are identified.
  - Just distal to this point, the tendon is tagged with a suture for later repair and then transected. The reflected head is separated from the capsule and detached from the ilium posteriorly to just beyond the most proximal point of the dislocated femoral head.
  - If the hip is not dislocated, the rectus femoris may be left intact as the innominate osteotomy is done just proximal to the insertion of the straight head into the anterior inferior iliac spine.
- If the innominate osteotomy is being done for dysplasia or mild subluxation, proceed to Step 7.

STEP 2 (WHEN HIP IS DISLOCATED)

- The capsule is cleared anteromedially of soft tissue, including the overlying iliopsoas, with a periosteal elevator.
- The periosteum previously stripped from the medial wall of the ilium overlying the iliopsoas muscle is incised longitudinally and its tendon separated from the surrounding muscle at the level of the pelvic brim. The tendon lies on the posterior surface of the muscle, so the muscle needs to be inverted with a retractor in order to expose the tendon prior to cutting it while leaving the muscle intact to bridge the recessed tendon.
- The capsule is now exposed from the level of the transverse acetabular ligament to the top of the femoral head (Fig. 6).

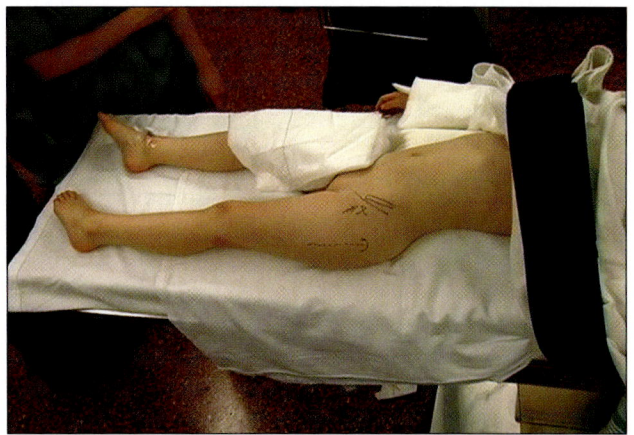

FIGURE 3

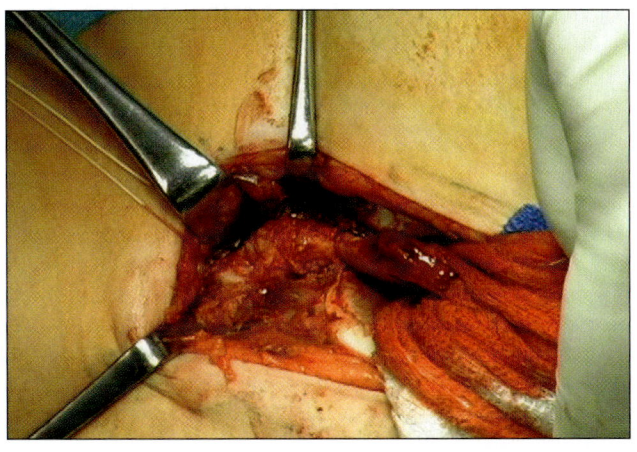

A
FIGURE 4

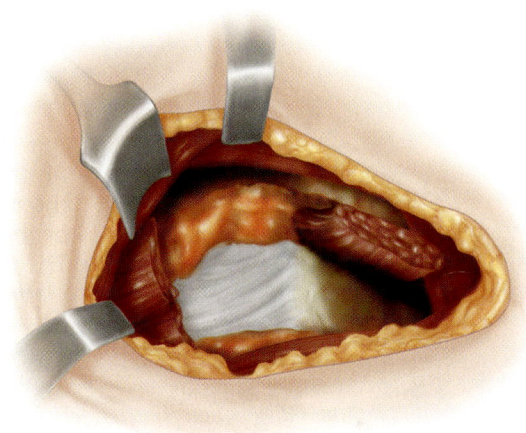

B

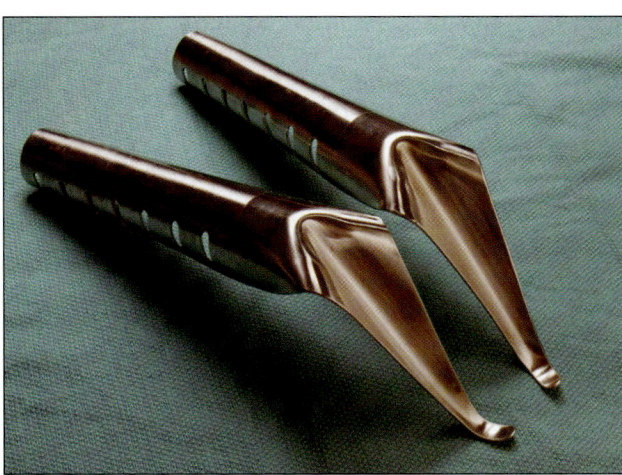

FIGURE 5

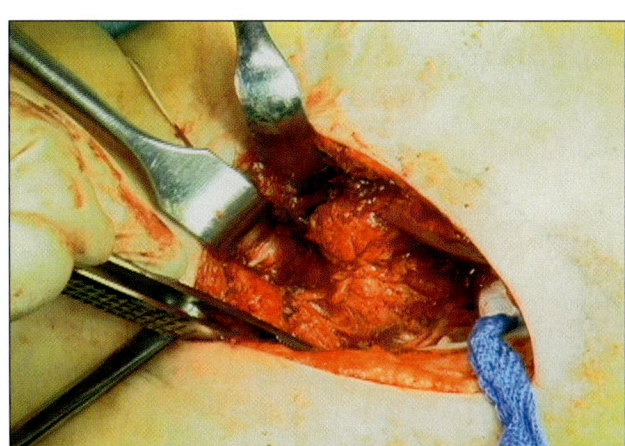

FIGURE 6

STEP 3

- A T-shaped capsulotomy is made with a scalpel (Fig. 7A).
- The horizontal limb is 1 cm distal to the margin of the acetabulum from the transverse acetabular ligament medially to the level of the most proximal portion of the femoral head laterally (Fig. 7B).
- The vertical limb commences lateral to the anterior inferior iliac spine and is perpendicular to the horizontal cut, extending along the length of the neck of the femur.

STEP 4

- The ligamentum teres is detached from the head of the femur with a scalpel, taking care to avoid injuring the articular cartilage.
- The ligamentum is grasped with a clamp and, while maintaining tension on it, this structure is removed from its medial attachment while also transecting the transverse acetabular ligament.
- A gentle trial reduction is attempted (Fig. 8). The acetabular labrum should not be cut or excised to achieve reduction as this will almost inevitably damage the lateral acetabular epiphysis, which is critical to the future development of the lateral portion of the acetabulum.
- If there is any resistance to reduction, the wound should be packed and the femur shortened through a separate incision.

STEP 5

- An 8- to 10-cm longitudinal incision is made from the base of the greater trochanter extending distally along the lateral aspect of the femur.
- The femur is exposed subperiosteally, and a four-hole straight plate of appropriate size is applied to the femur just distal to the greater trochanteric apophysis and fixed with two screws proximal to the site of the osteotomy.
- With the plate removed or in situ, a transverse osteotomy is made with an oscillating saw.
  - The femoral head is reduced into the acetabulum and the osteotomy allowed to overlap in order to estimate the amount of femoral shortening required (Fig. 9A). Typically 1.5 to 2.0 cm of shortening is required.
  - The distal femur is externally rotated to reduce excessive anteversion, if present.
- The plate is reapplied proximally if it has been removed to do the osteotomy, and the distal screws are inserted after closing the gap from the femoral osteotomy (Fig. 9B). The wound is closed and attention returned to the hip wound.

PITFALLS

- *Excessive shortening of the femur can lead to postoperative instability and re-dislocation of the hip.*

- *With intraoperative assessment of anteversion, there is the tendency to excessively derotate the femur, leading to posterior subluxation or dislocation after innominate osteotomy.*

- *Do not use an angled blade plate for the femoral osteotomy as medial displacement of the distal fragment may lead to abutment against the ischium and interfere with full medialization of the femoral head in the acetabulum. Typically, the seeming valgus of the femur seen on preoperative radiographs is due to external rotation of the dislocated femur and is more apparent than real. If there is true valgus of the neck of the femur, it seldom exceeds 10°, so a straight plate applied to the subtrochanteric curve of the femur will achieve some correction of the valgus, or the straight plate may be contoured to achieve the desired amount of varus of the proximal femur.*

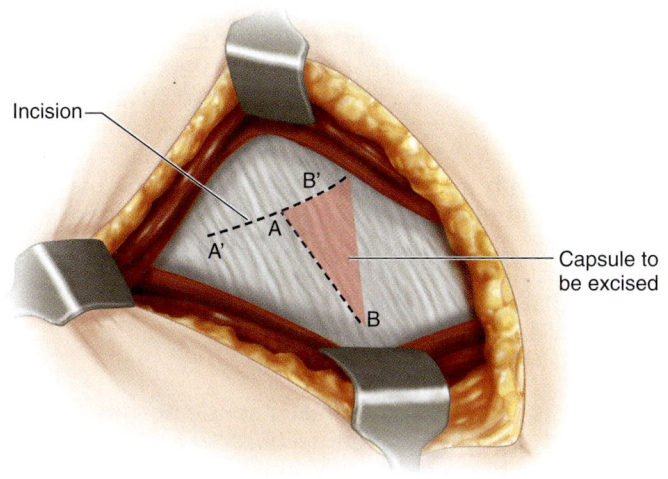

Incision

B'

A' A

B

Capsule to be excised

A

FIGURE 7

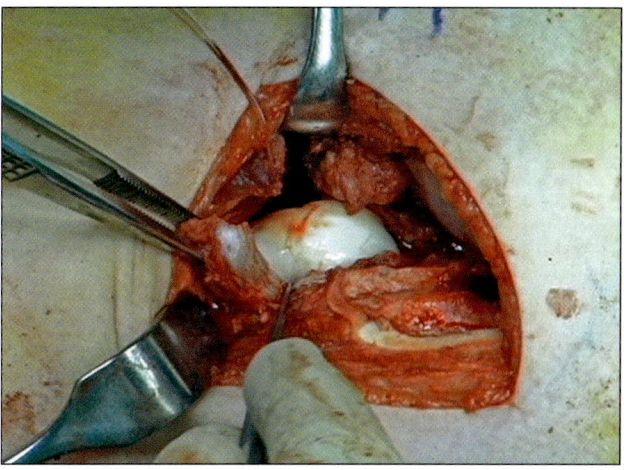

B

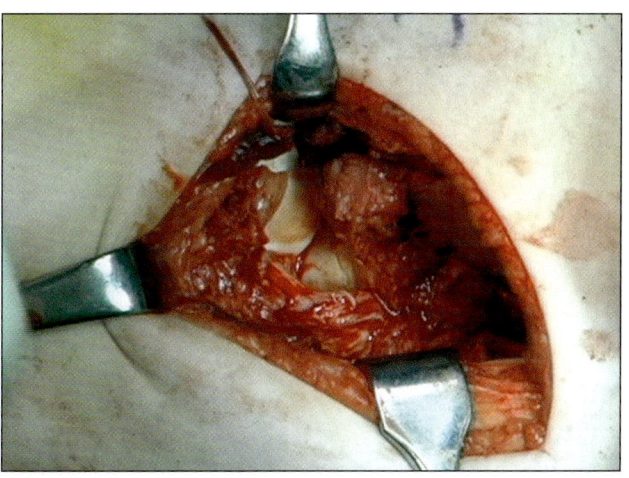

FIGURE 8

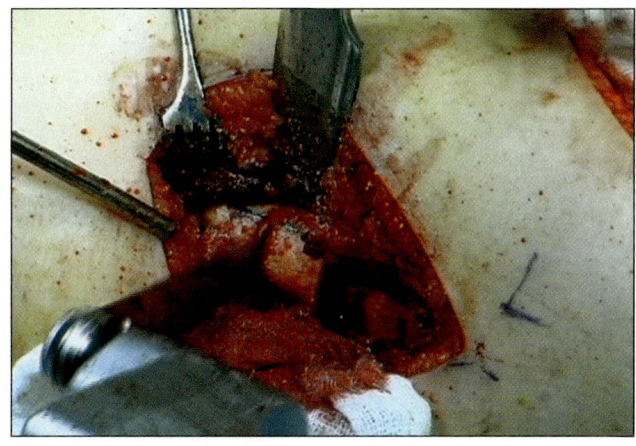

A

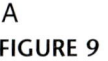

FIGURE 9

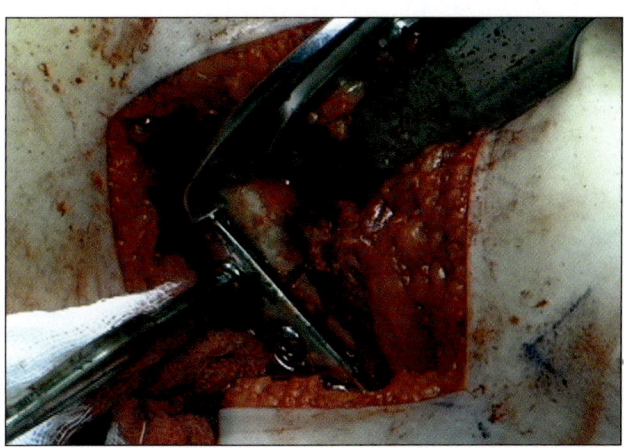

B

PEARLS

- *The capsulorrhaphy sutures are placed but not tied until after the innominate osteotomy is completed. If the hip is relocated and the sutures tied before the displacement of the acetabular fragment of the pelvis, posterior dislocation of the hip may occur and may not be recognized.*

PITFALLS

- *The osteotomy must be done perpendicular to the ilium rather than at a right angle to the patient or the operating room table. Failure to cut the ilium in the proper plane may lead to an oblique osteotomy, which is difficult to hold in the proper position while inserting the fixation pins.*

- *Cutting the ilium while the handles are not directed toward a point just proximal to the anterior inferior iliac spine may result in the osteotomy being made too proximally, leading to difficulty in moving the acetabulum into the desired position, or worse, the osteotomy being made too far distally such that the cut enters the hip joint.*

PEARLS

- *Packing a surgical sponge with a periosteal elevator in the sciatic notch posterior to the distal fragment prior to displacing the osteotomy will assist in preventing posterior displacement of the acetabular fragment.*

- *Insertion of a blunt periosteal elevator will assist in levering the acetabular side distally in line with the proximal fragment, and will free up the osteotomy and facilitate achieving the correct amount of displacement.*

PITFALLS

- *Pulling or levering the proximal fragment should be avoided as this could result in rotation through the sacroiliac joint with failure to displace the acetabular fragment and lead to inadequate correction of the acetabular dysplasia. Have an assistant stabilize the proximal ilium with a surgical rake or bone-holding forceps while the acetabular fragment is being placed in the correct position.*

STEP 6

- The hip is reduced and the capsulorrhaphy is prepared by excising the redundant capsule situated on the lateral portion of the T-shaped capsulotomy. The "T" is converted to a "V" by internally rotating the leg.
- Figure-of-8 nonabsorbable #1 sutures (Fig. 10A) are placed from medially to laterally, with the first suture placed from the medial aspect of the 1-cm cuff of capsule on the acetabulum to the junction of the horizontal and vertical limbs of the capsulotomy on the medial side of the distal capsulotomy (Fig. 10B). The sutures thus placed are not tied until after the innominate osteotomy is completed.

STEP 7

- The periosteum is stripped from the greater sciatic notch with a blunt elevator with a slightly curved tip (Bristow or Cobb elevator that has been blunted). Pushing the edge of a surgical sponge through the notch is recommended to safely avoid damaging the superior gluteal nerve and vessels.
- A pair of Rang sciatic notch retractors (see Fig. 5) are interlocked in the sciatic notch with the tip of the medial retractor resting on top of the lateral retractor.
- A Gigli saw is pushed from medial to lateral through the grooves of the retractors and attached to the saw handles (Fig. 11).
  - Alternatively, a curved forceps may be placed through the notch from medial to lateral and the saw threaded onto one arm of the curved forceps, which is clamped, and the saw pulled through the notch.
- The osteotomy is done with the saw handles separated and placed perpendicular to the plane of the ilium rather than perpendicular to the operating room table, which is a common pitfall leading to an oblique and unstable construct of the osteotomy. The osteotomy should exit the ilium just proximal to the anterior inferior iliac spine.

STEP 8

- After completing the osteotomy, a bone graft is taken from the ilium proximal to the osteotomy with an oscillating saw. The base of the triangular graft is the distance between the osteotomy and the anterior superior iliac spine.
- The distal fragment of the osteotomy is grasped with a towel clip or bone forceps just anterior to the sciatic notch, with the jaws of the forceps inside the osteotomy such that the acetabulum may be rotated distally in line with the proximal fragment.
  - It is critical that the osteotomy be levered open anteriorly but kept closed posteriorly so that anterolateral coverage of the head of the femur rather than transiliac lengthening is achieved.
  - Care must be taken to ensure that the distal fragment does not displace posteriorly. Thirty degrees of anterior opening is the correct amount of displacement.

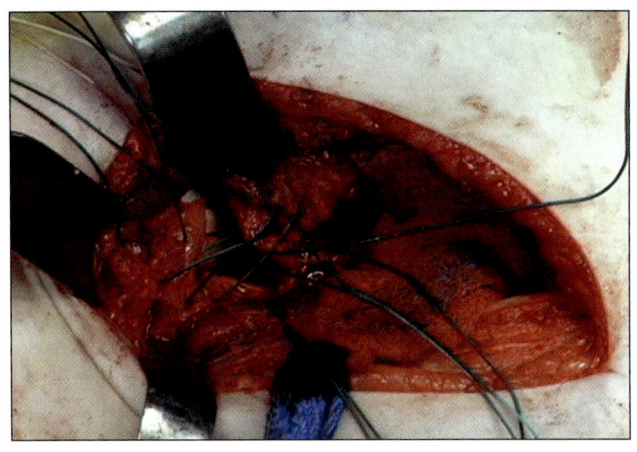

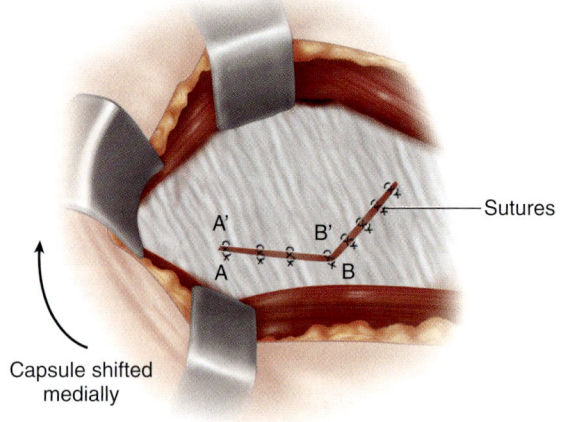

Sutures

Capsule shifted
medially

A

B

FIGURE 10

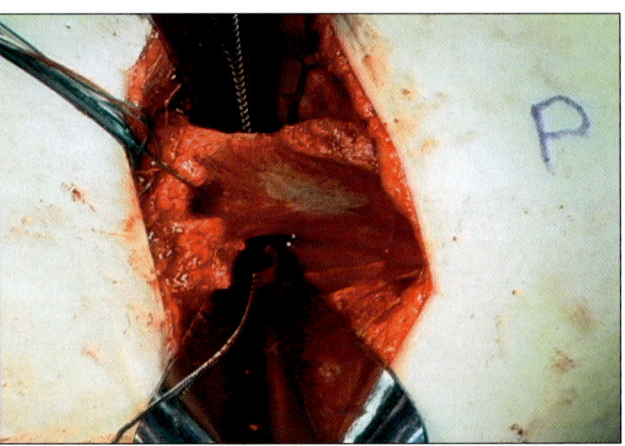

FIGURE 11

STEP 9

- While holding the acetabular fragment with a bone-holding forceps in 30–35° of correction, the triangular bone graft is inserted into the gap in the osteotomy site (Fig. 12).
- While still stabilizing the osteotomy, two threaded Kirschner pins (2.0 to 3.0 mm in diameter depending on the size of the child) are inserted from the iliac crest through the bone graft and into the distal fragment posterior and medial to the acetabulum, stopping just proximal to the triradiate cartilage.
- If the osteotomy is being done together with an open reduction, the tip of a finger is placed into the acetabulum to ensure that penetration of the hip joint has not occurred.
- If the osteotomy is being done for dysplasia and the joint capsule has not been opened, an intraoperative radiographic image should be obtained to confirm the proper position of the pins.

STEP 10

- The femoral head is reduced into the acetabulum and the previously placed sutures are tied from medial to lateral while an assistant holds the leg in 30° each of abduction, internal rotation, and flexion (Fig. 13).
- The distal stump of the rectus femoris is sutured to the proximal stump at the anterior inferior iliac spine with an absorbable suture.
- The two sides of the iliac apophysis are approximated over the crest with a towel clip and sutured with figure-of-8 absorbable #1 sutures.
- The fascia over the interval between the sartorius and tensor fascia femoris is closed with a continuous suture. The threaded pins are cut, leaving 4–5 mm protruding from the iliac crest for ease of later removal.
- The subcutaneous tissue and skin are also closed with continuous sutures.

STEP 11

- After applying sterile postoperative dressings, a single-hip spica cast is applied from the nipple line to just proximal to the ankle on the affected side with the hip in 30° each of abduction, internal rotation, and flexion (Fig. 14).
- If an open reduction of the hip has been done, the synthetic cast material is molded with the thenar eminence of the surgeon's hand over the greater trochanter.
- A generous hole in the cast is cut over the upper abdomen for comfort.

POSTOPERATIVE CARE AND EXPECTED OUTCOMES

- If a concurrent open reduction has been done, a limited axial cut computed tomography scan is done within 24 hours of the procedure to confirm maintenance of concentric reduction of the hip.
- The child is kept recumbent at home for 6 weeks after discharge from hospital. The cast is removed in the clinic thereafter and the child mobilized.
- Specific physiotherapy is not generally necessary as the child will ambulate spontaneously within several weeks and a full range of motion of the hip will return within 3 to 4 months.

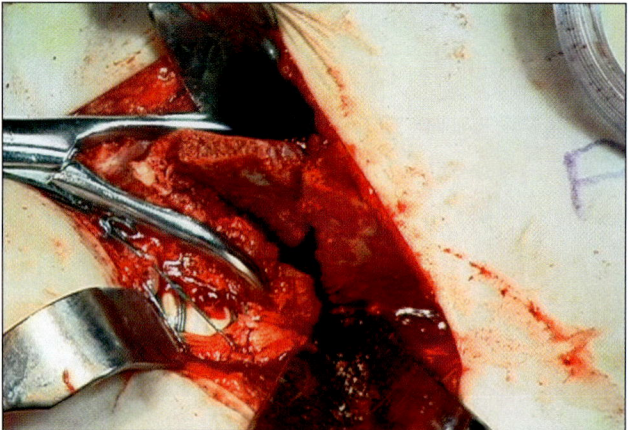

FIGURE 12

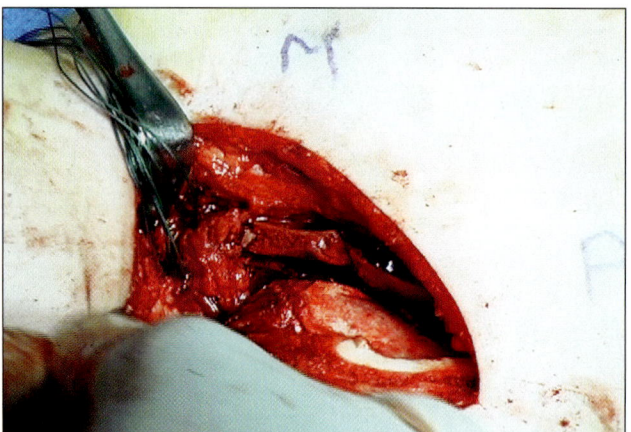

FIGURE 13

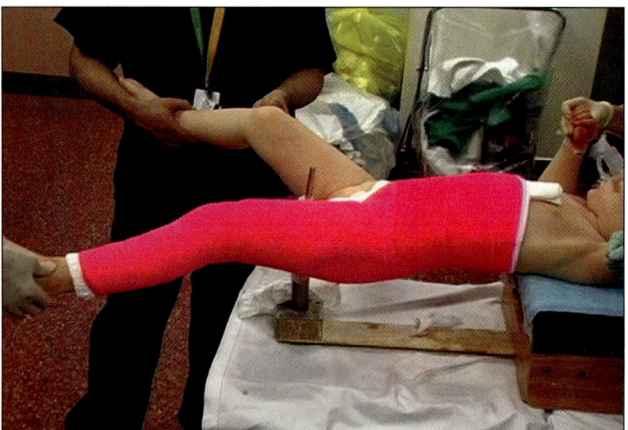

FIGURE 14

EVIDENCE

Salter RB. Innominate osteotomy in the treatment of congenital dislocation and subluxation of the hip. J Bone Joint Surg [Br]. 1961;3:518–39.

This paper provided the original description of this surgical procedure. (Level IV evidence)

Salter RB, Dubois JP. The first fifteen years personal experience with innominate osteotomy in the treatment of congenital dislocation and subluxation of the hip. Clin Orthop Relat Res. 1974;(98):72–103.

The results into adolescence of the original cohort of patients having this procedure were reported in this paper. Of particular note is that none of the patients required secondary osteotomies to correct residual subluxation or acetabular dysplasia. (Level IV evidence)

Thomas SR, Wedge JH, Salter RB. Outcome at forty-five years after open reduction and innominate osteotomy for late-presenting developmental dislocation of the hip. J Bone Joint Surg [Am]. 2007;89:2341–50.

This paper reported the long-term follow-up of 76 patients (101 dislocated hips), with the endpoint defined as having undergone hip replacement. None required replacement prior to 30 years and 86% had not been replaced at 40 years postoperatively. At 45 years after surgery, 19 patients (24 hips) had undergone hip replacement and 3 patients had died of unrelated causes. (Level III evidence)

Chiari Pelvic Osteotomy

Benjamin J. Shore and Brian Snyder

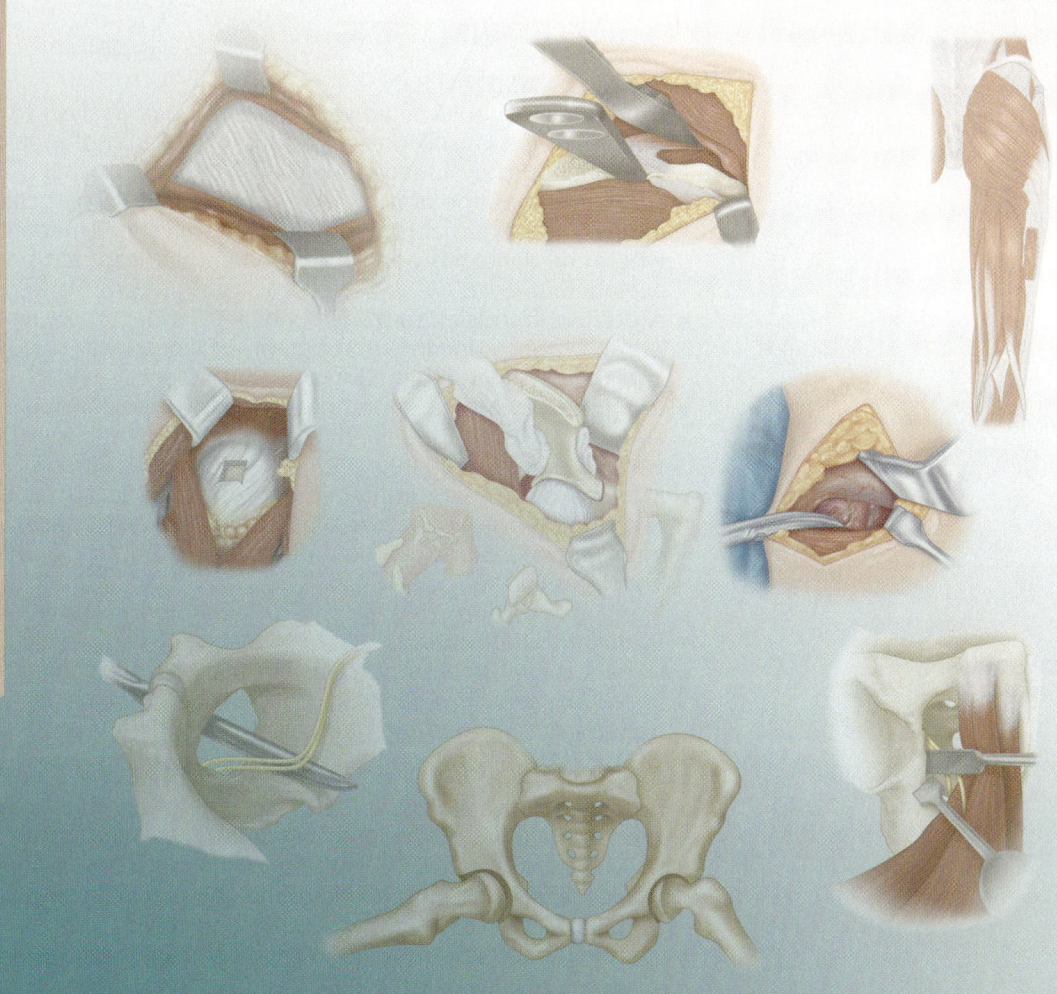

PITFALLS

- *Avoid in patients who already demonstrate with severe arthrosis.*

- *Avoid with significant proximal migration of the femoral head that prevents appropriate positioning of the osteotomy and insufficient projected cross section of ilium to form a "shelf" to cover the femoral head.*

- *Avoid with inability to cover at least 70% of the femoral head after the Chiari osteotomy.*

- *For successful results, the femoral head does not have to be completely reduced into the acetabulum.*

- *Redirectional and periacetabular osteotomies are unable to address femoral-acetabular incongruity and hence are contraindicated for these conditions.*

Controversies

- In the adult patient, a Chiari osteotomy can be utilized to create sufficient host bone on the acetabular side for subsequent total hip replacement.

- In nonambulatory patients with neuromuscular hip pathology, a Chiari osteotomy can be considered as an adjunct to a resection arthroplasty.

- If the patient has a weak gluteus medius muscle, the surgeon can consider combining a Chiari osteotomy with greater trochanteric advancement to improve tension and the overall gluteus medius moment arm.

INDICATIONS

- The Chiari pelvic osteotomy is a "salvage" procedure, which uses the ilium to form a "shelf" to cover over the femoral head and prevent subluxation. The osteotomy relies on metaplasia of the interposed hip capsule to form new fibrocartilage.
- This osteotomy is designed to treat acetabular dysplasia in the setting of painful hip subluxation and is considered in patients who demonstrate aspherical incongruity between the femoral head and dysplastic acetabulum.
- This osteotomy is particularly useful in neuromuscular hip pathology where acetabular deficiency is primarily posterolateral.

EXAMINATION/IMAGING

PHYSICAL EXAMINATION

- Examination should begin with observed gait analysis to document if a limp is present and if it is a result of antalgia or Trendelenburg dysfunction.
- A careful hip range of motion is documented; in particular, internal and external rotation limits can give information as to where the damaged portion of the femoral head and possibily acetabulum exist.
- A positive Trendelenburg's test indicates abductor weakness. It is important to document abductor weakness with side lying and the presence of an adductor contracture.
- In a positive anterior apprehension test, with extension and external rotation, the patient experiences apprehension, pain, or perceived hip instability.
- In a positive anterior impingement test, with flexion, adduction, and internal rotation of the hip, the patient experiences pain and discomfort; this can be indicative of labral tear or anterior labral pathology.
- The Galleazzi sign is significant for fixed hip instability and subluxation/dislocation.
- In patients with neuromuscular hip pathology, one may appreciate a positive Ortolani sign, where the hip actively may be reduced with varying degrees of discomfort.

IMAGING STUDIES

- Imaging studies are designed to document the congruency of the femoral head within the acetabulum, the amount of anterior and lateral acetabular coverage of the femoral head, and the reducibility of the femoral head into the native acetabulum.
  - Figure 1 shows preoperative anteroposterior (AP) (Fig. 1A) and lateral (Fig. 1B) radiographs of a patient with right hip Legg-Calvé-Perthes disease.
  - Figure 2 shows preoperative AP (Fig. 2A) and frog lateral (Fig. 2B) radiographs of a candidate for Chiari pelvic osteotomy.
- Imaging should include weight-bearing standing AP radiographs centered on both hips, false profile views of both hips, and a Von Rosen (maximal abduction and internal rotation) view of both hips.
  - The Von Rosen view can demonstrate the incongruous relationship between the femoral head and acetabulum and also demonstrate the reducibility of the femoral head within the acetabulum.
- Reconstructed computed tomography scans can aid surgeons in determining the three-dimensional relationship between the acetabulum and femoral head and identifying locations of acetabular deficiency (anterolateral vs. posterolateral).

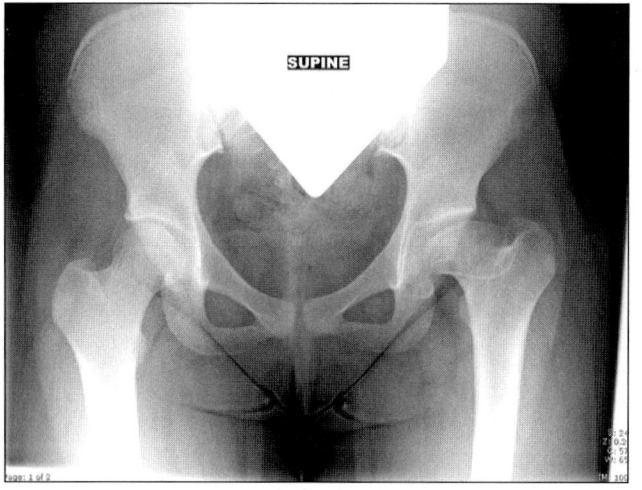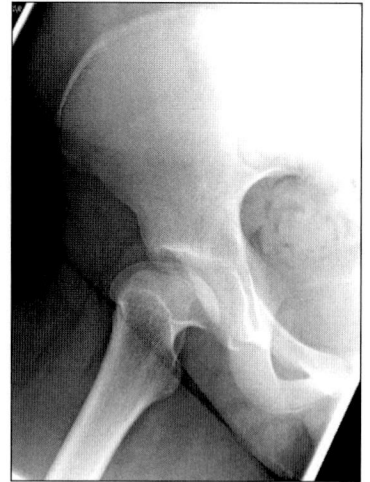

A

B

FIGURE 1

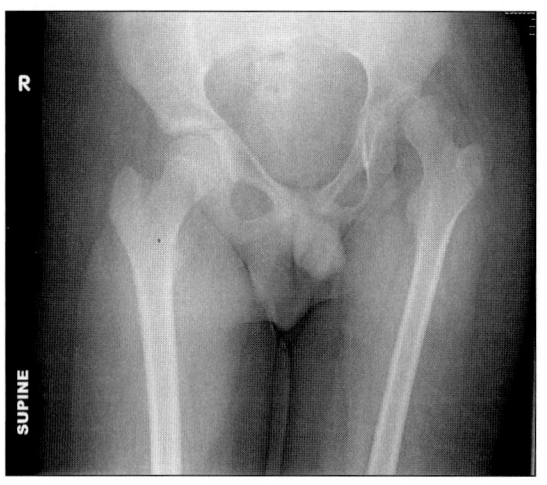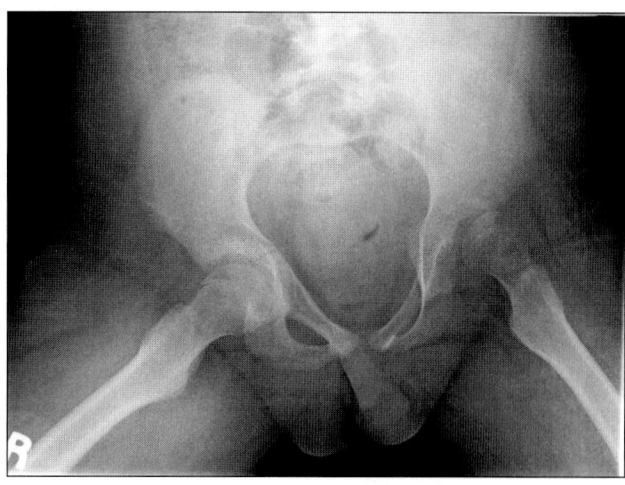

A

B

FIGURE 2

Treatment Options

- The "shelf" arthroplasty is another salvage pelvic osteotomy that can be considered for painful hip subluxation in the setting of an incongruous femoral head and acetabulum.

- If spherical congruency can be obtained, a periacetabular osteotomy is a viable option in children and young adults.

- In a nonambulatory young adult or older patient with a painful unstable hip, a resection arthroplasty has been described with varying degrees of long-term surgical success.

- In patients who demonstrate advanced arthrosis and significant joint space disease, reasonable treatment options would include a total joint arthroplasty or arthrodesis.

- Radial sequencing magnetic resonance imaging can aid surgeons in illustrating the condition and quality of the labrum and articular cartilage of the hip joint during the preoperative assessment.
- An intraoperative arthrogram is a useful study that demonstrates the dynamic stability of the hip and the relative congruency of the femoral head and acetabulum.

SURGICAL ANATOMY

- In the ilioinguinal approach to the hip, superficially the lateral femoral cutaneous nerve (LFCN) is at risk in the interval between the sartorius muscle medially and the tensor fascia lata (TFL) muscle laterally. By remaining in the compartment of the TFL, the LFCN is protected during the surgical approach.
- Deep in the interval between the direct head of the rectus femoris muscle and the gluteal muscles lie branches of the lateral femoral circumflex vessels. If necessary, these vessels can be ligated.
- The indirect head of the rectus femoris muscle can be a useful anatomic landmark. The indirect head is often stretched superolaterally with the subluxated femoral head. Often this structure can be seen deforming the subluxated lateral border of the femoral head over time. Once the indirect head is identified at the bifurcation from the direct head, it can be carefully dissected posterolaterally to its insertion on the lateral margin of the acetabulum. The insertion point helps the surgeon distinguish between the true acetabulum and the capacious "pseudoacetabulum," which lies just superior.
- The sciatic nerve is protected by meticulous subperiosteal dissection within the sciatic notch. Positioning of the knee in flexion can also take tension off the sciatic nerve when working around the sciatic notch.

POSITIONING

- The patient is positioned supine on a radiolucent operating room table.
- Often a bump is placed under the operative hip to achieve a "sloppy lateral" position.
- All bony prominences on the upper and lower extremities are padded.
- The ipsilateral arm is either draped across the chest in small children or in larger patients is forward flexed to 90° and supported on an elevated armholder.
- The operative extremity is draped free to the level of the costophrenic margin superiorly, medially to the ipsilateral border of the perineum, and laterally to the border of the buttocks. Figure 3 shows skin markings for a planned ilioinguinal approach and a direct lateral approach to the proximal femur for an additional intertrochanteric osteotomy.
- Epidural analgesia and Foley catheters are inserted preoperatively and when possible employed for 3 days postoperatively.
- A preoperative intravenous antibiotic is administered within an hour of the incision and repeated every 4 hours.
- Intraoperative fluoroscopy is employed from the contralateral side of the bed.

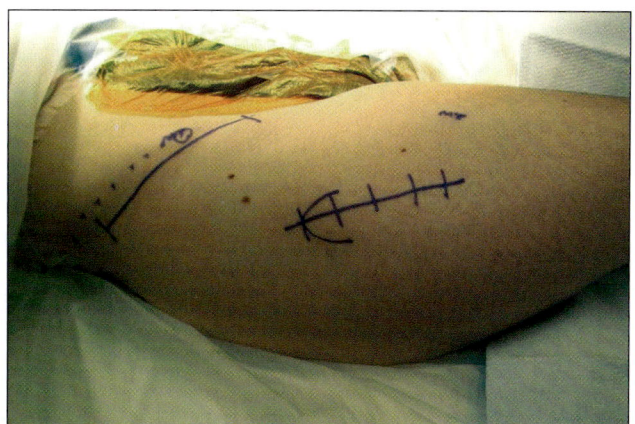

FIGURE 3

PORTALS/EXPOSURES

- The ilioinguinal approach is the exposure of choice for this osteotomy. In Figure 4, the iliac crest is marked with the direct head of the rectus femoris *(arrow)* deep to the TFL compartment (TFL retracted posteriorly).
- The incision begins approximately 1–2 cm below the iliac crest and extends medially 1.5–2 cm distal and medial to the anterior superior iliac spine (ASIS).
- The lateral fibers of the external oblique muscle overhang the lateral ilium and are reflected off the ilium with electrocautery or a #15 blade. Care is taken to clear the iliac apophysis of soft tissue and maintain meticulous hemostasis.
- Distally, the interval between the sartorius and TFL is identified. The TFL fascial compartment is opened and muscle is stripped directly off the intermuscular septum with a Cobb or periosteal elevator.
  - The TFL is retracted laterally and the intermuscular septum and sartorius muscle are retracted medially.
  - At this level, the LFCN of the thigh lies within the sartorial muscle compartment and is not visualized; however, the nerve lies under the fascia between the sartorius and TFL (Fig. 5), and care must be taken to avoid injury during the approach and when closing to avoid a painful neuroma.
- Blunt dissection of the TFL is continued proximally to the ilium and to the level of the anterior inferior iliac spine (AIIS).
- Subperiosteal dissection is continued anteriorly from the ASIS inferiorly to the AIIS.
  - Deep to the sartorius-TFL interval lies the direct and indirect heads of the rectus femoris, which insert onto the ASIS (Fig. 6). The direct head of the rectus femoris is identified inserting into the AIIS, and the bifurcation of the indirect head is located.
  - The indirect head is a key anatomic landmark to the edge of the true acetabulum posteriorly.

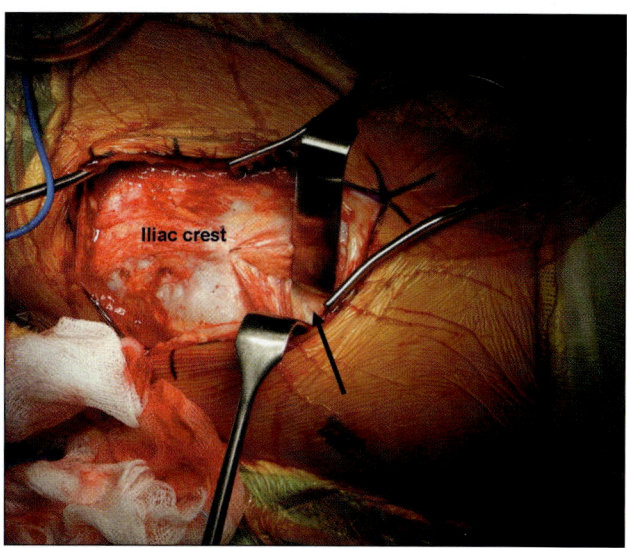

FIGURE 4

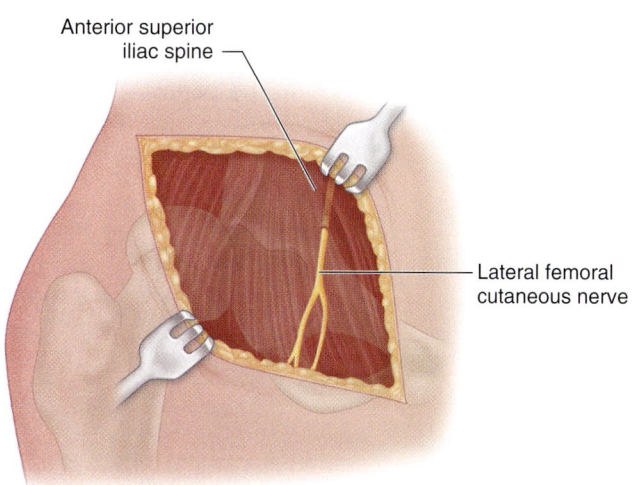

Anterior superior
iliac spine

Lateral femoral
cutaneous nerve

FIGURE 5

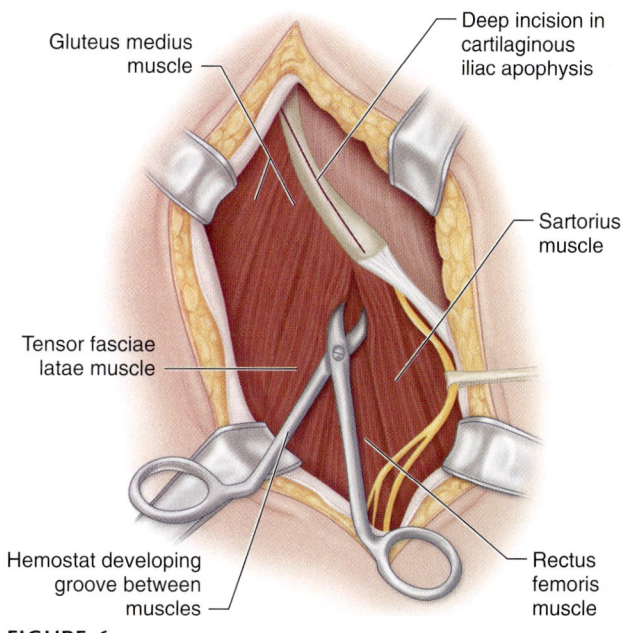

Gluteus medius
muscle

Deep incision in
cartilaginous
iliac apophysis

Sartorius
muscle

Tensor fasciae
latae muscle

Hemostat developing
groove between
muscles

Rectus
femoris
muscle

FIGURE 6

- Underneath the rectus femoris lie the capsule and the iliacus muscle. At this point, the outer table of the iliac apophysis is split in the midline to facilitate this portion of the dissection (Fig. 7). The glueal muscles are subperiosteally dissected off the outer table of the ilium, and the iliacus muscle is subperiosterally dissected off the inner table of the ilium. A moist sponge is packed tightly between the ilium and dissected muscles to aid in retraction and hemostasis.
- Now the outer table is subperiosteally dissected away from the abductor musculature inferiorly until firm resistance is met. This resistance indicates the insertion of the indirect head of the rectus femoris on the lateral aspect of the hip capsule.
- The surgeon now returns back to the bifurcation of the direct and indirect heads of the rectus femoris tendon. The indirect head is ligated at the bifurcation and followed posterolaterally to the suspected insertion into the lateral hip capsule.
- Dissection is continued posteriorly along the outer and inner tables of the ilium to the level of the greater sciatic notch. A Lane retractor is placed subperiosteally into the greater sciatic notch to elevate the superior gluteal artery and sciatic nerve away from the apex and anterior margin of the notch. This gives excellent visualization of the acetabular rim *(arrow)* all the way to the ischial spine (Fig. 8).
- The periosteum is incised along the superior border of the indirect head of the rectus femoris. This will allow subsequent release of the abductor minimus off the superior capsule to allow for proper chisel placement for the Chiari osteotomy.
- At this point, fluoroscopy is used to ensure that the surgeon has not been misled by a pseudoacetabulum and that the dissection has carried down to the acetabular margin. Visualization at this point of the operation is paramount.

PEARLS

- *In a subluxated or dislocated hip, the the indirect head of the rectus femoris and hip capsule are often adherent to the superolateral aspect of the outer table of the ilium, forming a pseudoacetabulum. These structures need to be dissected carefully off the outer table with a Cobb elevator to the level of the true acetabulum.*

- *Often the attenuated indirect head of the rectus femoris, once ligated, can be followed posterolaterally to an insertion point on the lateral aspect of the true acetabulum, inferior to the aforementioned pseudoacetabulum. This structure proves to be an important anatomic landmark during the dissection.*

- *Adequate exposure of the apex and anterior border of the sciatic notch along the posterior column of the acetabulum is necessary for initiating the cut into the posterior column of the acetabulum using a Mast or Ganz chisel.*

PITFALLS

- *A sponge can be packed in the sciatic notch to protect the superior gluteal artery and sciatic nerve during osteotomy.*

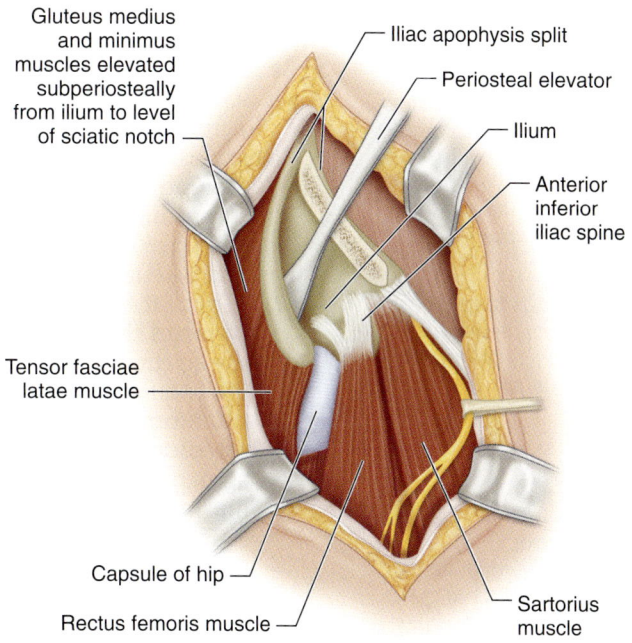

Gluteus medius and minimus muscles elevated subperiosteally from ilium to level of sciatic notch

Iliac apophysis split

Periosteal elevator

Ilium

Anterior inferior iliac spine

Tensor fasciae latae muscle

Capsule of hip

Rectus femoris muscle

Sartorius muscle

FIGURE 7

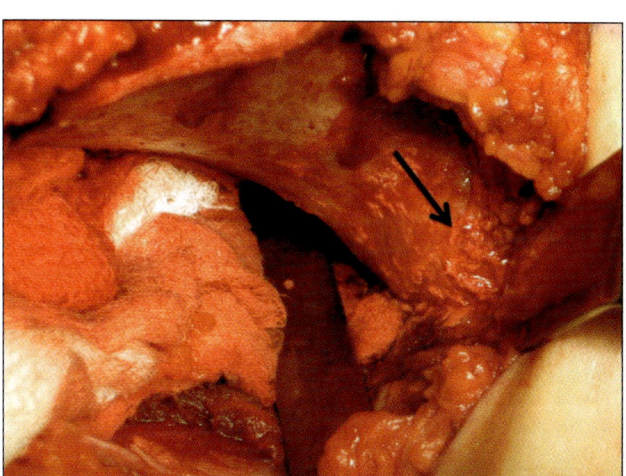

FIGURE 8

PROCEDURE

STEP 1: OSTEOTOMY

- Essentially the osteotomy is creating a transverse acetabular "fracture" in which both the anterior and posterior acetabular columns are cut and the ilium is displaced either anterolaterally (developmental dysplasia of the hip [DDH]) or posterolaterally (neuromuscular dysplasia) over the hip joint capsule, forming a shelf (Fig. 9).

  - The osteotomy is curvilinear in the supra-acetabular region. It begins at the anterior ilium at the level of the AIIS and traverses the capsular edge of the acetabulum to terminate at the sciatic notch.

  - We use a modification advocated by Hall wherein the osteotomy is truly curvilinear. The posterior limb of the osteotomy is curved distally, aiming a centimeter below the apex of the sciatic notch to increase posterior coverage, thus making the osteotomy more domelike in appearance.

  - In Figure 10A–C, Sawbones (Sawbones Inc, Vashon, WA) are used to demonstrate the planned supra-acetabular osteotomy using a combination of curved and dome-shaped osteotomes instead of a Gigli saw.

- The start of the osteotomy is determined anatomically and radiographically. Anatomically, the osteotomy is started anterior at the capsular margin. This point is double-checked with fluoroscopy to ensure that one is not within the false acetabulum.

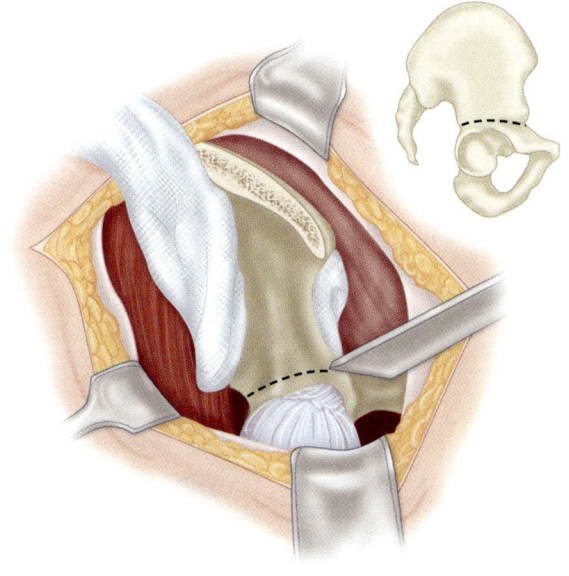

FIGURE 9

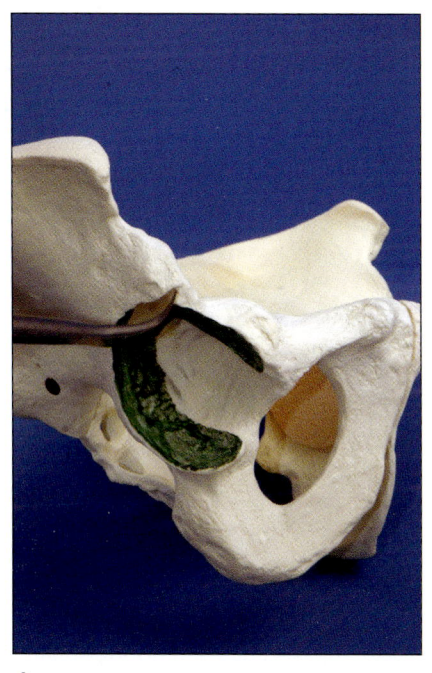

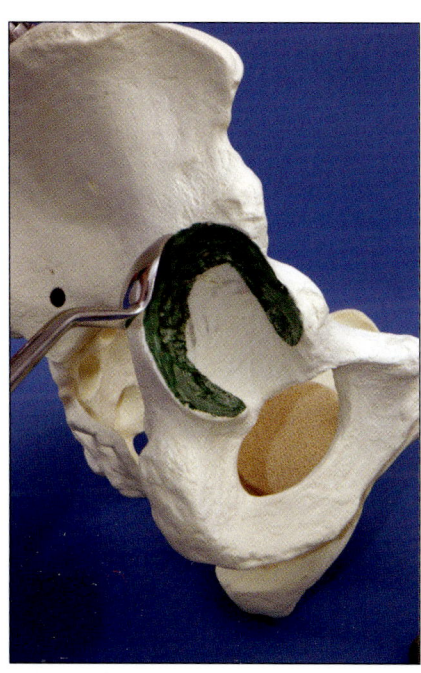

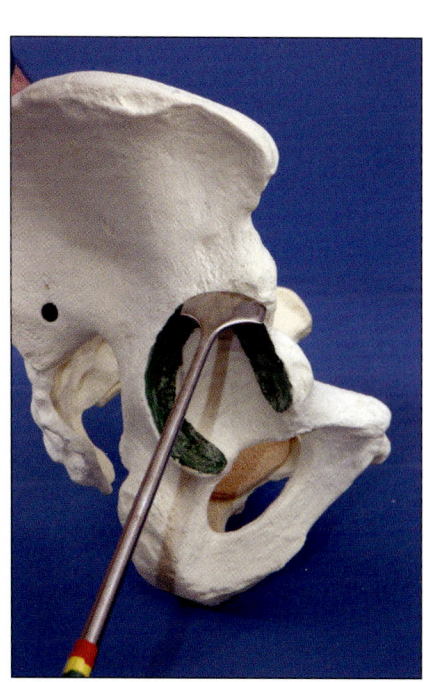

A

B

C

FIGURE 10

- Once the start point is verified, the curvilinear osteotomy is directed cranially and medial 10–15°, to faciliate sliding and displacement of the cut surface of the ilium over the hip joint capsule.
  - Figure 11 shows an AP fluoroscopic view of the right hip during osteotomy. Note that the osteotome enters at the edge of the acetabulum and is directed upward at an angle of approximately 10–15°.
  - The goal is to have the cut surface of the ilium in bony contact with the hip capsule, in continuity with the lateral acetabular bone margin.
- Conventially the osteomy is completed with a Gigli saw, with care taken to protect the important structures on the sciatic notch. We prefer making the osteotomy with the use of a series of curved or dome-shaped osteotomes and Ganz or Mast chisels.
  - Fluoroscopy is used to aid in the placement of the osteotomes.
  - The inner table of the ilium is often scored to prevent splintering of the inner table at completion of the osteotomy.
- Figure 12 shows the completed supra-acetabular osteotomy *(arrow)*.
- Figure 13 is a representation of the posterior aspect of the osteotomy; note the attempt to continue the osteotomy posterior to just above the ischial spine.

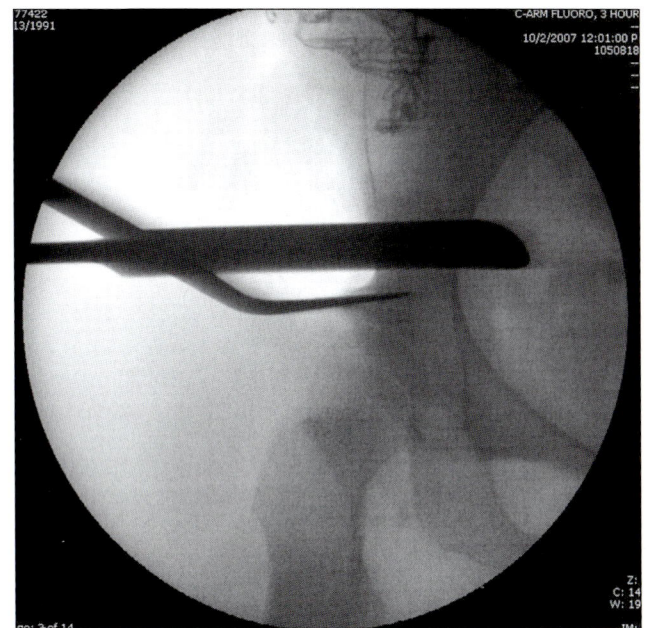

FIGURE 11

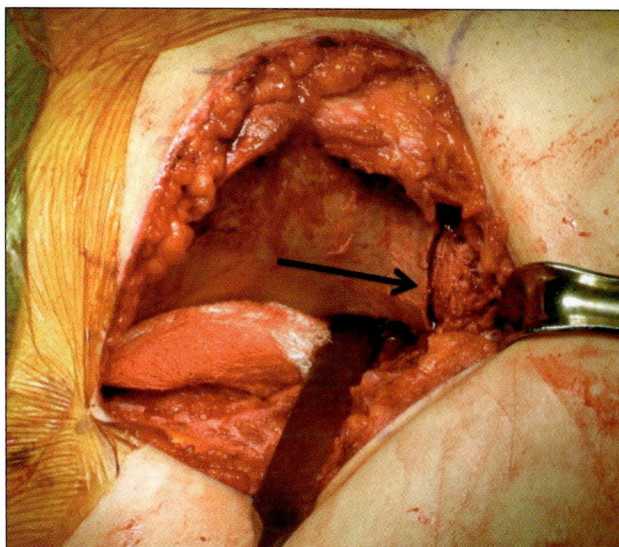

FIGURE 12

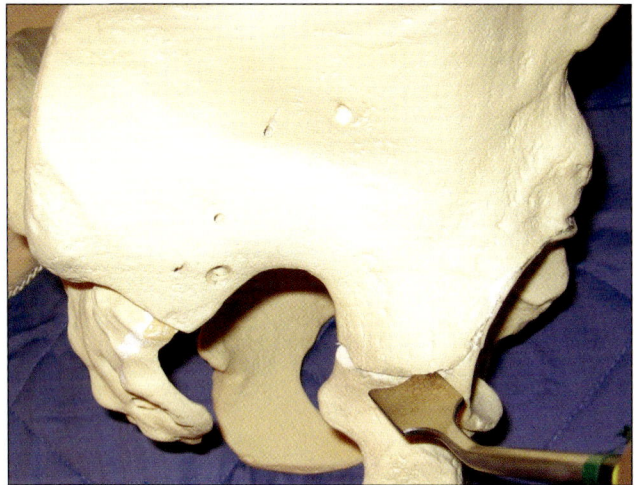

FIGURE 13

STEP 2: ACETABULAR DISPLACEMENT

- Often 100% displacement is required to facilitate appropriate coverage of the hip (Fig. 14A).
- The hip is abducted and axial force is applied to the leg as the femoral head is pushed medially to cause the acetabular fragment to displace medially underneath the ilium (Fig. 14B).
- Figure 14C is a view looking down from above, assessing the amount of superior coverage provided by the ilium. This also illustrates why augmenting with additional iliac graft may be required anteriorly.
- The amount of lateral displacement and relative anterior-posterior displacement is dependent on the degree of coverage that is required for the hip. Anterior deficiency is more common in DDH and posterior deficiency is more common in neuromuscular hip dysplasia.
  - When posterior coverage is required, the ilium is displaced posteriorly over the sciatic notch. However, extreme care must be taken to ensure that the sciatic nerve is not entrapped or compressed.
  - Anterior coverage with intimate contact of the ilium with the hip joint capsule can be difficult to attain. If additional coverage is necessary, the dome of the osteotomy can be contoured toward the anterior inferior margin of the AIIS.
- It is often necessary to use corticocancellous graft osteotomized from the inner table of the ilium to interpose between the anterior hip joint capsule and the ilium. This graft *(arrow)* is packed similar to a shelf-type procedure (Fig. 15), and needs to be secured with either a small Ethibond suture or a screw/threaded K-wire.

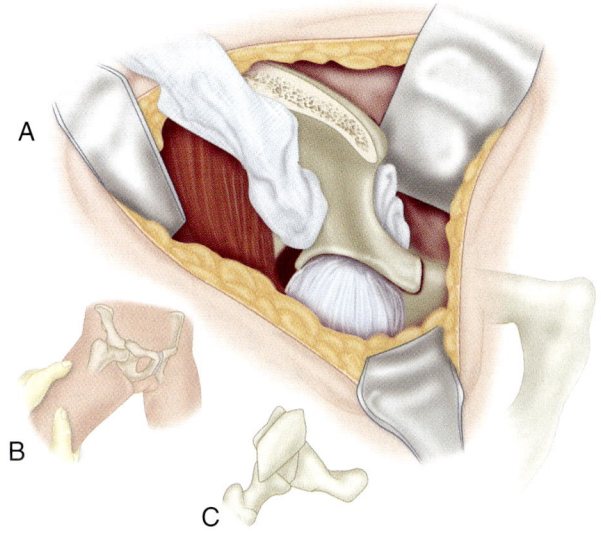

FIGURE 14

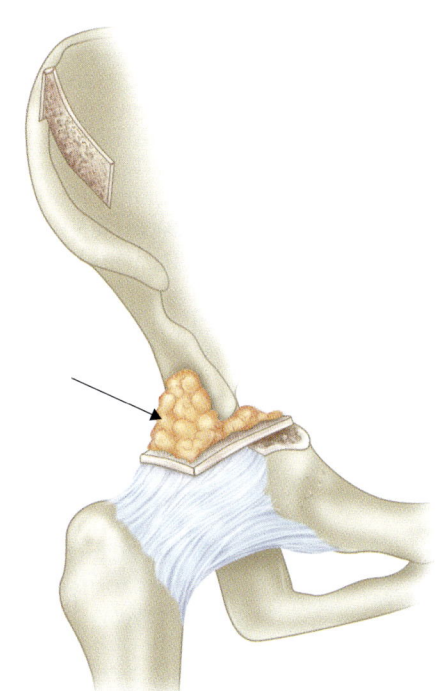

FIGURE 15

Instrumentation/ Implantation

- Long pelvic AO small-fragment screws or threaded Steinmann pins are used to fix the osteotomy.

STEP 3: FIXATION AND CLOSURE

- The osteotomy is fixed in place with either 3.5-mm or 4.5-mm cortical screws.
  - Traditionally these screws were placed along the iliac crest into the posterior column of the ischium. However, with 100% displacement of the distal fragment, solid screw fixation can be challenging.
  - We now prefer screw placement starting inferiorly from the ASIS on the outer table of the ilium and directed medially to facilitate more robust fixation into the ischium and distal fragment.
  - A significant amount of superior and posterior coverage can be attained even with 100% displacement (Fig. 16).
- These screws are placed under fluoroscopic guidance, and multiple views are necessary to ensure that there is no encroachment into the hip joint.
- Drains can be used in the superficial and deep tissues at the discretion of the surgeon.
- Wound closure involves repair of the iliac apophysis with heavy absorbable sutures in an interrupted figure-of-8 pattern.
- The remainder of the wound is closed in layers. In patients who are not toilet trained, we use Dermabond on the skin to provide a waterproof seal.
- Spica immobilization is not necessary; however, if uncertain about bone quality or fixation, or in a neuromuscular hip dysplasia patient, a one-legged pantaloon spica or bilateral long-leg casts with an A-frame bar are also acceptable if other procedures were performed simultaneously.
- Figure 17 shows postoperative AP (Fig. 17A) and frog-leg lateral (Fig. 17B) views of the right hip after fixation of the osteotomy and completion of an additional intertrochanteric osteotomy.
- Figure 18 shows postoperative AP (Fig. 18A) and frog-leg lateral (Fig. 18B) views of the procedure performed on a left hip.

POSTOPERATIVE CARE AND EXPECTED OUTCOMES

- Patients are allowed to sit up to 90° of hip flexion immediately. The operated leg is kept in approximately 30° of hip abduction. The patient is restricted to toe-touch weight bearing for 6 weeks.
- If no immobilization is employed, gentle range of motion from 0° to 70° is permitted. Gentle physical therapy in the first 6 weeks to maintain this range of motion can be employed if necessary.
- If the patient has been immobilized, the immobilization stays in place between 3 and 6 weeks, at which point the casts are removed and gentle physical therapy begins.

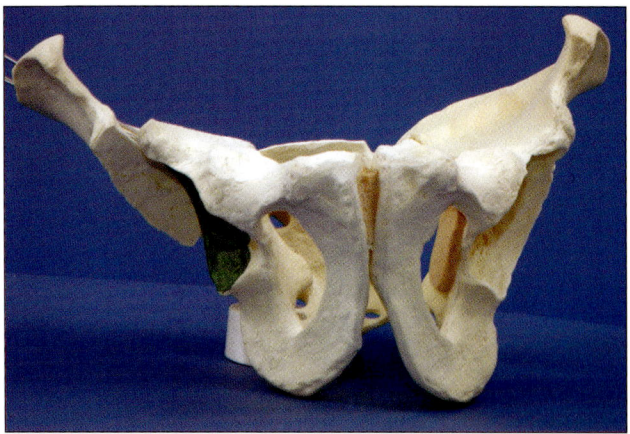

FIGURE 16

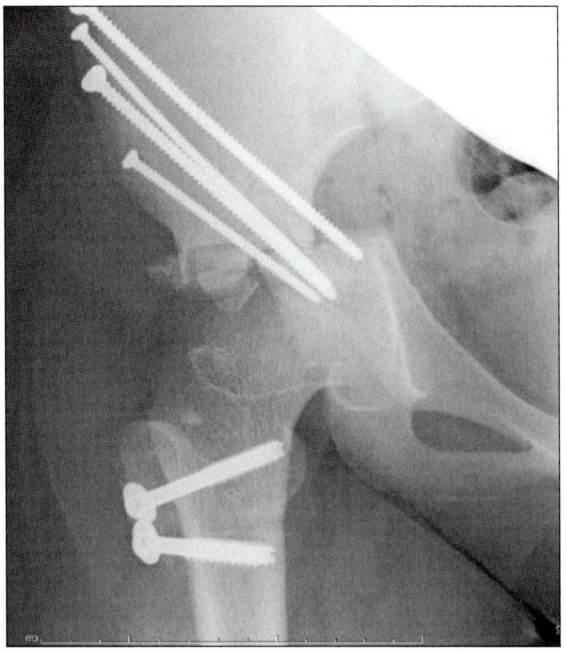

FIGURE 17 A

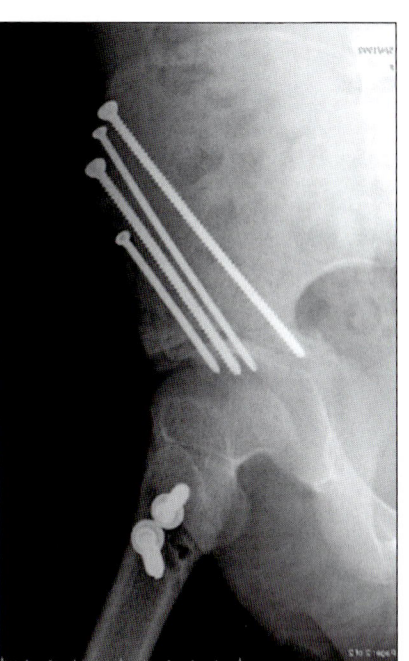

B

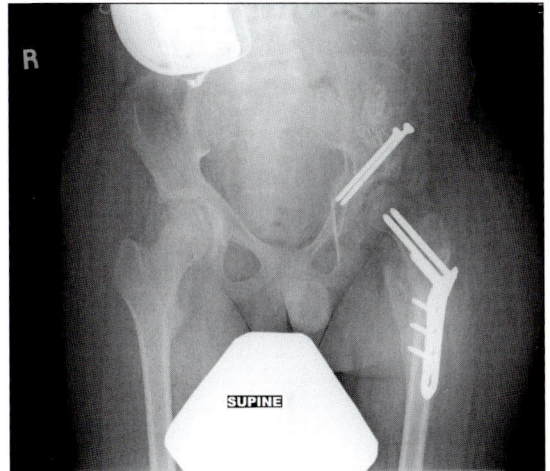

A

FIGURE 18

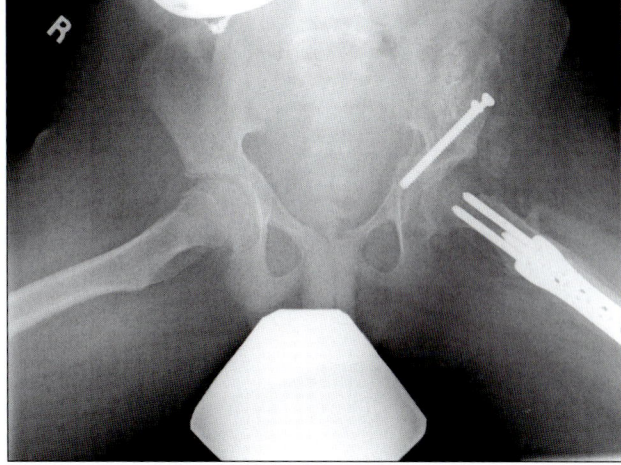

B

EVIDENCE

Bailey TE, Hall JE. Chiari medial displacement osteotomy. J Pediatr Orthop. 1985; 5:635–41.

Retrospective review of 36 Chiari medial displacement osteotomies. The most consistent results were observed in patients with congential hip dysplasia; less predictable results were observed in myelodysplasia, spasticity and Perthes disease. Authors concluded the Chiari is most suited for those individuals with painful hip subluxation where a concentric reduction is not possible. (Level IV evidence)

Debnath UK, Guha AR, Karlakki S, Vargese J, Evans GA. Combined femoral and Chiari osteotomies for reconstruction of the painful subluxation or dislocation of the hip in cerebral palsy: a long-term outcome study. J Bone Joint Surg [Br]. 2006;88:1373–8.

Retrospective review of 11 patients who underwent 12 combined femoral and Chiari pelvic osteotomies for the treatment of painful subluxation or dislocation secondary to cerebral palsy. Relief of pain, improvement in movement of the hip, and in sitting posture, and ease of perineal care were recorded in all, and were maintained at a mean follow-up of 13.1 years (8 to 17.5). The radiological migration index improved from a mean of 80.6% (61% to 100%) to 13.7% (0% to 33%) (p < 0.0001). The mean changes in center edge angle and Sharp's angle were 72° (56° to 87°; p < 0.0001) and 12.3° (9° to 15.6°; p < 0.0001), respectively. (Level IV evidence)

Delp SL, Bleck EB, Zajac FE, Bollini G. Biomechanical analysis of the Chiari pelvic osteotomy. Clin Orthop Relat Res. 1990;(254):189–98.

Biomechanical study which investigated how the Chiari osteotomy affects the function of hip abductor muscles. The biomechanical model analyzed postsurgery pelvic geometry and resulting hip abductor torque dependent on three surgical parameters: angulation of the osteotomy, distance of medial displacement, and angle of internal rotation. Simulated surgeries with high angulation and large medial displacement reduce gluteus medius abductor torque by up to 65%. Simulated horizontal osteotomies (0° to 10°) were found to best conserve both muscle length and abductor torque. (Level III evidence)

Ohashi H, Hirohashi K, Yamano Y. Factors influencing the outcome of Chiari pelvic osteotomy: a long-term follow-up. J Bone Joint Surg [Br]. 2000;82:517–25.

Retrospective review of 103 of 126 Chiari osteotomies from 1956 to 1987. Success of the Chiari was measured by time to development of advanced osteoarthritis. Advanced degenerative change developed in 33.7% and one hip required a total replacement arthroplasty (TRA), the mean survival time was 26.0 ± 2.5 years. Differences in survivorship curves related significantly to the severity of the preoperative OA, the shape of the femoral head and the level of osteotomy. The authors concluded that the Chiari osteotomy remains radiologically effective for about 25 years and is best suited for subluxated hips with round or flat femoral heads with early or no degenerative change. (Level IV evidence)

Windager R, Pongracz N, Shonecker W, Kotz R. Chiari osteotomy for congential dislocation and subluxation of the hip: results after 20 to 34 years follow-up. J Bone Joint Surg [Br]. 1991;73:890–5.

Retrospective review of 236 Chiari pelvic osteomies performed between 1953 and 1967 at the Orthopaedic University Clinic of Vienna for the treatment of congential dislocation and subluxation of the hip. The overall clinical results were excellent or good in 51.4%, fair in 29.8% and poor in 18.3%; with over 90% of the operations performed by Chiari himself. The results were worse with increasing age at operation. The addition of an intertrochanteric varus osteotomy in 36 cases did not achieve either better centering or better development of the acetabular roof. (Level IV evidence)

Triple Pelvic Osteotomy

Gleeson Rebello and Young-Jo Kim

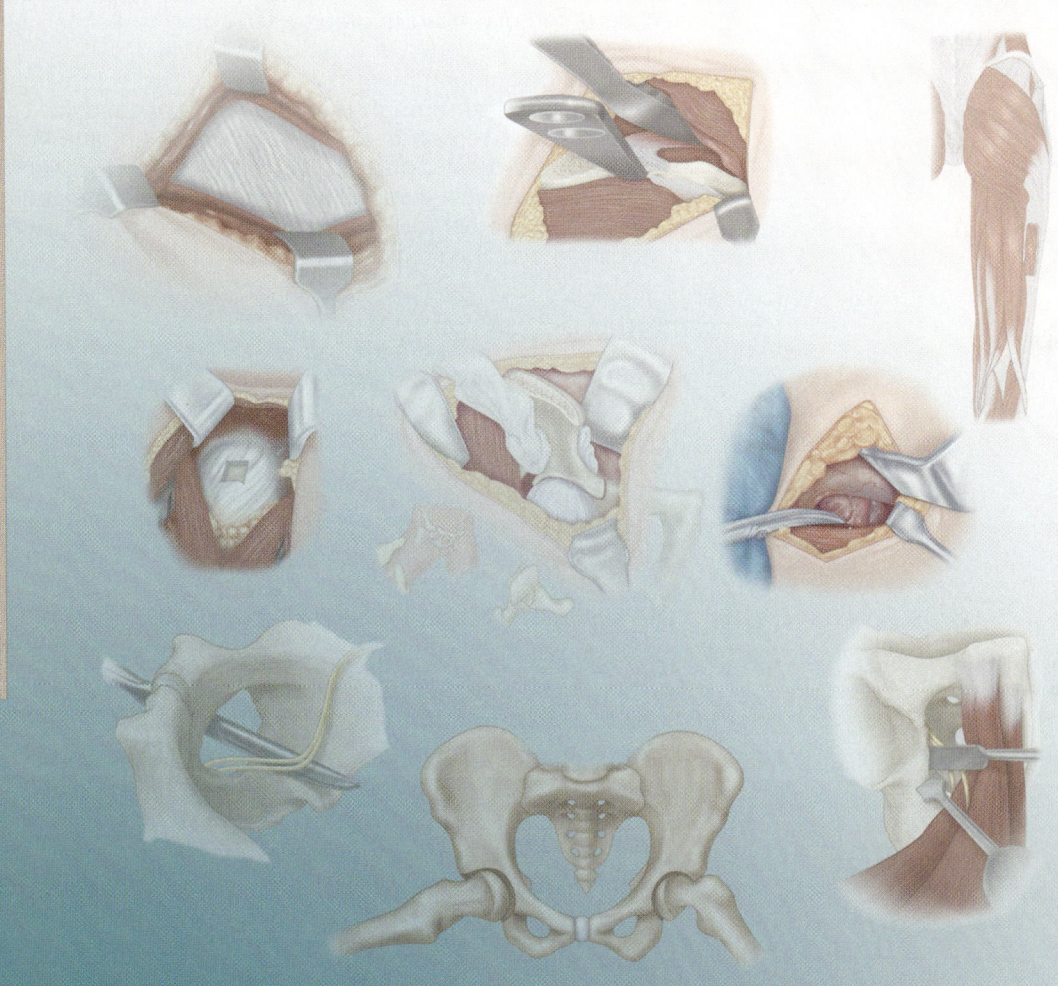

Controversies

- Performing a procedure of this magnitude in a profoundly handicapped patient with low or no ambulatory potential

Treatment Options

- Periacetabuloplasties (Roposch, Mubarak)

INDICATIONS

- Hip dysplasia in skeletally immature hips in which other pelvic osteotomies are ineffective, incomplete, or counterproductive. The use of this osteotomy is described in complex hip dysplasia secondary to neuromuscular and teratologic conditions.

EXAMINATION/IMAGING

- Plain anteroposterior (AP) radiographs of the pelvis and abduction/flexion/internal rotation view of the hips should be obtained. The surgeon should note the presence of triradiate cartilage and evaluate coverage of the femoral heads by measuring acetabular indices, lateral center edge angle of Wiberg, femoral head migration according to Reimer, Shenton's line, and the presence of a congruent joint.
- Computed tomography of the pelvis with both proximal femurs and a single slice through the distal femoral condyles can be used to assess version of the femoral neck (Kim and Wenger, 1997). Three-dimensional reconstructions help localize acetabular deficiency and allow for more specific planning concerning the degree of correction in each plane using a mobilized acetabular socket (Lee et al., 1991).

SURGICAL ANATOMY

- Smith-Petersen interval—superficial internervous plane between the sartorius (femoral nerve) and tensor fasciae latae (superior gluteal nerve) and deep internervous plane between the rectus femoris (femoral nerve) and gluteus medius (superior gluteal nerve).
- The lateral femoral cutaneous nerve should be preserved by incising the fascia of the tensor fasciae latae (TFL) from proximal to distal in an oblique fashion, remaining lateral to the anterior superior iliac spine (ASIS). Staying within the fascial sheath of the TFL will protect the lateral femoral cutaneous nerve because the nerve runs over the fascia of the sartorius. Cutting it can lead to a painful neuroma and diminished sensation on the lateral aspect of thigh.
- The large ascending branch of the lateral femoral circumflex artery crosses the operative field between the sartorius and TFL just below the ASIS and must be coagulated.
- Muscles either take origin from or insert into the iliac crest but do not cross it. Therefore, the crest offers a truly internervous plane. A part of the external oblique muscle attachment must be sharply incised to expose the underlying iliac apophysis for proximal extension of the approach. After sharply incising the iliac apophysis parallel to the crest, muscles attached to the crest may be stripped off the inner and outer wall of the ilium, always following the contour of the bone. Connecting this arm of the dissection to the Smith-Petersen interval provides excellent exposure.
- Contents of the greater sciatic foramen and lesser sciatic foramen—superior gluteal artery and nerve, inferior gluteal artery and nerve, pudendal nerve, internal pudendal vessels, nerve to the obturator internus, sciatic nerve, posterior femoral cutaneous nerve, nerve to the quadratus femoris. The internal pudendal vessels and nerve run in the lesser sciatic foramen along with the tendon of the obturator internus and nerve to the obturator internus. These structures passing through both foramens are at risk during the iliac and ischial osteotomy.

Equipment

- Radiolucent table
- C-arm

Instrumentation

- A Lane retractor helps in blunt dissection around the ischium in the first incision.

Controversies

- The ischium may be accessed through a medial extension of the bikini line incision and not need a separate medial longitudinal incision.

- Medial approach for ischial osteotomy—The anterior division of the obturator nerve passes through the obturator foramen between the adductor longus and brevis muscles. Tracing the nerve proximally will help locate the ischium, which borders the obturator foramen laterally.
- Pubic ramus osteotomy—While performing the pubic ramus osteotomy, the contents of the obturator foramen, which include the obturator nerve and vessels, have to be protected.

POSITIONING

- The patient is positioned supine on a radiolucent table with a small padding under both hips and shoulder to elevate the torso.

PORTALS/EXPOSURES

- First incision to obtain exposure for ischial osteotomy
  - The medial skin incision extends approximately 8 cm longitudinally along the posterior aspect of the adductor longus muscle.
  - First the fascia is incised in a line parallel to the skin incision and blunt dissection is used to elaborate the plane between the adductor longus and the brevis. This will expose the anterior division of the obturator nerve, which overlies the adductor brevis.
  - The nerve is traced proximally to the point at which it exits the obturator foramen, and a finger is then placed laterally in the foramen to identify the ischium.
  - The pectineus is retracted proximally and superficially to protect the femoral neurovascular bundle, which is just anterior to it. The ischium is cleared of soft tissue using blunt dissection. The surgeon must ensure that dissection is entirely extra-periosteal at this point.
- Second incision to obtain exposure for iliac and pubic ramus osteotomy
  - The "bikini line" skin incision begins just inferior to the ASIS and continues laterally to a point just beyond the summit of the iliac crest. This incision provides for a satisfactory cosmetic appearance.
  - The external oblique muscle is sharply elevated to the lateral half of its insertion on the iliac crest.
  - The iliac apophysis is incised sharply with a knife that runs bone deep through the middle of the iliac crest.
  - A Cobb elevator is utilized to elevate the apophysis of the medial aspect of the crest. Attention is then diverted to opening the Smith-Petersen interval between the TFL laterally and the sartorius medially.
  - The opening in the Smith-Petersen interval is connected to the incision in the iliac apophysis and, using blunt dissection, the sartorius along with the iliopsoas muscle is lifted off the inner table of the ilium while maintaining the lateral part of the apophysis that is attached to the abductors on the crest.
  - The iliopsoas is then elevated extra-periosteally all the way to the superior pubic ramus.

PROCEDURE

STEP 1: ISCHIAL OSTEOTOMY

- After exposing the area of the ischium just inferior and adjacent to the acetabulum, a Lane retractor is slid through the obturator foramen, hugging the periosteum (dissection is entirely extra-periosteal at this point) of the quadrilateral plate all the way to the ischial spine (Fig. 1A). The position of the Lane retractor is confirmed using fluoroscopic AP and false profile views (Fig. 1B). The Lane retractor is used to protect the contents of the sciatic notch.

- Under fluoroscopic control, a straight Ganz osteotome is used to make the ischial cut from a point just inferior to the margin of the acetabulum to a point above the proximal aspect of the ischial spine (Fig. 2A–C). Making the osteotomy cut at this level ensures that the ischio-spinous ligament that is attached to the ischial spine will not affect the mobility of the acetabular fragment.

- The maneuver is repeated on the lateral aspect by sliding the Lane retractor on the lateral aspect of the ischium. The retractor is used to protect the contents of the sciatic notch and complete the ischial cut laterally using the same osteotome.

- A few additional passes may need to be performed with the osteotome to ensure that the ischial cut is complete.

- When visualizing the ischial cut in its entirety in the AP plane, it is important to note that the cut is somewhat oblique, angling from proximal and medial to distal and lateral. The wound is then packed using moist gauze.

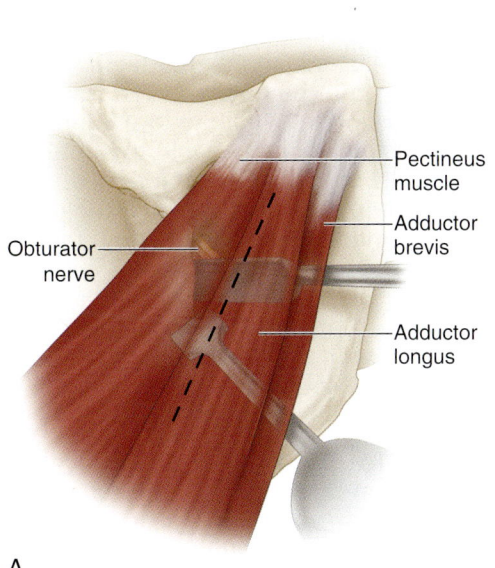

Obturator nerve

Pectineus muscle

Adductor brevis

Adductor longus

A

FIGURE 1

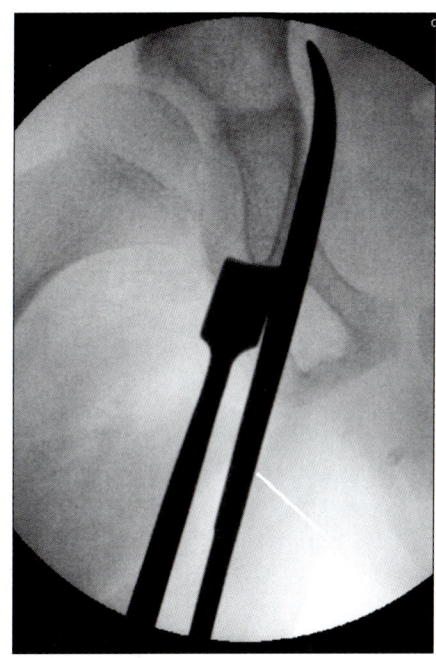

B

PEARLS

- *The thick periosteum of the ramus might need to be sharply incised to enhance the mobility of the acetabular fragment.*

PITFALLS

- *Ensure that the obturator nerve and vessels are not damaged during the pubic ramus osteotomy.*

PEARLS

- *Before angling the cut to the sciatic notch, a reverse Hohmann retractor is placed to protect the contents of the notch. The hip is kept extended to push the contents of the notch away from it. Also, look out for spontaneous foot movements that might indicate that the osteotomy is uncomfortably close to the sciatic nerve.*

Instrumentation/ Implantation

- A Ganz osteotome may be used to complete the iliac cut through the sciatic notch after using a power saw to cut down from the crest to the pelvic brim

STEP 2: SUPERIOR PUBIC RAMUS OSTEOTOMY

- The superior pubic ramus is exposed extra-periosteally by dissecting the iliopsoas muscle off it through the bikini line incision.
- A long, curved large hemostat, such as a Statinsky clamp, is inserted into the obturator formamen while staying extra-periosteal but close to the inferior aspect of the superior pubic ramus bone to avoid the obturator nerve and other contents of the obturator foramen.
- The clamp is used to thread a Gigli saw through the obturator foramen and around the ramus, and the saw is then used to make the superior pubic ramus cut. Before the Gigli saw is passed, the silk suture is pulled taut and, if the nerve is entrapped, the adductor musculature usually contracts.
- Alternatively, the superior pubic ramus cut can also be made with an osteotome.

STEP 3: ILIAC OSTEOTOMY

- The cut in the ilium is made in a manner similar to that used in the Bernese periacetabular osteotomy (Ganz et al., 1988). But, instead of angling it down through the posterior column, it is angled down into the sciatic notch (Fig. 3).
- This cut differs from the straight cut of a Salter-type osteotomy because of the angle of the cut, which increases supra-acetabular bone stock, thus facilitating stability and fixation.

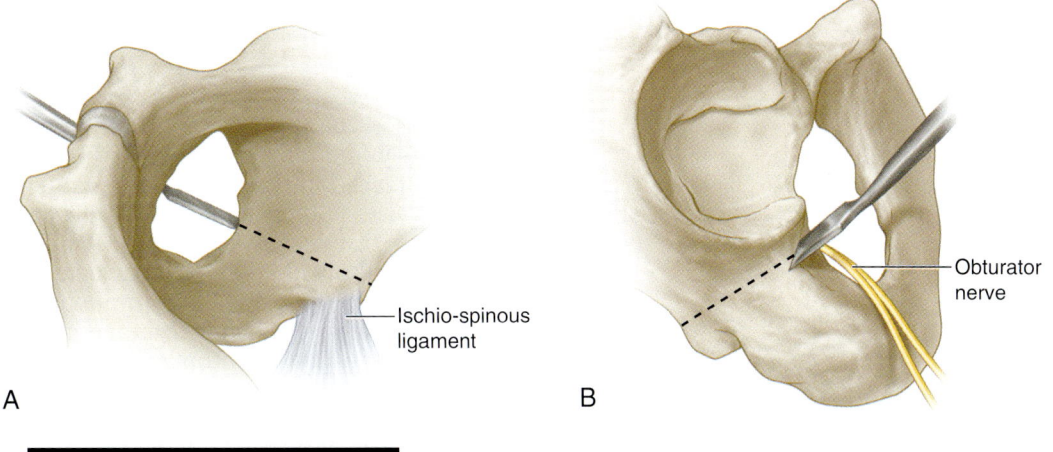

A

B

Ischio-spinous ligament

Obturator nerve

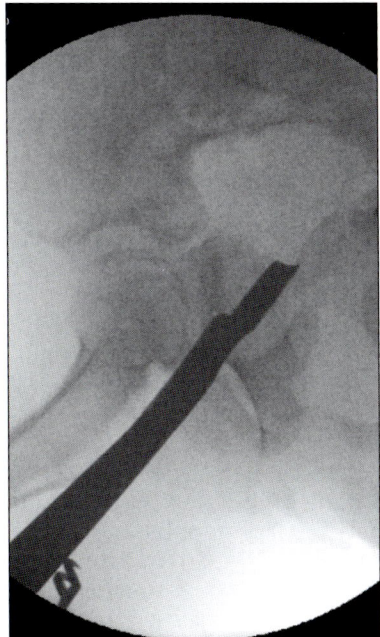

FIGURE 2 C

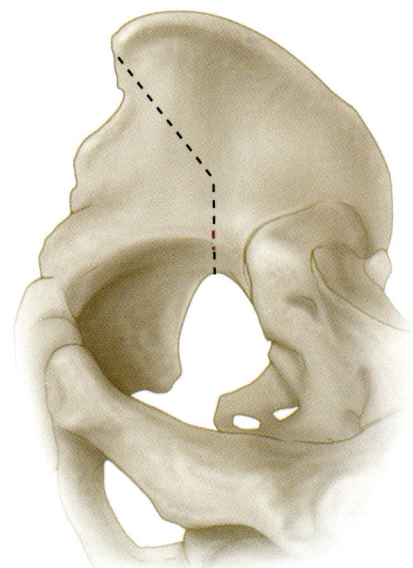

FIGURE 3

STEP 4: ACETABULAR FRAGMENT FIXATION

- The mobility of the acetabular fragment can be enhanced by revisiting all osteotomy cuts by insinuating a Cobb retractor into the gap between the bones. A few passes with an osteotome and nicks in the thick periosteum might be needed to completely free up the acetabular fragment. A 3.5-mm Schanz screw is placed in the acetabular fragment in the supra-acetabular region. Careful attention is then directed at accurately placing the fragment in the desired position.
- To address the issue of acetabular deficiency, which is usually posterolateral in hips with neuromuscular conditions, the acetabular fragment needs to be anteverted and adducted with respect to the iliac osteotomy (Rebello et al., 2009; Woolf and Gross, 2003) (Fig. 4).
- The fragment seldom needs to be extended as anterior coverage is usually not as badly compromised in these situations as it is in developmental dysplasia of the hip. The fragment is held in place with three to four 3/32-inch Kirschner wires (K-wires) drilled through the ilium into the acetabular fragment. Anteroposterior and false profile imaging is done with a C-arm to ensure the absence of violation of the hip joint and also the triradiate cartilage by the K-wires (Fig. 5A and 5B).
- The continuity in Shenton's line, the degree of acetabular coverage both in the AP and false profile views, the femoral head migration index, and the position of the teardrop and the sourcil are also noted. The hip joint is then ranged and its stability is determined.
- The need for a femoral osteotomy is determined based on the stability of the hip and the coverage of the femoral head. The acetabular fragment is stabilized by replacing the K-wires with three to four 3.5-mm long pelvic screws (Fig. 6A and 6B).
- Sharp edges in the acetabular fragment are trimmed and utilized as bone graft. The surgical wound is then thoroughly irrigated and the iliac apophysis is reapproximated with #1 Vicryl. The fascia of the Smith-Petersen interval is sutured with 3-0 Vicryl taking great care to avoid impaling the lateral cutaneous nerve. Skin is closed with subcuticular 3-0 Monocryl. A drain may or may not be utilized depending on local wound conditions prior to closure and surgeon preference.

POSTOPERATIVE CARE AND EXPECTED OUTCOMES

- Spica cast immobilization is done for 4 weeks with the hips in 30° of abduction and 20° of flexion.
- Sometimes a knee immobilizer that prevents excessive hip flexion and adduction is all that is necessary.

PEARLS

- In addition to careful clinical examination, postoperative follow-up should include serial radiographic follow-up.
- Complications that include persistent hip joint subluxation, nonunion of the osteotomy site, and premature closure of the triradiate cartilage should be assessed.

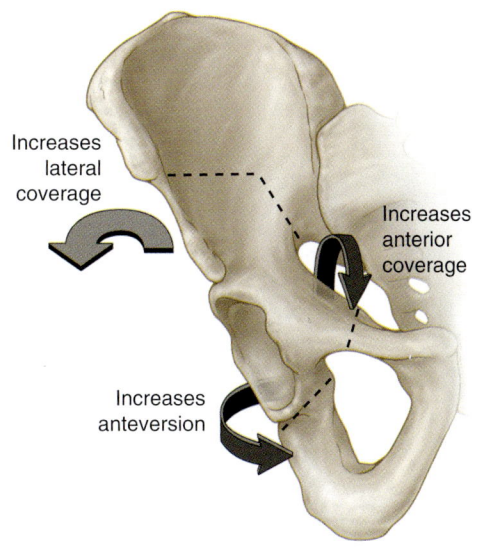

Increases
lateral
coverage

Increases
anterior
coverage

Increases
anteversion

FIGURE 4

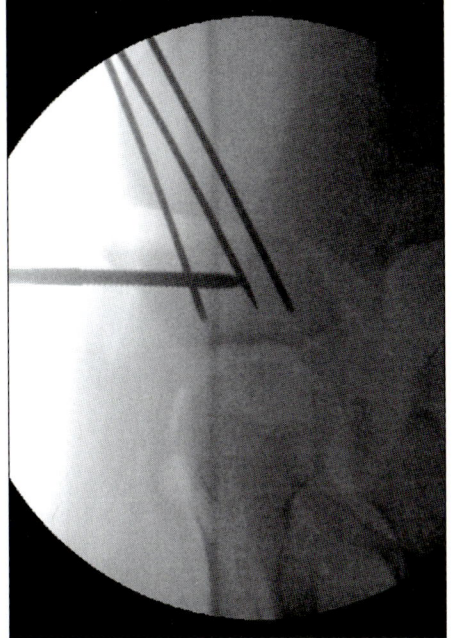

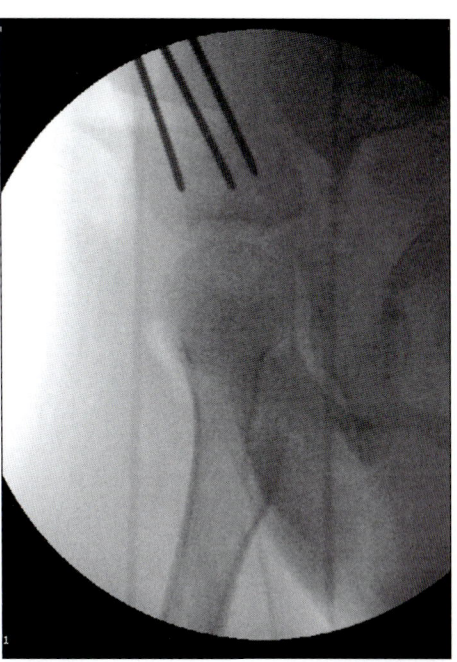

FIGURE 5 A

B

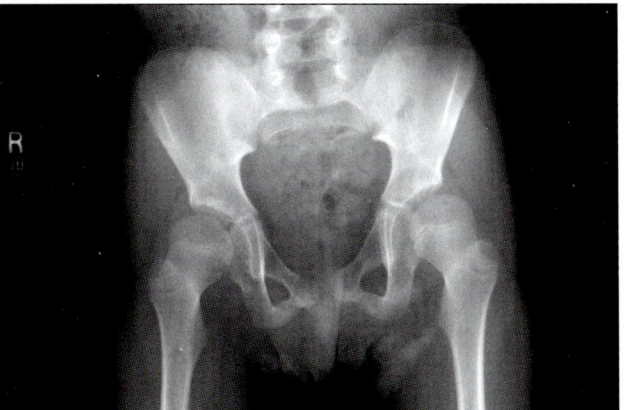

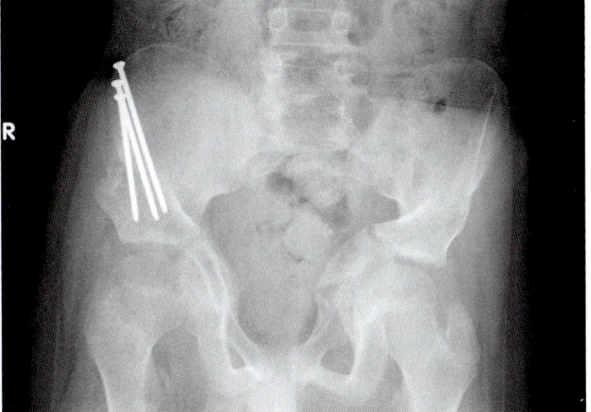

A

B

FIGURE 6

EVIDENCE

Ganz R, Klaue K, Vinh TS, et al. A new periacetabular osteotomy for the treatment of hip dysplasias: technique and preliminary results. Clin Orthop Relat Res. 1988;(232):26–36.

Kim HT, Wenger DR. Location of acetabular deficiency and associated hip dislocation in neuromuscular hip dysplasia: three dimensional computed tomographic analysis. J Pediatr Orthop.1997;17:143–51.

Lee DY, Choi IH, Lee CK, et al. Assessment of complex hip deformity using three-dimensional CT image. J Pediatr Orthop. 1991;11:13–9.

Rebello G, Zilkens C, Dudda M, Matheney T, Kim YJ. Triple pelvic osteotomy in complex hip dysplasia seen in neuromuscular and teratologic conditions. J Pediatr Orthop. 2009;29:527–34.

Woolf SK, Gross RH. Posterior acetabular wall deficiency in Down syndrome. J Pediatr Orthop. 2003;23:708–13.

Single-Incision Supraperiosteal Triple Innominate Osteotomy

Ira Zaltz

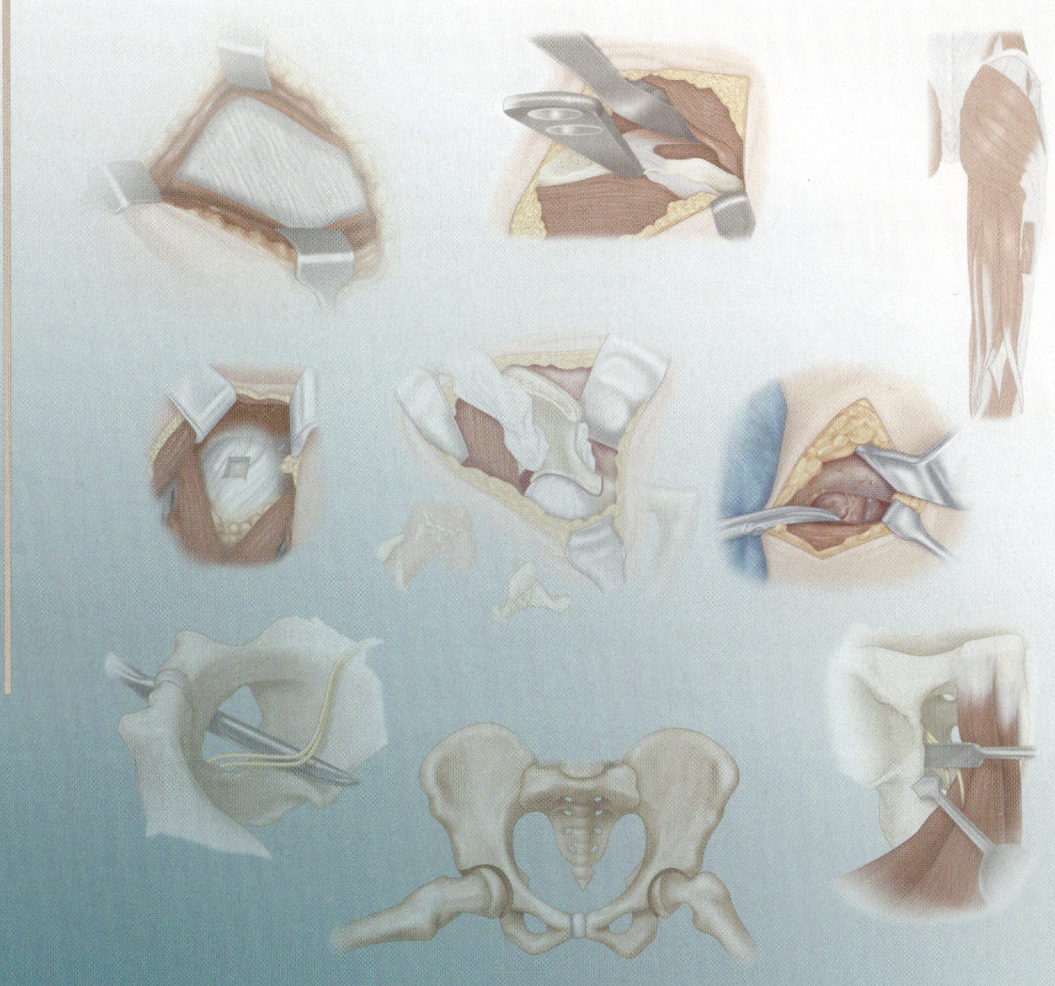

PITFALLS

- *Other osteotomies, including single innominate (Salter, Pemberton, or Dega), triple innominate (Steele, Tonnis), and Bernese periacetabular osteotomy, may be considered depending upon the familiarity of the surgeon, the age of the patient, and the degree and type of dysplasia.*
- *Simultaneous femoral osteotomy may be necessary in selected cases.*
- *Nonoperative treatment may allow further damage to the acetabulum and femoral epiphysis.*

Controversies

- Precise timing and necessity of corrective acetabular surgery in asymptomatic dysplasia in skeletally immature patients remains controversial.
- Children with symptomatic acetabular dysplasia, particularly those exhibiting either clinical or radiographic signs of hip joint dysfunction, are candidates for surgical reconstruction. Clinical signs include limb, signs of hip instability, and pain with provocative testing. Radiographic signs include any evidence of arthrosis (sourcil sclerosis, cyst formation, epiphyseal osteochondritis) and worsening dysplasia (progressive disruption of Shenton's line).

INDICATIONS

■ Correction of acetabular dysplasia in skeletally immature individuals in whom osteotomy through the triradiate cartilage may produce a growth arrest that may adversely affect continued acetabular growth and development.

EXAMINATION/IMAGING

■ A complete physical examination is necessary in the evaluation of children with developmental dysplasia of the hip. The patient's stature, spinal alignment, relative limb length, and neurologic examination must be assessed. In addition, a careful examination of the hip includes assessment of gait, and precise documentation of range of motion. A patient must have at least 20–30° of hip abduction in order to undergo acetabular reorientation.

■ Plain radiographs
  - Standard radiographs used in the evaluation of patients with acetabular dysplasia include anteroposterior (AP) pelvic (Fig. 1), frog-leg lateral (Fig. 2), false profile, and abduction and internal rotation views.
  - The diagnosis of dysplasia is established based upon plain radiographs. The acetabular version may not be determined due to skeletal immaturity. Upper femoral dysplasia and epiphyseal morphology are assessed on both AP and frog-leg views. Hip joint congruity and concentricity are established based upon the AP and abduction and internal rotation radiographs.

■ Computed tomography (CT)
  - Though not required for all patients, CT scanning can be useful to define acetabular anatomy in patients with neurologic or syndromic types of acetabular dysplasia, as nonstandard corrective maneuvering may be necessary during corrective surgery.
  - CT scanning with three-dimensional modeling is most helpful in defining the region of acetabular insufficiency.

■ Arthrographic evaluation is still the most accurate diagnostic method to establish hip joint congruency, and may be necessary to determine the position of congruity, particularly when the femoral epiphysis is significantly deformed.

■ Improvements in magnetic resonance imaging (MRI) technology have enabled visualization of the acetabular labrum and articular cartilage. Although its role in the assessment of skeletally immature patients is evolving, MRI is useful if significant intra-articular abnormality is suspected based upon the clinical scenario.

■ Arthroscopic hip joint assessment can be useful either as a staging study to evaluate articular surfaces or for concomitant treatment of either labral or chondral pathology. The role of simultaneous arthroscopic treatment of labral pathology with correction of acetabular dysplasia remains to be studied.

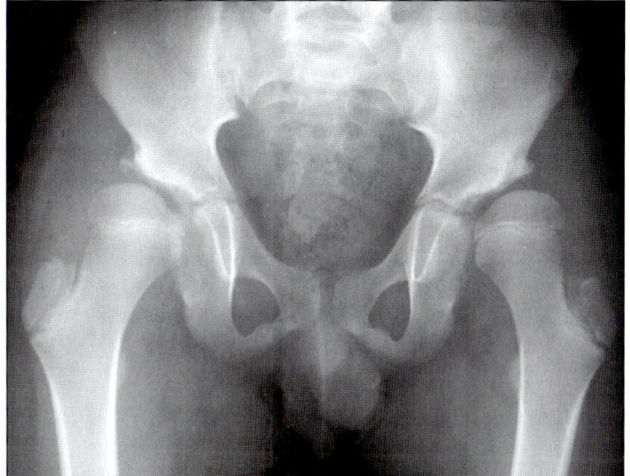

FIGURE 1

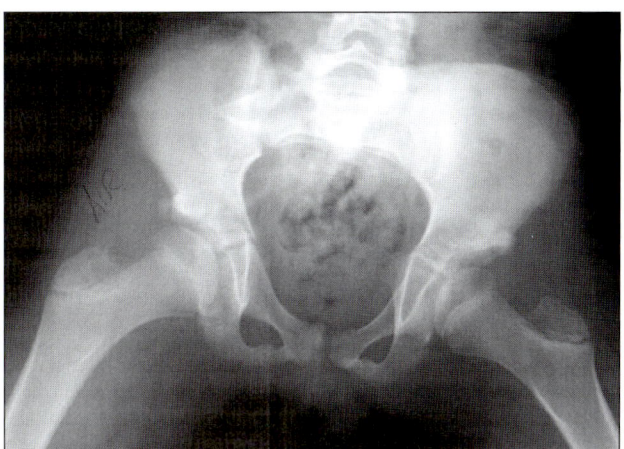

FIGURE 2

SURGICAL ANATOMY

- Preservation of the triradiate cartilage involves careful dissection of the pubis and medial ischium as well as anatomic knowledge of the location of the triradiate cartilage on the medial ilium, ischium and pubis.

POSITIONING

- The patient is positioned supine on a radiolucent operating table without a roll behind the ipsilateral pelvis in order to facilitate intraoperative evaluation of acetabular position (Fig. 3).
  - Care is taken to ensure that the frontal plane of the pelvis is horizontal, and a postpositioning AP pelvis radiograph is obtained to establish a baseline with which intraoperative acetabular alignment can be compared.
  - Positioning the contralateral arm over the chest on an armholder facilitates maneuvering of the fluoroscope.
- The surgeon stands on the side of the operative hip and the assistant stands opposite. A fluoroscope is positioned opposite the surgeon with the monitor at the patient's foot.
- The entire leg, hip, abdomen, and lower chest are included in the surgical field so that exposure is not compromised following draping.
- Following anesthetic induction, Foley catheterization is performed in order to protect the bladder during intrapelvic surgery.

PORTALS/EXPOSURES

- An oblique "bikini line" skin incision is made just distal to the anterior superior iliac spine.
- The subcutaneous tissue is divided in line with the incision. The external oblique muscle fascia is exposed proximal to the incision, and a subcutaneous flap is elevated distally in order to expose the distal tensor fascia lata–sartorius interval (Fig. 4).

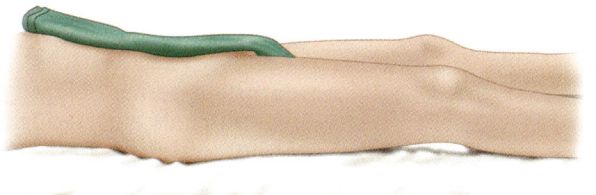

FIGURE 3

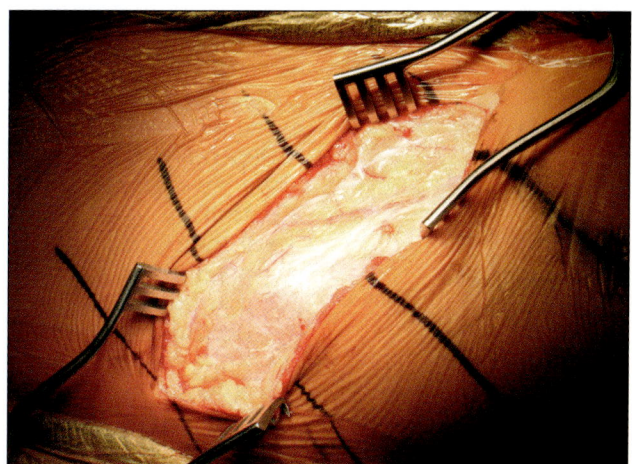

FIGURE 4

PROCEDURE

STEP 1: SUPERFICIAL DISSECTION

- The external oblique muscle fascia is incised laterally and the muscle is elevated from the iliac apophysis. The tensor-sartorius interval is opened longitudinally while protecting the lateral femoral cutaneous nerve.
- The iliac apophysis is incised along and in line with the iliac crest, and the medial table of the ilium is dissected in a subperiosteal fashion and the sciatic notch is identified. The tensor-sartorius interval medial flap is now continuous with the iliacus muscle.
- Within the tensor-sartorius interval, the rectus femoris is identified overlying the hip capsule, and the lateral fascia of the rectus is incised in order to facilitate medial retraction of the muscle (Fig. 5).
- The reflected head of the rectus femoris muscle is identified. Depending upon preoperative studies, one may elect to open the hip capsule in order to address labral or head-neck junction pathology.
  - If the surgeon plans to open the hip joint, then the reflected head of the rectus femoris and the direct head are released and the iliocapsularis muscle is reflected medially in order to expose the capsule.
  - If the surgeon does not plan to open the capsule, the anterior, largely chondral wall of the acetabulum must be clearly identifiable in order to estimate the degree of acetabular anteversion following corrective maneuvers. Placing a radiopaque instrument on the wall so as to locate it fluoroscopically facilitates identification of the anterior acetabular wall.
- The tensor fascia lata muscle can be elevated from the lateral ilium in order to identify the lateral sciatic notch. Depending upon whether the surgeon elects to use a Gigli saw or an osteotome, the iliac cut be performed using an abductor-sparing approach.

STEP 2: DEEP DISSECTION

- The rest of the pelvic dissection is performed in a supraperiosteal fashion, thus avoiding inadvertent periosteal stripping that can lead to formation of a growth arrest.
- The iliacus fascia is incised from the anterior superior iliac spine into the apex of the sciatic notch. It is helpful to carefully dissect the iliacus muscle from the periosteum so that the superior gluteal artery and sciatic nerve exiting the sciatic notch are protected. This is best accomplished using blunt dissection with either a small sponge or Kittner sponge.
- Once the periosteum of the iliacus muscle is incised, the muscle can be reflected from the periosteum and investing fascia, leaving the periosteum attached to the distal ilium. Figure 6 shows the iliacus muscle reflected medially with overlying periosteum. A retractor is within the sciatic notch, and a second retractor is exposing the psoas muscle distally and superficially.
- The hip and knee are now flexed to relax the iliopsoas. Slight adduction of the hip helps to facilitate medial retraction. Care must be taken to retract gently to prevent femoral neurapraxia.
- The iliacus muscle is easily dissected from the pubis, and the iliopectineal eminence is easily identified. The iliopectineal eminence is the anterior limb of the triradiate cartilage, and the periosteum must not be disturbed over this landmark.

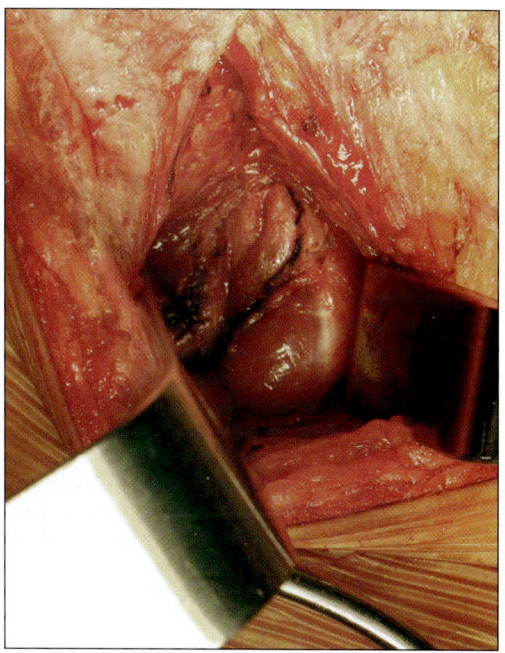

FIGURE 5

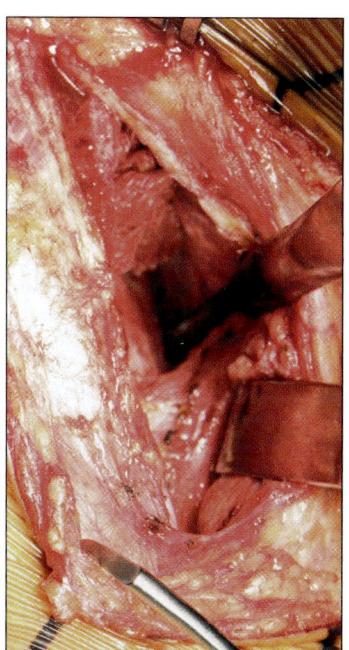

FIGURE 6

- Two similar surgical exposures can be employed to develop the interval between the psoas tendon and the hip capsule in order to access the anterior ischium.
  - The psoas sheath can be dissected from the medial hip capsule, the posteromedial periarticular fat identified, and the ischium identified. Alternately, the psoas sheath can be incised longitudinally and the posterior psoas sheath can be perforated and spread using dissecting scissors in order to access the anterior ischium.
  - Whichever technique is elected, the planes used to access the ischium and pubis must be contiguous or the acetabular mobility can be compromised by soft tissue tension.
- Once the anterior ischial plane is established, attention is directed to pubic and medial ischial supraperiosteal exposure. This exposure is not possible without releasing the iliopectineal fascia (medial fascia of the iliacus muscle) from its attachment to the iliopectineal line (medial ilium and posterior pubis). This is accomplished by gentle retraction on the iliacus muscle to reveal the fascia, followed by incision of the fascia. The fascia must be released up to the point of the pubic osteotomy. Excessive medial dissection places the femoral vessels at risk of injury.
- Once the iliopectineal fascia is released, the medial ischium and posterior pubis are accessible.
- Retroperitoneal fat is easily identified within the pelvis. A Deaver retractor is used to retract the iliopsoas complex. Often the obturator nerve is visible within the retroperitoneal fat and can be seen coursing distally and laterally toward the obturator foramen (Fig. 7). If the nerve within the fat is not visible, it is usually easily palpated. In order to protect the viscera and neurovascular structures, a Ray-Tec sponge is packed using a Hohmann retractor along the medial ischium.
- Last, the pubis is dissected supraperiosteally. The pubic osteotomy is performed using a Gigli saw that must be passed through the obturator foramen. This is best accomplished by using a large right-angle dissector to release the obturator fascia from the superolateral aspect of the medial pubis and ischium. Once released, a curved Satinsky clamp is passed from medial to lateral through the obturator foramen to facilitate passage of a suture that can be used later in order to pass a Gigli saw (Fig. 8). If the very thick periosteum of the pubis is not cut completely, movement of the acetabulum will be restricted. Of note, the pubic osteotomy is entirely medial to the iliopectineal eminence in order to avoid injuring the triradiate cartilage.

STEP 3: OSTEOTOMIES

- The ischial cut is performed using a curved Ganz osteotome.
  - The osteotome is maneuvered medial to the hip capsule and positioned at the level of the infracotyloid groove just distal to the acetabulum. A 50° cephalad–directed fluoroscopy image is used to confirm the position of the osteotome. The osteotome is directed into the lesser sciatic foramen.
  - Using 50° cephalad and 55° oblique fluoroscopic guidance, the ischium is cut in two passes. The medial ischium is cut before the lateral ischium, and the position of the osteotome is confirmed radiographically during the osteotomy. Figures 9 and 10 show a Ganz osteotome positioned adjacent to the infracotyloid groove and directed just distal to the ischial spine at the apex of the lesser sciatic foramen. Note the Ray-Tec sponge protecting neurovascular structures.

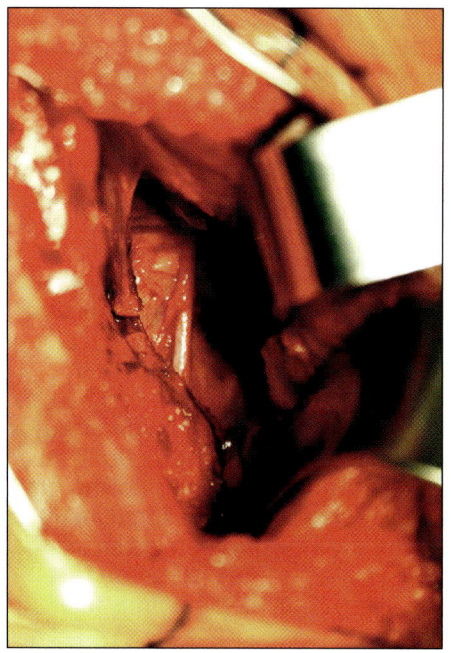

FIGURE 7

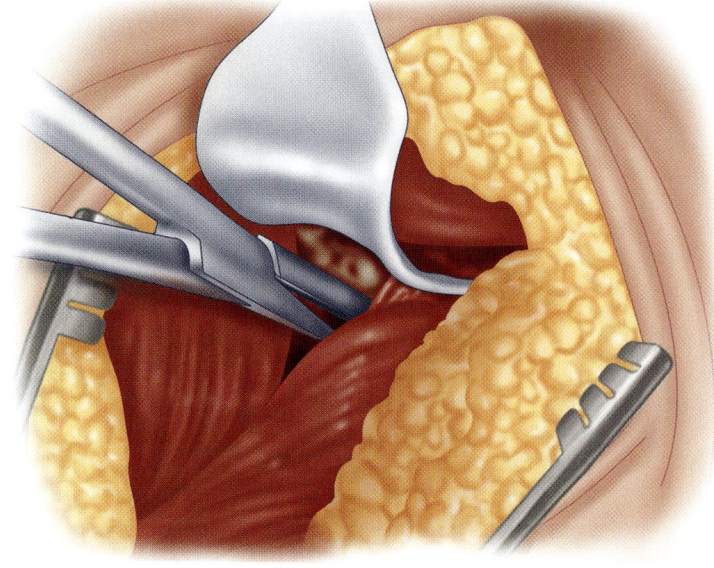

FIGURE 8

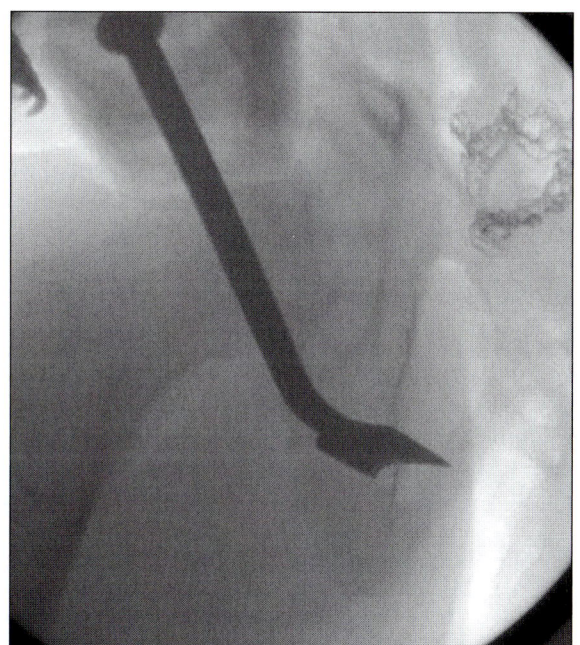

FIGURE 9

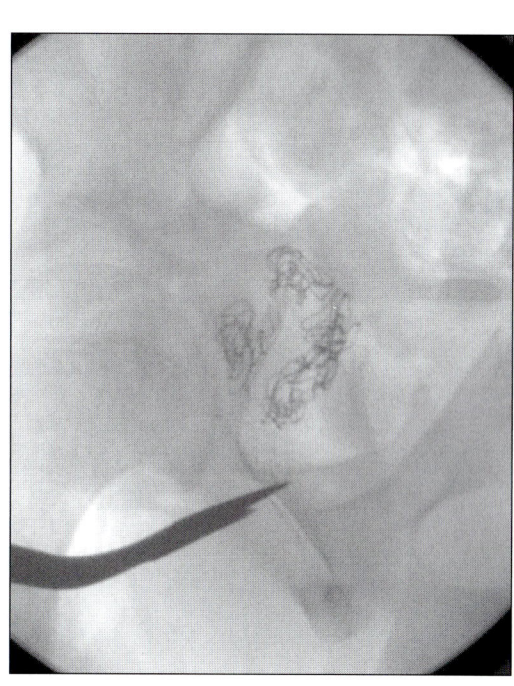

FIGURE 10

- The ischium is wider anteriorly than posteriorly, and the osteotome direction must be adjusted to avoid passing into the soft tissue posterolaterally. Rotating the osteotome and observing displacement of the ischium confirms completion of the osteotomy.

- The suture tape that was previously passed through the obturator foramen is then used to pass a Gigli saw. Rang retractors or a Hohmann retractor can be used to protect surrounding structures. The pubic osteotomy must pass entirely medial to the iliopectineal eminence. It is useful to angle the osteotomy approximately 30–45° relative to the long axis of the pubis and to incline the osteotomy from slightly medial to lateral to facilitate rotation of the acetabulum.

- The ilium can be cut in two ways: a Gigli saw can be used to make a Salter-like osteotomy, or the ilium can be osteotomized using an osteotome in a manner similar to the Bernese periacetabular osteotomy except continuing into the sciatic notch proximal to the posterior limb of the triradiate cartilage. The latter technique is employed if using an abductor-sparing approach.

- Following the third osteotomy, the acetabulum is freely mobile.

STEP 4: ACETABULAR POSITIONING AND FIXATION

- The acetabulum is maneuvered into position to correct the dysplasia. Although most cases are corrected by a combination of acetabular adduction, extension, and medial rotation, the correction is adjustable depending upon individual anatomic considerations.

- Two Kirschner wires are used to adjust the position of the acetabulum. One is inserted proximal to the acetabulum and a second medial to the acetabulum, in either the pubis or the medial acetabular wall. Since the bone is immature, it is less dense than adult bone and great care is used in manipulation. Excessive traction can disrupt the bone and compromise fixation.

- Once the acetabulum is appropriately corrected, provisional fixation is accomplished using Steinmann pins. An intraoperative AP pelvis radiograph taken with a marker on the anterior acetabular wall is used to assess the correction. In Figures 11 and 12, a Kirschner wire is positioned in the supra-acetabular ilium and used to maneuver the acetabulum into the desired position. Metzenbaum scissors are used to mark the anterior acetabular wall on both intraoperative false profile and AP projections.

- Stabilization is performed with Steinmann pins. Pin size should be appropriate to ensure adequate stability of the acetabulum. Depending upon the type and shape of the iliac osteotomy, a tricortical iliac graft is used to enhance stability. Allograft or autograft can be used depending upon the patient's bone size, prior surgery, and need for concomitant limb lengthening. Steinmann pins are cut to appropriate length and to facilitate easy removal. Figure 13 shows preoperative (Fig. 13A) and postoperative (Fig. 13B) views demonstrating final position and fixation of acetabulum.

- If additional intra-articular surgery is needed to address labral pathology or head-neck junction morphology, it can be performed after definitive fixation is secure.

- Closure is performed in a layered fashion. Suction drainage is not routinely employed. Spica casting is not routinely necessary.

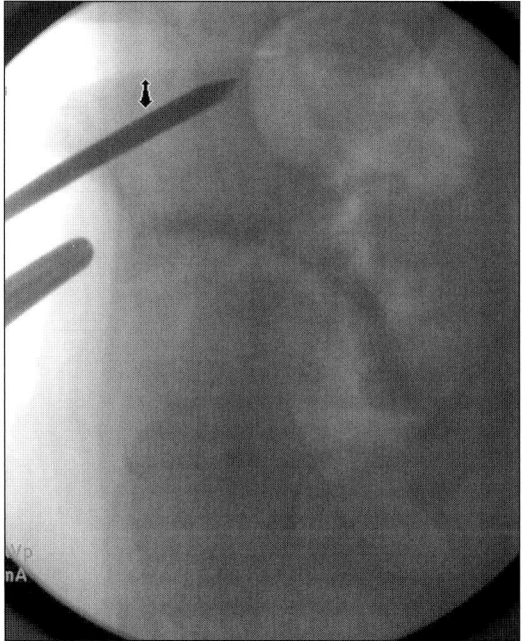

FIGURE 11

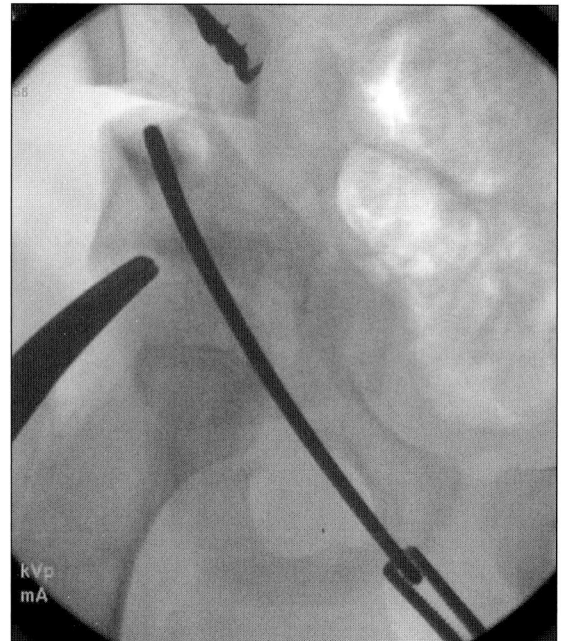

FIGURE 12

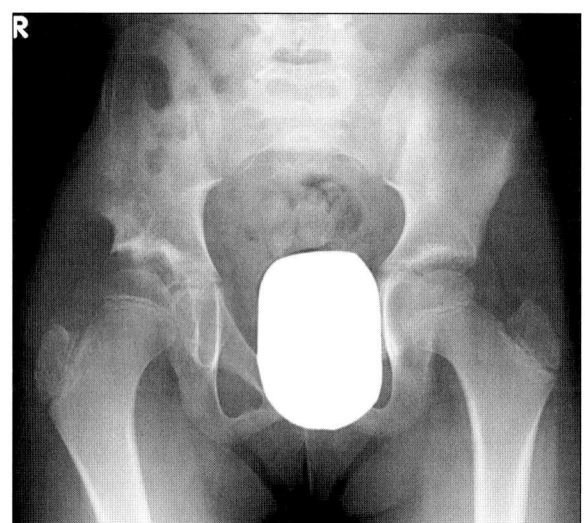

A
FIGURE 13

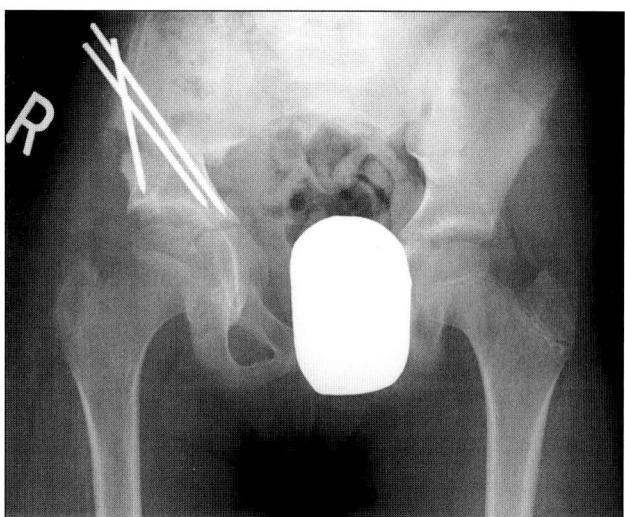

B

POSTOPERATIVE CARE AND EXPECTED OUTCOMES

- Patients are admitted to the hospital for analgesia and postoperative antibiotics.
- Weight bearing is restricted to toe-touch, and active hip motion is avoided for the first 6 weeks. Younger patients with poor muscular leg control following surgery are restricted to wheelchair transfers for 2–4 weeks.
- Once radiographic evidence of union is established, progressive weight bearing is permitted and muscle strengthening exercises are started under the direction of physical therapy.

EVIDENCE

Bucholz RW, Ezaki M, Ogden JA. Injury to the acetabular triradiate physeal cartilage. J Bone Joint Surg [Am]. 1982;64:600–9.

Dora C, Mascard E, Mladenov K, Seringe R. Retroversion of the acetabular dome after Salter and triple pelvic osteotomy for congenital dislocation of the hip. J Pediatr Orthop B. 2002;11:34–40.

Ganz R, Klaue K, Vinh TS, Mast JW. A new periacetabular osteotomy for the treatment of hip dysplasia. Clin Orthop Relat Res. 1988;(232):26–36.

Hailer NP, Soykaner L, Ackermann H, Rittmeister M. Triple osteotomy of the pelvis for acetabular dysplasia: age at operation and the incidence of nonunions and other complications influence outcome. J Bone Joint Surg [Br]. 2005;87:1622–6.

Hopf A. Huftpfannenverlagerung durch doppelte Beckenosteotomie zur Behandlung der Huftgelenksdysplasie und Subluxation bei Jugendlichen und Erwachsenen. Z Orthop. 1966;101:559–86.

Kim HT, Wenger D. Location of acetabular deficiency and associated dislocation in neuromuscular hip dysplasia: three-dimensional computed tomographic analysis. J Pediatr Orthop. 1997;17:143–51.

Kim HT, Wenger D. The morphology of residual acetabular deficiency in childhood hip dysplasia: three-dimensional computed tomographic analysis. J Pediatr Orthop. 1997;17:637–47.

Kumar D, Bache CE, O'Hara JN. Interlocking triple pelvic osteotomy in severe Legg-Calve-Perthes disease. J Pediatr Orthop. 2002;22:464–70.

Le Coeur MP. Revue de chirurgie orthopedique et reparatrice de l'appareil moteur. Rev Chir Orthop. 1965;51:211.

Lipton GE, Bowen JR. A new modified technique of triple osteotomy of the innominate bone for acetabular dysplasia. Clin Orthop Relat Res. 2005;(434):78–85.

O'Connor PA, Mullhall KJ, Kearns SR, Sheehan E, McCormack D. Triple pelvic osteotomy in Legg-Calve-Perthes disease using a single anterolateral incision. J Pediatr Orthop B. 2003;12:387–9.

Peters CL, Fukushima BW, Park T, Coleman SS, Dun HK. Triple innominate osteotomy in young adults for the treatment of acetabular dysplasia: a 9-year follow up study. Orthopedics. 2001;24:565–9.

Ponseti IV. Growth and development of the acetabulum in the normal child: anatomical, histological, and roentgenographic studies. J Bone Joint Surg [Am]. 1978;60: 575–85.

Roach J, Hobatho MR, Baker KJ, Ashman RB. Three-dimensional computer analysis of complex acetabular insufficiency. J Pediatr Orthop. 1997;7:158–64.

Salter RB. Inominate osteotomy in the treatment of congenital dislocation and subluxation of the hip. J Bone Joint Surg [Am]. 1965;47:65–86.

Steel HH. Triple osteotomy of the innominate bone. J Bone Joint Surg [Am]. 1973;55:343–50.

Tonnis D, Behrens K, Tscharani F. A modified technique of the triple pelvic osteotomy: early results. J Pediatr Orthop. 1981;1:241–9.

Tschauner C, Sylkin A, Hofmann S, Graf R. Painful nonunion after triple pelvic osteotomy. J Bone Joint Surg [Br]. 2003;85:953–5.

Repair of Proximal Hamstring Avulsion

Matthew Diltz and Mininder S. Kocher

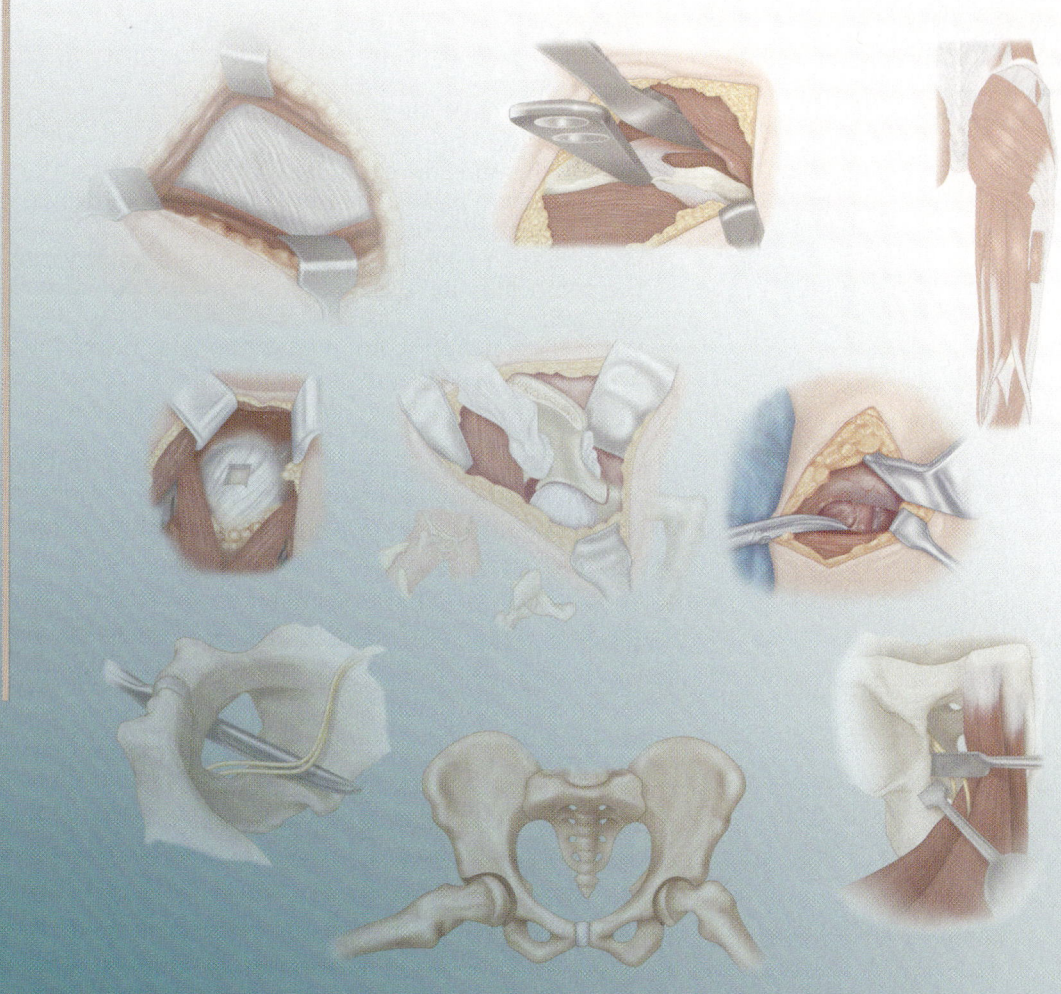

Controversies

• Nonoperative treatment of complete avulsion leads to poor results (Cohen and Bradley, 2007):

  ■ 60% return to sport
  ■ 60% hamstring muscle deficit
  ■ 90% return of hamstring muscle strength with repair
  ■ 60% return of strength with repair of chronic tears

Treatment Options

• Partial tears can be treated nonoperatively.

Equipment

• A beanbag can be used to place the patient in the decubitus position and manipulated to allow adequate exposure at the posterior thigh.

Controversies

• Some authors recommend the prone position. We have found that the lateral decubitus position provides adequate exposure, aids in retraction of the sciatic nerve out of the field, and facilitates general anesthesia.

INDICATIONS

■ Complete rupture of the origin of the hamstrings (semitendinosus, semimembranosus, and biceps femoris) in an active patient with functional disability
■ Chronic ruptures associated with sciatic nerve compression and pain
■ Large bony avulsion fragment causing discomfort with sitting

EXAMINATION/IMAGING

■ The patient will often report an eccentric load with an audible pop (e.g., "missed the soccer ball and hit the ground with my foot").
  • There is also an association with water skiing.
■ Patients can have difficulty with ambulation. They avoid hip and knee flexion.
■ There is point tenderness at the posterior thigh leading to difficulty with sitting.
■ A large ecchymosis develops 3 days to 1 week after the injury.
■ The sciatic nerve passes near the origin of the proximal hamstrings and can be injured acutely.
  • These tension injuries to the nerve have a tendency to affect the peroneal branch, leading to footdrop or weak inversion strength.
  • When there is a large fragment of bone associated with the avulsion, the callus formation during the body's attempt to heal the fracture can lead to entrapment of the nerve and paresthesias in the distribution of the sciatic nerve.
■ Radiographs can show the ischial avulsion fractures (Fig. 1).
■ Magnetic resonance imaging is the test of choice for differentiating partial and complete tears.

SURGICAL ANATOMY

■ The origin of the semimembranosus is at the inferiolateral aspect of the ischium (Miller and Webb, 2008).
■ The semitendinosus and the long head of the biceps femoris have a 2 × 3-cm common origin on the ischium. This is just medial to the semimembranosus.
■ The sciatic nerve lies 1.2 cm lateral to the lateral border of the ischium.
■ Figures 2 and 3 depict relevant anatomy.

POSITIONING

■ The patient is placed in the lateral decubitus position.
■ The involved leg is up. The knee is bent to approximately 30° to take tension off the hamstrings.
■ A U-shaped drape is placed at the groin and a bar drape is placed proximally.

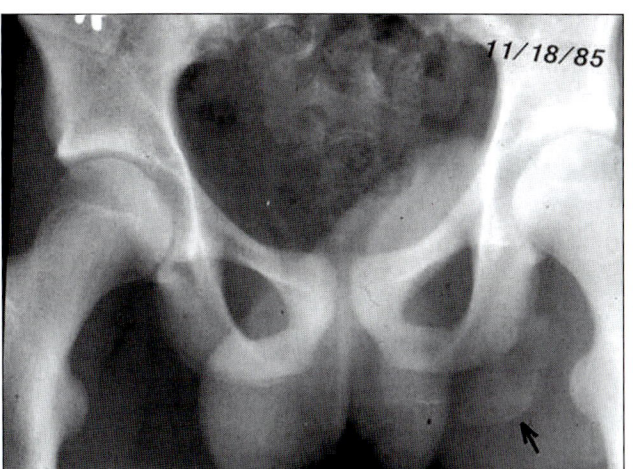

FIGURE 1

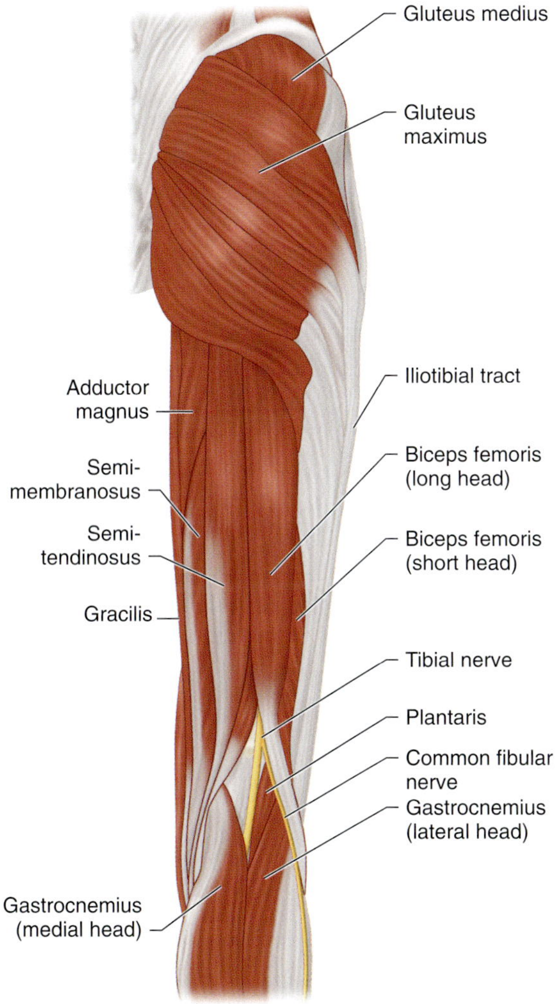

Gluteus medius

Gluteus maximus

Iliotibial tract

Biceps femoris (long head)

Biceps femoris (short head)

Tibial nerve

Plantaris

Common fibular nerve

Gastrocnemius (lateral head)

Adductor magnus

Semi-membranosus

Semi-tendinosus

Gracilis

Gastrocnemius (medial head)

FIGURE 2

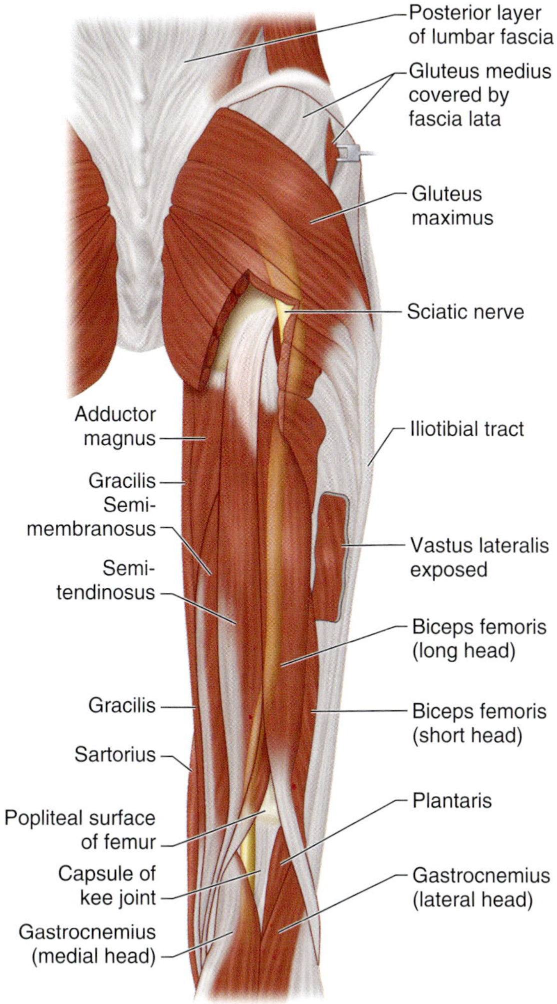

Posterior layer of lumbar fascia

Gluteus medius covered by fascia lata

Gluteus maximus

Sciatic nerve

Iliotibial tract

Vastus lateralis exposed

Biceps femoris (long head)

Biceps femoris (short head)

Plantaris

Gastrocnemius (lateral head)

Adductor magnus

Gracilis
Semi-membranosus

Semi-tendinosus

Gracilis

Sartorius

Popliteal surface of femur

Capsule of kee joint

Gastrocnemius (medial head)

FIGURE 3

PORTALS/EXPOSURES

■ For acute ruptures without sciatic symptoms, we use a vertical incision from the inferior aspect of the lateral ischium distally. For more chronic tears, particularly with sciatic nerve symptoms, an oblique incision aids in the exposure of the nerve.
■ After the initial skin incision, marcaine with epinephrine is injected to assist in hemostasis and postoperative pain control.
■ Sharp dissection is carried down to the gluteal fascia (Fig. 4).
■ A transverse incision is made in the fascia in order to expose the gluteus maximus (Fig. 5).
■ The fibers of the gluteus are spread with blunt dissection in line with the muscle (Fig. 6). Deep retractors are placed to expose the ischium and fascia of the proximal hamstrings.
■ In acute cases, the hematoma can often help delineate the proximal origin of the muscles. In more chronic cases, we recommend the presence of a microsurgeon to assist in the isolation of the sciatic nerve from surrounding scar tissue.

PROCEDURE

■ The repair of the proximal hamstrings is dependent on the type of injury.
■ For large avulsion fractures, the bone fragment should be reduced with fluoroscopic guidance and fixed in place.
■ Acute soft tissue avulsions and those involving only a minimal amount of the ischium are repaired primarily.
  • When there is a stump left at the origin or thick periosteum in our younger patients, #5 Ethibond or FiberWire is employed to reapproximate the tendons.
    ◆ The direct repair technique aids in the identification of the footprint of the tendons and correct restoration of the origins. A whipstitch is passed along the proximal aspect of the ruptured tendons. A free needle is then used to pass each limb of the suture in a mattress-type fashion.
    ◆ Once the tendons are reapproximated, the repair is reinforced with additional nonabsorbable suture.
  • In our patients with thinner periosteum, the surface of the ischium is exposed. Two to three double-loaded suture anchors are placed into the ischium. The more lateral sutures anchor is used to reapproximate the semimembranosus. The common origin of the biceps femoris and semitendinosus is repaired more medially.
■ For chronic injuries that have significant retraction, a fascia lata graft can be used to bridge the gap and make repair possible.

POSTOPERATIVE CARE AND EXPECTED OUTCOMES

■ A custom hip orthosis is employed to limit hip flexion to less than 15° for the first 2 weeks.
■ Toe-touch weight bearing is permitted for 2 weeks with crutches.
■ Active range of motion is begun at 4 weeks.
■ Use of the brace is discontinued at 6 weeks.

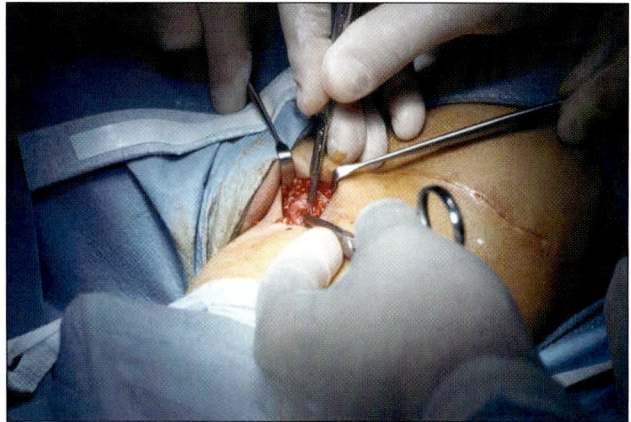

FIGURE 4

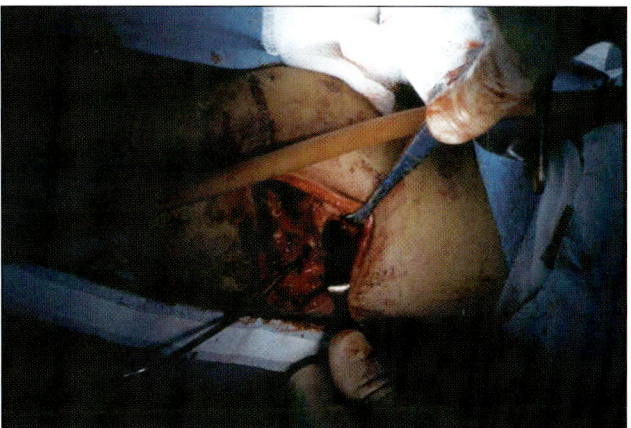

FIGURE 5

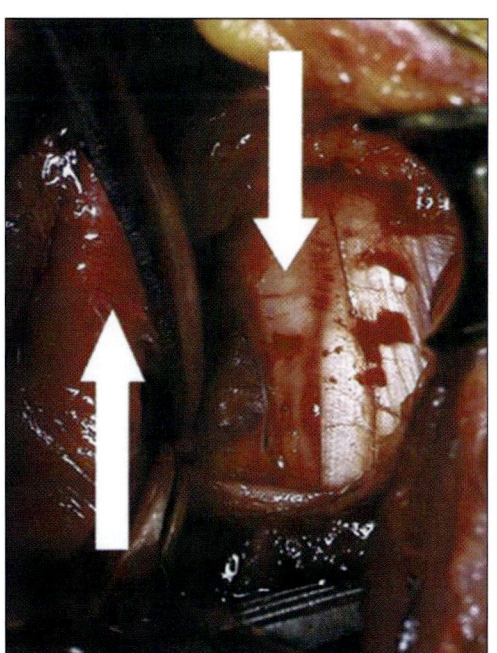

FIGURE 6

EVIDENCE

Cohen S, Bradley J. Acute proximal hamstring rupture. J Am Acad Orthop Surg. 2007;15:350–5.

This paper reviewed surgical and nonsurgical treatment of hamstring rupture.

Miller SL, Webb GR. The proximal origin of the hamstrings and surrounding anatomy encountered during repair: surgical technique. J Bone Joint Surg [Am]. 2008;90(Suppl 2 Pt 1):108–16.

The authors described their technique for proximal hamstring repair.

Miller SL, Gill J, Webb GR. The proximal origin of the hamstrings and surrounding anatomy encountered during repair: a cadaveric study. J Bone Joint Surg [Am]. 2007;89:44–8. (Erratum published in J Bone Joint Surg [Am]. 2007;89:637.)

The authors described the anatomy of the proximal origin of the hamstrings and its relationship to neurovascular and muscular structures.

Hip Pyarthritis

Jennifer C. Laine and Mohammad Diab

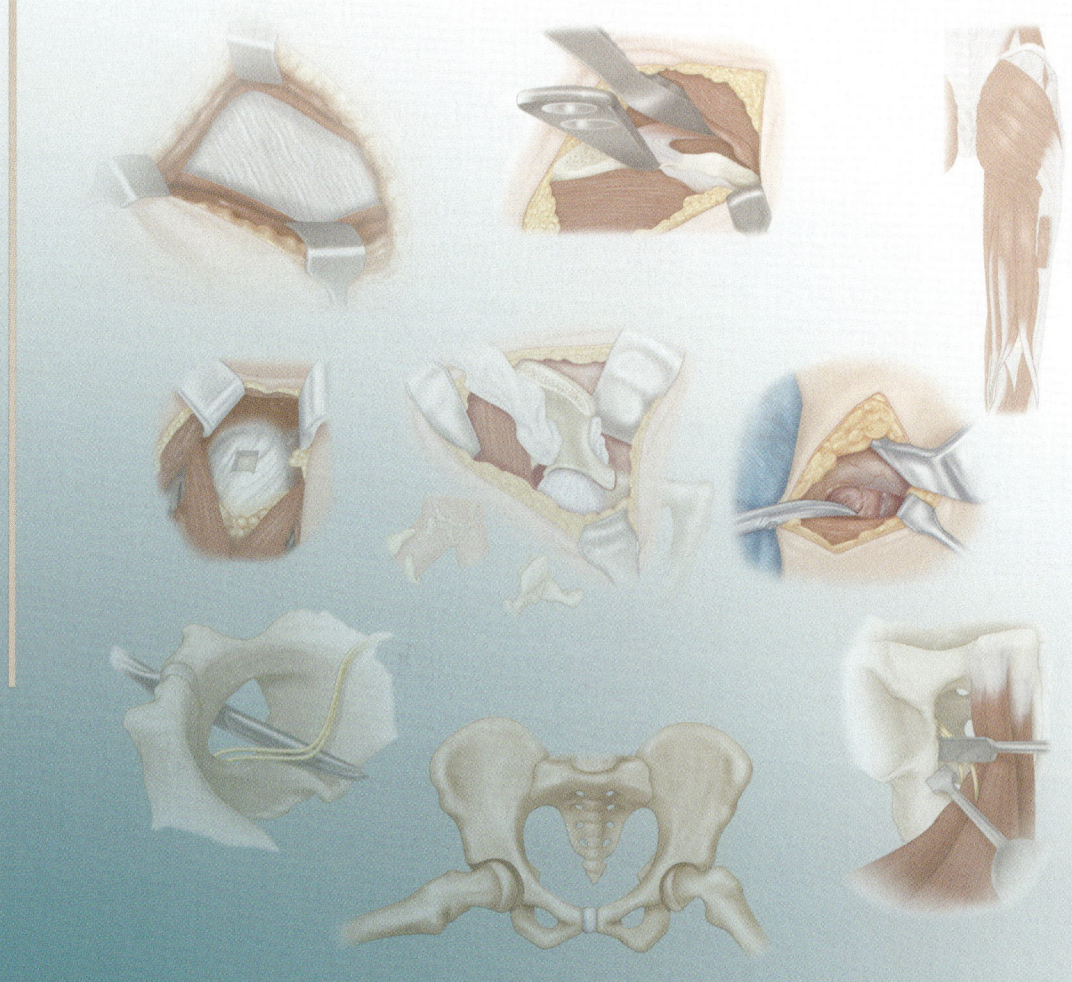

Controversies

- Because clinically poor outcome is associated with surgical treatment after 4 days from onset, observation up to 3 days may enter the management algorithm for equivocal presentations.

Treatment Options

- Joint evacuation is essential.

- Incision and drainage is recommended for central or axial joint infections, such as hip pyarthritis. Serial aspiration is accepted for peripheral or appendicular joint infections, such as ankle pyarthritis (Herndon et al., 1986). Having said this, no prospective randomized trials exist comparing the two methods for the two types of joints.

- Synovial fluid is sent for analysis before commencing antibiotics.

INDICATIONS

- Diagnosis of hip pyarthritis includes:
  - History of inability to bear weight
  - Presence of fever
  - A physical examination showing restricted and painful range of motion
  - Confirmatory laboratory data, including leukocyte count greater than 12,000, erythrocyte sedimentation rate ≥40 mm/hr and C-reactive protein greater than >2.0 mg/dl
- Taking into account ability to bear weight, fever, leukocyte count, and erythrocyte sedimentation rate, the predicted probability of septic arthritis is 3% for one predictor, 40% for two, 93% for three, and 99.6% for four (Kocher et al., 1999).
- C-reactive protein less than 1 mg/dl has an 87% negative predictive value (Levine et al., 2003).

EXAMINATION/IMAGING

- Imaging plays a relatively small role in the diagnosis of hip pyarthritis.
- Radiographs may show displacement of the proximal femoral epiphysis by effusion, as seen in the left proximal femoral subluxation in Figure 1. In addition, they may exclude other causes of hip pain and stiffness.
- Ultrasonography may determine quantitatively the presence and size of hip effusion, and qualitatively the nature of such an effusion (Zieger et al., 1987).
- Magnetic resonance imaging is useful for differential diagnosis of an extracoxal source of infection, such as psoas abscess. Figure 2 demonstrates an abscess within the left iliacus on coronal (Fig. 2A) and axial (Fig. 2B) magnetic resonance imaging.

SURGICAL ANATOMY

- The most common surgical approach is the anterior approach of Smith-Petersen (developed originally for arthroplasty).
- The superficial interval is between the sartorius and tensor fasciae latae (Fig. 3, *arrow*). The deep interval is between the rectus femoris and gluteus medius (Smith-Petersen, 1949).

POSITIONING

- The patient is positioned supine.
- The hindquarter is isolated.

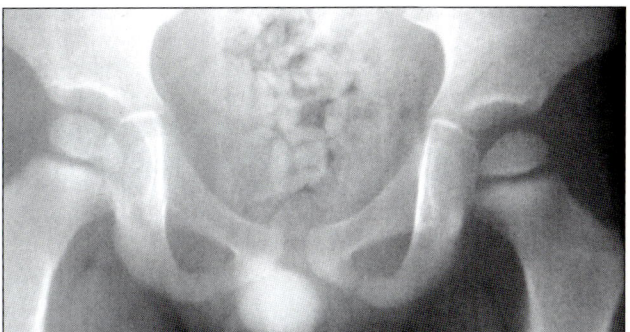

FIGURE 1

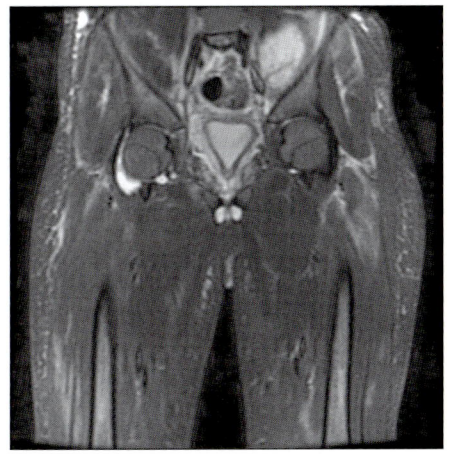

A

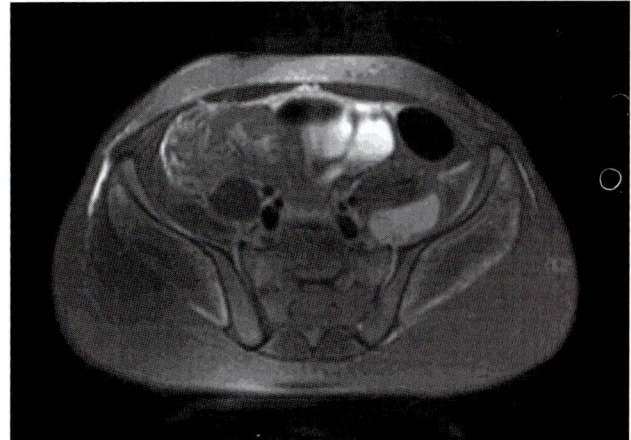

B

FIGURE 2

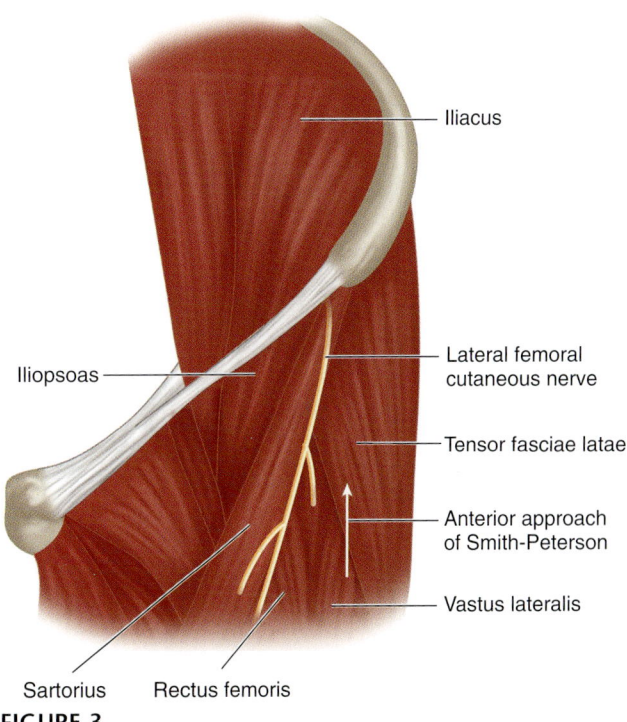

Iliacus

Iliopsoas

Lateral femoral
cutaneous nerve

Tensor fasciae latae

Anterior approach
of Smith-Peterson

Vastus lateralis

Sartorius   Rectus femoris

FIGURE 3

Instrumentation

- Blunt right-angled retractors are sufficient to maintain the surgical window.

PORTALS/EXPOSURES

- The incision has evolved from vertical as described by Smith-Petersen to oblique as modified by Salter (1961). The latter has been given the appellation "bikini line" incision (Fig. 4), because it may be covered by such a garment.
- The incision begins 2 fingerbreadths below the anterior superior iliac spine at the sartorius, and extends obliquely lateral-superior for 2–3 fingerbreadths in Langer's cutaneous lines.

PROCEDURE

STEP 1

- The superficial fascia is incised in line with the cutaneous incision.
- The fascia of the tensor fasciae latae is cut sharply in line with its fibers. The tensor is reflected from the medial sheath to gain access to the deep interval (Fig. 5).
- The deep interval between the rectus femoris and gluteus medius is developed bluntly. In Figure 6, the hip capsule can be seen between the gluteus medius and the rectus femoris muscles.

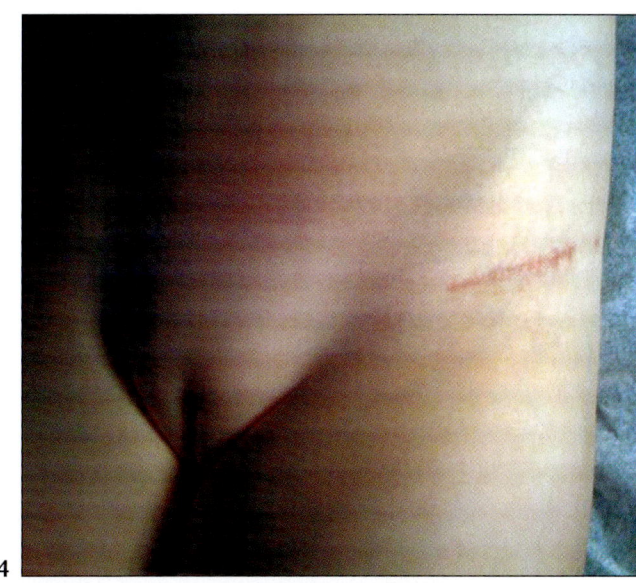

FIGURE 4

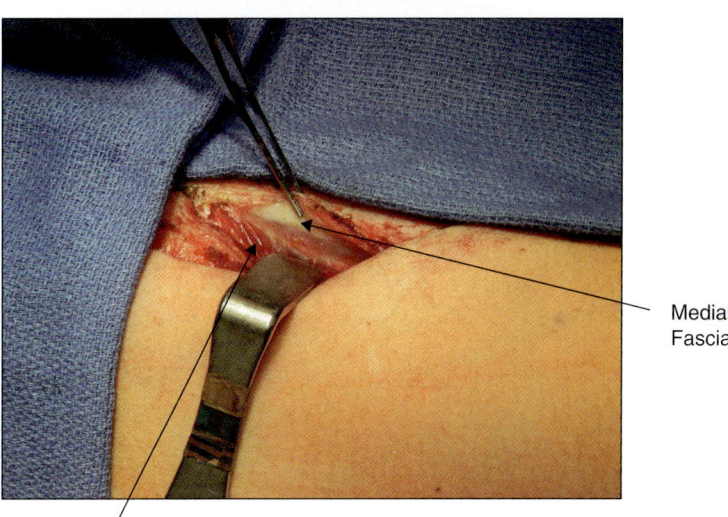

Medial
Fascia

FIGURE 5   Tensor Fasciae Lata

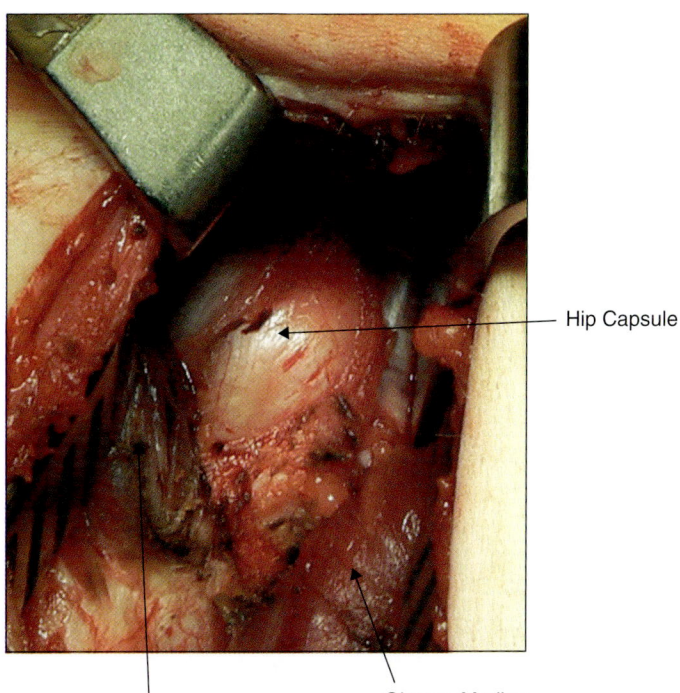

Hip Capsule

FIGURE 6   Rectus Femoris   Gluteus Medius

STEP 2

- Fat overlying the hip is swept away with a sponge and elevator.
- The distended hip joint capsule is secured with a clamp, and a 1-cm^2 window is excised to allow spontaneous drainage (Fig. 7).
- Fluid from the hip joint is sent for cell count, Gram stain, and culture and sensitivity, after which intravenous antibiotics may be administered.
- The hip joint is irrigated thoroughly with crystalloid, putting the joint through a full range of motion to break up any loculations.
- A drain is placed inside the hip joint around the neck of the femur. It is brought out proximally through a separate stab incision in line with the cutaneous incision, and is left to bulb suction.

STEP 3

- The structures of the deep and superficial intervals are allowed to fall together spontaneously.
- The skin is closed loosely with interrupted nonabsorbable monofilament suture.

POSTOPERATIVE CARE AND EXPECTED OUTCOMES

- The patient is restricted to bed rest until the wound is dry, then activity as tolerated. No other immobilization is necessary.
- The drain is removed when the wound is dry.
- Antibiotics are tailored according to culture results, although these are productive in only half of cases.
  - Intravenous antibiotics are given until clinical and laboratory response is achieved. The former is defined as normal body temperature, significant diminution in pain, and a dry wound. The latter is defined as a normal leukocyte count and a downward-trending C-reactive protein to less than 2 mg/dl.
  - After adequate clinical and laboratory response, the patient is converted to oral antibiotics. These are continued on an outpatient basis until the erythrocyte sedimentation rate is less than 20 mm/hr.

PITFALLS

- *Inadequate clinical and laboratory response by 72 hours after drainage is an indication for further intervention. This may include further imaging, alteration in antibiotic administration, and repeat incision and drainage.*

Controversies

- The window for intravenous antibiotics, and for total duration of antibiotics, is narrowing. Duration determined by clinical and laboratory response is preferable to an arbitrary period such as the traditional 6 weeks.

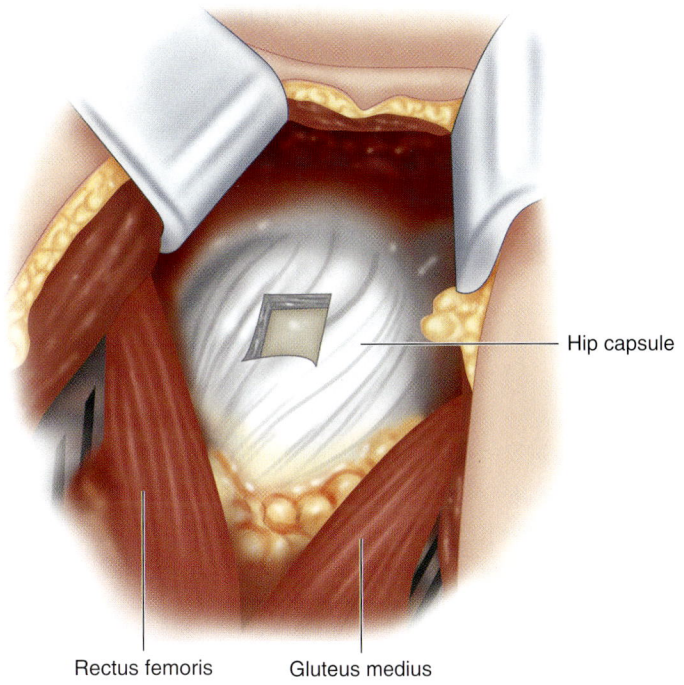

Hip capsule

Rectus femoris   Gluteus medius

FIGURE 7

EVIDENCE

Choi IH, Pizzutillo PD, Bowen JR, Dragann R, Malhis T. Sequelae and reconstruction after septic arthritis of the hip in infants. J Bone Joint Surg [Am]. 1990;72:1150–65.

Herndon WA, Knauer S, Sullivan JA, Gross RH. Management of septic arthritis in children. J Pediatr Orthop. 1986;6:576–8.

Kocher MS, Zurakowski D, Kasser JR. Differentiating between septic arthritis and transient synovitis of the hip in children: an evidence-based clinical prediction algorithm. J Bone Joint Surg [Am]. 1999;81:1662–70.

Levine MJ, McGuire KJ, McGowan KL, Flynn JM. Assessment of the test characteristics of C-reactive protein for septic arthritis in children. J Pediatr Orthop. 2003;23:373–7.

Luhmann SJ, Jones A, Schootman M, Gordon JE, Schoenecker PL, Luhmann JD. Differentiation between septic arthritis and transient synovitis of the hip in children with clinical prediction algorithms. J Bone Joint Surg [Am]. 2004;86:956–62.

Salter RB. Innominate osteotomy in the treatment of congenital dislocation and subluxation of the hip. J Bone Joint Surg [Br]. 1961;43:518–39.

Smith-Petersen MN. Approach to and exposure of the hip joint for mold arthroplasty. J Bone Joint Surg [Am]. 1949;31:40–6.

Zieger MM, Dorr U, Schulz RD. Ultrasonography of hip joint effusions. Skeletal Radiol. 1987;16:607–11.

Surgical Dislocation of the Hip

Wudbhav N. Sankar and Michael B. Millis

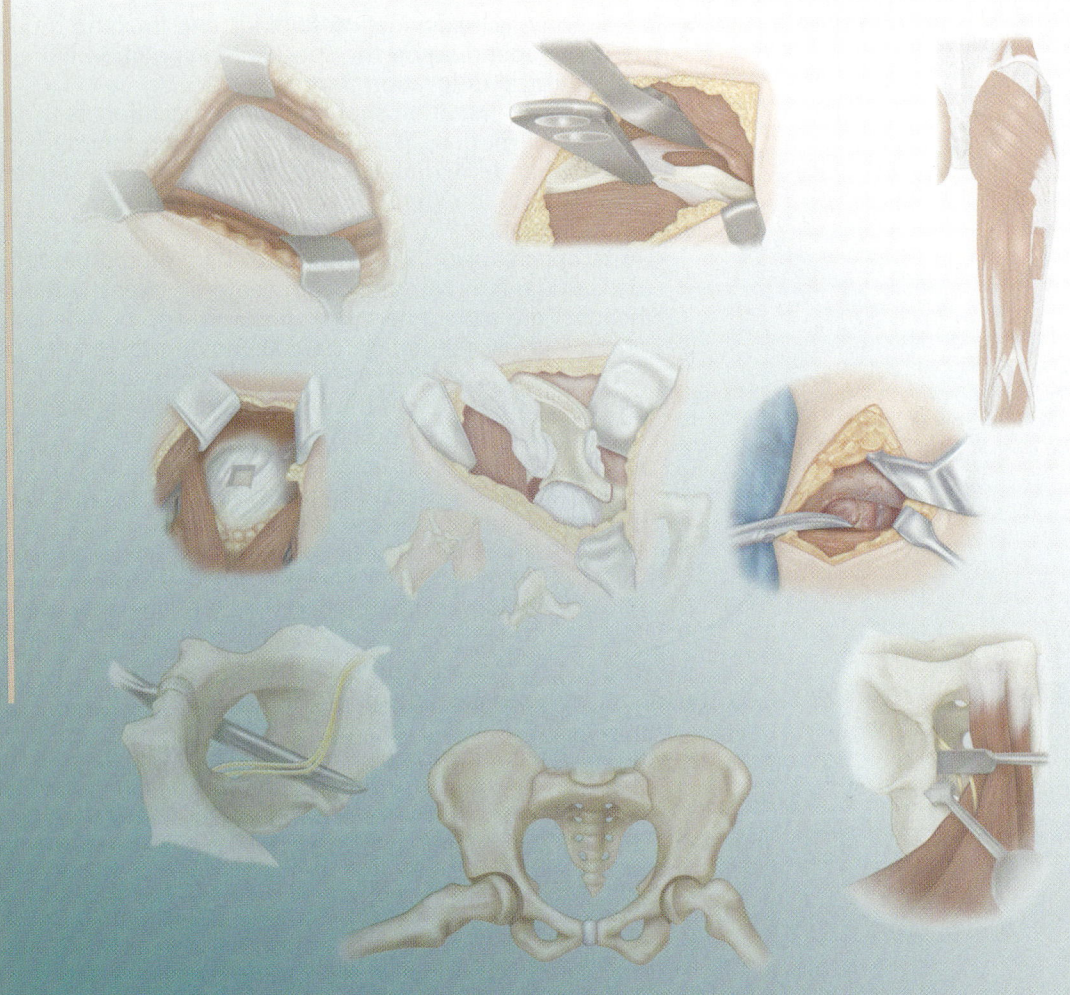

Treatment Options

- A direct anterior approach via the Smith-Petersen interval allows excellent visualization of the anterior head-neck junction without the need for a trochanteric osteotomy; however, circumferential visualization is much more limited. Circumferential visualization is impossible.

- The Watson-Jones approach between the gluteus medius and tensor fascia lata provides excellent access to the anterior neck and intertrochanteric region but limited access to the femoroacetabular articulation.

INDICATIONS

- Femoroacetabular impingement caused by (CAM) and/or pincer-type mechanisms (may be idiopathic or due to Perthes' disease, slipped capital femoral epiphysis, etc.)
- Subcapital realignment of unstable slipped epiphyses
- Intra-articular lesions such as pigmented villonodular synovitis or synovial chondromatosis
- Femoral head and neck fractures
- Any other procedure requiring full exposure of the femoral head, femoral neck, or acetabulum

EXAMINATION/IMAGING

- Specific physical examination findings and imaging modalities may vary depending on the specific hip condition being treated by the surgical dislocation approach.
- In general, examination should include a careful assessment of hip range of motion, including flexion, extension, abduction, adduction, and internal and external rotation. The latter should be tested both in extension and 90° of hip flexion.
- Plain radiographs
  - Anteroposterior (AP) views of both hips should be obtained on a single film with the beam centered over the femoral heads. Care should be taken to ensure appropriate pelvic tilt and avoid pelvic rotation. Lateral center-edge angles can be measured to assess lateral acetabular coverage.
  - On false profile views of both hips, anterior coverage can be evaluated by measuring an anterior center-edge angle.
  - Frog-leg lateral, cross-table lateral, or modified Dunn lateral views have all been used to assess femoral head-neck offset, but many cam lesions can still be missed.
  - Figure 1 shows AP (Fig. 1A) and frog-leg lateral (Fig. 1B) views of the pelvis in a 28-year-old male with cam- and pincer-type femoroacetabular impingement. Note the decrease in femoral head-neck offset, the large cam deformity, and the right rim fracture caused by impingement.
- Magnetic resonance imaging (MRI): diGEMRIC with radial sequences
  - diGEMRIC MRI is the best imaging study to evaluate the soft tissues of the hip, including the labrum, ligamentum teres, and extracapsular musculature.
  - diGEMRIC sequences are especially useful for evaluating the health of the articular cartilage and identifying chondral flaps.
  - Radial cuts taken circumferentially around the femoral head and neck allow better identification of subtle cam lesions. In a 20-year-old female with right hip pain, a plain AP radiograph is somewhat suggestive of a cam deformity, but the findings are subtle (Fig. 2A). Radial sequence MRI of the same hip, however, clearly shows the cam morphology (Fig. 2B).

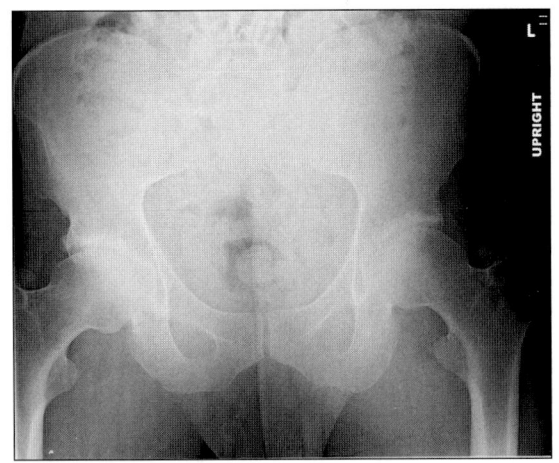

A
FIGURE 1

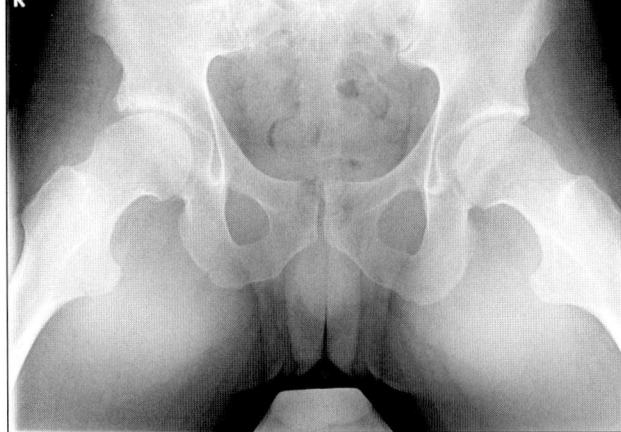

B

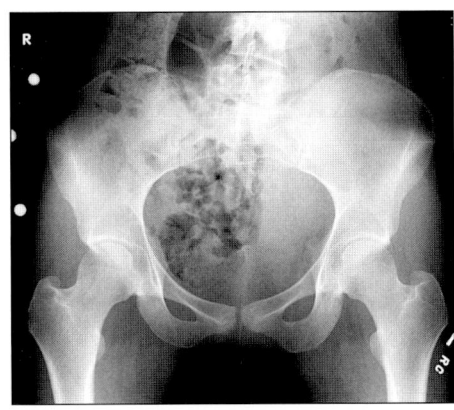

A
FIGURE 2

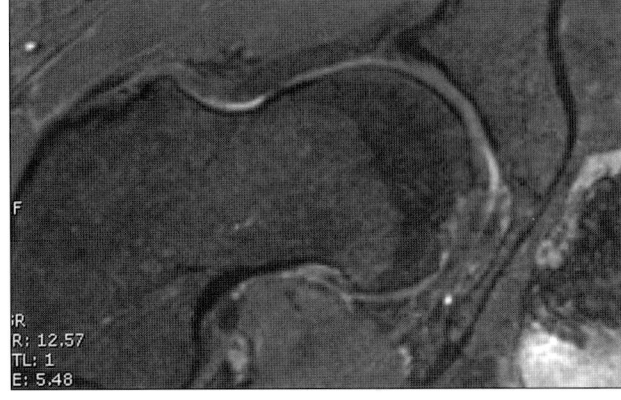

B

Equipment

• Pegboard and gel-lined pegs

• "Pillow-tunnel" or standard bed pillows

• Cardiac armholder

SURGICAL ANATOMY

■ The main blood supply to the femoral head arises from branches of the medial femoral circumflex artery (MFCA), and preservation of this blood supply is critical to achieving safe surgical dislocation of the hip (Fig. 3).

■ The trochanteric branch of the MFCA does not contribute appreciably to the perfusion of the femoral head but is a constant landmark that will guide the surgeon to the level of the obturator externus.

■ The deep branch of the MFCA is the largest contributor to femoral head perfusion. It crosses posterior to the obturator externus and anterior to the tendons of the superior gemellus, obturator internus, and inferior gemellus. It perforates the capsule of the hip just proximal to the insertion of the tendon of the superior gemellus and distal to the tendon of the piriformis.

■ During dislocation of the hip, this vessel is protected by the intact obturator externus muscle.

POSITIONING

■ The patient is placed in a lateral decubitus position on a radiolucent table (Jackson, Steris, etc.) using a pegboard.
  • We prefer the use of a pegboard, but other positioning aids are equally effective.

■ The ipsilateral arm is placed in a safe position using a cardiac armholder.

■ A special pillow placed over the down leg to protect it also provides a good working surface on which to lay and position the operative leg (Fig. 4). Alternatively, standard pillows can be used over the down leg.

■ A plastic hip drape is used that will allow placement of the leg into a sterile bag during the anterior dislocation maneuver.

PORTALS/EXPOSURES

■ A longitudinal incision is made over the lateral aspect of the femur, centered over the anterior third of the greater trochanter.
  • The proximal extent of the incision is just distal to the iliac crest, and the distal end of the incision is 6–8 cm past the vastus ridge. The average incision length is 20–25 cm.
  • The Gibson approach starts with a straight incision centered over the anterior third of the greater trochanter (Fig. 5).
  • Alternatively, the cephalad limb of the incision can be curved posteriorly for the Kocher-Langenback approach.

■ The subcutaneous tissues are divided sharply down to the level of the iliotibial band and the fascia over the gluteus maximus muscle. The gluteus maximus should be released at its anterior edge. The anterior border of the gluteus maximus can be located by identifying the perforating branches of the inferior gluteal artery (Fig. 6, A). These blood vessels are constant and mark the anterior edge of the muscle.

■ The fascia overlying the gluteus maximus should be preserved and the muscle can be released along its anterior edge. Distally, the fascia lata can be split in line with the femur.

■ The fatty tissue overlying the gluteus medius should be cleared off and the bursa should be reflected anteriorly to fully expose the vastus ridge and the trochanteric branch of the MFCA.

■ The fascia of the vastus lateralis should be incised in line with the femur just anterior to the posterior edge, and the muscle fibers should be dissected off of the lateral femur extraperiosteally.

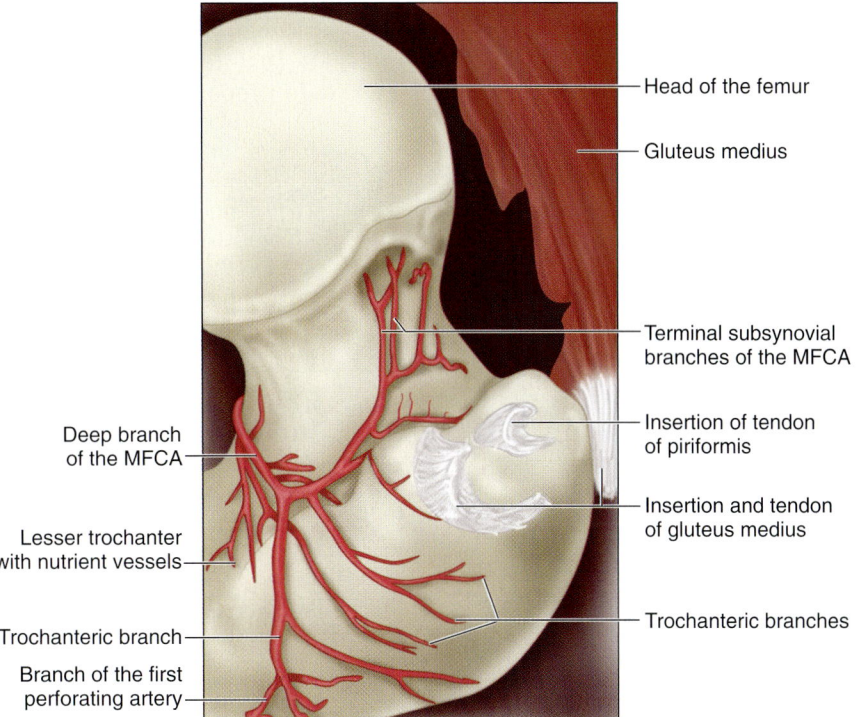

Head of the femur

Gluteus medius

Terminal subsynovial
branches of the MFCA

Insertion of tendon
of piriformis

Insertion and tendon
of gluteus medius

Deep branch
of the MFCA

Lesser trochanter
with nutrient vessels

Trochanteric branch

Branch of the first
perforating artery

Trochanteric branches

FIGURE 3

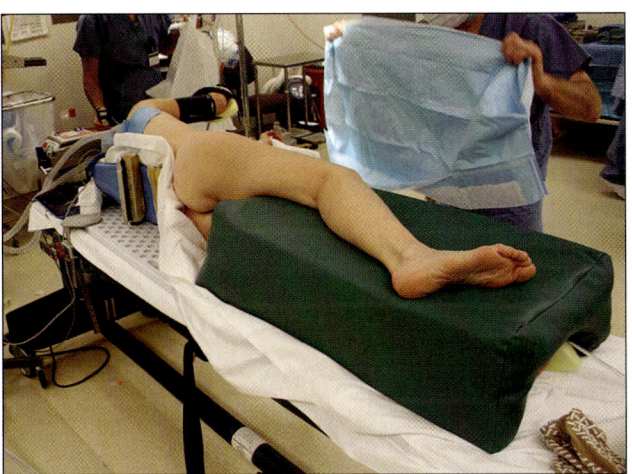

FIGURE 4

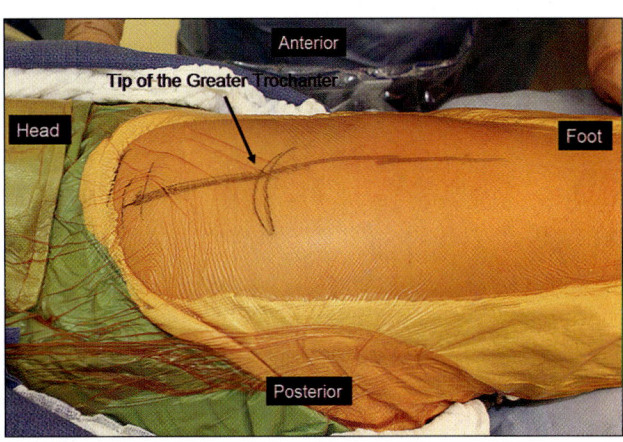

FIGURE 5

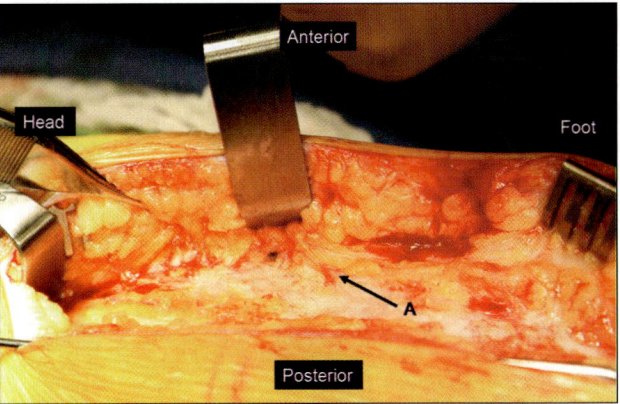

FIGURE 6

PEARLS

- *The goal of the trochanteric osteotomy is to keep the insertions of the gluteus medius, gluteus minimus, and vastus lateralis on the trochanteric fragment.*

- *The majority of the piriformis should stay with the proximal femur (the piriformis tendon protects the deep branch of the MFCA).*

PITFALLS

- *An osteotomy that is too deep, extending into the base of the neck, risks osteonecrosis of the femoral head.*

- *A trochanteric fragment that is too thin may fracture during attempted fixation.*

PEARLS

- *Staying superior to the piriformis during the capsular exposure protects the anastomosis between the inferior gluteal artery and the MFCA, which runs along the distal border of the tendon.*

- *Preservation of the short external rotators provides protection to the MFCA.*

PITFALLS

- *The sciatic nerve runs in close proximity to the piriformis muscle and is at risk if the capsular exposure is performed distal to the tendon. This risk is even higher for those rare patients who have anomalous branching of the sciatic nerve such that it encloses the piriformis tendon.*

PEARLS

- *Branches of the lateral femoral circumflex artery often need to be cauterized during the inferomedial capsulotomy. These do not contribute appreciably to the perfusion of the femoral head.*

- *A small cuff of tissue should be left on the inferior neck during the inferomedial capsulotomy to facilitate later closure of the capsule.*

PITFALLS

- *The inferomedial limb of the capsulotomy must remain anterior to the lesser trochanter to avoid any damage to the main branch of the MFCA.*

PROCEDURE

STEP 1: TROCHANTERIC OSTEOTOMY

- To prepare the hip for the trochanteric osteotomy, the hip should be extended and internally rotated 20–30° and the posterior border of the gluteus medius should be identified.
- The periosteal incision for the trochanteric osteotomy is made from the posterior-superior edge of the greater trochanter to the posterior border of the vastus lateralis ridge (Fig. 7, *dotted line A–B*). Use of Bovie electrocautery allows cauterization of the trochanteric branch of the MFCA.
- At its proximal end, the osteotomy should exit just anterior to the most posterior insertion of the gluteus medius.
- The trochanteric osteotomy is made using an oscillating saw from posterior to anterior (Fig. 8). Alternatively, an osteotome can be used. The maximum thickness of the trochanteric fragment should be approximately 1.5 cm. Irrigation is often used to cool the blade.
- A Hohmann retractor is placed over the anterior edge of the osteotomy and the trochanteric fragment is flipped anteriorly. Remaining fibers of the gluteus medius and vastus lateralis that are attached to the stable trochanter may need to be released.

STEP 2: CAPSULAR EXPOSURE

- Posteriorly, the capsule is approached through the interval between the gluteus minimus (Fig. 9, *A*) and the piriformis tendon (Fig. 9, *B*).
- The minimus and the overlying flap are retracted superiorly and anteriorly. The muscle should be sharply dissected from the underlying posterior extension capsule.
- This action is facilitated by extension and internal rotation of the hip.
- Anteriorly, the remaining fibers of the vastus lateralis and vastus intermedius are sharply elevated from the anterior and inferior capsule.
- To facilitate this dissection, the leg should be flexed, abducted, and externally rotated.

STEP 3: CAPSULOTOMY

- After completing the capsular exposure, the capsule is first incised longitudinally along the axis of the anterior femoral neck while taking care not to injure the articular cartilage of the femoral head or the labrum.
- Next, the capsulotomy is continued inferomedially parallel to the intertrochanteric line.
- The final limb of the capsulotomy is performed by incising the capsule along the superior acetabular rim heading posteriorly toward the piriformis.
- The final appearance of the capsulotomy is Z-shaped for a right hip and "reverse" Z-shaped for a left hip (Fig. 10).
- To dislocate the hip, the femoral head is first subluxed by flexing and externally rotating the hip. The use of a bone hook around the femoral neck facilitates this maneuver (Fig. 11, *A*).
- Curved scissors are then inserted into the joint and used to cut the ligamentum teres (see Fig. 11, *B*).
- The hip can now be fully dislocated and the foot and leg can be placed into the anterior sterile bag.

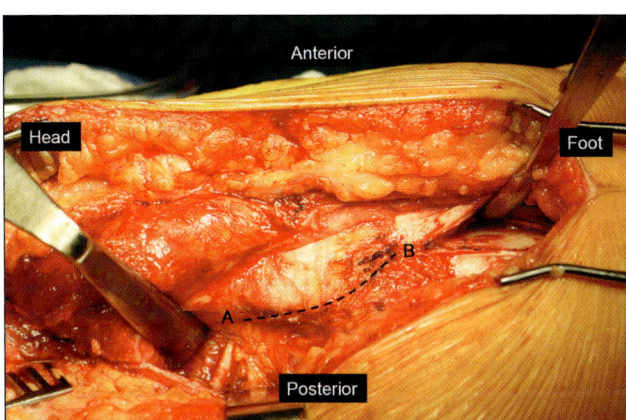

FIGURE 7

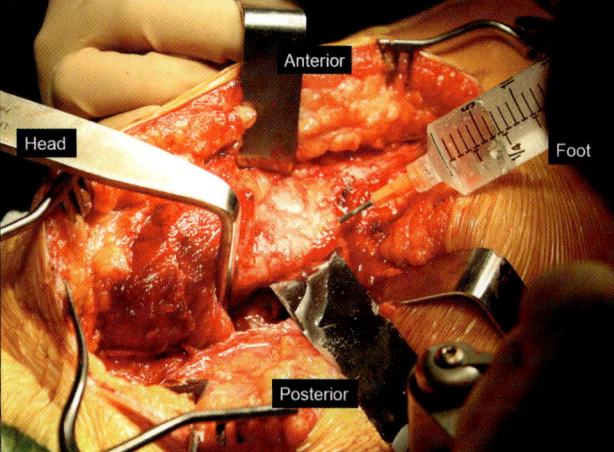

FIGURE 8

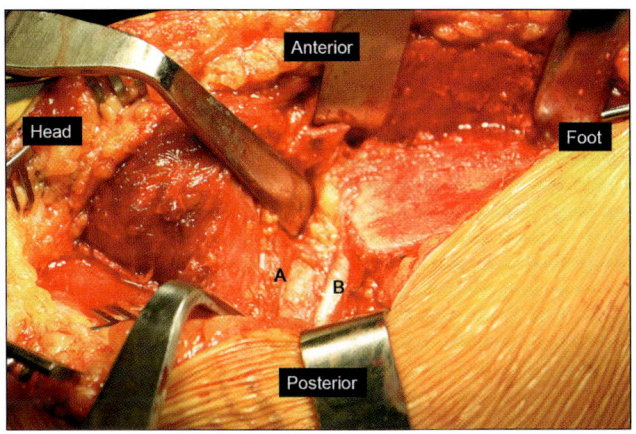

FIGURE 9

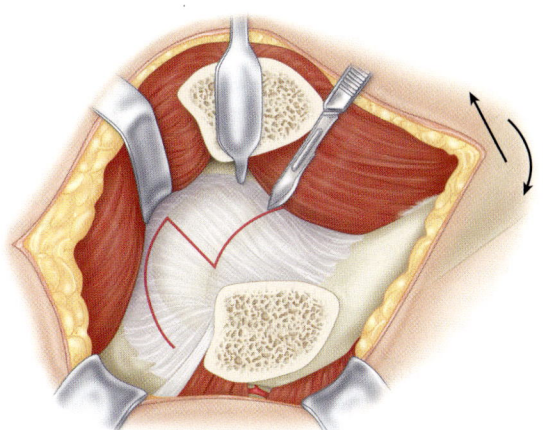

FIGURE 10

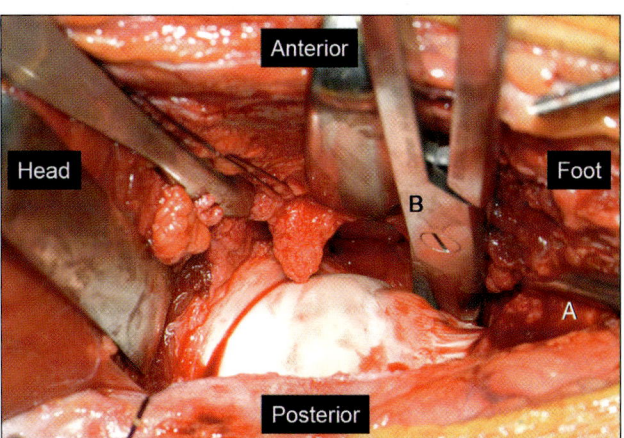

FIGURE 11

STEP 4: INTRA-ARTICULAR SURGERY

- Regardless of the goals of the specific procedure, any hip that has been surgically dislocated should undergo a thorough inspection of both the acetabulum and the femoral head
- The acetabulum can be better visualized by using angled Hohmann retractors around the rim and a bone hook to retract the proximal femur out of the way (Fig. 12, *A* and *B*).
  - Use of a nerve hook can facilitate inspection of the labrum and articular cartilage (see Fig. 12, *C*).
  - If more extensive acetabular work is necessary, as for a rim trim, a spiked Hohmann can be placed anteriorly over the anterior inferior iliac spine and a second can be placed more proximally in the ilium above the acetabular dome.
  - Chondrolabral dissociations and chondral flaps, when present, are generally located superior and anterior within the joint
- The femoral head is easily visualized.
  - Any remaining ligamentum teres should be transected at the level of the fovea and removed.
  - In cases of cam-type femoroacetabular impingement, the prominent area is easily identified by its contour and the abnormal bruising of the articular surface (Fig. 13, *arrow*). Spherometers can be useful to localize the area of asphericity (Fig. 14).
  - Osteoplasties of the head-neck junction are performed by first using a scalpel to circumscribe the lesion; a curved osteotome and a burr are then used to remove the cam lesion and re-establish adequate femoral head-neck offset (Fig. 15). Spherometers are again useful to confirm the adequacy of the osteoplasty (Fig. 16).

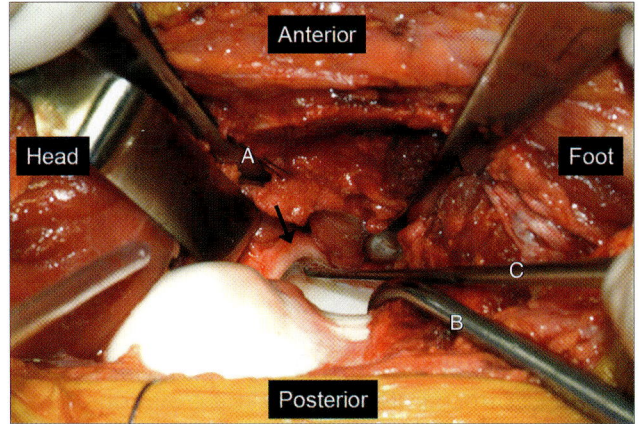

FIGURE 12

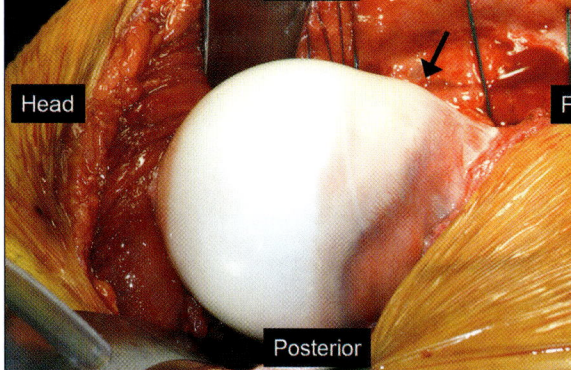

FIGURE 13

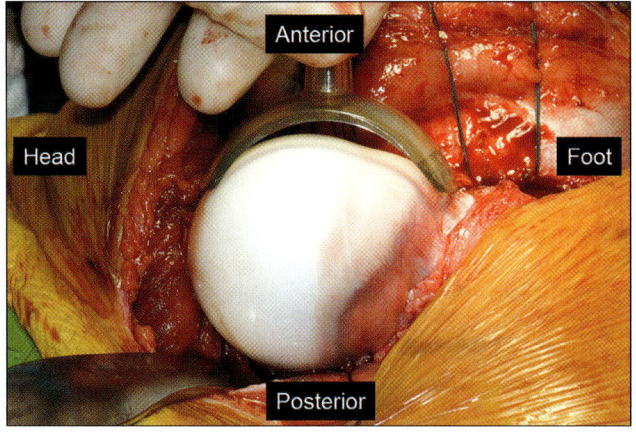

FIGURE 14

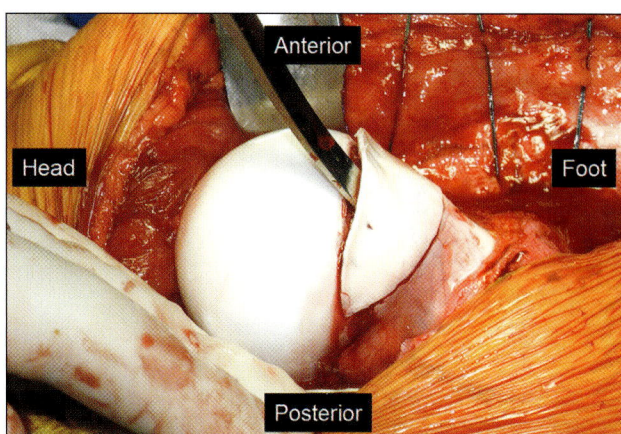

FIGURE 15

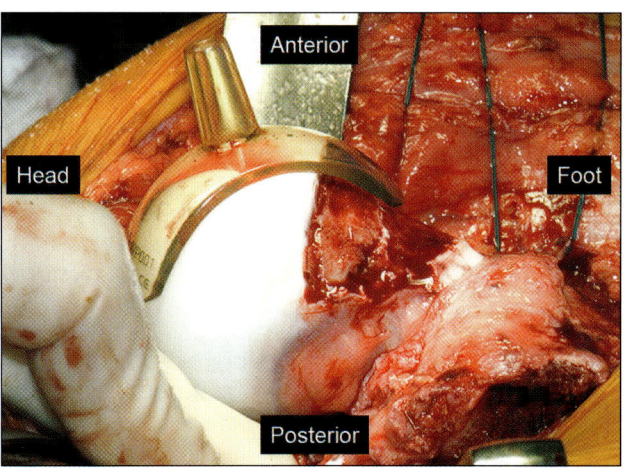

FIGURE 16

PEARLS

- *The capsule does not need to be closed watertight. The risks of postoperative dislocation are minimal as long as flexion, adduction, and external rotation are avoided in the first few weeks after surgery.*

PITFALLS

- *The trajectory of the trochanteric screws should be from proximal to distal. If the screws are inserted in a transverse fashion, the tips of the screws may cause a stress riser at the base of the femoral neck.*

PEARLS

- *The use of indomethacin, ketorolac, or other potent nonsteroidal anti-inflammatory drugs during the early postoperative period may limit the regrowth of bone after an osteoplasty.*

PITFALLS

- *During the healing phase of the trochanteric osteotomy, abductor function can be compromised. Weight bearing too early without the use of one or two crutches can lead to a painful Trendelenburg gait, or worse, a trochanteric nonunion.*

Controversies

- There is no evidence to support the use of CPM after surgical dislocations of the hip. Anecdotally, however, we have found that CPM limits the amount of scar formation after open dislocation and preserves range of motion.

STEP 5: FIXATION OF THE TROCHANTERIC OSTEOTOMY AND CLOSURE

- After completion of the intra-articular portion of the surgery, the joint is irrigated copiously and the femoral head is gently relocated. The hip is put through a full range of motion to ensure that it is free of impingement.
- The flaps of the capsule are reapproximated and loosely closed using interrupted 2-0 Vicryl stiches (Fig. 17). The capsule does not need to be closed watertight.
- The trochanteric fragment is reduced to its original position and fixed to the proximal femur using three 4.5-mm cannulated screws or small fragment screws (Fig. 18). The general trajectory of the screws is from lateral and proximal to medial and distal (i.e., toward the lesser trochanter), as seen in the intraoperative fluoroscopic view in Figure 19.
- The vastus lateralis fascia is repaired using a running absorbable suture.
- The fascia lata is closed with a running heavy Vicryl suture. A deep drain may be placed if desired by the surgeon.
- The subcutaneous tissues and skin are closed in a layered fashion using absorbable suture.

POSTOPERATIVE CARE AND EXPECTED OUTCOMES

- Patients are placed into a standard lower extremity continuous passive motion (CPM) machine with settings of 30–80°. Motion is started in the postanesthesia recovery unit and continued during the inpatient stay. After discharge, we recommend that the CPM machine be used approximately 8 hours a day for 4 weeks.
- Pain is generally managed postoperatively with intravenous patient-controlled analgesia. If more extensive bone work has been done (e.g., intertrochanteric osteotomy), we generally prefer epidural and general analgesia.
- Patients are generally mobilized by physical therapy on postoperative day 1–2.
- Patients are allowed to bear one sixth of their body weight on the operative side, and use crutches to ambulate.
- Flexion-extension range of motion is limited to 30–80° for the first four weeks primarily for patient comfort.
- Active abduction is limited for the first 4–8 weeks after surgery to facilitate healing of the trochanteric osteotomy.
- If an osteoplasty has been performed, patients are discharged on an oral regimen of indomethacin (generally, 25 mg PO tid) for 4 weeks as prophylaxis against bone regrowth.
- Anticoagulation may be necessary depending on the age of the patient and associated risk factors.
- At the 4-week postoperative appointment, patients are progressed to full weight bearing with one crutch if radiographs show satisfactory healing of the trochanteric osteotomy.
- Most patients are able to discontinue walking aids and bear weight normally by 8 weeks after surgery.

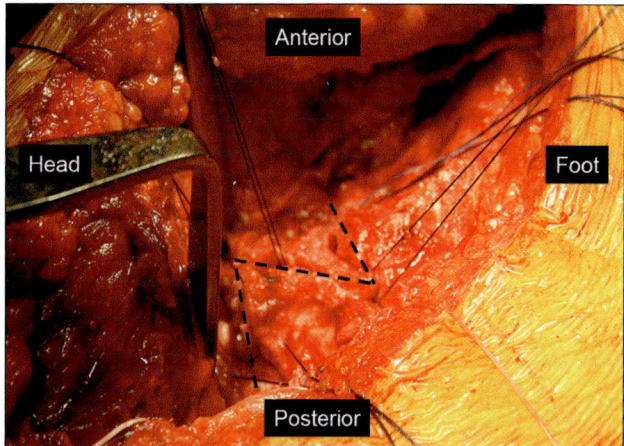

FIGURE 17

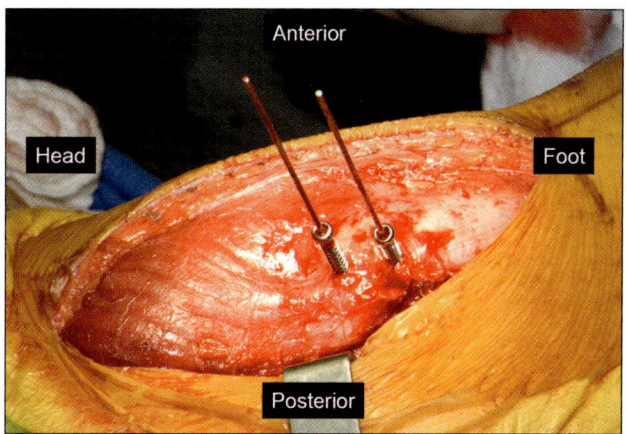

FIGURE 18

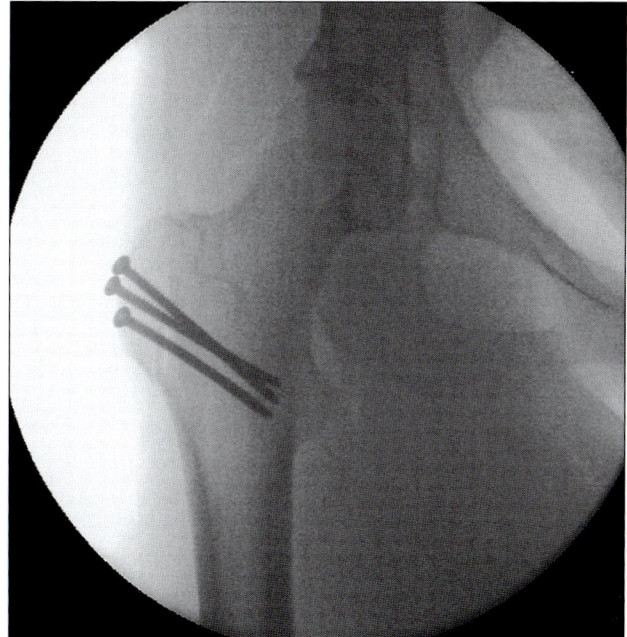

FIGURE 19

EVIDENCE

Surgical dislocation of the hip is a relatively new procedure. As a result, the literature is limited to retrospective case series (i.e., Level IV evidence).

Beck M, Leunig M, Parvizi J, Boutier V, Wyss D, Ganz R. Anterior femoroacetabular impingement: part II. Midterm results of surgical treatment. Clin Orthop Relat Res. 2004;(418):67–73.

This study was a retrospective review of 19 adults treated for femoroacetabular impingement with surgical dislocation and creation of offset. Five of 19 patients failed treatment and eventually required total hip arthroplasty; most had greater than grade I osteoarthrosis of the hip prior to treatment. The authors concluded that surgical dislocation and osteoplasty was an effective treatment option for correcting impingement in patients with limited degenerative changes. (Level IV evidence)

Espinosa N, Beck M, Rothenfluh DA, Ganz R, Leunig M. Treatment of femoro-acetabular impingement: preliminary results of labral refixation. Surgical technique. J Bone Joint Surg [Am]. 2007;89(Suppl 2 Pt 1):36–53.

The authors presented an excellent discussion of the surgical technique, as well as a retrospective review of 60 hips treated for cam- and (predominantly) pincer-type femoroacetabular impingement. Patients who underwent rim trim and labral refixation had superior long-term outcomes compared to those who had trimming of their acetabular rim and débridement of their labrum. (Level IV evidence)

Ganz R, Gill TJ, Gautier E, Ganz K, Krugel N, Berlemann U. Surgical dislocation of the adult hip: a technique with full access to the femoral head and acetabulum without the risk of avascular necrosis. J Bone Joint Surg [Br]. 2001;83:1119–1124.

This paper was one of the original descriptions of the surgical dislocation technique from the group in Bern, Switzerland. In a series of 213 hips treated with this technique for various indications, no cases of avascular necrosis were found. Two cases of partial sciatic nerve palsies were reported, as well as three patients who required refixation of their trochanteric osteotomy for nonunion. (Level IV evidence)

Gautier E, Ganz K, Krugel N, Gill T, Ganz R. Anatomy of the medial femoral circumflex artery and its surgical implications. J Bone Joint Surg [Br]. 2000;82:679.

This foundational anatomic study on 24 human cadavers described the perfusion of the femoral head and provided the anatomic background for the safe surgical dislocation technique.

Kim YJ, Millis MB. Safe surgical dislocation of the hip. Oper Tech Orthop. 2005;15:338–344.

The authors provided a detailed discussion of the surgical technique, and also included a retrospective series of 80 hips treated with surgical dislocation. Mean WOMAC pain scores decreased from 7.4 to 3.8, and complications were limited. (Level IV evidence)

Rebello G, Spencer S, Millis MB, Kim YJ. Surgical dislocation in the management of pediatric and adolescent hip deformity. Clin Orthop Relat Res. 2009;(467):724–731.

This retrospective review of a large series of patients with various pediatric hip conditions included patients with slipped capital femoral epiphysis, Perthes' disease, avascular necrosis, and other diagnoses. In general, WOMAC pain scores improved after surgical dislocation. Four cases of osteonecrosis were reported: three after concomitant femoral neck osteotomy and one after concomitant intertrochanteric osteotomy (both performed through the surgical dislocation approach). (Level IV evidence)

Percutaneous in situ Cannulated Screw Fixation of Slipped Capital Femoral Epiphysis

Benjamin J. Shore and Michael B. Millis

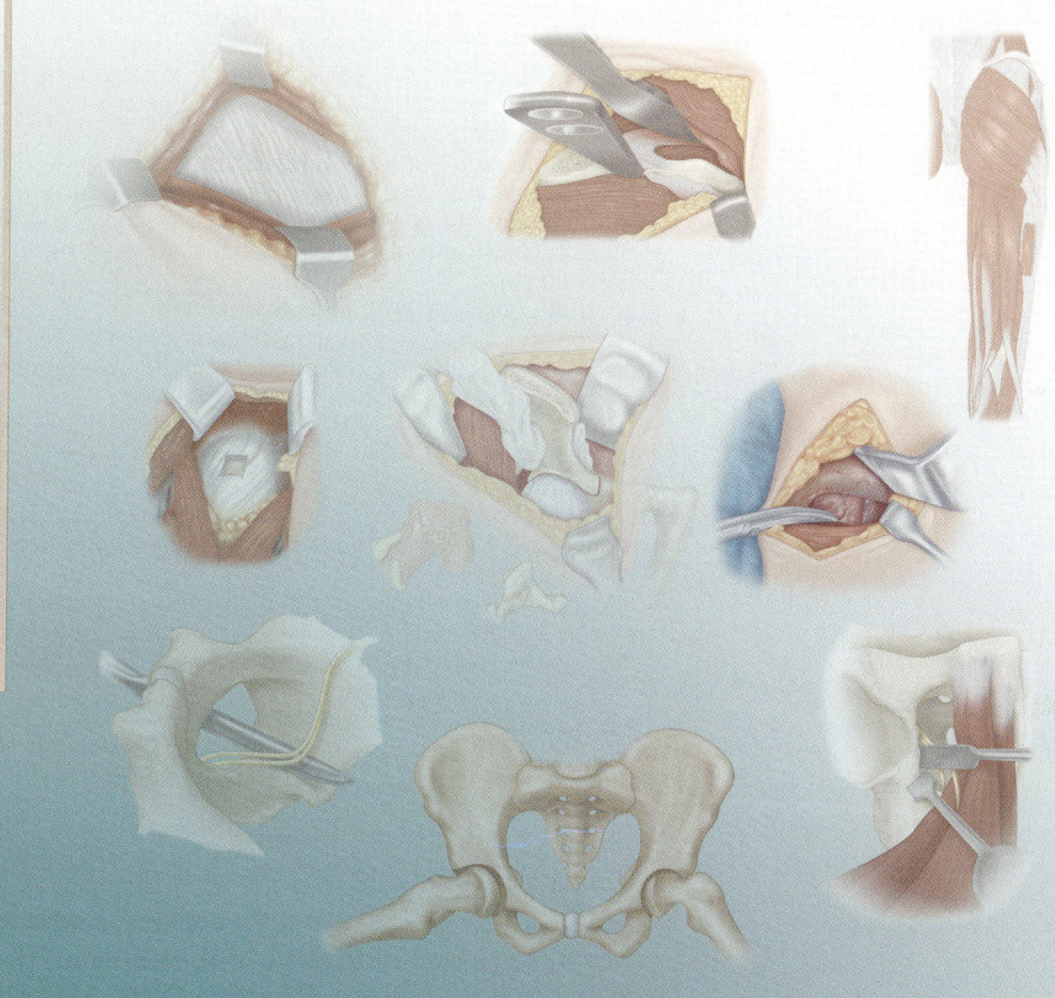

Controversies

• Consider prophylactic pinning of the contralateral side in children presenting at a young age (< 10 years), obese children and those with underlying endocrinopathy such as hypothyroidism, growth hormone deficiency, or secondary hyperparathyroidism, and in children in whom orthopedic follow-up will be challenging.

• Forceful reduction of a displaced SCFE is contraindicated and is related to increased rates of avascular necrosis (AVN). "Inadvertent reduction" with positioning of the patella anteriorly without excessive force is a commonly practiced alternative, with relatively low but not zero risk of AVN.

INDICATIONS

■ A child with a slipped capital femoral epiphysis (SCFE) and an open capital femoral physis.
■ In North America, the "gold standard" treatment for stable SCFE is percutaneous in situ cannulated screw fixation.
■ Orthogonal radiographs are sufficient to diagnose SCFE.

EXAMINATION/IMAGING

■ Symptoms and physical findings vary according to the stability of the physis, chronicity of presentation, and severity of the slip.
■ In the acute and unstable scenario, the patient holds the leg in an externally rotated position on the stretcher and will not tolerate active or passive range of motion and is unable to bear weight on the affected extremity.
■ Patients with stable SCFE exhibit a spectrum of clinical findings.
   • Gait is variably antalgic with a universal external foot progression angle component.
   • Passive hip range of motion reveals a decrease in flexion and internal rotation, with variable reduction in abduction.
   • In moderate and severe SCFE, terminal flexion is coupled with obligate external rotation (as a result of anterior neck impingement).
■ Both anteroposterior (AP) and lateral radiographs are essential for diagnosis. Slips first displace posteriorly, where the AP radiographic findings may be subtle. A line drawn tangential to the superior femoral neck on the AP radiograph (Klein's line) will intersect a smaller portion of the capital epiphysis (Fig. 1A) or not intersect at all (Trethowan's sign; Fig. 1B) compared to the uninvolved hip.
■ Southwick classified the degree of slippage by measuring the femoral head-shaft angle on the AP (Fig. 2A) or frog-leg lateral (Fig. 2B) view.
■ Radiographic examination of the contralateral hip in AP (Fig. 3) and frog-leg lateral (Fig. 4) views at the time of surgery is critical as the incidence of bilateral involvement at initial presentation is at least 25%.
■ Three-dimensional computed tomography scanning is a useful in assessment of deformity of the proximal femur and acetabulum in the setting of SCFE.

Treatment Options

• Pinning in situ is the gold standard for the treatment of stable SCFE.

• Currently, some surgeons are electing to treat moderate and severe slips with open capital reduction, and fixation through either an anterior or trans-trochanteric approach.

• Primary compensating flexion osteotomy through the intertrochanteric area can also be considered in addition to stabilization of the physis.

• The metaphyseal prominence can be removed easily through a limited anterior approach at the time of in situ pinning.

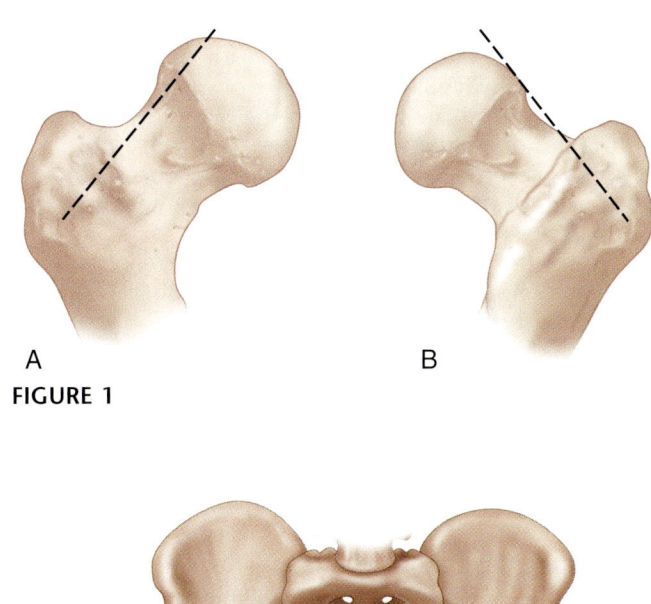

A   B

FIGURE 1

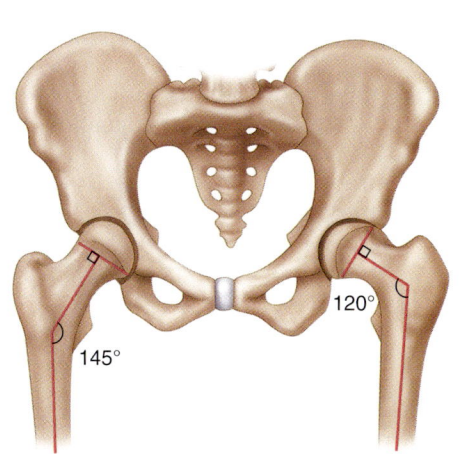

145°   120°

Normal   Slip side

A

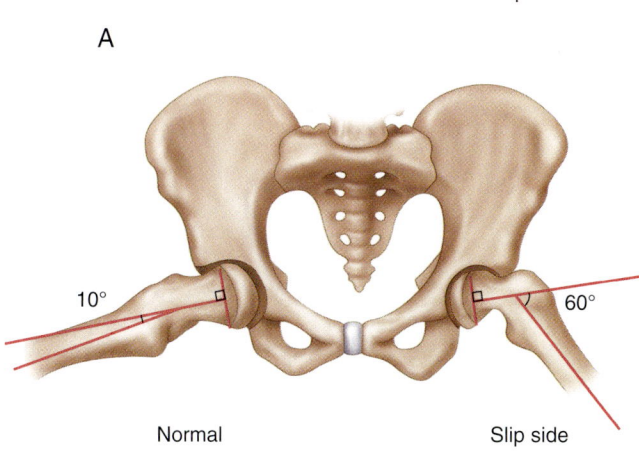

10°   60°

Normal   Slip side

B

FIGURE 2

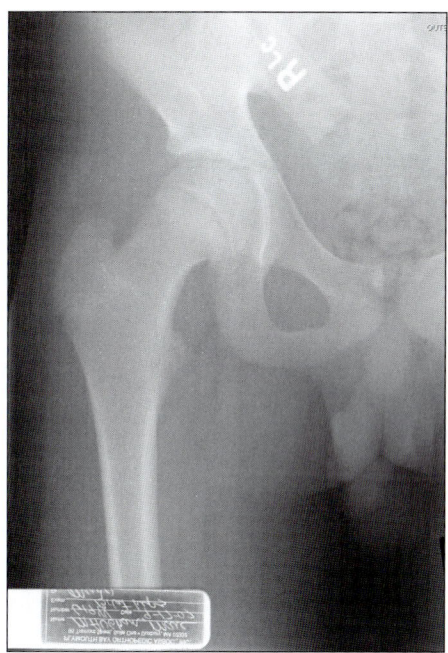

FIGURE 3

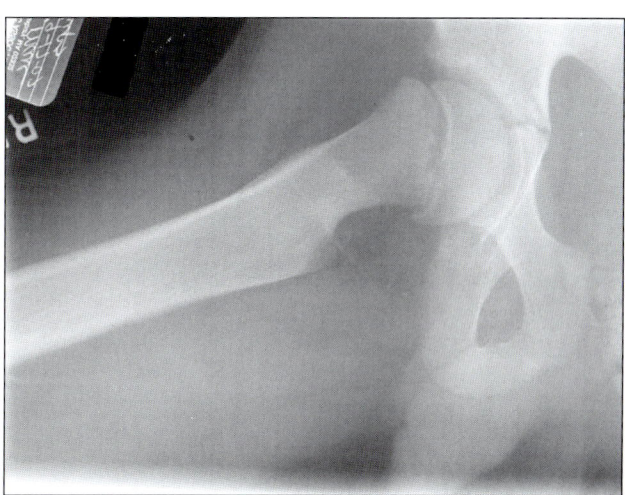

FIGURE 4

SURGICAL ANATOMY

- The capital epiphysis always slips in a posterior direction as the neck moves anteriorly and the femur externally rotates. Vascular structures in the femoral head and neck are shown in Figure 5.
- The correct screw placement for in situ pinning occurs at the anterior capsular junction of the femoral neck at or proximal to the intertrochanteric line.
- Hemorrhage associated with unstable SCFE may increase intracapsular pressure and necessitate arthrotomy of the anterior capsule to decrease the rate of AVN.

POSITIONING

- The position of choice is supine on a radiolucent operating table.
- Great care must be taken to position the patient with an unstable slip.
- Once on the fracture table, position the ipsilateral arm across the body to give the C-arm the greatest space for operation (Fig. 6A–C).
- An experienced radiographer controlling the C-arm is vital to obtaining well-penetrated orthogonal images.

PEARLS

- *Prior to prepping the patient, check with fluoroscopy to ensure that the appropriate orthogonal images can be obtained.*

- *In chronic situations, osteopenia of the femoral head makes it difficult to visualize flouroscopically, and in these situations an arthrogram with a small amount of dye may be helpful.*

PITFALLS

- *For obese children on a radiolucent table, avoid positioning the leg for a frog-leg lateral radiograph. Instead, use the C-arm to "frog" and obtain lateral views.*

  - *If soft tissue tension on the wire is present, a small incision over the wire rectifies this problem.*

- *Excessive internal rotation of an unstable SCFE should be avoided to prevent damage to the remaining intact posterior periosteum and blood supply to the femoral head.*

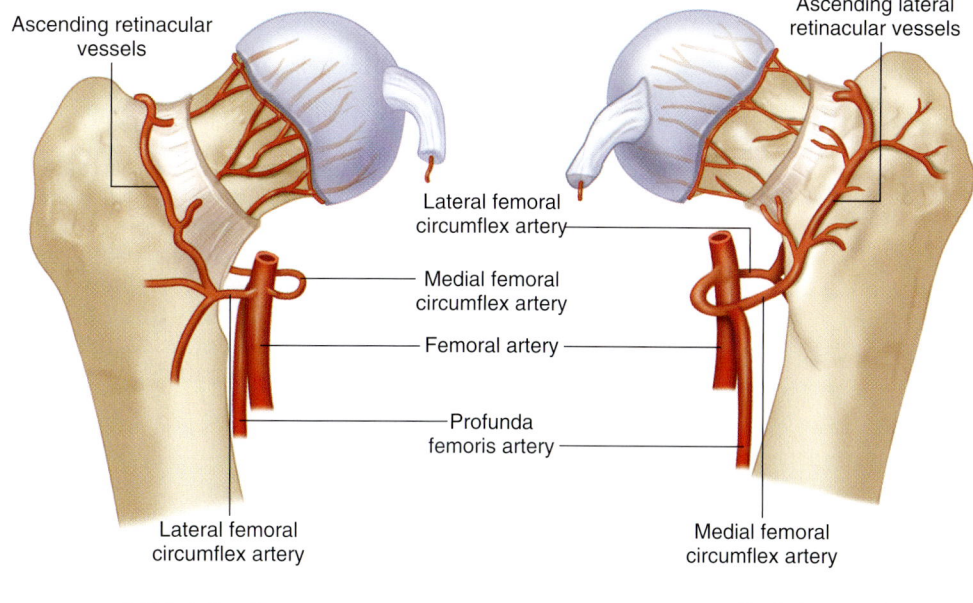

Ascending retinacular vessels

Ascending lateral retinacular vessels

Lateral femoral circumflex artery

Medial femoral circumflex artery

Femoral artery

Profunda femoris artery

Lateral femoral circumflex artery

Medial femoral circumflex artery

Anterior aspect

Posterior aspect

FIGURE 5

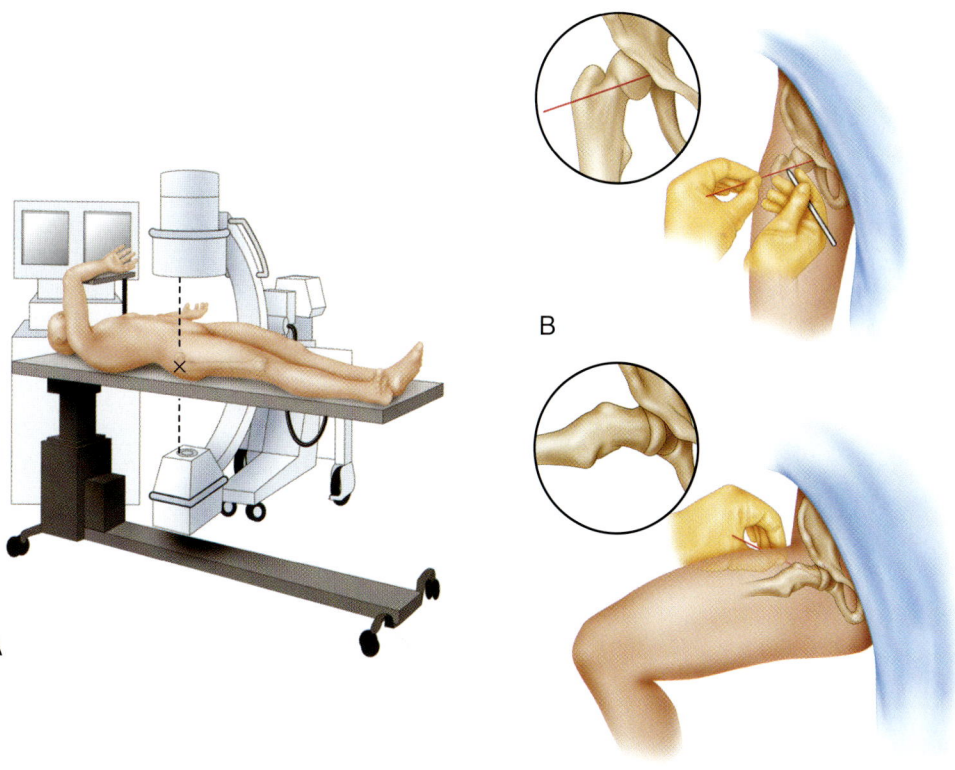

A

B

C

FIGURE 6

PITFALLS

- *The outline of the epiphyseal plate, femoral head, and articular subchondral bone must be visualized radiographically in the AP and lateral planes before surgery is started.*

PORTALS/EXPOSURES

- Each hip is free-draped separately for sterility.
- A guidewire is rested against the skin in the AP and lateral views and the ideal trajectory is marked on the skin with a marking pen (Figs. 7 and 8).
  - The meeting of the two virtual lines marks the incision site. However, the ideal starting point may be slightly proximal to the intersection based on the girth of the patient.
- Make a small (2- to 3-cm) incision extended cranially from the intersection of the virtual lines.
- Blunt dissection occurs through skin, subcutaneous tissue, and anterior comparment fascia before the anterior cortex of the femoral neck is palpated.

Controversies

- Frogging the leg for intraoperative lateral radiographs is commonly performed (Figs. 9 and 10), but should be avoided for fear of bending guidewires and causing damage to the femoral head

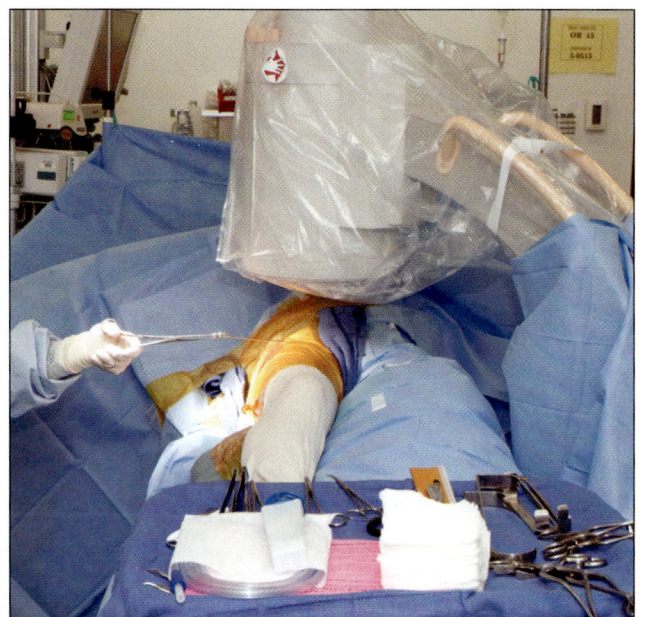

FIGURE 7

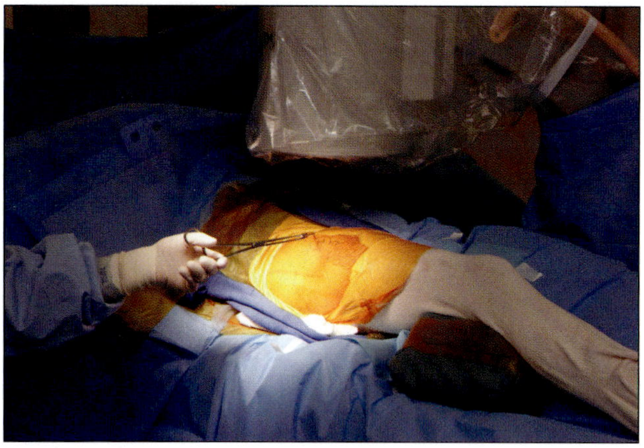

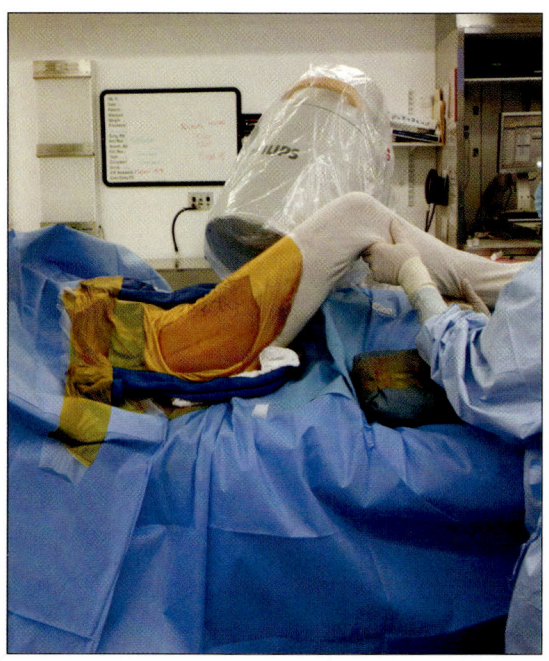

FIGURE 8

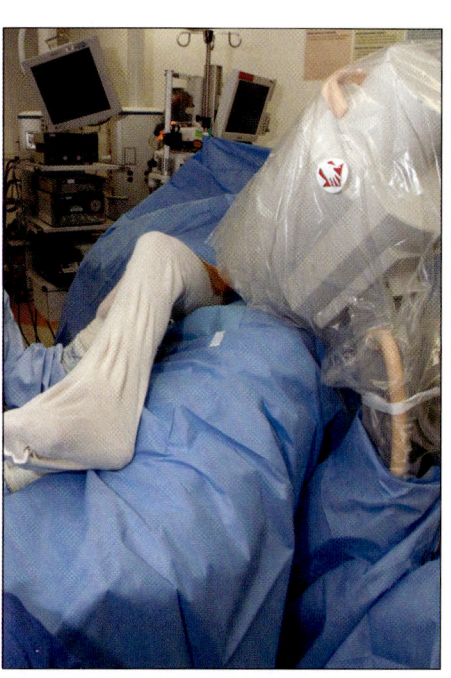

FIGURE 9

FIGURE 10

PROCEDURE

STEP 1

- The ideal position for screw fixation is perpendicular to the capital physis and in the center of the head and neck.
- Fluoroscopy is used to obtain the desired biplanar trajectory (Figs. 11 and 12).
- Once the wire trajectory is satisfactory on the AP view, the threaded guide pin is advanced 1–3 cm into the bone and the trajectory on the lateral view is assessed.
- It may take several attempts to get the correct trajectory in both planes, but once the trajectory is acceptable, the threaded guide pin is carefully driven across the physis to the level of the subchondral bone (Figs. 13 and 14).
- For unstable slips, the surgeon should endeavor to have two screws that are perpendicular to the physis. Therefore, a second guide pin is inserted directed inferomedially to avoid the rich blood supply superolaterally in the femoral head-neck junction.

PEARLS

- *A mallet can be used to tap the guidewire into a starting position that has some stability while alternating between the AP and lateral views if having difficulty setting your angle.*

- *Once the trajectory on the AP view is acceptable, the entry hole can be overdrilled slightly to give greater degrees of freedom to achieve the appropriate lateral guide pin trajectory.*

- *If having difficulty with establishing a new path for the threaded guide pin, try drilling on reverse to establish a new trajectory.*

PITFALLS

- *Avoid a subtrochanteric starting point for guidewire insertion, since this will create a stress riser and risk subtrochanteric fracture.*

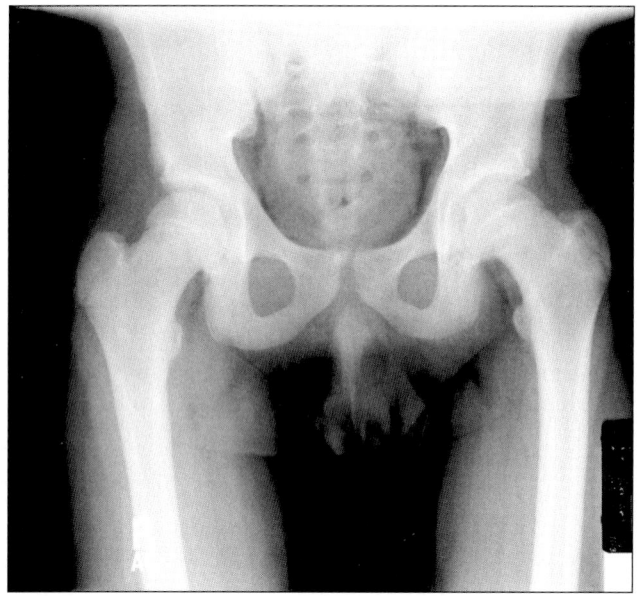

FIGURE 11

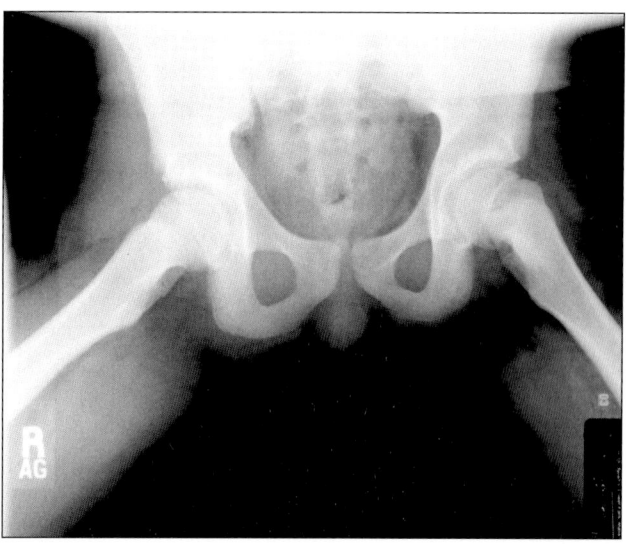

FIGURE 12

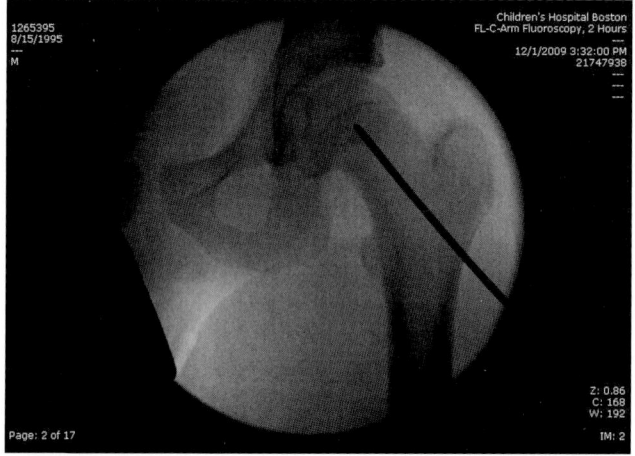

FIGURE 13

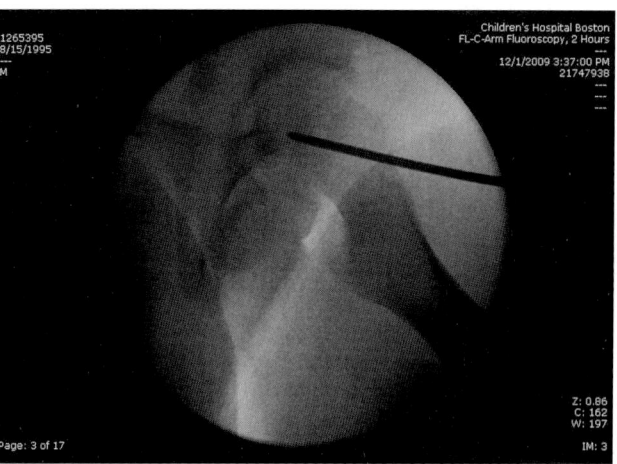

FIGURE 14

STEP 2

- The appropriate depth of the guidewire is measured and a *fully threaded* screw(s) is selected.
- The guide pin is carefully overdrilled, leaving the last 5–10 mm of the length of the guidewire undrilled. When removing the drill, the surgeon should serially check with fluoroscopy to confirm that the guidewire is not being removed simultaneously.
- The self-tapping, fully threaded cannulated screw is passed over the guidewire and checked with fluoroscopy to ensure that the appropriate length has been chosen (Fig. 15).
- The surgeon should endeavor to have as many threads as possible across the physis while avoiding intra-articular penetration. At least three full screw threads must cross the physis (Fig. 16).
- Multiplanar fluoroscopy is used to ensure that the screw is not intra-articular on any view.
- The superficial tissues are irrigated and closed in layers with absorbable suture.

Instrumentation/Implantation

- 6.5-mm or 7.3-mm fully threaded self-tapping cannulated screws are preferred.
- Partially threaded cannulated screws are difficult to remove and frequently break in situ, making hardware removal difficult and traumatic for both patient and surgeon.
- Titanium screws are attractive because of their magnetic resonance imaging compatability; however, we prefer stainless steel screws because of their increased modulus of elasticity.

Controversies

- Multiple smooth Kirschner wires are an acceptable alternative to for fixation of the mild, stable SCFE. The theoretical advantage is permission of further physeal growth; however, this is offset with a potential for loss of fixation due to overgrowth or migration.

POSTOPERATIVE CARE AND EXPECTED OUTCOMES

- Crutch walking is taught in the postoperative period.
- Patients with stable slips are mobilized with weight bearing as tolerated with crutches, while those with unstable slips are restricted to toe-touch weight bearing for 6 weeks.
- For those patients who appear to have difficulty with crutches, strict wheelchair transport for the first 6 weeks is preferred.
- The patient returns to the clinic regularly for assessment of range of motion, confirmation of physeal closure, and surveillance of the contralateral hip in cases in which bilateral pinning was not performed.
- Return to sporting activities is considered at 3 months' follow-up.

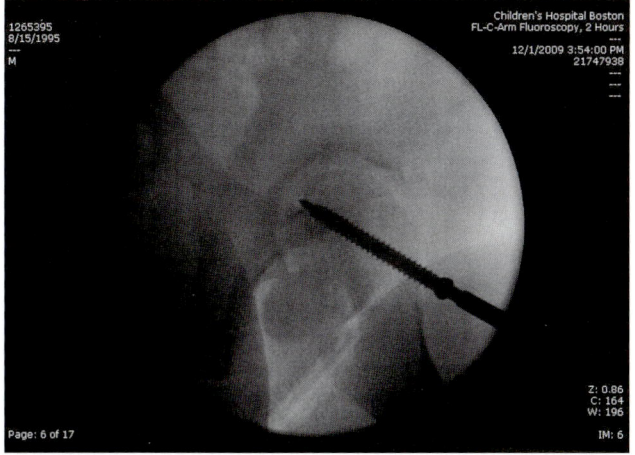

FIGURE 15

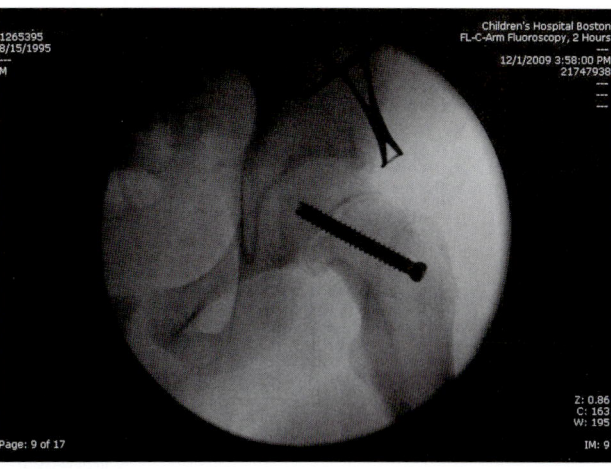

FIGURE 16

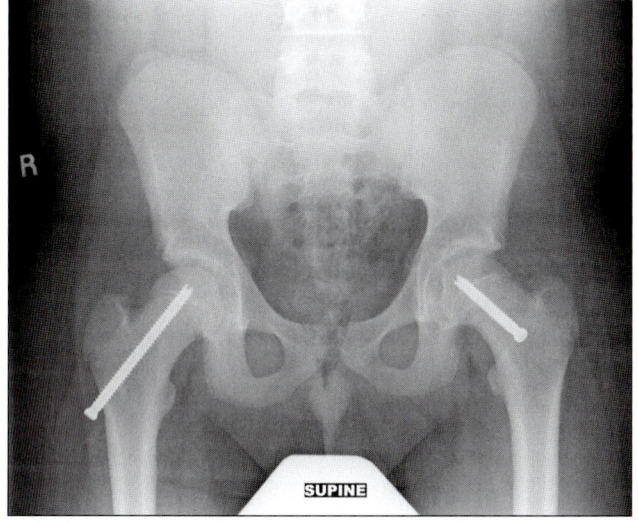

FIGURE 17

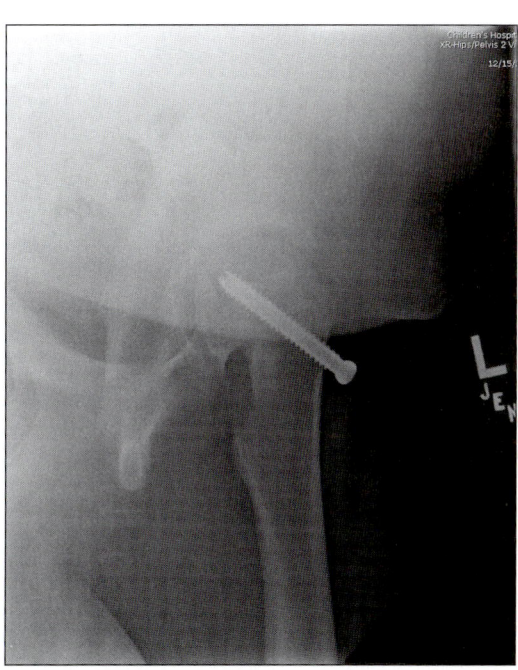

FIGURE 18

EVIDENCE

Diab M, Hresko MT, Millis MB. Intertrochanteric versus subcapital osteotomy in slipped capital femoral epiphysis. Clin Orthop Relat Res. 2004;(427):204–12.

A retrospective review of 15 flexion intertrochanteric osteotomies and 11 subcapital osteotomies for the treatment of severe slipped capital femoral epiphysis. The authors found minimal differences in radiographic correction and complications between the two groups; however, a higher reoperation rare was found in the supcapital osteotomy group. The authors concluded that flexion intertrochanteric osteotomy is a safe, effective and reproducible realignment osteotomy for treatment of severe, stable SCFE. (Level IV evidence)

Klein A, Joplin RJ, Reidy JA, Hanelin J. Roentgenographic features of slipped capital femoral epiphysis. Am J Roentgenol Radium Ther. 1951;66:361–74.

Retrospective review of 68 patients with 81 cases of slipped capital femoral epiphysis treated at Massachusetts General Hospital from 1933 to 1949. Found that the most constant roentgenographic indication was a widened epiphyseal plate and capital slipping. (Level IV evidence)

Kocher MS, Bishop JA, Hresko MT, Millis MB, Kim YJ, Kasser JR. Prophylactic pinning of the contralateral hip in slipped capital femoral epiphysis. J Bone Joint Surg [Am]. 2004;86:2658–65.

An expected-value decision analysis designed to investigate the optimal management strategy for treatment of the contralateral hip in slipped capital femoral epiphysis. Twenty-five adolescent male patients without SCFE were questioned to formulate the decision tree and optimal treatment predictions. In comparing prophylactic pinning versus observation, they concluded that the optimal decision was observation. However, in cases where the probability of contralateral SCFE exceeds 27% or in cases where reliable follow-up is not feasible, pinning of the contralateral hip is favored. (Level III evidence)

Loder RT, Richards BS, Shapiro PS, Reznick RR, Aronson DD. Acute slipped capital femoral epiphysis: the importance of physeal stability. J Bone Joint Surg [Am]. 1993;75: 1134–40.

A retrospective study to test the classification system of slipped capital femoral epiphysis. Fifty-four patients presenting with SCFE were classified according to their radiographs and symptoms as unstable or stable. Slips were considered to be unstable when the patient had such severe pain that weight-bearing was not possible even with crutches. Slips were considered to be stable when the patient could bear weight, with or without crutches. All slips were treated with internal fixation. Avascular necrosis developed in fourteen (47%) of the unstable hips and in none of the stable hips. (Level IV evidence)

Morrissey RT. Slipped capital femoral epiphysis: technique of percutaneous in-situ fixation. J Pediatr Orthop. 1990;10:347–50.

The technique for percutaneous in situ fixation of chronic slipped capital femoral epiphysis (SCFE) is described. The technique utilizes a cannulated screw, which obviates the need for an incision and allows variation of the starting point of the screw depending on the degree of slippage. (Level V evidence)

Southwick WO. Slipped capital femoral epiphysis. J Bone Joint Surg [Am]. 1984;66:1151.

Editorial review of two articles describing the results of biplanar high-femoral neck osteotomy for the treatment of deformity associated from slipped capital femoral epiphysis. (Level V evidence)

Ziebarth K, Zilkens C, Spencer S, Leunig M, Ganz R, Kim YJ. Capital realignment for moderate and severe SCFE using a modified Dunn procedure. Clin Orthop Relat Res. 2009;(467):704–16.

A retrospective review of 40 patients, followed for 3 years, treated with capital reorientation for slipped capital femoral epiphysis. The surgical technique for capital reorientation and surgical dislocation is described. There were no cases of osteonecrosis or chondrolysis. Articular cartilage damage, full-thickness loss, and delamination were observed at the time of surgery, especially in the stable slips. The authors conclude that this technique appears to have an acceptable complication rate and ability for full correction of moderate to severe slipped capital femoral epiphyses with open physes. (Level IV evidence)

Bernese Periacetabular Osteotomy

Travis Matheney, Justin M. LaReau, and Michael B. Millis

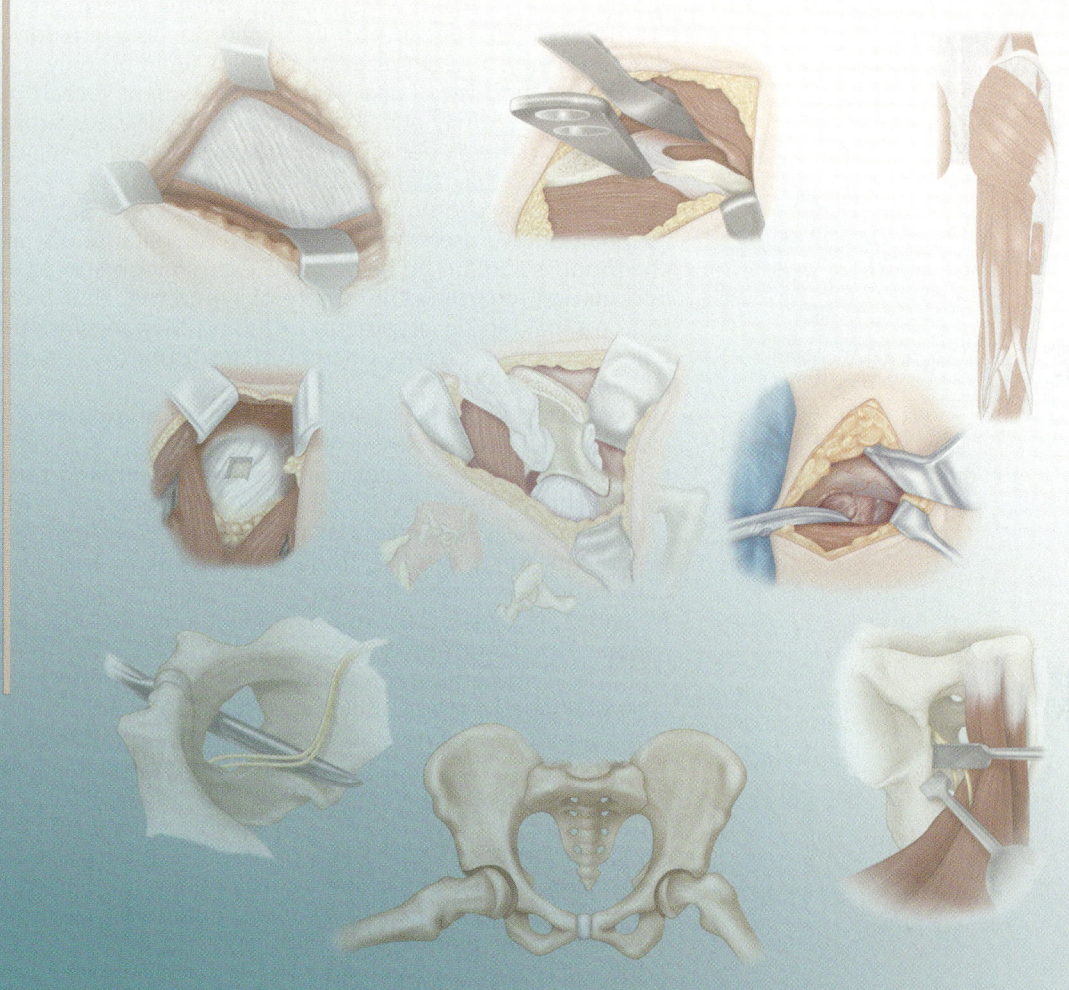

INDICATIONS

- Congruent hip dysplasia in skeletally mature patients with well-preserved articular cartilage

EXAMINATION/IMAGING

- Symptoms of hip dysplasia are commonly overlooked, leading to significant delays in diagnosis. Seemingly benign complaints of pain overlying the inguinal structures, greater trochanter, and buttocks are frequently dismissed by patients and physicians alike. Complaints of weakness, instability, locking, or catching are often noted. Referred pain to the ipsilateral knee and lumbosacral spine should be investigated appropriately.
- Family history remains a vital aspect of clinical evaluation. Strong evidence supports an underlying genetic link for dysplasia and subsequent arthrosis. Not uncommonly, evaluation and history of a young adult patient reveals parents and extended family affected by late-stage disease. Similarly, children of patients demonstrating symptoms of dysplasia should be carefully evaluated.
- Medical history should include careful review for prior hospitalizations, use of corticosteroids, neonatal sepsis, and childhood trauma. The history and examination should elicit information regarding the variety of syndromes that predispose to abnormal hip development, including Marfan syndrome, Ehlers-Danlos syndrome, Charcot-Marie-Tooth disease, trisomy 21, and cerebral palsy.
- Systematic, thorough physical examination is imperative to evaluation of the dysplastic hip.
  - Examination should begin with review of standing posture with careful attention to limb-length discrepancy, pelvic tilt, and weakness in single-limb stance. Gait evaluation for an abductor lurch, positive Trendelenburg's sign, and dynamic rotational alignment is essential.
  - Seated and recumbent examination should include careful neurologic and musculoskeletal assessment, with attention to subtle asymmetry in limb size (thigh circumference), sensation, and motor function. While complete examination should include all muscle groups, focus upon hip abductor strength and fatigue is paramount. Evaluation of iliopsoas tendon tenderness, snapping, and function should be included.
  - Range-of-motion testing and provocative maneuvers remain a mainstay of clinical evaluation. At a minimum, testing should include evaluation for hip flexion contractures, rotational profiles in flexion and extension, and provocative tests for instability and impingement. The apprehension test, anterior and posterior impingement tests, and evaluation for tenderness overlying the piriformis muscle are helpful tools to investigate symptoms of discomfort.
- Standard workup should include an anteroposterior (AP) pelvis radiograph centered on the femoral heads, the frog-leg lateral and false profile views popularized by Lequesne, and abduction-internal rotation views as described by Von Rosen. Careful attention should be paid to measurement of the Tönnis angle, anterior and lateral center-edge angles, femoral head sphericity as described by Nötzli, head-neck offset, acetabular version, the presence of a posterior wall sign, and joint congruity.
  - Figure 1 shows a standing bilateral AP radiograph of the hips. On the left hip, the lateral center-edge angle of Wiberg is drawn. On the right hip, the Tönnis acetabular roof angle is drawn. Note that the edge line is drawn to the end of the edge of the weight-bearing sourcil.

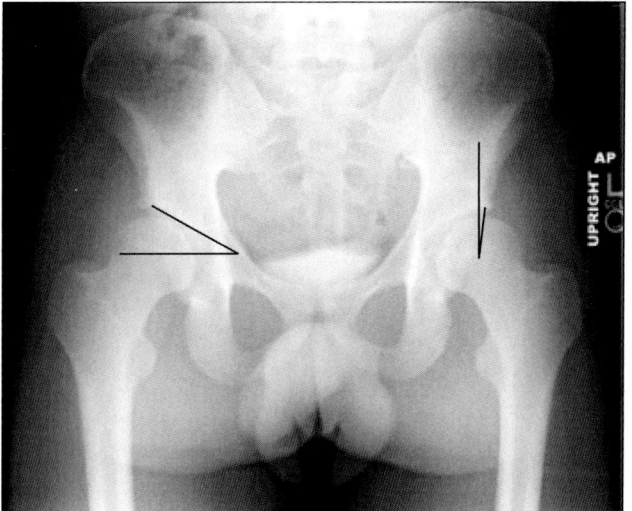

FIGURE 1

Treatment Options

- Hip arthroscopy may be indicated in patients with very mild dysplasia with concomitant labral pathology. A hypertrophic acetabular labrum is frequently encountered in patients with hip dysplasia.

- Chiari osteotomy may be indicated in patients with poorly congruent articular surfaces when the existing acetabular cartilage is well preserved.

- Total hip arthroplasty may be indicated in patients with advanced degenerative changes in the articular cartilage.

- Figure 2 shows a standing false profile view of the hip. The anterior center-edge angle of Lequesne is drawn. Note that the edge line is drawn to the end of the edge of the weight-bearing sourcil.
- Figure 3 shows a supine AP radiograph of the pelvis with the hips in abduction and internal rotation. This is to simulate what the hip would look like following reorientating periacetabular osteotomy (PAO). Congruency is measured on this view preoperatively and on the standing AP radiograph postoperatively.

- Advanced imaging modalities, including magnetic resonance imaging (MRI; Fig. 4), computed tomography, and ultrasound, offer valuable insights for perioperative planning. Recent investigations have detailed the valuable prognostic utility of intravenous gadolinium–enhanced MRI for patients being considered for Bernese PAO.

SURGICAL ANATOMY

- The lateral femoral cutaneous nerve should be protected throughout the procedure. The tensor-sartorius surgical interval may be approached by entering the tensor fascia lata just distal and lateral to the anterior superior iliac spine (ASIS). Once the fascia is incised in line with its fibers, blunt dissection may be carried out medially to enter the appropriate interval. Patients should be counseled preoperatively regarding possible neurapraxia.
- The sciatic nerve is at risk primarily during the osteotomy of the posterior column. The osteotomy of the posterior column should initially be performed to, but not through, the lateral cortex. The osteotomy may be carefully completed with a Ganz osteotome just prior to correction of the acetabular fragment.
- The femoral nerve is at heightened risk during osteotomy of the ischium. Tension should be relieved by placing a large bump underneath the operative extremity, thereby flexing the hip and reducing tension on the nerve.
- The medial femoral circumflex artery can potentially be injured during distal dissection along the ischium in preparation for osteotomy. Care should be taken not to dissect distal to the obturator externus tendon during preparation for this cut, which begins in the infracotyloid groove just distal to the transverse acetabular ligament.

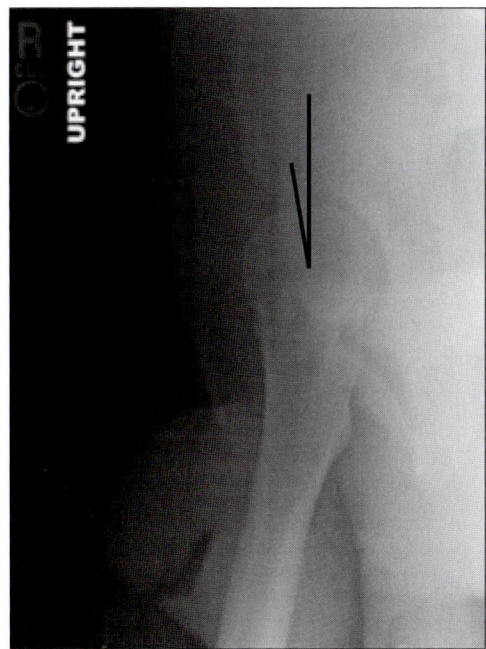

FIGURE 2

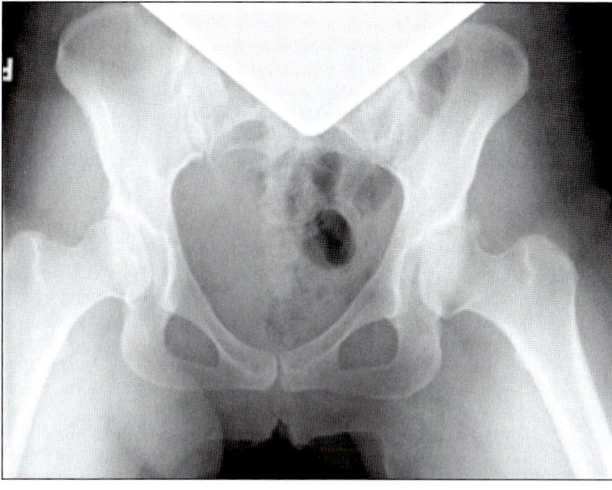

FIGURE 3

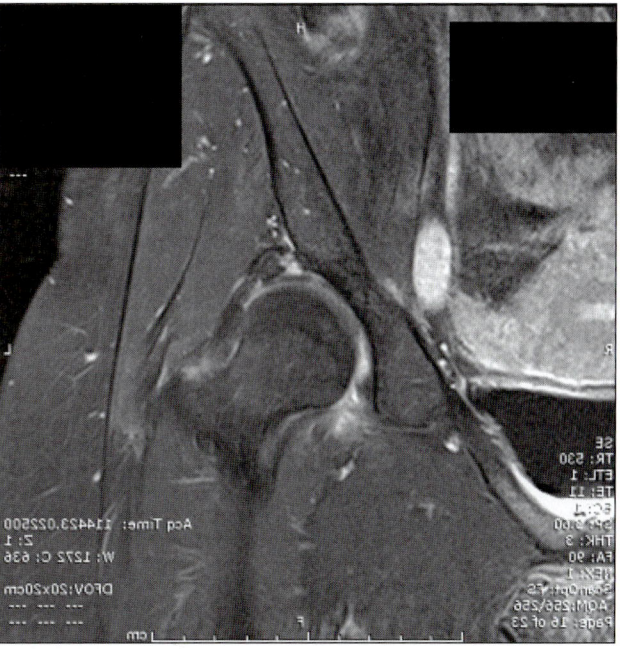

FIGURE 4

PITFALLS

- *Care should be taken to assure that the surgical field is prepped proximally to the costal margin, posteriorly to the posterior third of the ilium, and medially to the umbilicus.*

Equipment

- The fluoroscope and monitor should be placed on the contralateral side.
- A padded Mayo stand may assist in positioning the hip in an abducted position.

PEARLS

- *A longitudinally extended iliofemoral incision may be particularly helpful in muscular male patients.*
- *Identification of the reflected head of the rectus femoris may be achieved by careful dissection along the Smith-Petersen interval proximally until the "prow" of bony pelvis is reached just lateral to the anterior inferior iliac spine (AIIS).*

POSITIONING

- The patient is positioned supine on a radiolucent Jackson table. A preoperative supine radiograph is helpful for correlation with intraoperative correction.
- Epidural analgesia is commonly used for perioperative pain management.
- The shoulder of the operative side may be gently positioned in abduction and external rotation to facilitate surgical access to the operative site, with care taken to avoid excessive traction on the brachial plexus.
- The entire lower extremity should be prepped and draped freely to facilitate intraoperative assessment of joint motion.

PORTALS/EXPOSURES

- Surgical technique relies on a modified iliofemoral approach. While an extended skin incision curving longitudinally may improve access, poor wound healing and cosmesis may result. More limited incisions paralleling the ilioinguinal ligament and iliac wing may provide sufficient exposure and improved wound healing.
- A "bikini line" incision is used after administration of local anesthetic. A mixture of normal saline with epinephrine may be injected to reduce blood loss. The incision varies in size with patient body habitus. Typical incisions are 12–14 cm in length, paralleling but just distal to the iliac crest, terminating medially 1–2 cm beyond the palpated tensor-sartorius interval (Fig. 5).
- The initial exposure relies on the creation of two windows.
  - The first window is created proximally by dissection of the external oblique fascia off the iliac crest. Subperiosteal dissection of the iliacus along the inner table of the pelvis should ensue.
  - In the second, more distal window, the compartment of the tensor fascia lata is entered and the muscle bluntly dissected off the septum with the sartorius muscle. This is in an effort to protect the lateral femoral cutaneous nerve. The floor of this compartment is identified proximally until the anterior ilium is palpated. Dissection along the deep interval between the rectus femoris and gluteus medius includes division of the reflected head of the rectus femoris (Fig. 6). Once this dissection has been carried down to the hip capsule, the two windows are connected through an osteotomy and reflection of the ASIS with its attached sartorius muscle.

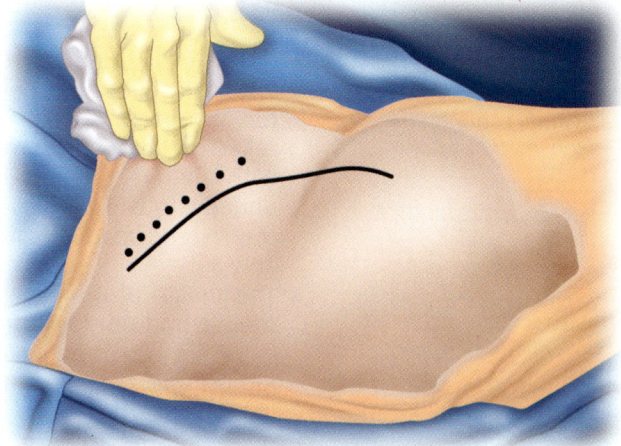

FIGURE 5

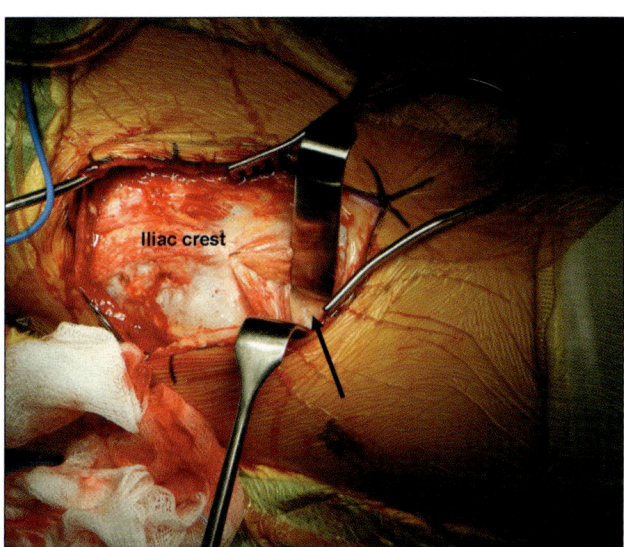

Iliac crest

FIGURE 6

PROCEDURE

STEP 1: DEEP DISSECTION

- The deep dissection begins with flexion and adduction of the hip to take tension off the anterior hip musculature. The reflected head of the rectus femoris is divided at its junction with the direct head. The direct head of the rectus femoris and underlying capsular iliacus are elevated as a unit and reflected distally and medially off the underlying joint capsule (Figs. 7 and 8).

- The sheath of the psoas may be opened longitudinally and its muscle and tendon retracted medially. One may also achieve exposure by subperiosteal release of the psoas sheath from the ramus, and separating the sheath from the capsule in an effort to avoid scarring of its contents. Dissection should be carried out along the anterior superior pubic ramus medial to the iliopectineal eminence, an important landmark denoting the medial extent of the bony acetabulum.

- The interval between the medial joint capsule and iliopsoas tendon is created and sequentially dilated using the tip of a long Mayo scissors and/or Lane bone levers. The tips of the scissors and Lane retractors are also used to palpate the anterior ischium at the infracotyloid groove. Proper placement is confirmed with an image intensifier. The goal is to place them superior to the obturator externus tendon (Fig. 9).

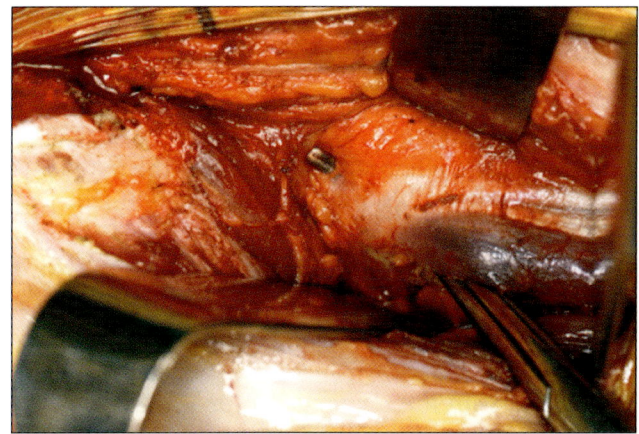

FIGURE 7

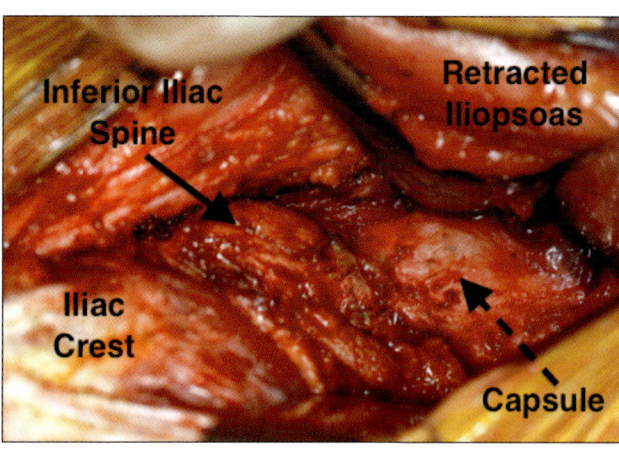

Inferior Iliac Spine

Retracted Iliopsoas

Iliac Crest

Capsule

FIGURE 8

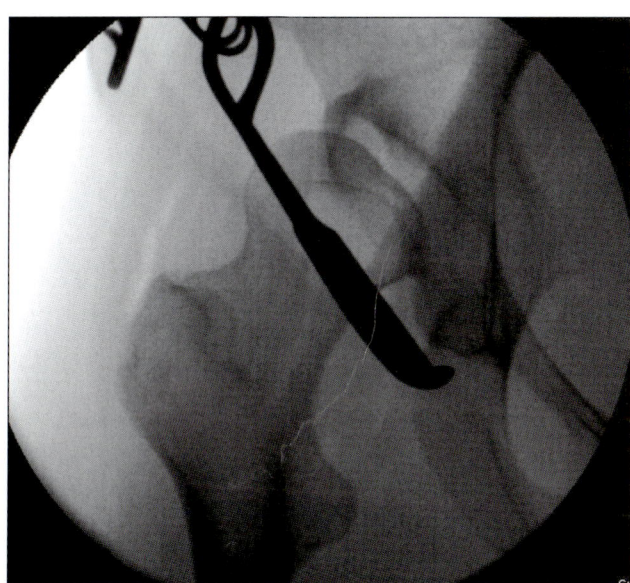

FIGURE 9

STEP 2: ANTERIOR ISCHIAL OSTEOTOMY

- The hip is flexed 45° and slightly adducted. A 30° forked, angled bone chisel (Synthes, USA; 15- or 20-mm blade widths) is inserted through the previously created interval between the medial capsule and psoas tendon to place its tip in contact with the superior portion of the infracotyloid groove of the anterior ischium, just superior to the obturator externus tendon (Fig. 10A–C). Staying proximal to the obturator externus helps to prevent injury to the nearby medial femoral circumflex artery.
- The medial and lateral aspects of the anterior ischium are gently palpated with the chisel and position confirmed with image intensifier in both the AP and iliac oblique views. The proper position of the chisel is approximately 1 cm below the inferior lip of the acetabulum, with the tip aimed at, or slightly above, the ischial spine (as seen on the oblique view in Fig. 10C).
- The chisel is impacted to a depth of 15–20 mm through *both the medial and lateral cortices* of the ischium.
- The ischial osteotomy may be extended posteriorly by using a nonforked 30° aesculap chisel along the inferior aspect of the quadrilateral surface.
- Care should be taken not to drive the osteotome too deeply through the lateral cortex as the sciatic nerve is in close proximity, especially with the leg flexed and adducted.

PEARLS

- *The hip must be flexed and slightly adducted to allow access through this interval.*
- *Dilating the interval before attempting to place the osteotome is beneficial to allow easier passage of the forked osteotome.*
- *A more superficial bony landmark for the anterior ischium is the iliopectineal eminence.*

PEARLS

- *The key to this osteotomy is to stay medial to the iliopectineal eminence to avoid intra-articular osteotomy.*

STEP 3: SUPERIOR PUBIS OSTEOTOMY

- The hip remains flexed and adducted. The psoas tendon and medial structures are gently retracted medially. Retraction may be aided by impacting either the tip of a spiked Hohmann retractor or a large-gauge Kirschner wire into the superior ramus just beyond the medial-most extent of the dissection.
- The periosteum over the superior pubic ramus is incised along its axis and careful circumferential subperiosteal dissection performed. This can be aided by making a transverse periosteal incision 1–2 cm medial to the iliopectineal eminence and working to continue the previous subperiosteal dissection of the inner iliac table into the lateral obturator foramen.
- Either blunt Hohmann or Rang retractors or Lane bone levers are placed anteriorly and posteriorly around the superior ramus into the obturator foramen to protect the obturator nerve and artery.

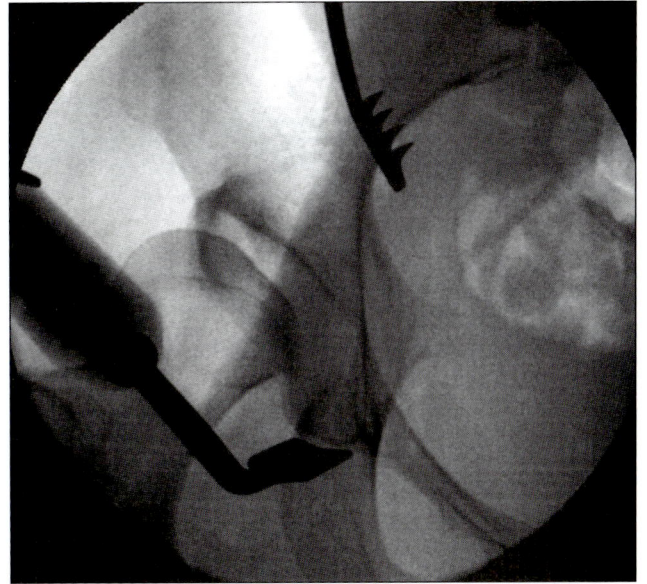

A

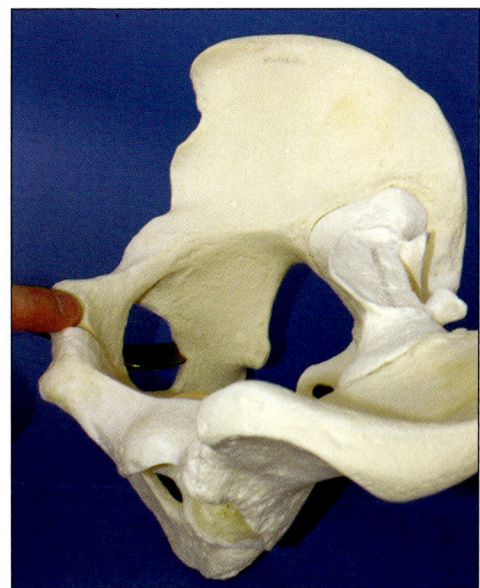

B

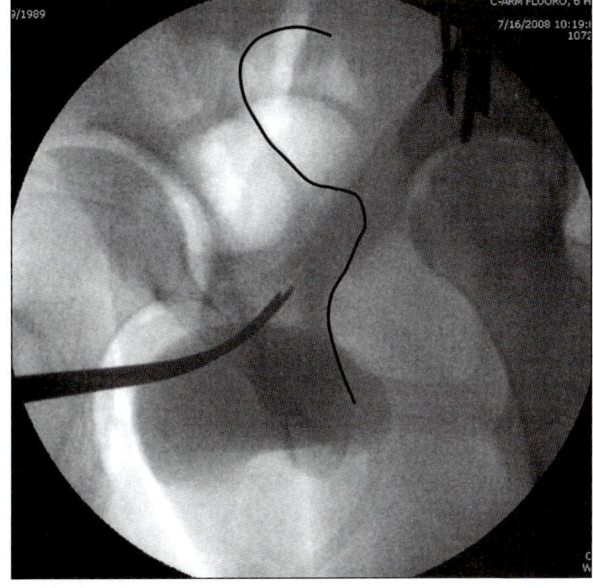

C

FIGURE 10

- The surgeon should note any leg spontaneous adduction that may be caused by stretching or irritation of the obturator nerve.
- The superior ramus osteotomy is perpendicular to the long axis when viewed from above and oblique from proximal-lateral to distal-medial when viewed from the front.
  - It may be made either by passing a Gigli saw around the ramus and sawing upward *away* from the retractors or by impacting a straight osteotome just medial to the iliopectineal eminence (Fig. 11).
  - In the former method, the Gigli saw is passed with a Satinsky vascular clamp.

STEP 4: ARTHROTOMY AND INTRACAPSULAR INSPECTION

- An arthrotomy may be performed if there is concern for intra-articular pathology such as torn labra, femoral neck "cam" lesions, or loose bodies.
- A T-shaped arthrotomy is performed centered on the anterior lateral femoral neck to avoid injury to the retinacular vessels running along the posterior superior femoral neck.
  - Make this limb of the arthrotomy first to allow visualization of the labrum while making the portion that runs along the acetabular rim.
- Labral tears may be either repaired if full thickness or débrided if at the free edge.
- Femoral neck cam lesions can be resected with either curved and straight osteotomes or a high-speed burr.
- Adequacy of resection can be assessed clinically with range of motion and/or a lateral view on the image intensifier.
- The arthrotomy is closed loosely with simple, interrupted absorbable sutures before proceeding with the remainder of the osteotomies.

STEP 5: SUPRA-ACETABULAR ILIAC OSTEOTOMY

- An approximately 1.5- to 2-cm subperiosteal window is started beneath the anterior abductors just distal to the ASIS without disturbing the abductor origin.
- The leg is slightly abducted and extended to allow atraumatic subperiosteal dissection using a narrow elevator posteriorly toward, but not into, the apex of the greater sciatic notch.
  - A narrow, long, spiked Hohmann retractor is placed in this window.
  - Correct placement is confirmed with an image intensifier; in the lateral projection, the spike of the Hohmann retractor should point toward the apex of the sciatic notch (Fig. 12A and 12B).
- The iliacus is retracted medially with a reverse Hohmann retractor whose tip is placed on the quadrilateral surface.
- Under direct vision, the iliac osteotomy is performed with an oscillating saw and cooling irrigation in line with the Hohmann retractor until reaching a point approximately 1 cm above the iliopectineal line (well anterior to the notch) (Fig. 12C).
- The surgeon must confirm that both the lateral and medial cortices are cut before proceeding. This endpoint of the iliac saw cut represents the posterior superior corner of the PAO. This corner is also the starting point of the posterior column osteotomy, which will be midway between the sciatic notch and posterior acetabulum.
- At this point, a 3.2-mm drill is used to create a passage for a single Schanz screw on a T-handled chuck. The Schanz screw is inserted into the acetabular fragment distal and parallel to the iliac saw cut, well above the dome of the acetabulum.

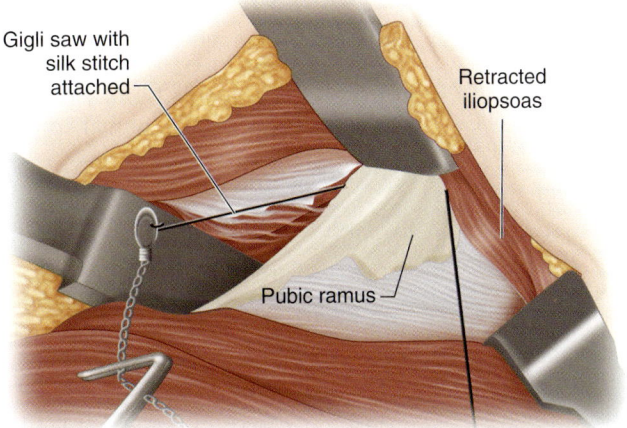

Gigli saw with silk stitch attached

Retracted iliopsoas

Pubic ramus

FIGURE 11

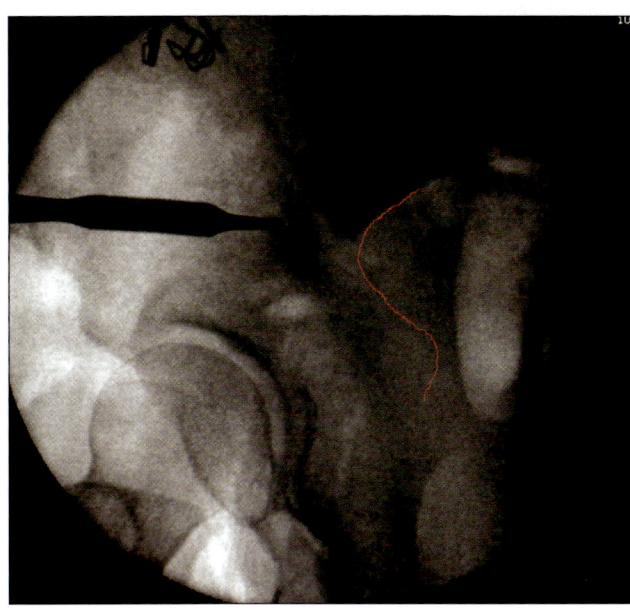

A

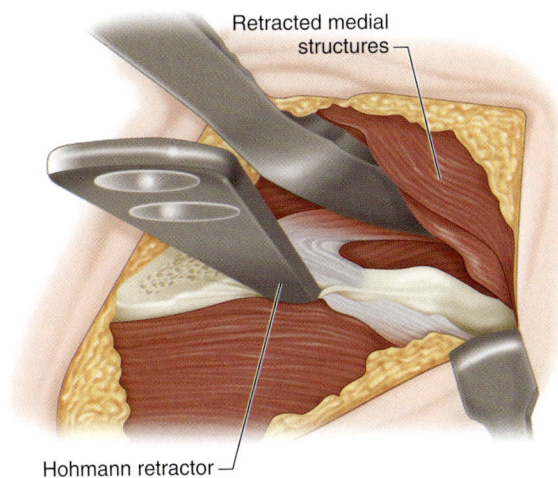

Retracted medial structures

Hohmann retractor

B

FIGURE 12

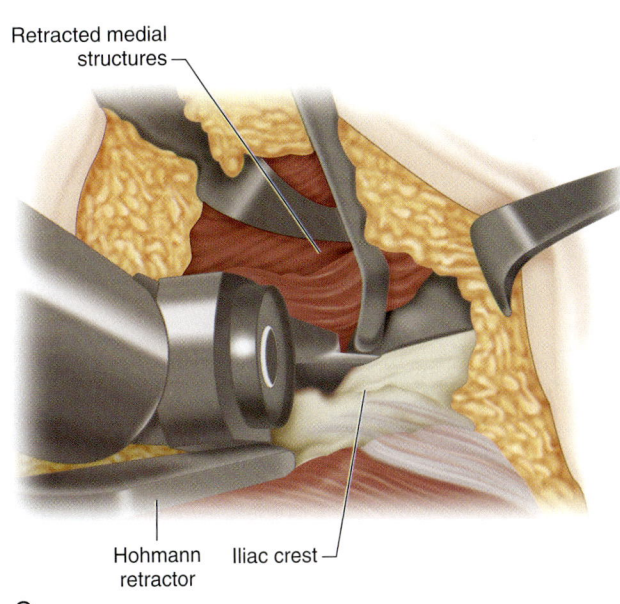

Retracted medial structures

Hohmann retractor

Iliac crest

C

PEARLS

- *Extend and abduct the hip slightly to move the sciatic nerve away as much as possible without overly tensioning the iliopsoas and making access to the medial acetabulum difficult.*

- *Confirm that the iliac osteotomy is complete through the lateral ilium, where it will eventually meet the posterior column cut.*

STEP 6: POSTERIOR COLUMN OSTEOTOMY

- The leg is once again flexed and adducted to relax the medial soft tissues.
- A reverse blunt Hohmann retractor is placed medially with the tip on the ischial spine. Dissection into the sciatic notch is not necessary.
- The osteotomy is made through the medial cortex with a long, straight 1.5-cm osteotome. It extends from the posterior end of the iliac saw cut, passing over the iliopectineal line, through the medial quadrilateral plate, parallel to the anterior edge of the sciatic notch on iliac oblique fluoroscopy, and is directed toward the ischial spine (Fig. 13). This posterior cut is made first through the medial, then second through the lateral wall of the ischium.
  - The osteotome is not set perpendicular to the medial quadralateral plate. Instead, the free medial edge of the osteotome should be tipped 10–15° *away* from the sciatic notch to create a more true coronal plane osteotomy, perpendicular to the *lateral* cortex of the posterior column (Fig. 14A and 14B).
- The surgeon must confirm that the medial and lateral cortices of the posterior column are completely cut. A Ganz osteotome may be used to connect the medial and lateral cortices beginning at the proximal posterior column. This must be done very carefully so as no™t to injure the sciatic nerve and other structures leaving the sciatic notch.
- The final osteotomy is a completion osteotomy of the posteroinferior medial corner of the quadrilateral plate connecting the anterior and posterior ischial cuts. A 30°-angle long-handled chisel is used to contect these two prior osteotomies (Fig. 15A and 15B).

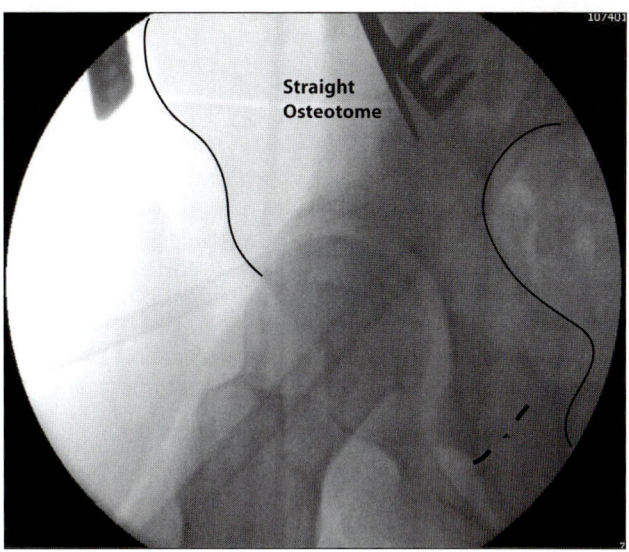

FIGURE 13

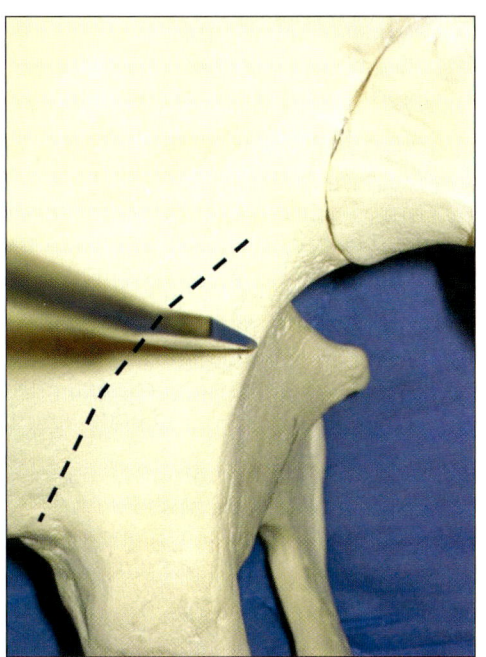 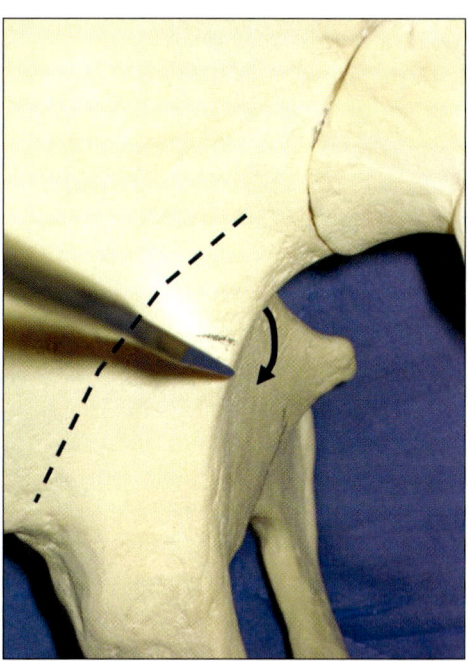

FIGURE 14 A   B

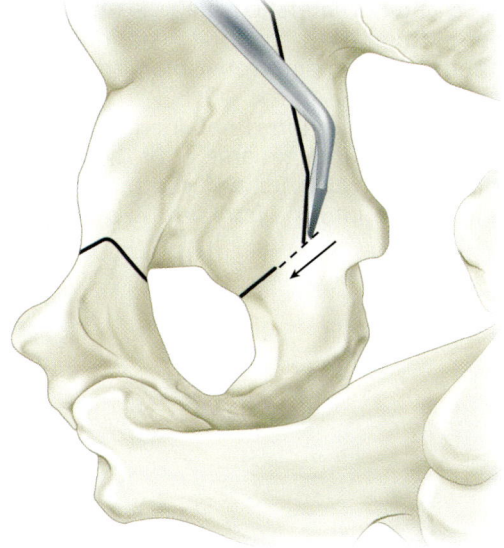

A
FIGURE 15

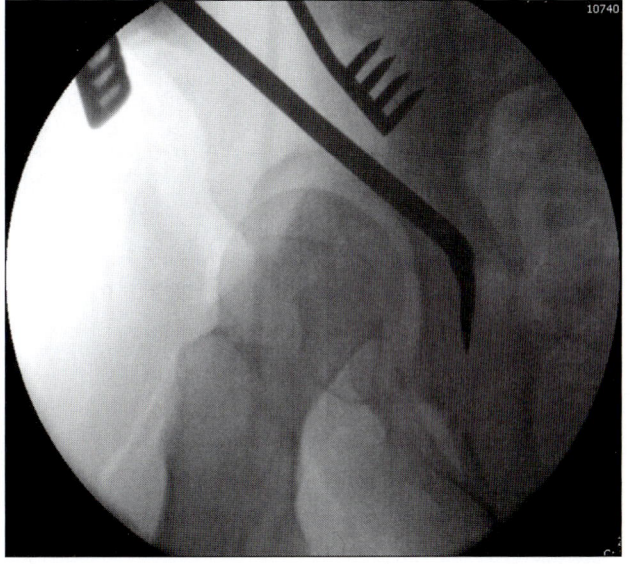

B

Step 7: Acetabular Displacement

- We define the acetabular displacement in reference to the iliac osteotomy.
- A 1-inch straight Lambotte chisel is placed into the supra-acetabular iliac saw cut to both confirm completion of the lateral cortex osteotomy and protect the cancellous bone above the acetabulum during displacement.
- The tines of a Weber bone clamp are placed onto the superior ramus portion of the acetabular fragment in such a way as to place its handle anterior and in contact with the Schanz screw.
- A lamina spreader is placed into the iliac osteotomy between the posterior superior intact ilium and the Lambotte chisel anteriorly (Fig. 16). While gently opening the lamina spreader, the Schanz screw/Weber clamp are used to mobilize the acetabular fragment.
  - It is important to ascertain whether the posterior and anterior osteotomies are complete; otherwise, the fragment will not freely rotate and the common outcome will be distal and lateral displacement as one hinges on the lateral, intact cortices. These cuts can be inspected with a narrow or broad 30° chisel (see Fig. 11).
- Once the fragment is completely free, it may be positioned to obtain the desired correction.
  - As previously noted, the most common deficiency is anterior and lateral. Therefore, the most commonly used maneuvers are as follows: lift the acetabular fragment slightly toward the ceiling, creating an initial displacement followed by a three-step movement of lateral, distal, and internal rotation. Another way of describing this would be internally rotating the fragment to antevert, extending the fragment to get anterior coverage, and adducting the fragment to get lateral coverage.
  - When performed properly, the posterosuperior corner of the acetabular fragment should be impacted slightly into the superior intact iliac cut and the prominent superior tip of the acetabular fragment should be roughly in line with the superior intact iliac crest (Fig. 17).
- Note: The radiographic "teardrop" and its relation to the femoral head after fragment positioning should be elevated and tilted laterally, or adducted, commensurate with the amount of lateral correction.
- It is commonly necessary to medialize the acetabular fragment a little once the desired anterior/lateral coverage is obtained to re-create the proper position of the femoral head in relation to the medial pelvis. This will maintain proper biomechanical position of the femur in relation to the pelvis.
- Once the desired acetabular position is obtained, smooth Kirschner wires (of the approximate diameter of the planned drill bit to be used for later fixation) are placed proximal to distal through the ilium and into the fragment in a divergent pattern.

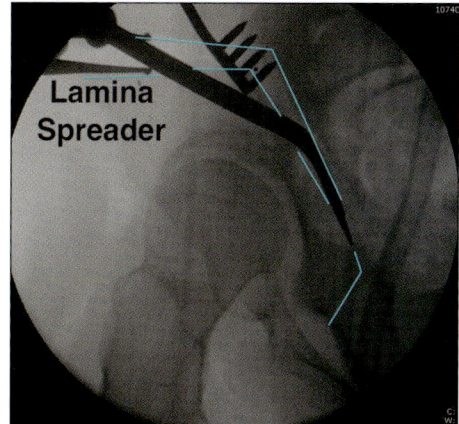

FIGURE 16

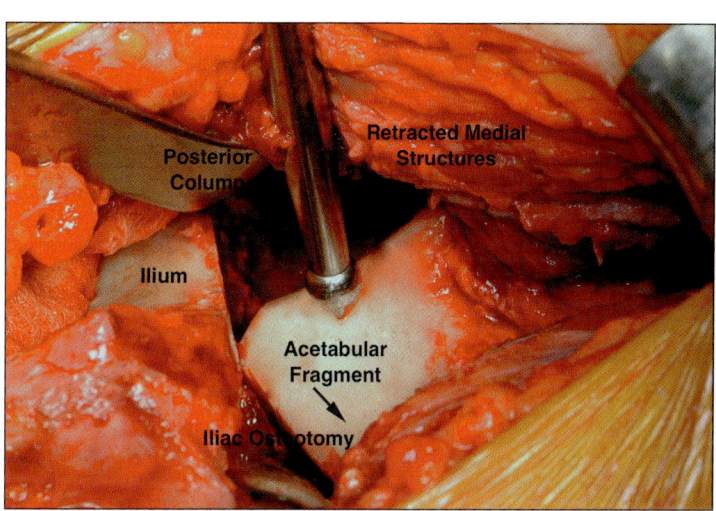

FIGURE 17

- At this point, we perform a final fragment position check in the AP and false profile views. In the false profile view, it is important to check the anterior femoral head coverage in full extension and at 100° of flexion (Fig. 18A-C).
  - In the AP view, the proper position of the sacrococcygeal junction in relation to the pubic symphysis should be seen, the sourcil should be roughly horizontal, the femoral head should be well covered, the posterior acetabular wall should overlap the center of the femoral head, the anterior wall shadow should not overlap the posterior wall, and Shenton's line should be intact.
  - The false profile view is to confirm that we have neither overcovered the femoral head nor created impingement from a femoral-sided deformity.
- The Kirschner wires are measured for depth and length and then replaced with either 3.5- or 4.5-mm cortical screws. An image intensifier is used to confirm extra-articular placement of all screws (Fig. 19A and 19B).
- An additional "home run" screw may be placed anterior to posterior from the AIIS posteriorly into the inferior ilium if required for stability (especially in patients who are ligamentously lax, have a neuromuscular condition, or have poor bone quality). We prefer not to utilize this screw unless necessary as it is our practice to remove these screws once bony healing is confirmed or in case MRI is to be performed at a later point.
- The anterior iliac prominence of the acetabular fragment is trimmed and used for bone graft.

STEP 8: CLOSURE

- All sponges are removed and wounds are irrigated copiously.
- The direct head of the rectus femoris is repaired with heavy nonabsorbable sutures.
- Suction drains are placed under the iliacus.
- The ASIS osteotomy (if performed) is either reattached with a 3.5-mm, partially threaded cancellous screw and washer or sewn back with heavy, absorbable sutures through thinner wafer.
- Careful attention is paid to proper, tight closure over the iliac crest. This is accomplished by predrilling holes in the iliac crest to facilitate passage of heavy, absorbable sutures to reattach the abductor, iliacus, and external oblique musculature.
- The remainder of the wound is closed in layers.

POSTOPERATIVE CARE AND EXPECTED OUTCOMES

- Postoperative analgesia is maintained with an epidural catheter for 72 hours postoperatively. Patients are transitioned to oral pain medications as they begin to mobilize.
- Weight bearing is permitted to one sixth of the patient's body weight on the affected limb for 6–8 weeks.
- Sitting is permitted on postoperative day 2.
- A continuous passive motion machine (CPM) is utilized for all cases in which an arthrotomy is performed to address intra-articular pathology.
- Range of motion is limited to 90° of flexion, 10° from full extension, and 10° of adduction, abduction, and rotation for the first 6 weeks.
- Resistive exercises are avoided for 3 months.
- Patients older than 16 years are given either low-molecular weight heparin or warfarin for 4–6 weeks.
- Nonsteroidal anti-inflammatory drugs are avoided.

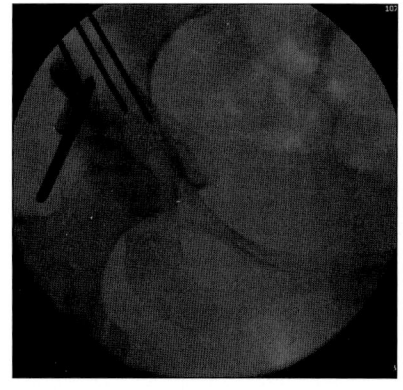 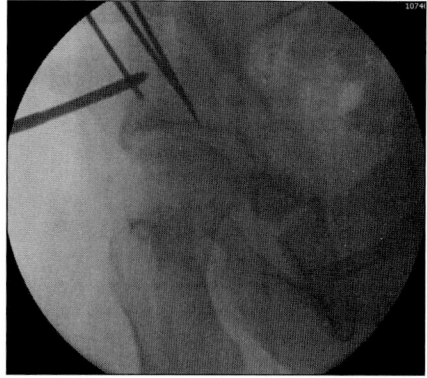 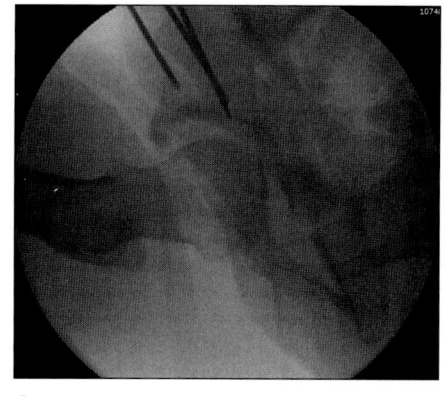

A

FIGURE 18

B

C

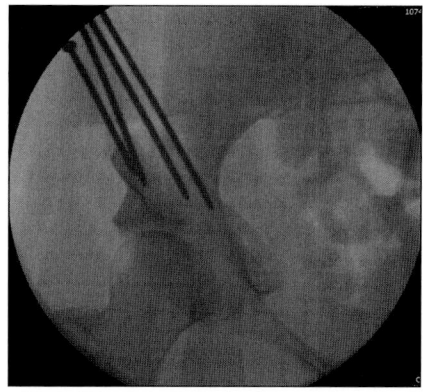 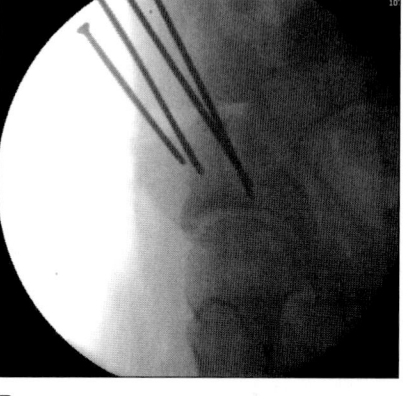

A

FIGURE 19

B

EVIDENCE

Clohisy JC, Barrett SE, Gordon JE, Delgado ED, Schoenecker PL. Periacetabular osteotomy for the treatment of severe acetabular dysplasia. J Bone Joint Surg [Am]. 2005;87:254–9.

Sixteen hips with severe acetabular dysplasia (Severin IV and V) were evaluated before and after PAO. The authors found at an average of 4.2 years' follow-up that correction of the severely dysplastic hip was possible with overall very good results. (Level IV evidence)

Clohisy JC, Carlisle JC, Beaule PE, Kim YJ, Trousdale RT, Sierra R, Leunig M, Schoenecker PL, Millis MB. A systematic approach to the plain radiographic evaluation of the young adult hip. J Bone Joint Surg [Am]. 2008;90:47–66.

The authors reviewed and described the most commonly used radiographs to assess hip dysplasia.

Cunningham T, Jessel RH, Zurakowski D, Millis MB, Kim YJ. Delayed gadolinium enhanced MRI of cartilage (dGEMRIC) as a predictor of early failure after bernese periacetabular osteotomy for hip dysplasia. J Bone Joint Surg [Am]. 2006;88:1540–8.

Forty-two hips were evaluated and the preoperative dGEMRIC value was found to be predictive of postoperative PAO failure, defined as high pain score, loss of minimum joint space on radiograph, and/or requiring total hip replacement. (Level II evidence)

Ganz R, Klaue K, Vihn TS, Mast JW. A new periacetabular osteotomy for the treatment of hip dysplasias: technique and preliminary results. Clin Orthop Relat Res. 1988;(232):26–36.

This paper was the original description of this newer technique for reorientation of the acetabulum in such a way as to preserve a portion of the posterior column. (Level IV evidence)

Matheney TH, Kim YJ, Zurakowski D, Matero C, Millis MB. Intermediate to long-term results following the Bernese periacetabular osteotomy and predictors of clinical outcome. J Bone Joint Surg [Am]. 2001;91:2113–23.

At an average 9-year follow-up of 135 hips following PAO, the authors found two independent predictors of osteotomy failure, defined as higher pain score or requiring total hip arthroplasty: age greater than 35 years and poor or fair preoperative joint congruency. (Level II evidence)

Millis MB, Kain M, Sierra R, Trousdale R, Taunton MJ, Kim YJ, Rosenfeld S, Kamath G, Schoenecker P, Clohisy JC. Periacetabular osteotomy for acetabular dysplasia in patients older than 40 years. Clin Orthop Relat Res. 2009;(467):2228–34.

This preliminary study suggested that PAO will give satisfactory functional and pain scores in patients over age 40 having dysplastic hips with mild or no arthrosis. (Level IV evidence)

Murphy SB, Millis MB. Periacetabular osteotomy without abductor dissection using direct anterior exposure. Clin Orthop Relat Res. 1999;(364):92–8.

This paper was a follow-up to the original surgical technique described by Ganz et al. (1988) with the modification that a subperiosteal window be made instead of completely taking down the hip abductor musculature. (Level IV evidence)

Steppacher SD, Tannast M, Ganz R, Siebenrock KA. Mean 20-year follow-up of bernese periacetabular osteotomy. Clin Orthop Relat Res. 2008;466:1633–44.

In a follow-up study of Ganz's initial cohort of 75 hips following PAO, the authors' findings at an average of 20 years identified six factors predicting poor outcome: age at surgery, preoperative Merle d'Aubigné and Postel scores, positive anterior impingement test, limp, osteoarthrosis grade, and the postoperative extrusion index. (Level II evidence)

Stevenson DA, Mineau G, Kerber RA, Viskochil DH, Roach JW. Familial predisposition to developmental dysplasia of the hip. J Pediatr Orthop. 2009;29:463–6.

Data suggested a genetic contribution to developmental dysplasia of the hip, with a 12-fold increase in risk for first-degree relatives. Better phenotypic characterization and classification will be critical for future genetic analyses.

Anteromedial Approach to a Developmentally Dislocated Hip

Stuart L. Weinstein

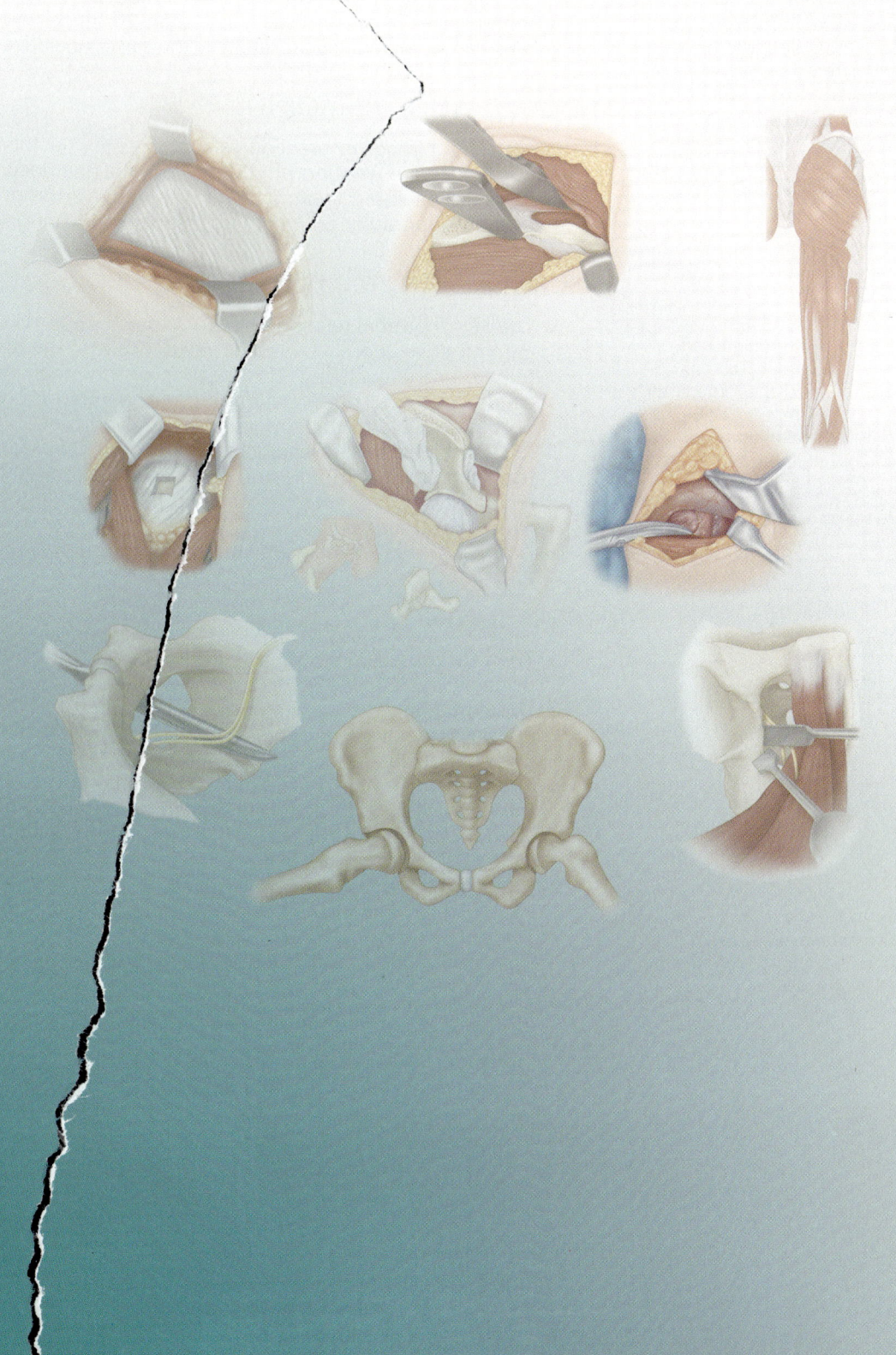

Controversies

- Criticism of this approach generally centers around several issues: poor visibility, inability to perform secondary procedures, and higher incidence of aseptic necrosis. If the interval between the pectineus and the femoral neurovascular bundle is used, excellent visualization of all structures is easily attained.

- In children younger than 2 years, particularly those younger than 18 months, it is rarely necessary to perform a secondary procedure. Complication rates of aseptic necrosis using this approach have been comparable to those of other series reported in the literature.

Treatment Options

- Other approaches to open reduction in the late-diagnosed developmentally dislocated hip case include a pure medial approach as described by Ferguson (1973) or a standard anterolateral approach as described by Salter, among others, through a "bikini line" incision.

- If the physician is considering other procedures such as femoral shortening or acetabular procedures, the standard anterior approach is indicated.

PEARLS

- *If both hips are to be openly reduced, the author uses clear plastic adhesive tape to occlude the rectum and vaginal area and preps out this area. Thus, in bilateral cases, both lower extremities and hemipelvis are prepped and draped free to allow full motion of the hip and knee during the procedure.*

INDICATIONS

- The indication for the anteromedial approach in a developmentally dislocated hip is when concentric reduction cannot be obtained or maintained by closed methods.
- It is ideal for children under 18–24 month of age, although the author has used it in older patients when open reduction is the only procedure planned.
- The advantages of this particular approach are avoidance of injury to the hip abductor muscles and to the growth plate of the iliac crest, and a scar that is well hidden.
- Blood loss is minimal, usually less than 20 ml per hip, and both hips can be operated on safely in the same operative session.

EXAMINATION/IMAGING

- No special imaging procedures are necessary for this specific approach. The treating physician will have had documentation of failure of closed treatment via plain films, arthrograms, and/or ultrasonography or magnetic resonance imaging.

SURGICAL ANATOMY

- The key anatomic relationships to understand in the anteromedial approach are the relationship of the neurovascular bundle to the pectineus; the location of the medial femoral circumflex vessels; the relationship of the anterior branch of the obturator nerve to the adductor longus and brevis; the relationship of the lesser trochanter and the iliopsoas tendon to the neurovascular bundle and the pectineus; and finally the relationship of the anteromedial hip joint capsule to the overlying structures.
- Figure 1 shows the relevant surgical anatomy for this procedure.

POSITIONING

- The procedure is performed with the patient in the supine position.
- The entire lower extremity, including the hemipelvis on the involved side, is draped free to allow full motion of the hip and knee during the procedure.
- The hip is then flexed to about 70° in unforced abduction while the neurovascular bundle is identified and the superior and inferior borders of the abductus longus are palpated.

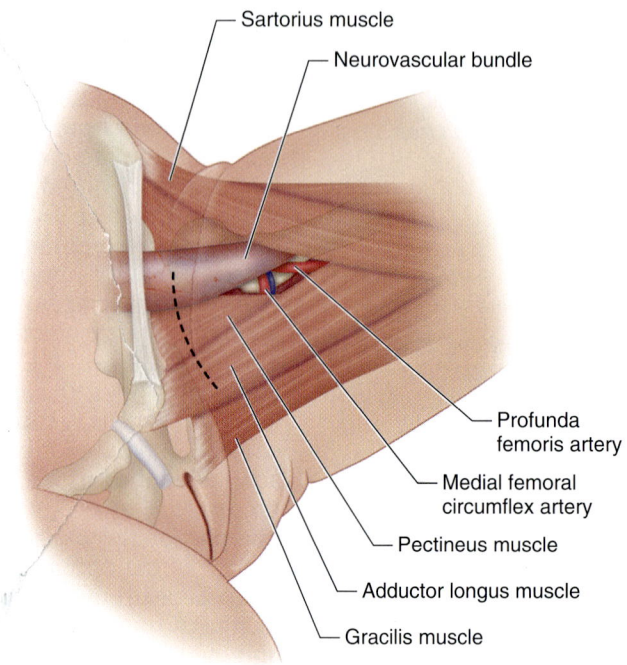

FIGURE 1

PEARLS

- *The author uses Kuji blunt retractors to maintain exposure, one placed anteriorly and one posteriorly.*

- *Exposing the interval between the pectineus and the femoral vein should be done with a dissecting scissors but always in line with the pectineus muscle fibers and the femoral vein.*

- *The lesser trochanter must be palpated in the wound; the leg is externally rotated until the lesser trochanter is easily palpable in the operative field. This position is then maintained while the iliopsoas is identified and sectioned.*

- *Retraction should never be in both directions at the same time. When exposing the capsule superiorly, the femoral neurovascular bundle can be retracted. When exposing it inferomedially, the pectineus side can be retracted.*

PITFALLS

- *Care must be taken not to injure the medial femoral circumflex vessels during the exposure; it should be identified and protected throughout the procedure. However, occasional injury to these vessels has not resulted in a higher incidence of aseptic necrosis.*

- *As the exposed area is quite small and vital structures are being retracted, the author only pulls on one retractor firmly at a time to avoid tearing vital structures.*

PORTALS/EXPOSURES

- The groin crease is identified as well as the superior and inferior borders of the adductor longus in the groin crease. The incision should extend from just inferior to the femoral neurovascular bundle in the groin crease to the inferior border of the adductor longus. The skin and subcutaneous tissues are incised sharply down to the deep fascia. This fascia is incised longitudinally with a #15 blade along the adductor longus in the direction of the muscle fibers for about 2–3 cm.

- The adductor longus is isolated using dissecting scissors (Fig. 2). The anterior branch of the obturator nerve is seen on the anterior surface of the adductor brevis muscle below the adductor longus; this nerve should be protected. The adductor longus muscle is sectioned close to its insertion with bipolar cautery. The anterior branch of the obturator nerve is once again identified as it crosses the adductor brevis muscle and protected.

- The pectineus muscle is next identified by following the anterior branch of the obturator nerve proximally to its entrance into the thigh beneath the pectineus muscle. The thin fascia over the pectineus muscle is incised with a #15 blade. Both the superior and inferior boarders of the muscle should be carefully identified.

- The interval between the pectineus muscle and the femoral neurovascular bundle is then identified and bluntly dissected using scissors (Fig. 3). Great care must be taken in this dissection to avoid injury to the medial femoral circumflex artery, which courses in a superior-to-inferior direction in the operative field. Retraction on the femoral neurovascular bundle must be gentle to avoid injury to the femoral vein, which is directly under the retractor. Just distal to the medial femoral circumflex artery, the iliopsoas tendon can be palpated. This is greatly facilitated by externally rotating the leg until the lesser trochanter is easily palpable in the operative field.

- The iliopsoas tendon is then isolated with a curved hemostat and sectioned sharply at the insertion on the lesser trochanter. With gentle retraction on the femoral neurovascular bundle superiorly and on the pectineus muscle inferiorly, the hip joint capsule is isolated with blunt dissection (Fig. 4).

- It is important to visualize the entire hip joint capsule completely in the field before proceding with the open reduction. The capsule will be visualized both medially and laterally to the medial circumflex vessels in the surgical field. In high dislocations, the capsule must be separated carefully from the femoral neurovascular bundle so that the incision may be extended along the posterior superior rim of the acetabulum.

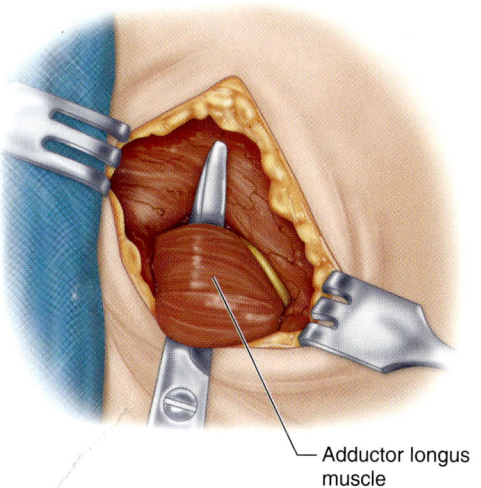

Adductor longus
muscle

FIGURE 2

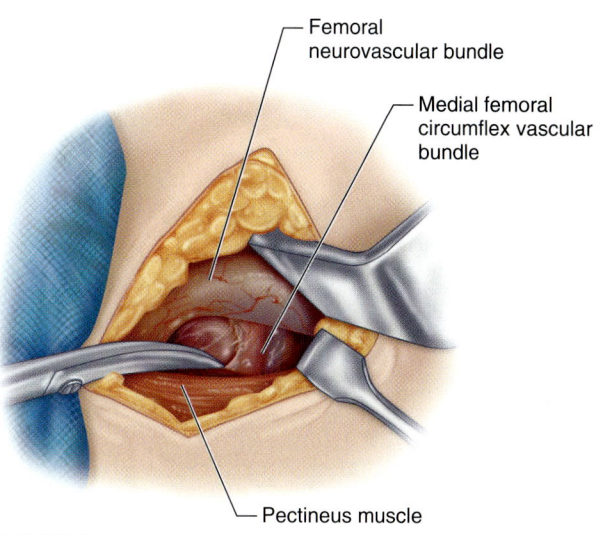

Femoral
neurovascular bundle

Medial femoral
circumflex vascular
bundle

Pectineus muscle

FIGURE 3

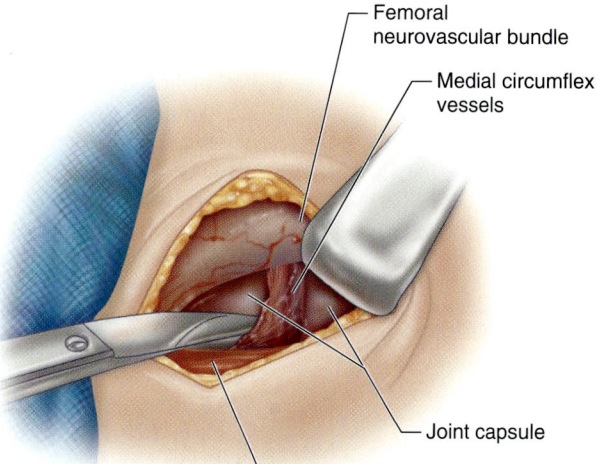

Femoral
neurovascular bundle

Medial circumflex
vessels

Joint capsule

Pectineus muscle

FIGURE 4

PROCEDURE

STEP 1

- The actual open reduction is accomplished by first making a small incision in the anteromedial hip joint capsule parallel to the anterior acetabular margin.
- Through the capsular opening, the ligamentum teres can be visualized. It is grasped with a Graham hook and delivered into the wound. The capsular incision is then further extended along the ligamentum teres to locate the ligament's insertion on the femoral head. The leg can be rotated to facilitate bringing the head into the operative field.
- The ligamentum teres is detached sharply from the femoral head using a #15 blade (Fig. 5).
- The stump of the ligamentum teres is grasped with a hemostat and the interval between the ligamentum teres and the anteroinferior medial aspect of the joint capsule identified. A dissecting scissors is placed between the ligamentum teres and the anteromedial joint capsule. A #15 blade is then used to extend the capsular incision to the base of the acetabulum (Fig. 6).
- After the entire anteromedial capsule is incised, the ligamentum teres, along with the transverse acetabular ligament, is excised sharply either with a knife or dissecting scissors. The acetabulum can now be completely visualized.
- The fibrofatty tissue of the pulvinar can be removed with pituitary rongeurs and the posterior, superior, and inferior walls of the acetabulum inspected (Fig. 7).

STEP 2

- Now that the anatomic obstacles to reduction have been removed, the head can be reduced directly into the acetabulum (Fig. 8).
  - Occasionally it is necessary to "T" the joint capsule in high long-standing dislocations. In this case, the "T-ing" of the capsule is very similar to that done in the anterior approach, extending from the anterior inferior spine distally.
- After the head is reduced, stability is assessed. The surgeon must assess the safe zone. In most cases the hip is very stable up to almost neutral abduction-adduction in 90° of flexion. The stability is naturally affected by the severity of the hip dysplasia in the superior and posterior walls of the acetabulum.
- The hip is held reduced by an assistant while closure is completed. The usual position is in 90–100° flexion and 30–40° abduction

STEP 3

- No drains are used, and the hip capsule is left open. Only the deep fascia of the thigh is approximated with a running 2-0 absorbable suture. Subcutaneous tissues are closed with a 2-0 absorbable suture, and the skin is closed with a subcuticular 3-0 absorbable suture. The wound is dressed with a bio-occlusive dressing.
- The patient is placed in a postoperative well-molded one-and-one-half leg spica cast extending from the nipple line to just above the ankle on the involved side and just above the knee on the noninvolved side. The cast must be well molded dorsal to the greater trochanters to prevent re-dislocation.
- We send the patient directly to the computed tomography (CT) scanner from the operating room to get a single-cut CT scan through the triradiate cartilage to document reduction.

PEARLS

- *The entire anteromedial joint capsule must be completely opened down to the base of the acetabulum and the transverse acetabular ligament must be excised in order for the femoral head to be located in its anatomic position.*

- *We have never had to take a patient back to the operating room to re-reduce the hip. However, if the postoperative CT scan showed that the femoral head was not in the desired location, we would take the child back to the operating room to re-reduce and reapply a new spica cast with the hip in the correct position.*

PITFALLS

- *No peripheral acetabular tissue should ever be excised or the patient will without doubt have hip dysplasia, as the surgeon is excising growth cartilage.*

- *The hip must be stabilized in the desired position by an assistant while the hip spica cast is applied.*

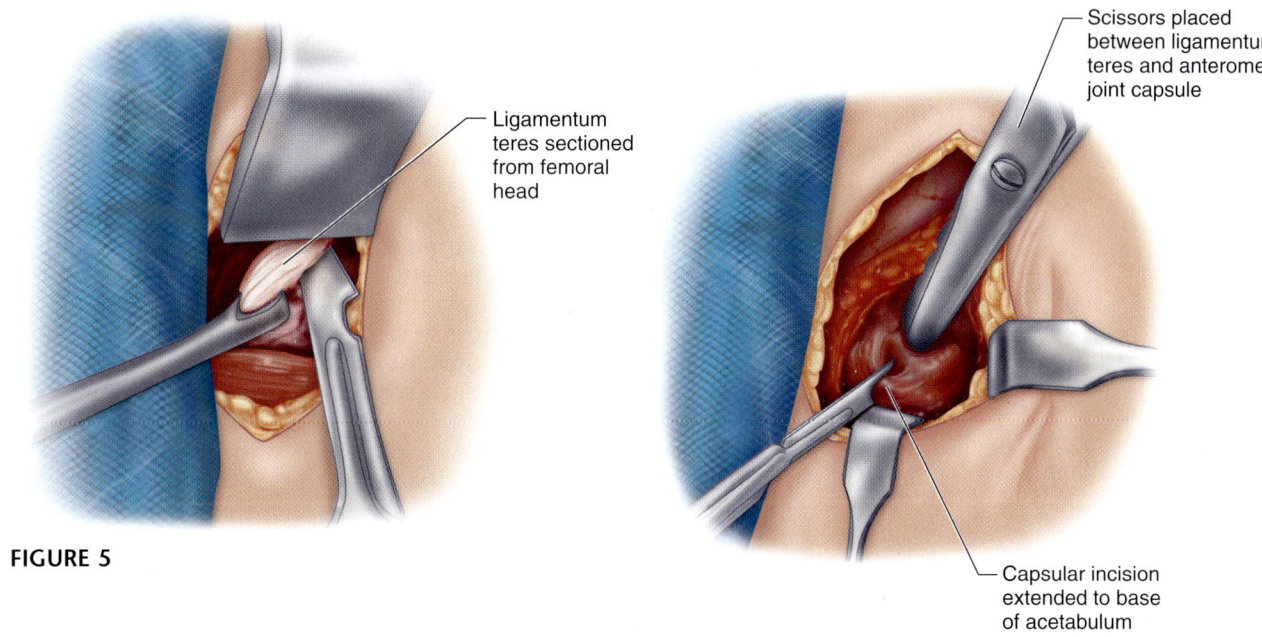

Ligamentum teres sectioned from femoral head

FIGURE 5

Scissors placed between ligamentum teres and anteromedial joint capsule

Capsular incision extended to base of acetabulum

FIGURE 6

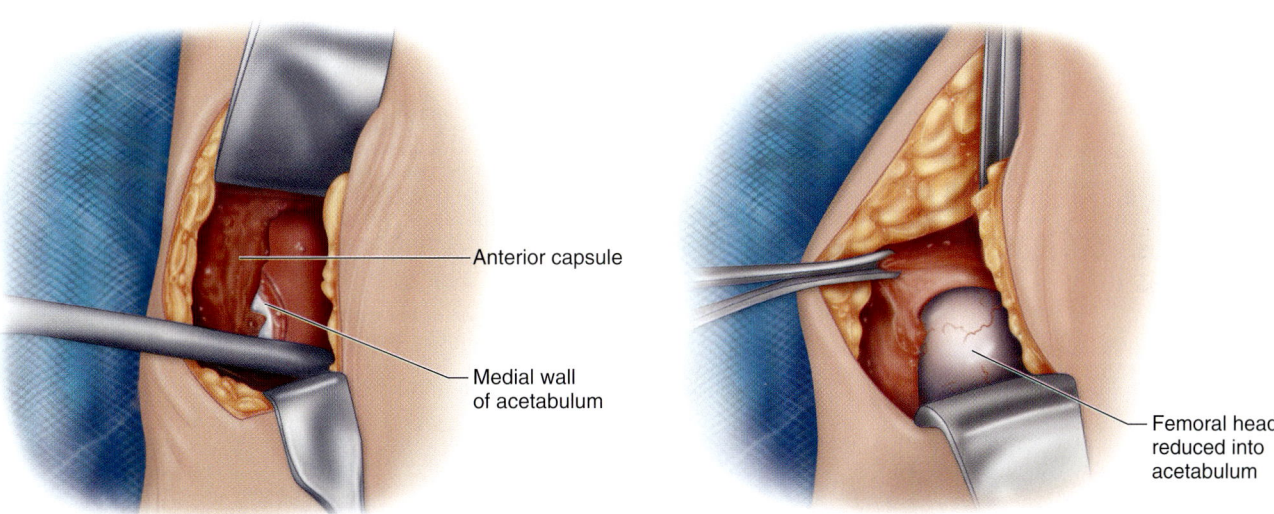

Anterior capsule

Medial wall of acetabulum

FIGURE 7

Femoral head reduced into acetabulum

FIGURE 8

POSTOPERATIVE CARE AND EXPECTED OUTCOMES

- Patients are usually discharged on the day after surgery or on the same day. Parents are instructed on cast care. It is essential for them to know that it is the cast that is maintaining the reduction attained at surgery. Most patients require little analgesia postoperatively. We generally recommend that the patients are nursed in a sitting position during the day as well as at night. The parents are encouraged to pick the child up not under the arms, but rather under the cast to prevent "shucking," which may cause cast sores.
- Six weeks after surgery, the cast on the involved side distal to the knee is removed to allow some motion of the knee and some rotation at the hip.
- Three months after surgery, the entire cast is removed and an abduction brace is applied that is structured to maintain the hip in the same position that it was in while in the plaster cast. Patients wear this abduction orthosis full time except while bathing (during which time the hips are kept in abduction).
- At about 5 months after surgery, the patient is gradually weaned from the brace to wearing it only at night and nap time until acetabular development is normal.
- The brace is usually worn for an average of 11–23 months after surgery.
- Patients are then followed to maturity, assessing progress in acetabular development and possible need for further surgical interventions.

EVIDENCE

Ferguson AB Jr. Primary open reduction for congenital dislocation of the hip using a median adductor approach. J Bone Joint Surg [Am]. 1973;55:671–89.

Kalamchi A, Schmidt TL, MacEwen GD. Congenital dislocation of the hip: open reduction by the medial approach. Clin Orthop Relat Res. 1982;(169):127–32.

Ludloff K. The open reduction of the congenital hip dislocation by an anterior incision. Am J Orthop Surg. 1913;10:438–54.

Morcuende JA, Meyer MD, Dolan LA, et al. Long-term outcome after open reduction through an anteromedial approach for congenital dislocation of the hip. J Bone Joint Surg [Am]. 1997;79:810–7.

Simons GW. A comparative evaluation of the current methods for open reduction of the congenitally displaced hip. Orthop Clin North Am. 1980;11:161–81.

Weinstein SL, Ponseti IV. Congenital dislocation of the hip: open reduction through a medial approach. J Bone Joint Surg [Am]. 1979;61:119–24.

FEMUR

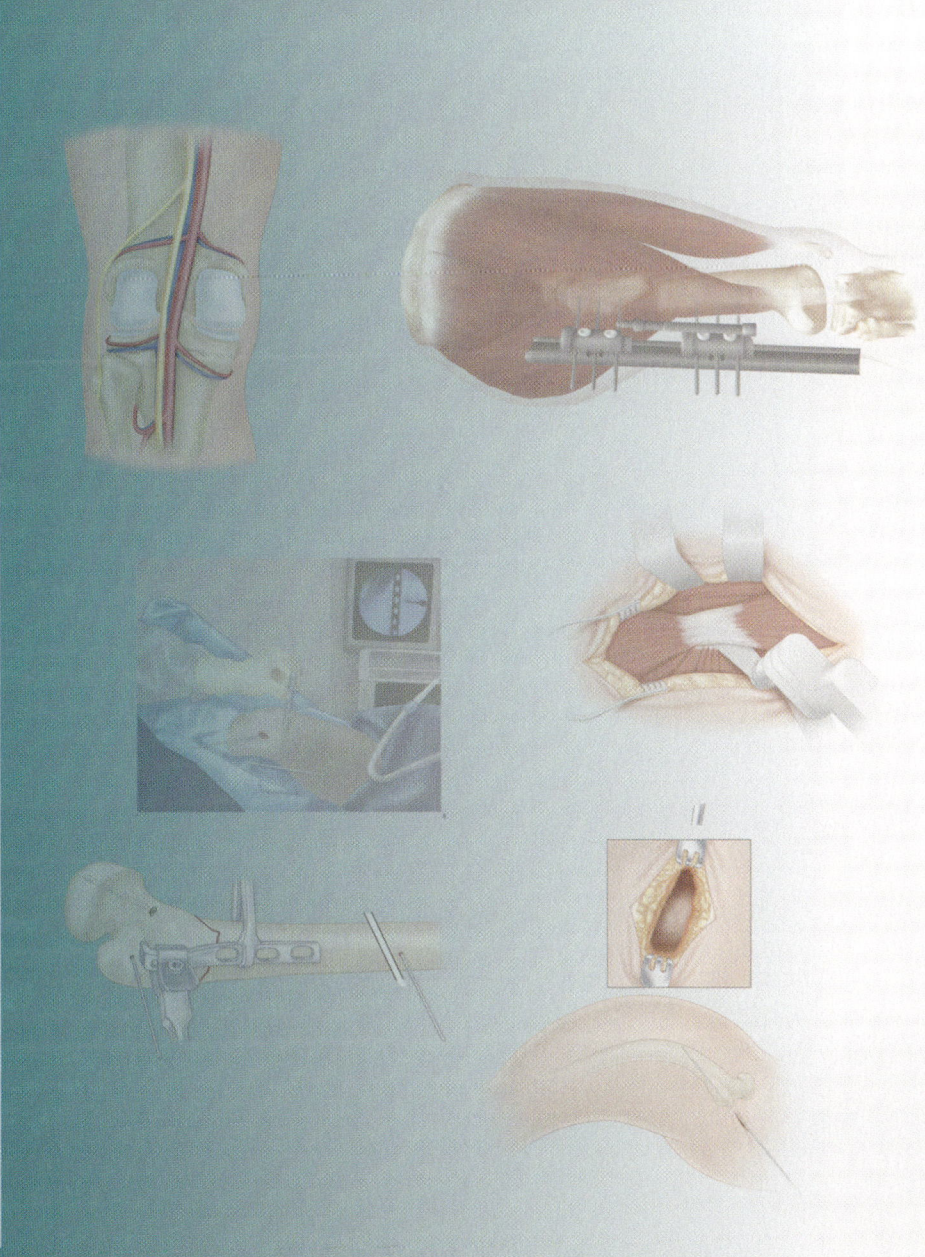

Femur Fracture: Flexible Intramedullary Nailing

Purushottam Arjun Gholve and John M. Flynn

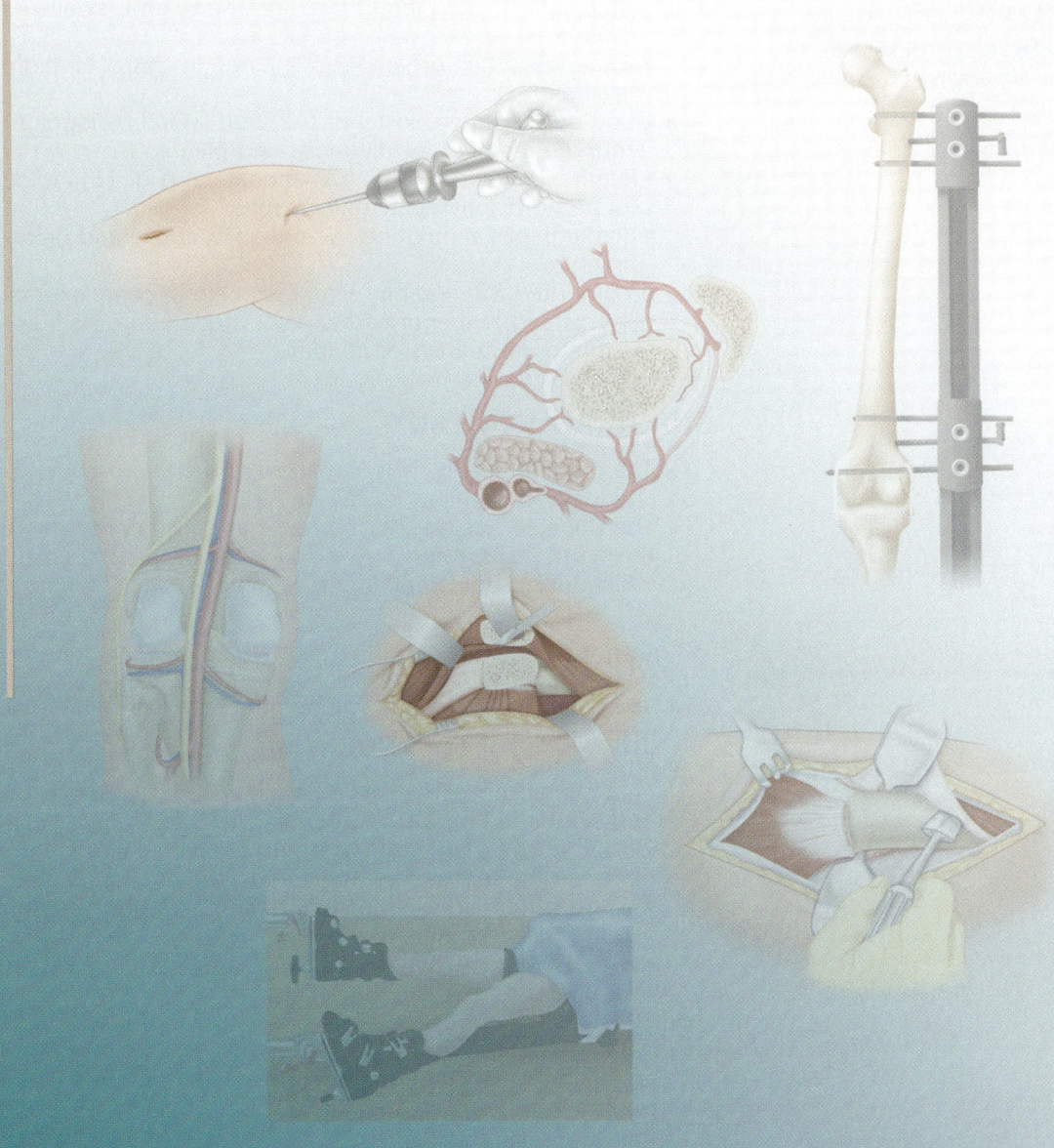

Treatment Options

• Closed reduction under sedation with spica cast

• If greater than 2 cm of shortening, initial traction followed by spica cast after 3 weeks

• Enders nail

INDICATIONS

- Children 5 to 12 years old (younger or older child is not a true contraindication)
- Length-stable fractures with minimum or no comminution
- Middle 70% of the diaphysis
- Weight less than 50 kg

EXAMINATION/IMAGING

- A thorough physical examination is conducted.
  - Note the mechanism of injury.
  - Examine the skin, surrounding soft tissue, and neurovascular status. In isolated femur fracture, the thigh is swollen and bruised.
  - Examine other organs and injuries in cases of high-energy trauma.
- Good-quality anteroposterior (AP) and lateral radiographs of the femur are required for diagnosis and planning.
  - Figure 1 shows AP (Fig. 1A) and lateral (Fig. 1B) radiographs of a mid-diaphyseal femur fracture.
  - Radiographs should include one joint above and below the fracture.
- A computed tomography scan may help in complex fracture patterns and to identify other associated injuries such as stress fracture or intra-articular injuries.

SURGICAL ANATOMY

- The distal femoral physis is marked under fluoroscopy to avoid any inadvertent injury to the physis.
- The popliteal vessels and the nerve are posterior to the femur at the surgical site (Fig. 2). Avoid slippage of the drill posteriorly while drilling the lateral and medial holes.

Equipment

• Functioning fracture table with all attachments

POSITIONING

- The patient is positioned supine on a radiolucent table or a fracture table (our preference).
- Smaller children (usually < 8 years old) may be better positioned on a radiolucent table, while bigger children (>8 years old) are best positioned on a fracture table.
- On the fracture table, the foot of the affected extremity is placed in the foot holder attached to the traction device.
  - The affected leg is abducted 15–30°, allowing working on both sides of the femur (Fig. 3).
  - The *white arrow* between the legs in Figure 3 depicts the position of the image intensifier.
- The unaffected foot is placed in a similar foot holder with the hip in extension (scissor position of the well leg) or 15° of abduction. Due to reports of compartment syndrome, we avoid positioning the unaffected leg in a flexed, abducted position of the hip over the patient.
- If it is not possible to place traction through the foot of the affected extremity, a traction pin may be inserted in the proximal tibia.

PORTALS/EXPOSURES

- Two 2-cm incision are made medially and laterally over the distal femoral physis.

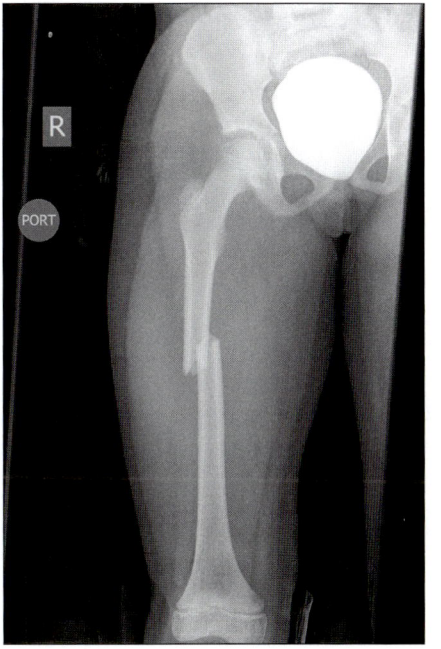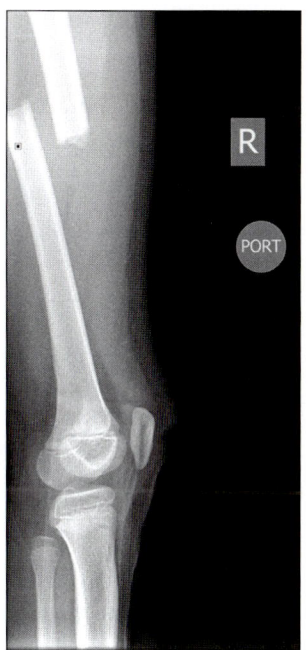

A   B

FIGURE 1

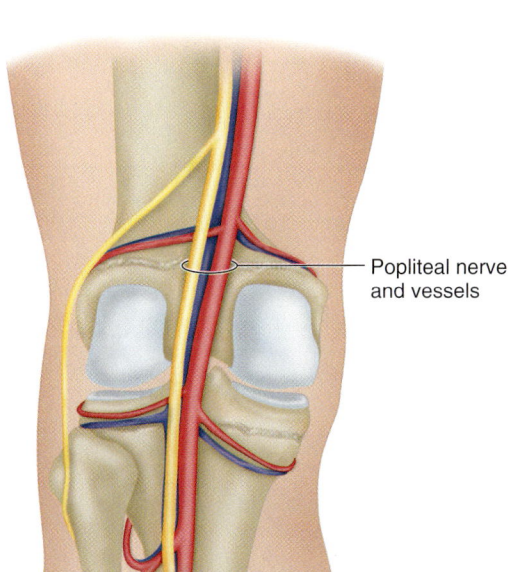

Popliteal nerve and vessels

FIGURE 2

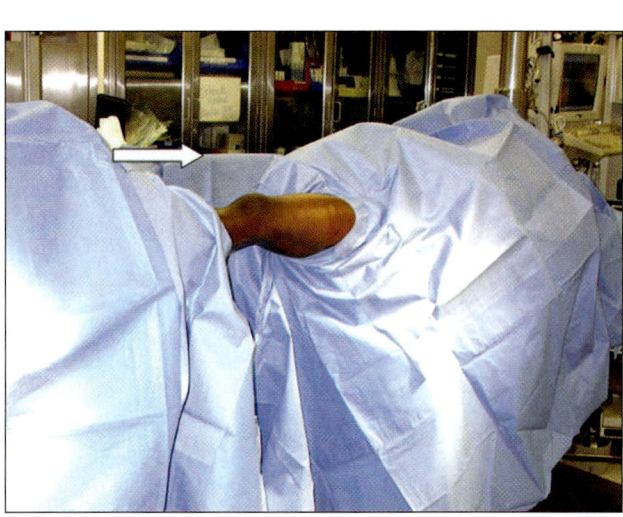

FIGURE 3

PEARLS

- *The drill hole should be oblique in the cephalad direction.*

PITFALLS

- *Avoid deep dissection/subperiosteal exposure directly over the physis.*

PROCEDURE

STEP 1

- After adequate positioning of the patient on a fracture table, the fracture is reduced as best as possible. The leg is prepared and draped in a standard manner either on the fracture table or on a radiolucent table.
- The distal femoral physis is identified under an image intensifier (Fig. 4), and the nail entry sites are marked 2 cm proximal to the physis on the medial and lateral distal femoral metaphyses.
- Two 2-cm skin incisions are made medially and laterally extending distally from the nail entry point toward the physis (Fig. 5).
- The incisions are carried through the deep tissue and quadriceps musculature using a Bovie.
- For each nail, a drill with a drill sleeve is placed at the nail entry site (2 cm proximal to the physis and midway between the anteroposterior cortex) (Fig. 6). The size of drill is usually 5 mm larger than the size of the nail to be used.
- Immediately on breaching the near cortex, the drill is angulated vertically in a cephalad direction to create an oblique path for nail entry (Fig. 7A). The fluoroscopic view in Figure 7B shows the oblique path of the drill for the nail entry.

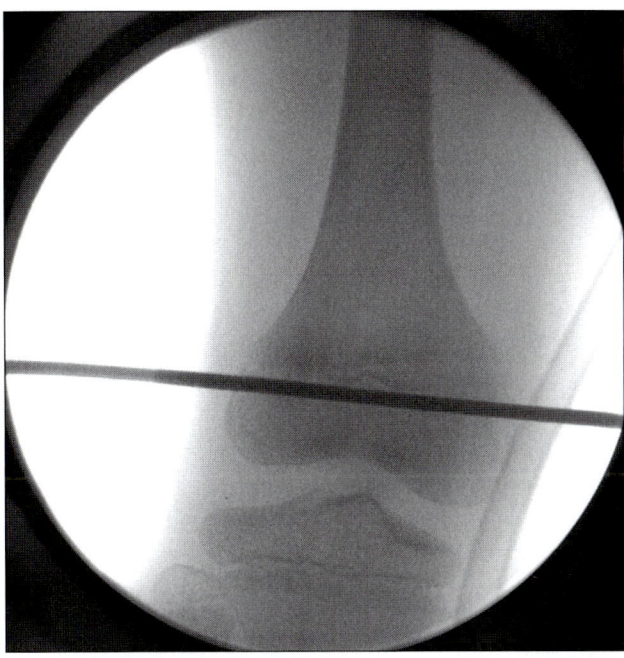

FIGURE 4

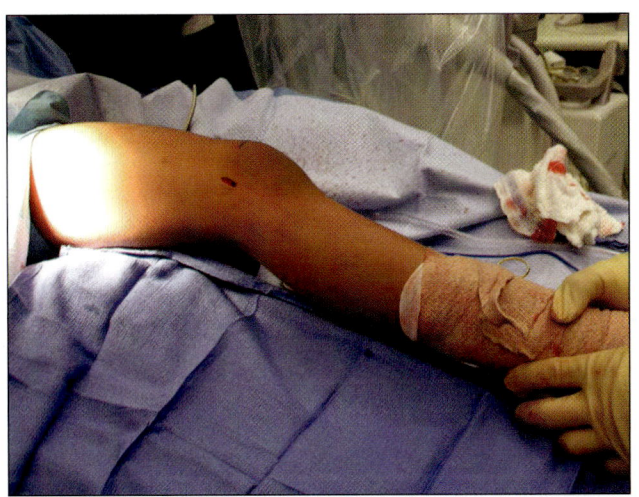

FIGURE 5

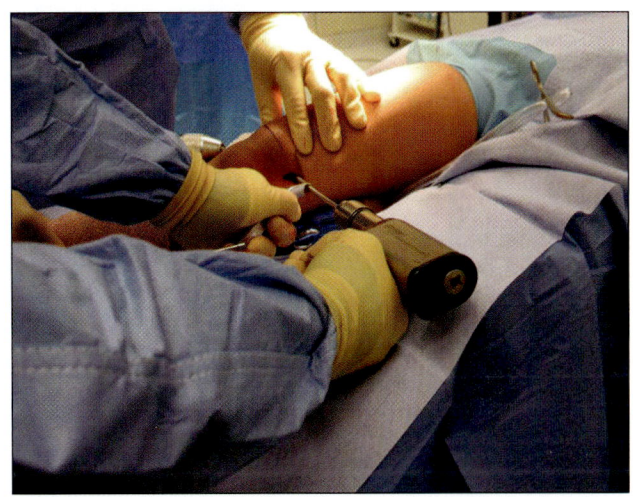

FIGURE 6

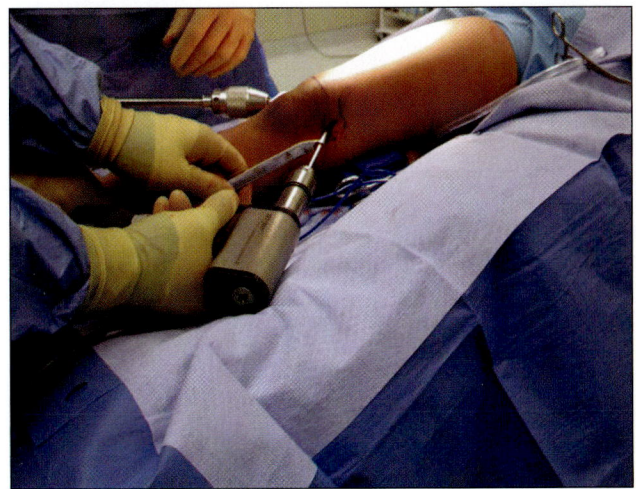

A

FIGURE 7

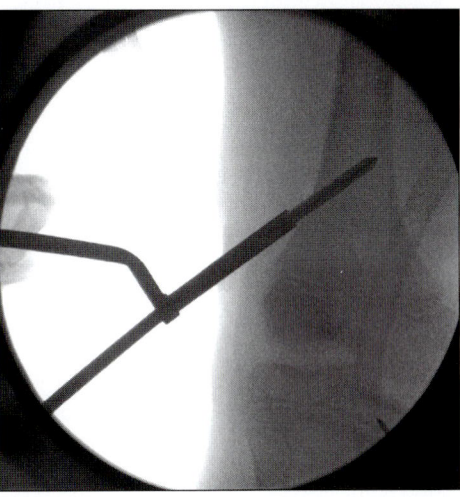

B

Instrumentation/ Implantation

- Flexible nails
  - Prebend the nails in C shape.
  - Both nails should be of the same diameter.

STEP 2

- The flexible nails are prebent in a C shape before insertion.
- The nail size is predetermined by measuring the isthmus of the femoral shaft. The nail of choice is usually 40% of the narrowest diameter (e.g., if the isthmus measures 1 cm, then a 4-mm nail is used). Thus two nails of the same diameter fill 80% of the isthmus.
- The first nail is introduced through one of the drill holes and advanced up to the fracture site under image intensifier guidance (Fig. 8A). Gentle tapping is all that is necessary to advance the nail.
- Another same-diameter nail is introduced through the other drill hole and advanced up to the fracture site (Fig. 8B).

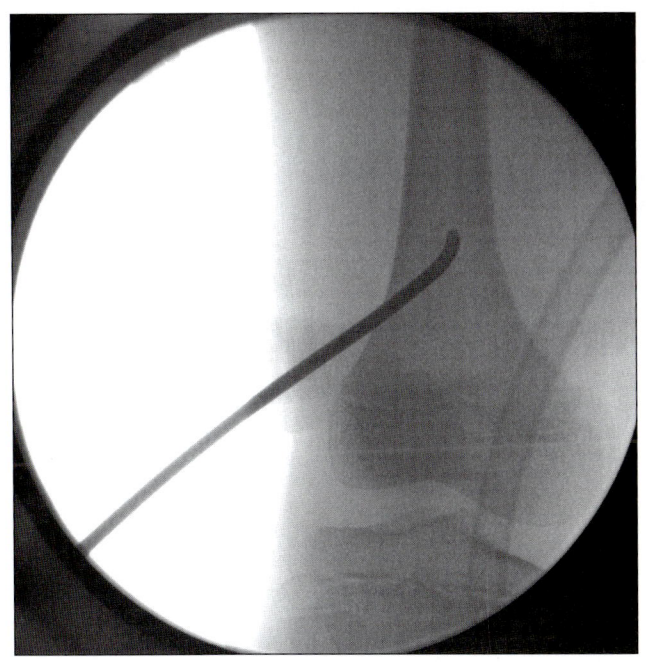 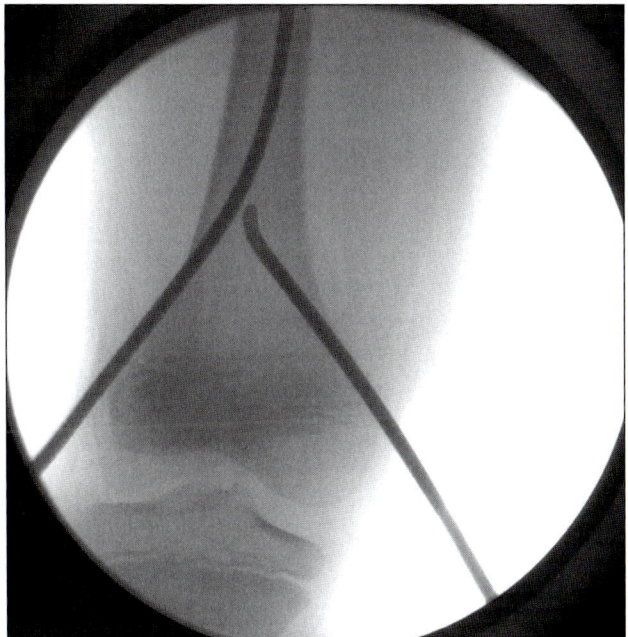

A

B

FIGURE 8

Instrumentation/ Implantation

- F tool (see Fig. 9B)

Step 3

- The fracture is best reduced by manipulating with an "F" tool (Fig. 9A and 9B) or free hands.
- The nail that is more difficult to pass across the fracture site is advanced first.
  - The tip of the nail is hooked in the proximal fragment (Fig. 10A).
  - The nail is rotated 180° to aid the fracture reduction (Fig. 10B).
  - Patience, gentle manipulation and tapping, and judicious use of AP and lateral fluoroscopy assist in the reduction of the fracture and passage of the first nail.
- Once the first nail is across the fracture site, the other nail is similarly advanced across the fracture.

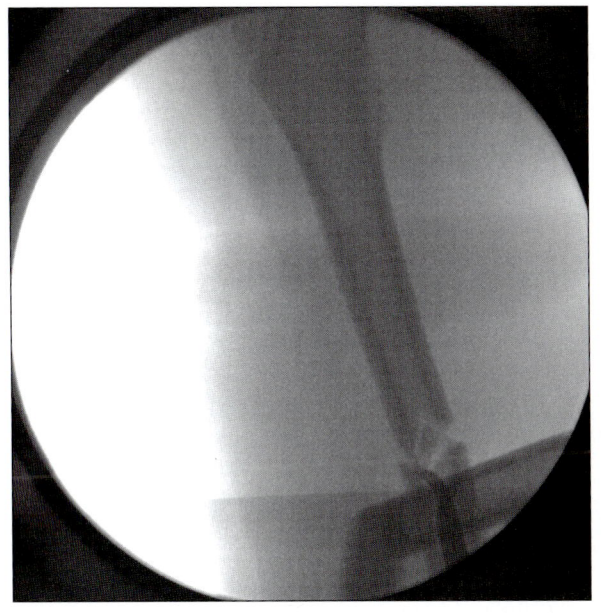

A

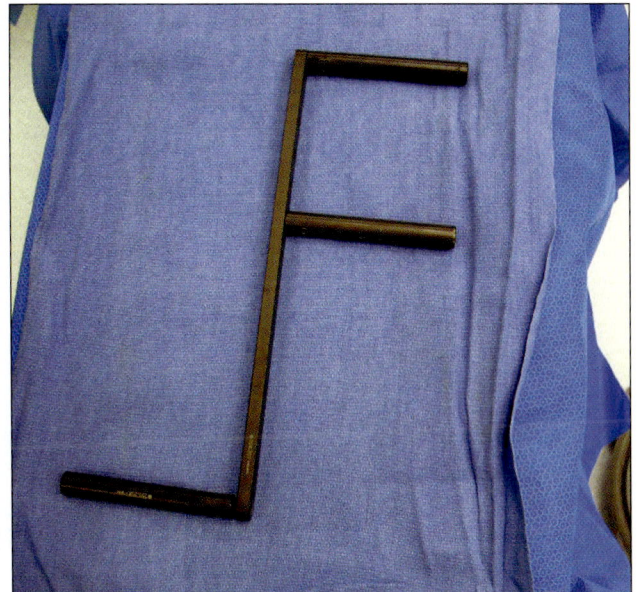

B

FIGURE 9

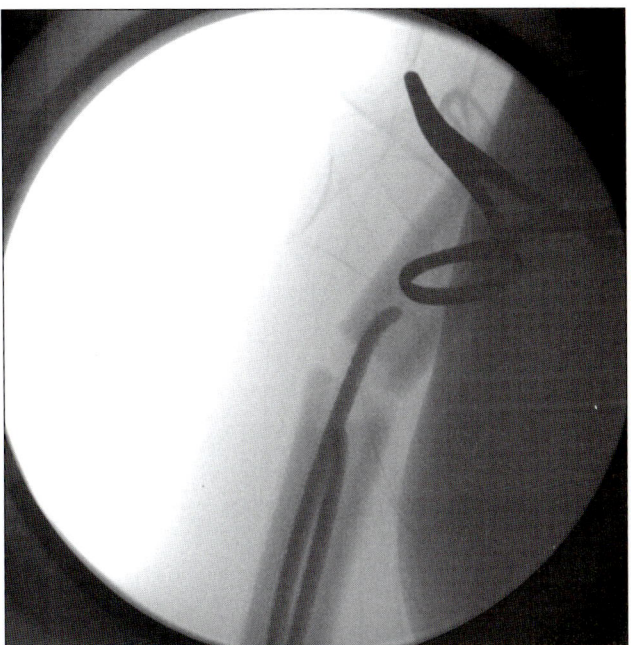

A

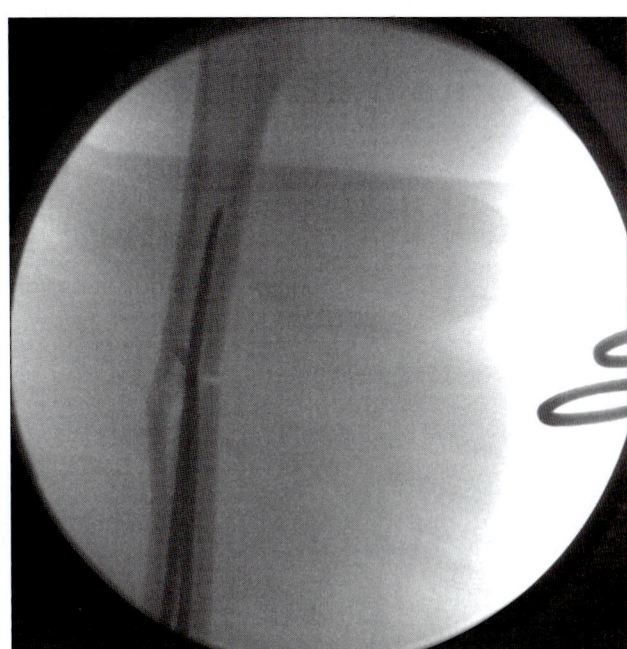

B

FIGURE 10

Complications

• Skin irritation at the insertion site if the nail is bent outward or cut too proud

• Nonunion, delayed union, or malunion (rotational or angular deformity)

• Leg length discrepancy

• Compartment syndrome or neurovascular injury

• Implant-related complication (retrograde pullout of the nail, breakage)

STEP 4

■ Once both the nails have crossed fracture site, they are advanced gradually to their final position (Fig. 11).

■ The nail entering laterally stops just beneath the greater trochanteric apophysis while the medial nail is advanced up to the medial calcar of the femoral neck (Fig. 12).

■ Both the nails are withdrawn 2 cm and cut at appropriate length (Fig. 13A). The nails are tapped back to their final position such that the cut tip is 5–10 mm from the femoral cortex (Fig. 13B).

■ If there is significant distraction at the fracture site, the traction is released and the fracture is impacted.

■ Figure 14 shows immediate postoperative AP (Fig. 14A) and lateral (Fig. 14B) radiographs of a repaired femur.

■ The wound is closed in layers.

POSTOPERATIVE CARE AND EXPECTED OUTCOMES

■ The leg is immobilized in a knee immobilizer for comfort and support for about 2 weeks.

■ Partial or full weight bearing as tolerated is commenced immediately postoperatively.

■ Analgesics are administered for pain on an as-needed basis.

■ Radiologic healing is observed in 8–12 weeks.

■ Nail removal is usually done 6 months after fracture healing.

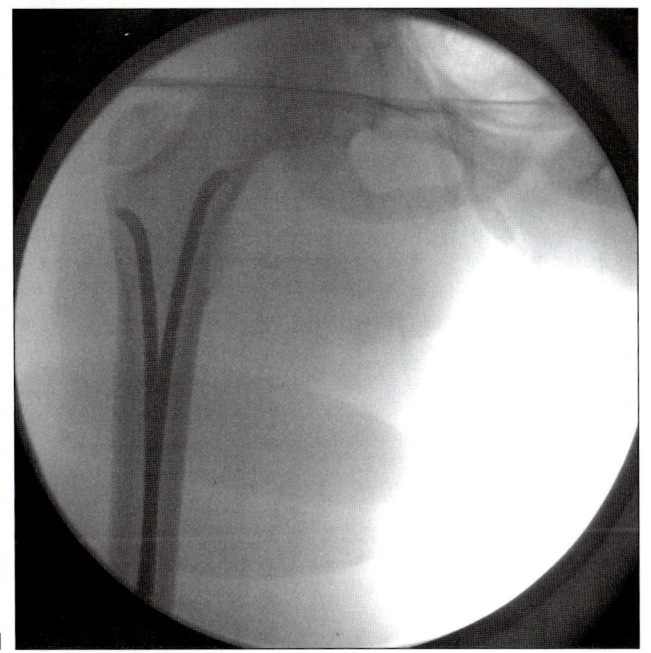

FIGURE 11

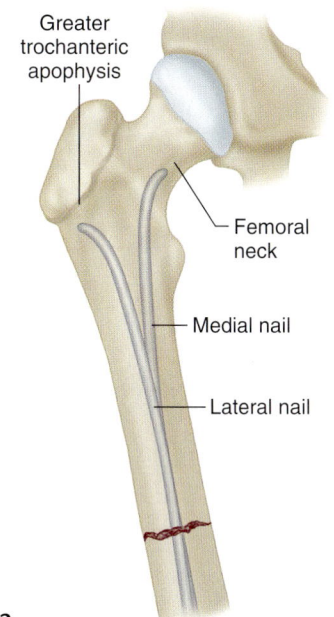

Greater
trochanteric
apophysis

Femoral
neck

Medial nail

Lateral nail

FIGURE 12

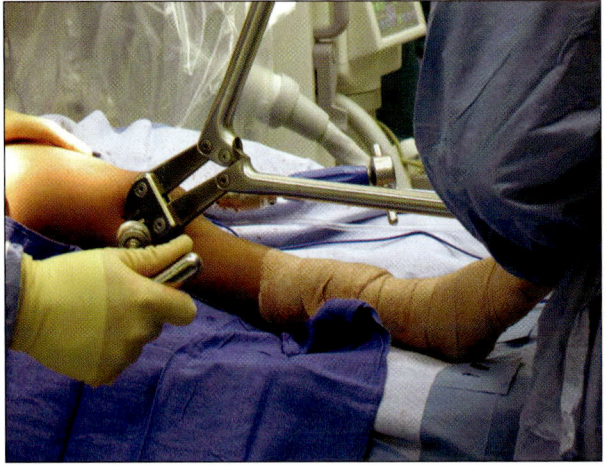

A

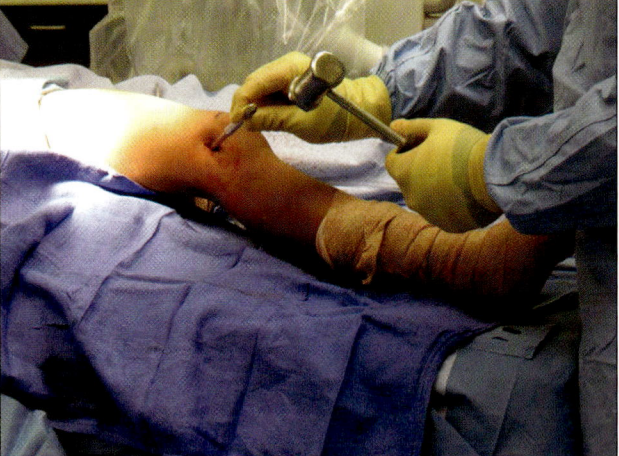

B

FIGURE 13

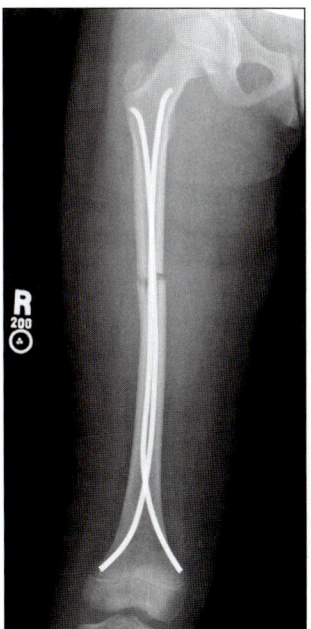

FIGURE 14 A

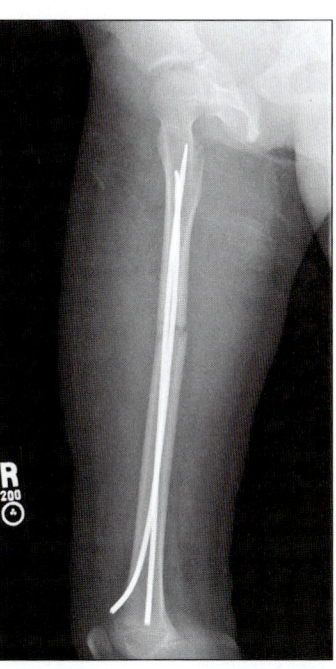

B

EVIDENCE

Bopst L, Reinberg O, Lutz N. Femur fracture in preschool children: experience with flexible intramedullary nailing in 72 children. J Pediatr Orthop. 2007;27:299–303.

In this study, preschool children treated with flexible intramedullary nailing benefited from a short hospital stay and early weight bearing and mobilization. Complications included early distal nail backout and femur overgrowth. (Level IV evidence)

Flynn JM, Hresko T, Reynolds RA, Blasier RD, Davidson R, Kasser J. Titanium elastic nails for pediatric femur fractures: a multicenter study of early results with analysis of complications. J Pediatr Orthop. 2001;21:4–8.

Flynn JM, Luedtke L, Ganley TJ, Pill SG. Titanium elastic nails for pediatric femur fractures: lessons from the learning curve. Am J Orthop. 2002;31:71–4.

Flynn JM, Schwend RM. Management of pediatric femoral shaft fractures. J Am Acad Orthop Surg. 2004;12:347–59.

In these papers, the authors discussed the use of flexible nails for school-age children. Potential complications included angular or rotational deformity, delayed union, and skin irritation at the nail entry site. (Level IV evidence)

Flynn JM, Luedtke LM, Ganley TJ, et al. Comparison of titanium nails with traction and a spica cast to treat femoral fractures in children. J Bone Joint Surg [Am]. 2004;86-A(4):770–7.

In this prospective cohort study of 83 consecutive femoral fractures, the data reveal that children treated with flexible nails recover the milestones faster and that the complication rate is similar. There were no cost differences in the nail versus traction/spica groups. (Level III evidence)

Goodwin R, Mahar AT, Oka R, et al. Biomechanical evaluation of retrograde intramedullary stabilization for femoral fractures: the effect of fracture level. J Pediatr Orthop. 2007;27:873–6.

The authors determined that distal femoral fractures could be best treated with C- or S-shaped titanium nails placed via an antegrade approach. (Level IV evidence)

Ho CA, Skaggs DL, Tang CW, Kay RM. Use of flexible intramedullary nails in pediatric femur fractures. J Pediatr Orthop. 2006;26:497–504.

In this study of 94 femur fractures treated with flexible nails, the complication rate was higher in patients age 10 years or more (34%) as compared to younger patients (9%). Postoperative hip and knee range of motion improved rapidly with loss of 4° by 6 months. (Level IV evidence)

Moroz LA, Launay F, Kocher MS, et al. Titanium elastic nailing of fractures of the femur in children: predictors of complications and poor outcome. J Bone Joint Surg [Br]. 2006;88:1361–6.

In this multicenter retrospective study of 234 femoral fractures treated with a titanium nail, only 10% had poor outcome, including leg length discrepancy, bad angulation, and failure of fixation in one patient. Children greater than 11 years of age and greater than 49 kg of weight were more prone to poor outcomes. (Level III evidence)

Morshed S, Humphrey M, Corrales LA, et al. Retention of flexible intramedullary nail following treatment of pediatric femur fractures. Arch Orthop Trauma Surg. 2007;127:509–14.

In this retrospective case series of 24 children treated with a flexible nail for femoral fractures, 25% required surgery due to persistent discomfort at the nail entry site. About 50% had residual nondebilitating pain at the nail entry site 2–5 years postinjury regardless of the presence of hardware. (Level IV evidence)

Sink EL, Gralla J, Repine M. Complications of pediatric femur fractures treated with titanium elastic nails: a comparison of fracture types. J Pediatr Orthop. 2005;25:577–80.

In this study of 39 consecutive femur fractures treated with titanium elastic nails, eight patients (21%) required unplanned surgery. Six of the eight patients had length-unstable fractures (long oblique or comminuted fractures). (Level IV evidence)

Guided Growth— Hemiepiphysiodesis

Peter M. Stevens

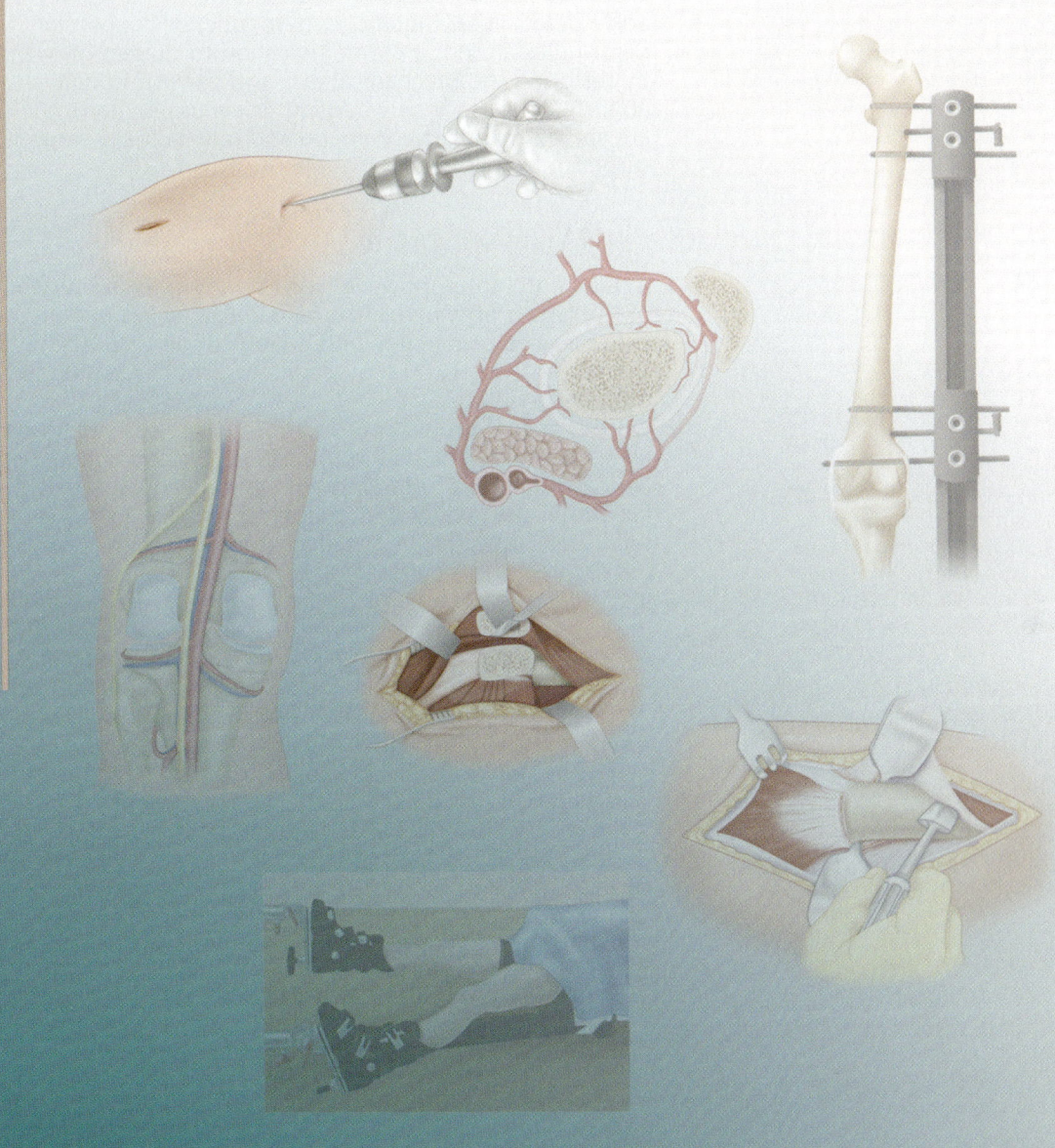

Contraindications

- Physiologic deformities (such as genu varum < age 2 and genu valgum < age 6)
- Physeal bar (unresectable)
- Skeletal maturity

Controversies

- One does not necessarily have to resort to osteotomy in order to effect improvement in relative length and correct rotation. The priority should be to correct the angular deformity first and then reassess the limb lengths and torsional profile. There may be concomitant improvement in secondary deformities, and even in joint laxity, as the mechanical axis is restored to neutral.

Treatment Options

- Phemister permanent epiphysiodesis (open vs. percutaneous)—While no hardware is implanted, this is an unforgiving and irreversible technique whereby the physis is surgically ablated. Errors in timing or follow-up may result in iatrogenic deformity requiring an osteotomy for salvage.

- Blount staples—Practiced for 6 decades, problems with staple migration, bending, and breakage have led to its declining popularity.

- Metaizeau (PETS) procedure—This uneccessarily violates the physis with large (6.5-mm) screws that may be difficult to remove. This is inapplicable in younger children and may not be reversible. It is not feasible to correct sagittal or oblique plane deformities.

- Osteotomy—Considered the "gold standard" for the previous century, this is much more invasive, requiring immobilization and deferred weight bearing. There are associate risks, including infection, under- or overcorrection, neurovascular injury, nonunion, and secondary growth disturbance. Osteotomy should be considered a salvage procedure when limb lengthening is required, or reserved for skeletally mature patients.

INDICATIONS

- Any angular deformity of the extremities, as long as the physis is still open
  - Age range: 18 months to 18 years
  - Size range: 12–200 kg
- Any etiology: posttraumatic, developmental, metabolic, genetic, dysplasias, neuromuscular etc.
- Guided growth is the most recent and refined treatment available. Reversible in nature, the 8-plate is removed upon achievement of the desired neutral alignment.
- The most common application for guided growth is for correction of frontal plane deformities of the knee. However, it is also useful for oblique or sagittal deformities as well as for ankle deformities. Metabolic, dysplastic, or congenital deformities are not a contraindication to guided growth. In fact, by restoring the mechanical axis and correcting gait abnormalities (such as waddling or circumduction), the physes are spared cumulative damage and may actually respond surprisingly well.

EXAMINATION/IMAGING

- A full-length anteroposterior (AP) standing teloroentgenogram of the legs is obtained with the patellae facing forward and the pelvis leveled as needed with a block under the foot of the shorter leg (Fig. 1). The other side is properly positioned with the patella neutral.
- On this frontal projection, the mechanical axis should bisect the knee, or at least fall within the central two quadrants (Fig. 2A). Dividing the knee into quadrants, the mechanical axis should fall within the central two quadrants (± zone 1). Zones 2 and 3 represent indications for guided growth to restore the axis to (or slightly past) neutral (Fig. 2B).
- Also, AP and lateral views of the hip, knee, or ankle are obtained to see the details of the physes of interest.
  - Figure 3A demonstrates a 12-year-old female presenting with unilateral Blount disease, including lateral ligamentous laxity and thrust. There is no concomitant femoral valgus or varus deformity.
  - Twelve months following guided growth of the tibia, her mechanical axis is neutral, the lateral laxity and thrust are resolved, and the 8-plate was removed (Fig. 3B).
- Fluoroscopic views orthogonal to the physis (such as in Blount disease) may be obtained to rule out a physeal bar.
- An intraoperative arthrogram (in young children) may be obtained to outline the chondroepiphyses and facilitate targeting/postition of implants.

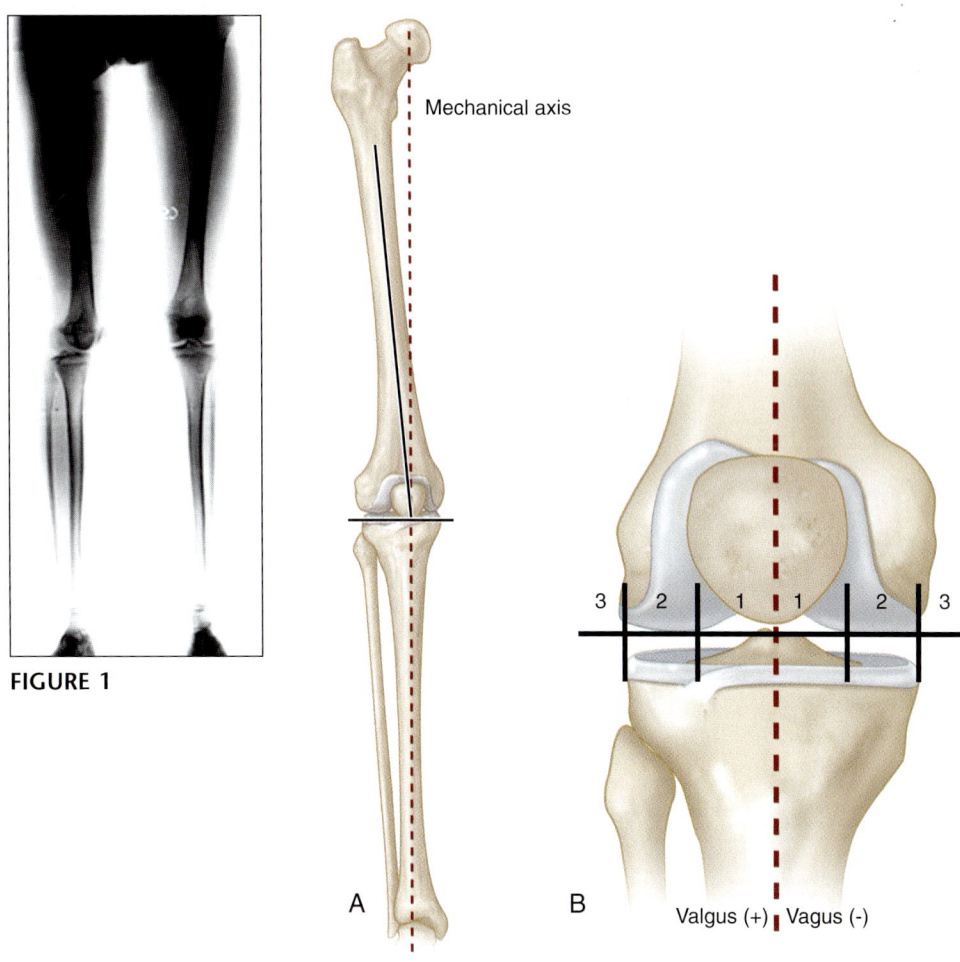

FIGURE 1

Mechanical axis

Valgus (+) Vagus (-)

A   B

FIGURE 2

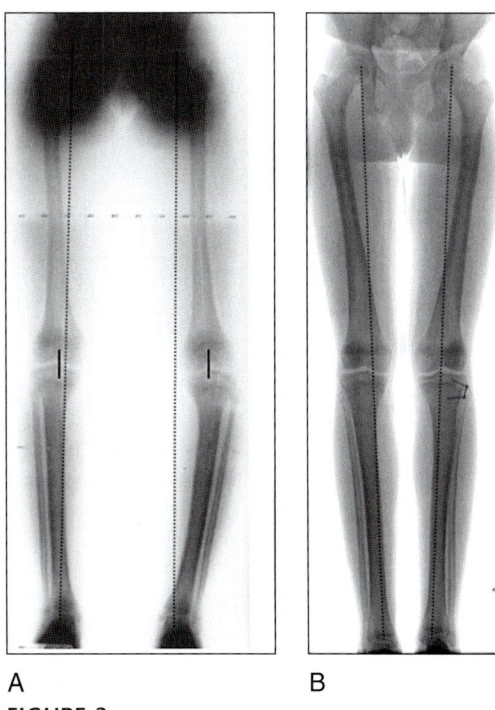

A   B

FIGURE 3

SURGICAL ANATOMY

- Fortunately, most physes are virtually subcutaneous and readily approached. They are also remote from important neurovascular structures, which generally are not visualized during the surgical approach.
- To preserve a horizontal knee, the femur and tibia may both require attention.
- The adductor tubercle medially and the lateral epicondyle laterally represent the perimeter of the physis of the femur.
- The medial and lateral physeal ridges of the tibia are relatively prominent and easy to identify, allowing the skin to be marked under fluoroscopic guidance.
- The 8-plate is typically positioned at the apex of a given deformity.

POSITIONING

- The patient is placed supine on a radiolucent table.
- An image intensifier is positioned on the opposite side of the tabel for unilateral cases, or may be placed at the foot of the table for bilateral cases.

PORTALS/EXPOSURES

- The skin is marked at the level of the physis.
- Subcutaneous tissues are infiltrated with 0.25% Marcaine/epinephrine.
- A 2- to 3-cm incision is centered over the physis of interest.
- Upon splitting the overlying fascia, muscles and tendons are retracted, leaving the periosteum and perichondrial ring undisturbed.

PEARLS

- *Preserve the perisoteum to avoid physeal closure.*

PROCEDURE

STEP 1

- A subfascial/submuscular approach is used to place the implants.
- A Keith needle is inserted into the physis parallel to its course (note that it will not cause harm to the physis).
- The position of the needle is checked fluoroscopically (AP and lateral projections), readjusted as needed, and rechecked.

STEP 2

- The 8-plate is applied with the center hole over the Keith needle.
  - The 8-plate (Orthofix, Inc.) (Fig. 4A) is a nonlocking, titanium plate that comes in two dimensions: 12 and 16 mm (center hole to center hole). The screws can diverge approximately 30° before contracting the plate, whereupon the precontoured plate may reverse bend with continued growth.
  - The cannulated screws (Fig. 4B) come in 3 lengths: 16, 24, and 32 mm. The solid screws (circled tips) come in 2 lengths: 24 and 36 mm. the latter are useful for length inhibition and some patients with Blount's disease.
- Smooth 1.6-mm guide pins are inserted (epiphyseal first, then metaphyseal).
- The cortex is predrilled to a depth of 5 mm to avoid shear stress upon screw insertion.
- Two cannulated screws are inserted (solid screws are used for Blount disease).

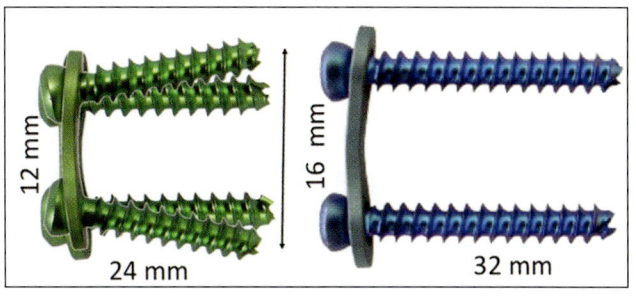

A

FIGURE 4

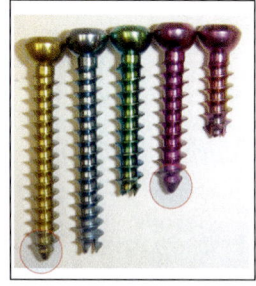

B

Controversies

- Rebound growth/recurrence—this reflects the natural history of a given condition; it is not iatrogenic. However, it highlights the need for biannual follow-up after explantation.

- Repeat guided growth is safe and well tolerated, but it is best to forewarn the parents of the possibility at the outset.

- Screw length and hardware position are rechecked by fluoroscopy.
- The guide pins are removed.
- The screws are alternately tightened/countersunk to avoid three-point bending stress that could lead to screw fracture.

STEP 3

- The wound is closed in layered fashion.
- Steri-Strips with OpSite spray or a Tegaderm dressing is used to close the skin.
- A soft compression dressing is applied; no splint is required.

POSTOPERATIVE CARE AND EXPECTED OUTCOMES

- Showering is permitted at 2 days, and bathing and swimming at 7 days.
- Immediate mobilization and weight bearing are encouraged.
- Crutches are optional, and may be used as needed for comfort.
- Physical therapy is optional, and can be used if the patient is slow to mobilize.
- Return to activities and sports is permitted as tolerated.
- Follow-up after implant removal should be continued until skeletal maturity. Routine follow-up is done at 3-month intervals. Correction occurs in 12 ± 3 months (average); radiographs are obtained only when clinical correction is achieved.
- In the event that there is rebound growth causing recurrent deformity, guided growth may safely be repeated and is still preferable to an osteotomy. Figure 5 depicts the rebound growth trend. Timely $\pm$ repeated intervention, correcting the mechanical axis to or slightly past neutral, should suffice to manage most deformities without resorting to osteotomy.

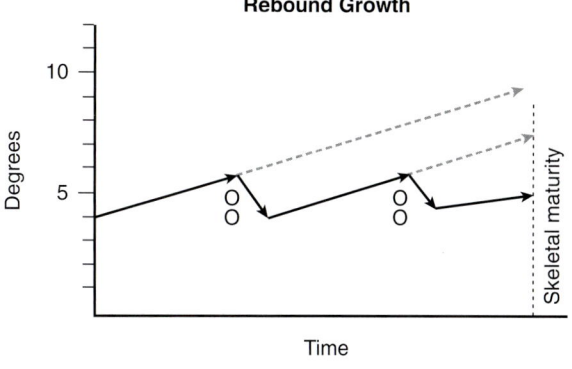

FIGURE 5

EVIDENCE

Grover J, Noonan K. Mechanical behavior of the lamb growth plate in response to asymmetrical joint loading: a model for Blount disease. J Pediatr Orthop. 2007; 27:485–92.

(Level III evidence)

Klatt J, Stevens PM. Guided growth for fixed knee flexion deformity. J Pediatr Orthop. 2008;28:626–31.

(Level III evidence)

Machen MS, Stevens PM. Should full-length standing anteroposterior radiographs replace the scanogram for measurement of limb length discrepancy? J Pediatr Orthop B. 2005;14:30–7.

(Level III evidence)

Mast N, Brown NAT, Brown C, Stevens PM. Validation of a genu valgum model in a rabbit hind limb. J Pediatr Orthop. 2008;28:375–80.

(Level III evidence)

Novais E, Stevens PM. Hypophosphatemic rickets: the role of hemiepiphysiodesis. J Pediatr Orthop. 2006;26:238–44.

(Level III evidence)

Stevens PM, Klatt JB. Guided growth for pathological physes: radiographic improvement during realignment. J Pediatr Orthop. 2008;28:632–9.

(Level III evidence)

Stevens PM. Guided growth for angular correction: a preliminary series using a tension band plate. J Pediatr Orthop. 2007;27:253–9.

(Level III evidence)

Stevens PM. Guided growth: 1933 to the present. Strategies Trauma Limb Reconstr. 2006;1:29–35.

(Level III evidence)

Stevens PM, Pease F. Hemiepiphysiodesis for posttraumatic tibial valgus. J Pediatr Orthop. 2006;26:385–92.

(Level III evidence)

Stevens PM, MacWilliams B, Mohr RA. Gait analysis of stapling for genu valgum. J Pediatr Orthop. 2004;24:70–4.

(Level III evidence)

Femoral Lengthening with External Fixation

Shawn C. Standard and John E. Herzenberg

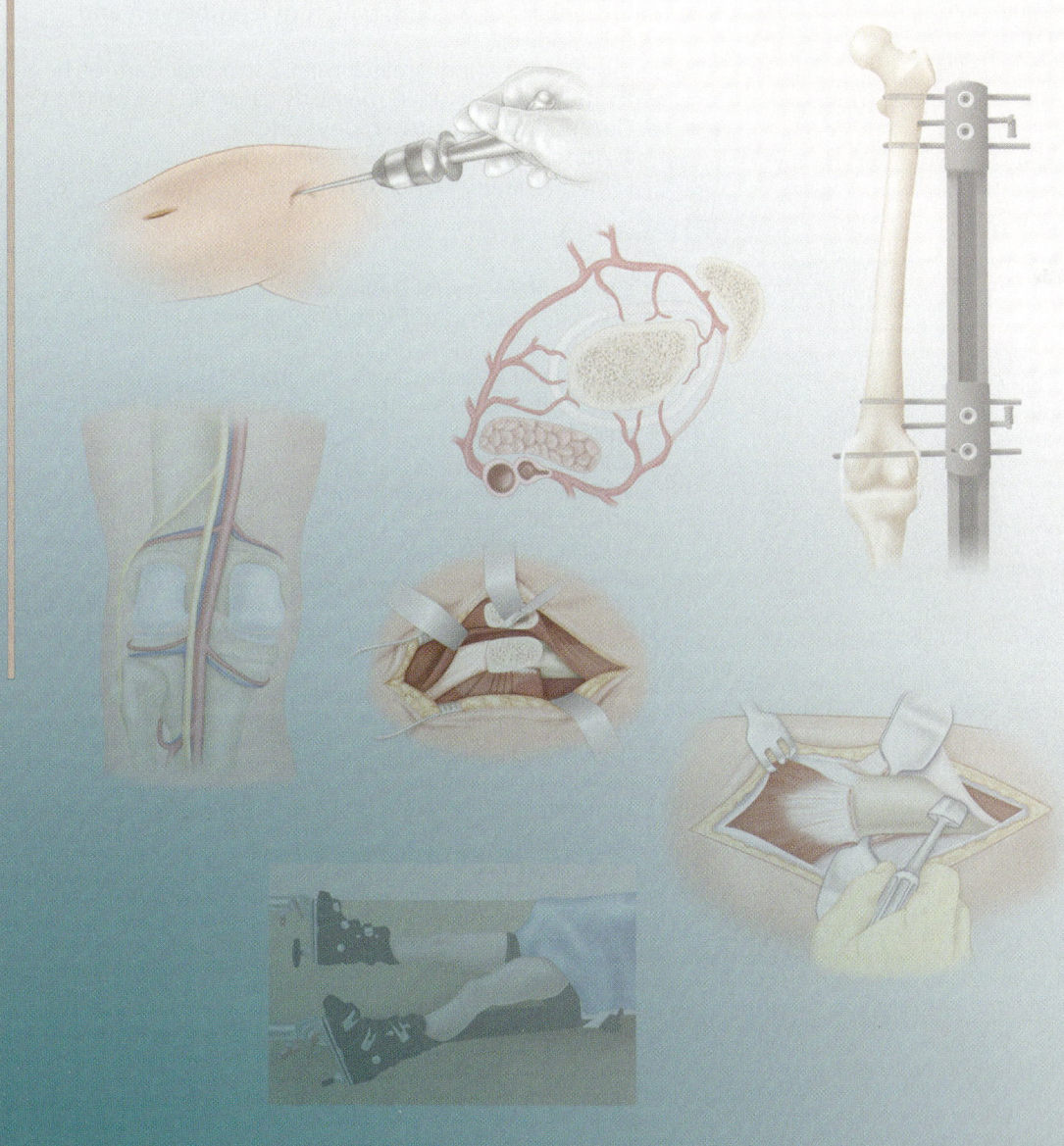

Continued

PITFALLS

- *Congenital femoral deficiency*

  - *Severe concurrent deformities of the hip and knee—Joint realignment and reconstruction prior to lengthening.*

  - *Intrinsic soft tissue contractures—Release of the rectus femoris tendon and excision of the ITB prior to lengthening.*

  - *Concurrent instability of the hip and knee joints—The hip joint requires correction of the concurrent acetabular dysplasia with a pelvic osteotomy prior to lengthening. The knee joint should always be bridged with a hinged external fixation component during the lengthening of the congenitally deficient femur.*

- *Russell-Silver syndrome*

  - *Difficult to predict the final limb-length inequality during growth.*

  - *Wait until skeletal maturity to equalize limb lengths. May proceed with initial lengthening if leg length discrepancy (LLD) is greater than 5 cm; parents must be warned to expect possible recurrence and need for further treatment.*

- *Juvenile rheumatoid arthritis*

  - *Type V growth pattern with upward slope–plateau–downward slope with improvement without intervention.*

  - *Final LLD should be assessed at skeletal maturity and then corrected.*

- *Achondroplasia*

  - *Premature limb lengthening at ages less than 8 years can result in growth inhibition.*

  - *Greater than 6–7 cm of femoral lengthening in a skeletally immature patient can result in growth inhibition.*

- *Hemihypertrophy: Klippel-Trénaunay syndrome*

  - *Avoid acute shortening of the involved side secondary to potential venous malformations.*

INDICATIONS

- Femoral shortening with or without concurrent limb deformity
  - Acute deformity correction can be performed with subsequent gradual distraction for lengthening at the same osteotomy site.
  - Double femoral osteotomies can be performed for deformity correction at one site and lengthening at the second site.
  - Figure 1 shows an example of a patient with congenital femoral deficiency that is undergoing a femoral lengthening. A double-level osteotomy has been performed for acute deformity correction both proximally and distally with concurrent lengthening at the distal osteotomy site.
- Femoral shortening greater than 7–8 cm will require sequential lengthenings or a combination of lengthening and epiphysiodesis.
- Femoral shortening greater than 3 cm that cannot be treated with more conservative methods (shoe lifts or epiphysiodesis)
  - Contraindications to epiphysiodesis:
    - Abnormal predicted overall height
    - Inadequate growth remaining

ETIOLOGIES

- Congenital
  - Congenital femoral deficiency
    - Proximal femoral focal deficiency
    - Congenital short femur
    - Postaxial hypoplasia of the limb
  - Fibular hemimelia with concurrent femoral shortening
  - Hemihypertrophy
    - Neurofibromatosis
    - Beckwith-Wiedemann syndrome
    - Idiopathic
    - Proteus syndrome
    - Klippel-Trénaunay syndrome
  - Hemiatrophy
  - Congenital banding syndrome (Streeter's dysplasia)
- Neuromuscular
  - Hemiplegic cerebral palsy
  - Polio
  - Myelomeningocele
  - Sciatic nerve injury
- Traumatic
  - Malunion
  - Growth arrest
  - Bone loss
- Infection
  - Septic arthritis
    - Growth arrest or bone loss
    - Neonatal
  - Osteomyelitis
    - Growth arrest or bone loss
  - Meningococcal septicemia
- Developmental
  - Developmental dysplasia/dislocation of the hip
  - Slipped capital femoral epiphysis
  - Legg-Calvé-Perthes disease
  - Ollier's enchondromatosis
  - Multiple hereditary exostosis
  - Russell-Silver syndrome
  - Melorheostosis
  - Rickets

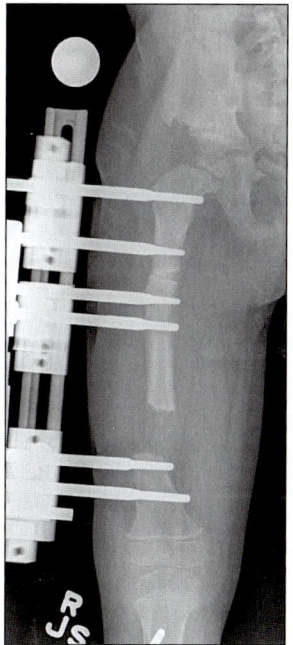

FIGURE 1

PITFALLS—cont'd

- *Polio*

  - *Delayed regenerate bone formation and healing—Consider decreased rate of distraction.*

  - *Must maintain full knee extension or slight hyperextension for patients with decreased quadriceps strength. Residual knee flexion contractures eliminate the patient's ability to lock the knee during ambulation and result in brace requirement for supported ambulation.*

- *Developmental dysplasia/dislocation of the hip, slipped capital femoral epiphysis, and Legg-Calvé-Perthes disease*

  - *LLD resulting from residual hip deformity may be treated with proximal femoral/hip osteotomies that impart length with concurrent realignment: proximal femoral valgus osteotomy (Wagner osteotomy); femoral neck lengthening osteotomy (Morscher osteotomy); surgical hip dislocation with subcapital osteotomy.*

Treatment Options

- LLD less than 2 cm
  - No treatment
  - Shoe lift

- LLD less than 5 cm
  - Shoe lift
  - Epiphysiodesis
  - Acute shortening

- Extreme LLD
  - Limb ablation with prosthetic reconstruction: used when LLD predicted to be greater than 30–35 cm, or with severe dysplasia or absence of associated joints (hip and knee)

- Renal osteodystrophy
- Skeletal dysplasia/achondroplasia
- Osteogenesis imperfecta
- Juvenile rheumatoid arthritis

Controversies

- LLD less than 2 cm
  - Considered within normal variation
  - Easily treated with internal shoe lift
  - No evidence of long-term sequelae

- Severe deformities requiring extensive lengthening
  - Reconstruction with lengthening should be performed at specialized centers.
  - Limb ablation with prosthetic reconstruction can be considered if total predicted LLD is greater than 30–35 cm. Associated joints are not amendable to reconstruction.

- LLD less than 5 cm in the skeletally immature patient
  - Long-leg epiphysiodesis if adequate growth remains and height prediction is within normal range

- LLD less than 5 cm in the skeletally mature patient
  - Femoral shortening of long leg; requires significant rehabilitation for quadriceps strength recovery

EXAMINATION/IMAGING

PHYSICAL EXAMINATION

- Range of motion of the hip, knee, and ankle joints
  - Concurrent contractures or joint/bony abnormalities must be documented.
    - Special consideration must be given to knee fixed flexion deformity. The cause (soft tissue contracture vs. bony deformity) must be determined.
  - Concurrent joint instabilities and ligamentous deficiencies must be documented.
    - The majority of congenital femoral deficiencies have concurrent absence of anterior and posterior cruciate ligaments.
- Clinical alignment
  - Coronal plane: varus deformity vs. valgus deformity
  - Sagittal plane: recurvatum vs. procurvatum
- Rotational profile
  - The presence of internal or external femoral torsion must be determined.
- Clinical limb-length assessment
  - One-centimeter blocks are placed under the short leg until the pelvis is level.
- Neurologic examination
  - The patient's strength, sensation, and reflexes should be noted.

RADIOGRAPHIC EXAMINATION

- Anteroposterior (AP) and lateral standing long-leg radiographs are obtained (taken at a distance of 10 feet using a 51-inch cassette) (Figs. 2 and 3).
  - Malalignment and malorientation tests are performed to determine concurrent deformity and location of deformity.
  - Limb lengths are assessed (the pelvis should be leveled with blocks and the number of blocks noted on the radiograph).

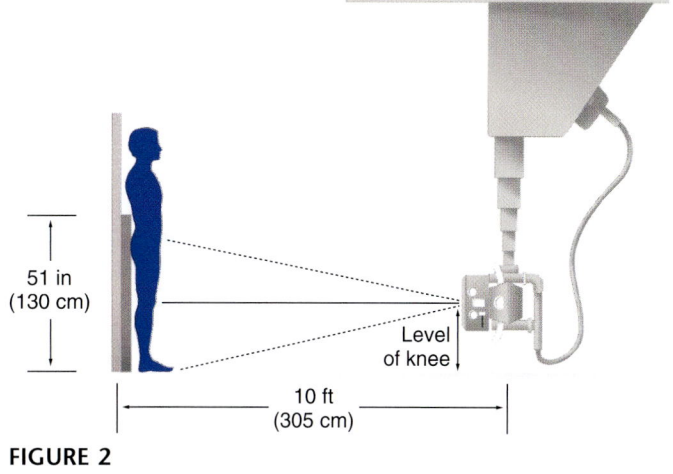

FIGURE 2

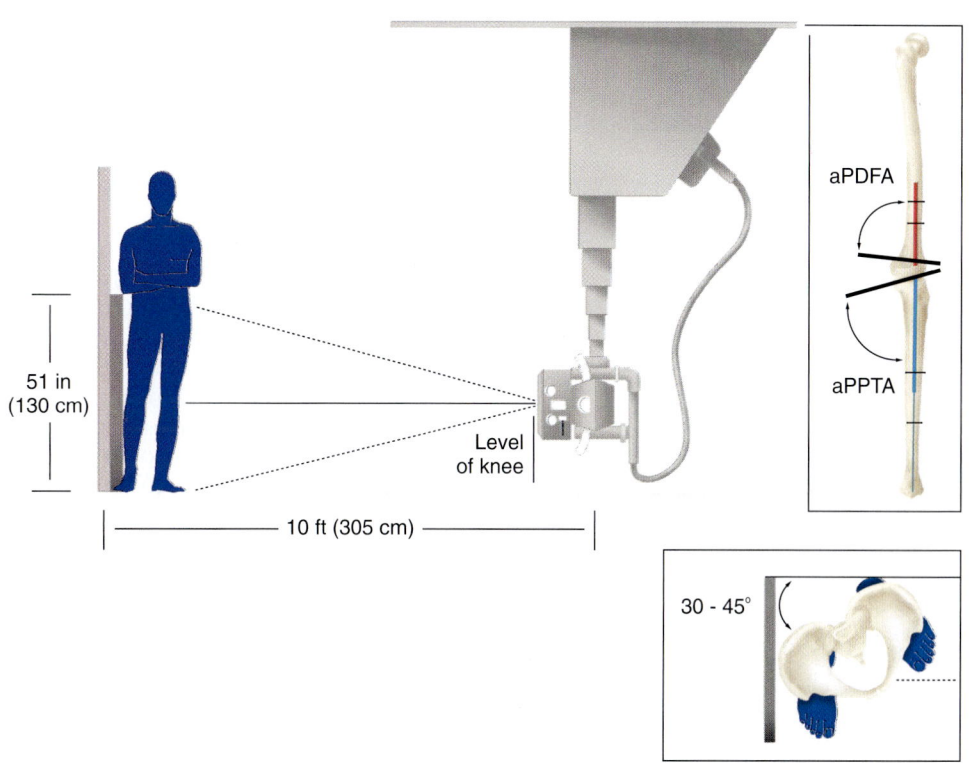

FIGURE 3

■ Standing long-leg lateral radiographs (with maximum knee extension) are obtained (Fig. 4).
  • The radiographs are checked for fixed flexion deformity of the knee.
  • A malorientation test is performed to determine the presence and location of sagittal plane deformity.
  • The radiographs are checked for joint subluxation (significant anterior-posterior instability).
■ Significant joint or limb deformity should be assessed on a separate radiograph centered on the joint or limb segment of interest.
■ A supine AP pelvis radiograph should be obtained prior to lengthening to assess the integrity of the hip joint (center-edge angle and appearance of the sourcil).

SURGICAL ANATOMY

■ Acetabulum
  • Significant dysplasia will result in increased risk of hip dislocation.
    ◆ Up-slanting sourcil
    ◆ Abnormal center-edge angle
  • Significant dysplasia requires pelvic osteotomy prior to femoral lengthening (Dega osteotomy, triple osteotomy, periacetabular osteotomy).
■ Tensor fascia lata/iliotibial band (ITB)
  • This structure will be penetrated by the laterally placed half-pins.
    ◆ At the end of the procedure, the knee must be maximally flexed to stretch/tear the fascia lata around the half-pins.
    ◆ If the fascia lata is not stretched, a postoperative knee extension contracture will result with minimal knee flexion.
  • If a preoperative contracture is present, then a prophylactic release is required at the time of surgery.
    ◆ Congenital femoral deficiency lengthening requires an excision of the ITB prior to lengthening.
    ◆ Achondroplasia requires a prophylactic release of the distal ITB prior to the second femoral lengthening (if performed).
■ Sciatic nerve/peroneal nerve
  • These nerves are not directly at risk during the external fixation application or osteotomy.
  • Rapid lengthening or concurrent deformity correction can place tension on the neural elements.
    ◆ The sciatic nerve is tethered as the common peroneal nerve enters the lateral compartment of the lower leg.
    ◆ Peroneal nerve tension or irritation initially will result in pain on the anterior aspect of the lower leg and dorsum of the foot and altered sensation in the first web space. Late findings include weakness of dorsiflexors or footdrop. Young patients will often hold the toes up with their hands or continuously rub their foot. Treatment involves slowing the rate of distraction, allowing the hip to extend and the knee to flex, and decompression of the peroneal nerve.

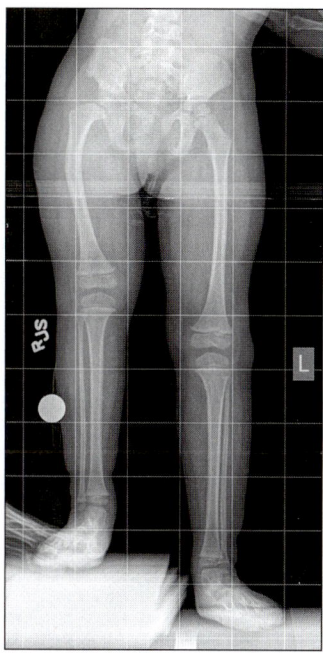

FIGURE 4

Equipment

- The use of sterile bumps to elevate the distal thigh and lower leg will allow lateral fluoroscopic visualization of the operative leg.
- A radiopaque grid is placed under the OR table pad for intraoperative alignment.

- Knee joint
  - Significant instability will result in increased risk of joint subluxation or dislocation.
    - A contracted ITB will result in rotatory subluxation of the knee joint with concurrent knee flexion contracture and patella dislocation.
    - Contracted hamstrings will result in posterior subluxation/dislocation of the knee joint.
  - Severe knee instability should be addressed with ligamentous reconstruction and patella realignment prior to femoral lengthening.
- Figure 5 illustrates the neurovascular structures of the proximal anterior thigh region that are located medial to the sartorius muscle (Fig. 5A) and the typical placement of the monolateral external fixator for femoral lengthening (Fig. 5B). Note that the external fixation pins are placed from the lateral position posterior to the tensor fascia lata muscle and away from the neurovascular elements.

POSITIONING

- The patient is placed supine on a radiolucent table that allows visualization from the hips to the ankles.
- The fluoroscopy machine is placed on the opposite side of the operating room (OR) table and perpendicular to the involved extremity.
- A small bump is placed under the ipsilateral sacrum to allow the lower extremity to rest in a patella-forward position.
- The entire lower extremity is prepped and draped to include the groin area, gluteal region, and iliac crest to the subcostal margin.
  - This allows the extremity to be manipulated during the procedure.
  - All aspects of the hip, femur, and knee are accessible.
- Figure 6 shows a patient with fibular hemimelia with significant concurrent congenital femoral deficiency (Fig. 6A). The patient's lower extremity is draped to allow entire access from the pelvis to the foot (Fig. 6B and 6C).

PROCEDURE: EXTERNAL FIXATOR PLACEMENT

STEP 1

- The limb is held patella forward and the patient is adjusted so a line on the radiopaque grid runs through the center of the hip joint.
- The limb is adducted or abducted to center the ankle on the same radiopaque line that runs through the hip.
  - This marks the limb's mechanical axis.
  - If the mechanical axis runs through the center of the knee joint, then a straight lengthening can be performed without concurrent deformity correction.
  - If an abnormal mechanical axis is present, then preoperative planning is required to determine the level of the deformity.
    - The osteotomy site will be influenced by the level of the center of rotation of angulation (CORA) of the deformity.
    - Deformity correction with concurrent lengthening can be performed through either a single or double osteotomy.

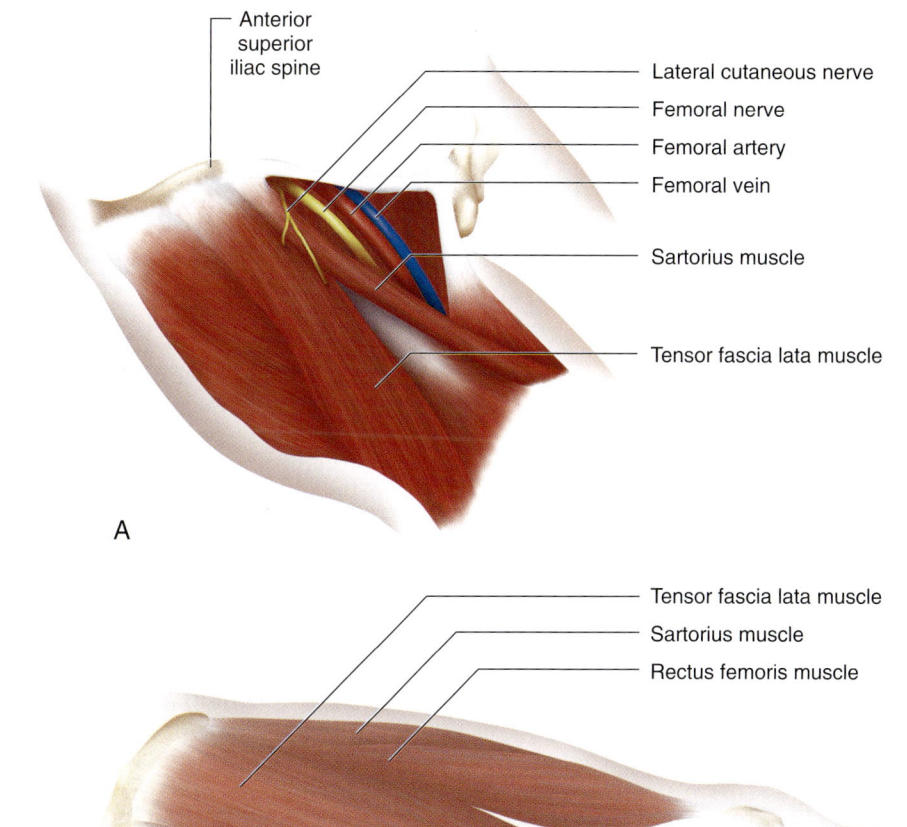

Anterior superior iliac spine

Lateral cutaneous nerve
Femoral nerve
Femoral artery
Femoral vein
Sartorius muscle
Tensor fascia lata muscle

A

Tensor fascia lata muscle
Sartorius muscle
Rectus femoris muscle

FIGURE 5 B

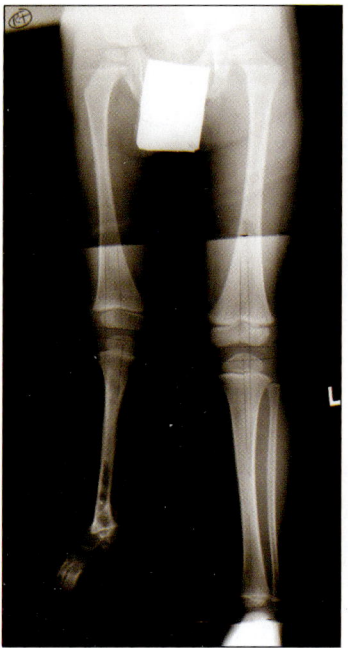

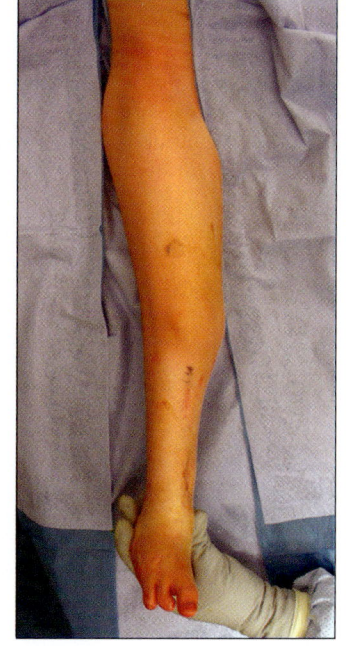

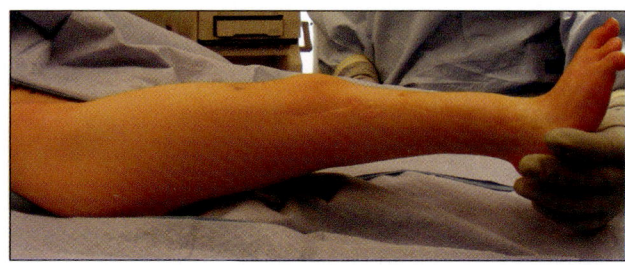

A

FIGURE 6

B

C

STEP 2

- A 1.8-mm Ilizarov wire is placed percutaneously at the base of the greater trochanter and driven perpendicular to the mechanical axis (Fig. 7A).
  - The limb is held patella forward.
  - The wire should be parallel to the horizontal plane/floor.
- A lateral fluoroscopic view is taken to ensure the wire is placed in the center of the bone.
- If the wire is in proper position, a small incision (5 mm) is made at the wire site and the soft tissues are gently spread with a straight hemostat.
- The wire is overdrilled with a 4.8-mm cannulated drill bit and a 6-mm hydroxyapatite (HA)-coated half-pin is inserted. This is termed the cannulated drill technique for half-pin placement.
- The initial half-pin is the reference half-pin that determines the lengthening axis.
  - The lengthening axis is perpendicular to the initial/reference half-pin.
  - The lengthening axis should be parallel to the mechanical axis of the limb segment or of the entire limb.
  - If the lengthening axis is not parallel to the mechanical axis, then a secondary deformity will result during the gradual lengthening (Fig. 7B).
    - A lengthening axis that is parallel to the *anatomic* axis of the limb will drive the knee in a medial direction and force the mechanical axis in a lateral direction, resulting in a valgus deformity at the knee.
    - For every centimeter of lengthening down the anatomic axis, the mechanical axis is driven laterally by 1 mm.
- Half-pin size is determined by the diameter and location of pin placement.
  - Half-pin diameter should be approximately one-third the diameter of the bone.
  - In pediatric femurs, the metaphyseal ends of the bone can accommodate larger half-pins (5 mm and 6 mm).
- All half-pins are HA coated.

Instrumentation/Implantation

- Ilizarov wires (1.8 mm and 1.5 mm)—Smith and Nephew
- Drill bits:
  - 4.8-mm and 3.2-mm cannulated—Orthofix
  - 3.8-mm cannulated—Smith and Nephew
- Half-pins:
  - 6.0-mm HA-coated pins—Orthofix and Smith and Nephew
  - 4.5-mm HA-coated pins—Smith and Nephew
  - 3.5- to 4.5-mm tapered HA-coated pins—Orthofix

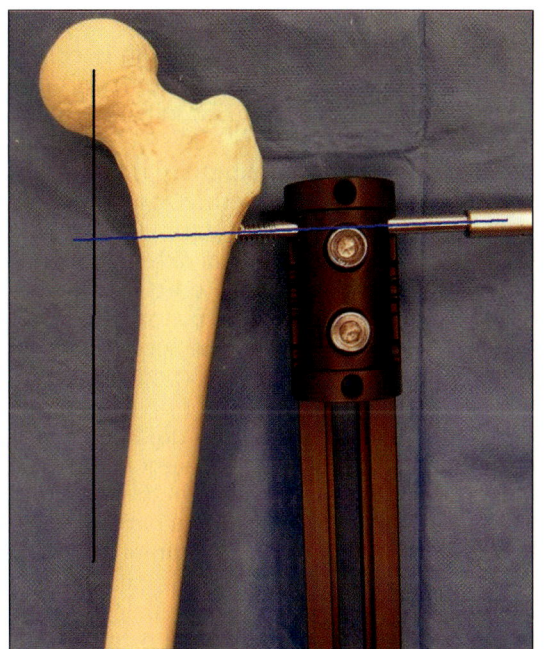

A

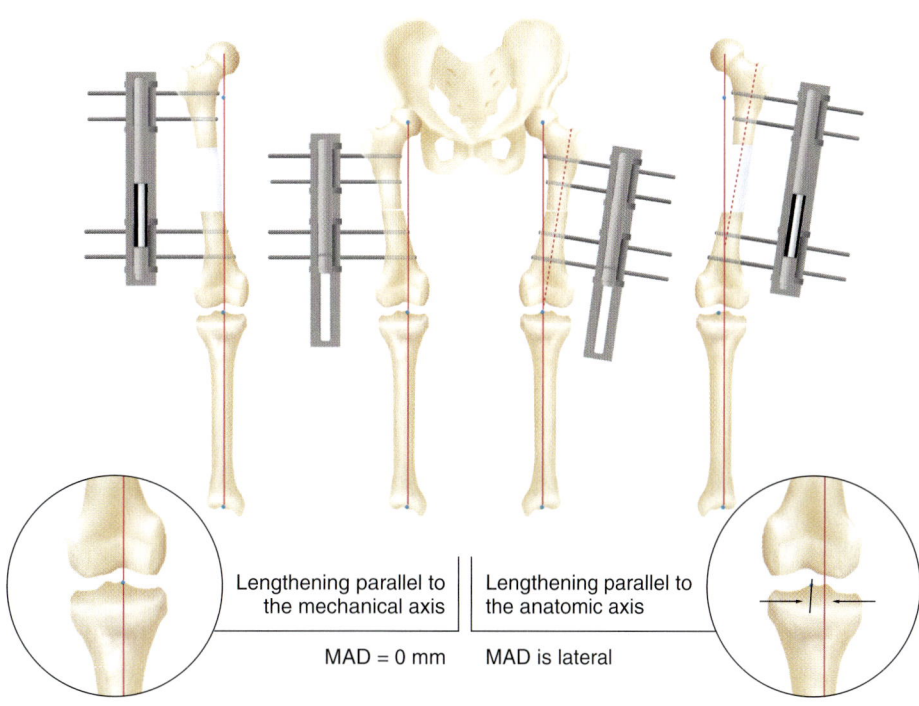

Lengthening parallel to
the mechanical axis

Lengthening parallel to
the anatomic axis

MAD = 0 mm

MAD is lateral

B

FIGURE 7

STEP 3

- The initial proximal pin becomes the reference pin for the remainder of the external fixation application for a straight lengthening (i.e., initial normal mechanical axis of the lower limb).
- The lower extremity is manipulated until the proximal half-pin is parallel to the horizontal grid lines under fluoroscopy and held still by the assistant.
- The monolateral external fixator (Orthofix LRS—pediatric or adult) is placed onto the proximal half-pin.
  - The external fixator consists of a proximal and distal pin clamp that can accommodate five half-pins (adult size) or three half-pins (pediatric size).
  - With the fixator on the proximal half-pin, the external fixator becomes a pin guide or template (Fig. 8).
- A guidewire is placed into the distal pin clamp and the clamp is translated proximal or distal along the rail until the distal pin fixation level is reached.
  - For proximal femoral osteotomies, the distal pin level should be at the junction of the middle and distal thirds of the femur.
  - For distal femoral osteotomies, the distal pin level should be placed as far distal as possible, being limited by the knee joint or the distal femoral physis.
- A 1.8-mm Ilizarov wire is placed through the guidewire in the *most distal pin option* of the *distal pin clamp.*
  - The wire is inserted percutaneously and the femur is palpated with the tip of the wire.
  - The external fixator is raised and lowered, allowing the anterior and posterior aspects of the femur to be palpated with the wire.
  - The wire is placed in the center of the femur and driven through the bone.
    - This guidewire should be parallel to the proximal half-pin and the horizontal grid lines.
- The wire is then overdrilled with the appropriate-size cannulated drill to complete the cannulated drill technique for half-pin placement.
  - This includes the small skin incision at the pin site and spreading of the soft tissues with a straight hemostat.
- The half-pin is then inserted through the small skin incision.

Instrumentation/Implantation

- Our preference for monolateral external fixation devices is the Orthofix Limb Reconstruction System (LRS; pediatric or adult size).

- Wire guides, drill guides, and drill bits are contained in the Orthofix Instrument Tray.

- Although the external fixator and wire guides can be used as a guide, the instruments are not rigidly fixed, meaning that care still needs to be taken to keep all wires and pins in the same plane.

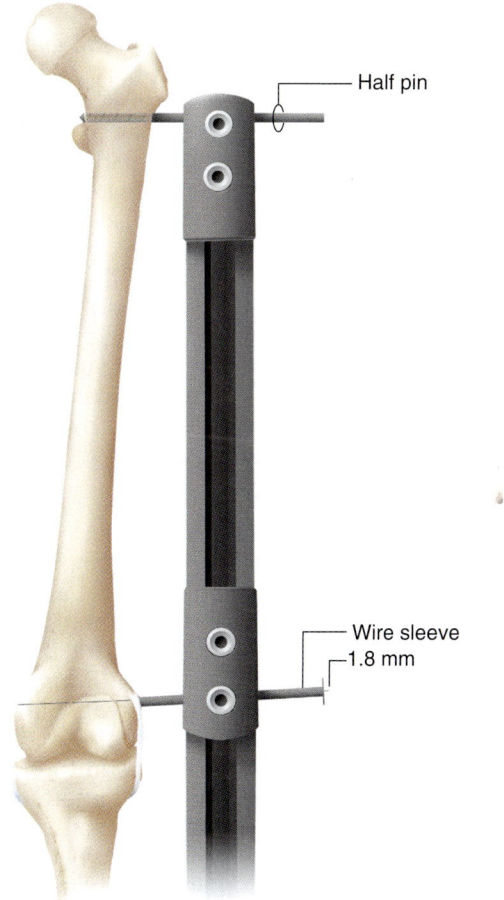

Half pin

Wire sleeve
1.8 mm

FIGURE 8

STEP 4

- The monolateral external fixator is placed over the proximal and distal half-pins
  - The fixator should slide easily onto the pins if the half-pins were inserted parallel (Fig. 9).
- Two wire guides are inserted into the pin clamps.
  - The first wire guide is inserted into the distal-most pin option of the proximal pin clamp.
  - The second wire guide is inserted into the proximal-most pin option of the distal pin clamp.
- Two 1.8-mm Ilizarov wires are inserted through the wire guides into the femur.
  - The wires' positions are checked on AP and lateral fluoroscopy.
- The wires are overdrilled with a cannulated drill and half-pins are inserted.

STEP 5

- Two solid drill sleeves are placed in the center pin options of the proximal and distal pin clamps (Fig. 10).
- The drill sleeves are pressed gently against the skin to leave a minimal indentation.
  - This marks the area for incision.
  - Two small (5-mm) skin incisions are made and the tissues gently spread with straight hemostats.
- A solid drill bit is inserted through the drill sleeves and the femur is drilled through the proximal and distal pin clamps.
- Half-pins are inserted through the newly drilled pin sites.
- The pin insertion is now complete.
  - Typical external fixator configuration requires three fixation points per bone segment.

Instrumentation/Implantation

- Ilizarov wires (1.8 mm and 1.5 mm)—Smith and Nephew
- Drill bits:
  - 4.8-mm and 3.2-mm cannulated—Orthofix
  - 3.8-mm cannulated—Smith and Nephew
- Half-pins:
  - 6.0-mm HA-coated pins—Orthofix and Smith and Nephew
  - 4.5-mm HA-coated pins—Smith and Nephew
  - 3.5- to 4.5-mm tapered HA-coated pins—Orthofix

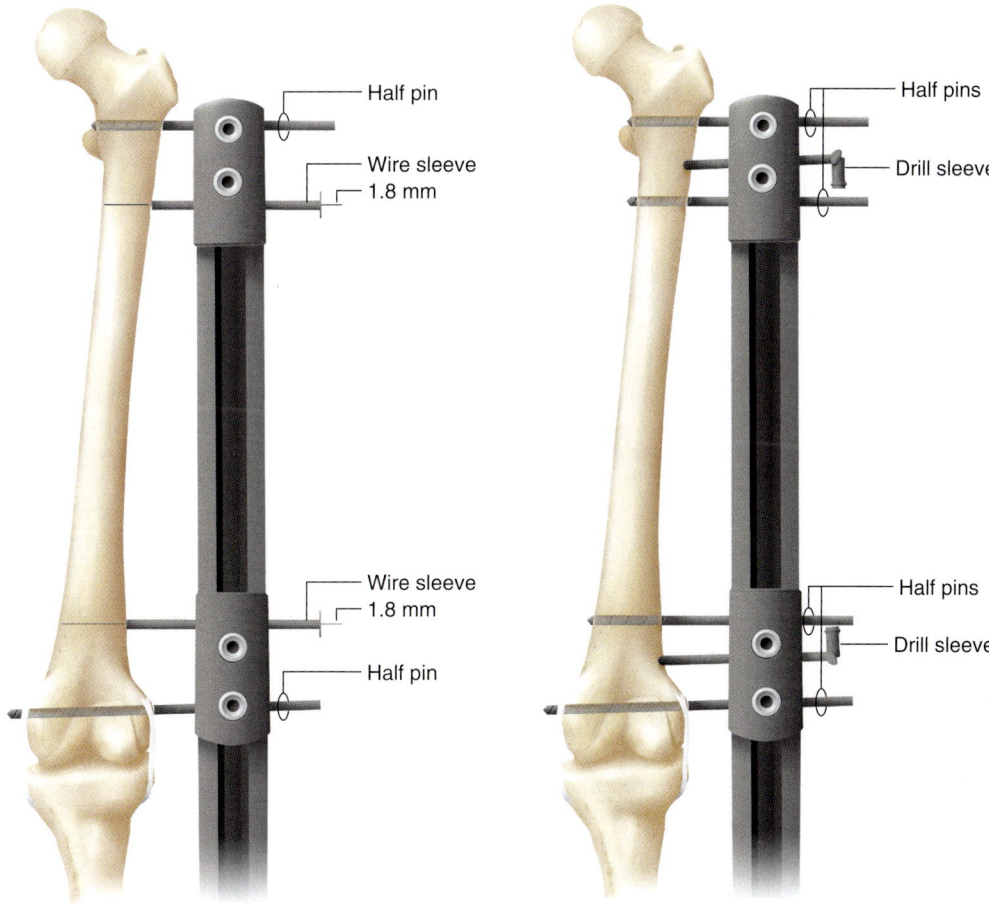

Half pin

Wire sleeve
1.8 mm

Wire sleeve
1.8 mm

Half pin

FIGURE 9

Half pins

Drill sleeve

Half pins

Drill sleeve

FIGURE 10

Step 6

- The external fixator is removed from the pins.
- The preoperatively determined osteotomy site is identified.
- A small stab incision (5–10 mm) is performed on the anterior lateral thigh and the soft tissues are spread with a straight hemostat.
- A 4.8-mm solid drill is inserted into the incision and multiple drill holes are created at the level of the osteotomy (Fig. 11A).
- The osteotomy is then completed with an osteotome and mallet (Fig. 11B).
    - After the osteotome is driven across the diameter of the femoral shaft, the osteotome is twisted 90°, completing the osteotomy.
- Level of osteotomy is determined by the level for optimal bone formation or the CORA for concurrent deformity correction.
    - Proximal femoral osteotomy
        - Subtrochanteric region
        - Typical level for majority of straight femoral lengthenings
        - Proper level for femoral derotational osteotomies
    - Distal femoral osteotomy
        - Correct level for lengthening in congenital femoral deficiency.
        - Proximal osteotomies in congenital femoral deficiency produce very poor regenerate bone.
        - Required level to correct concurrent distal femoral deformities.

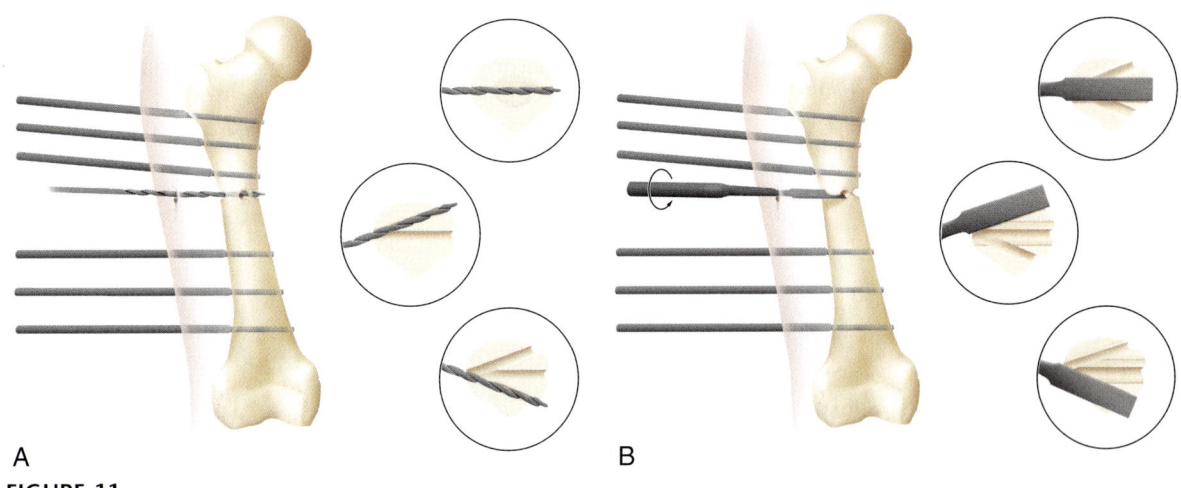

A

B

FIGURE 11

PEARLS

- *When reapplying the external fixator device after the osteotomy, ensure that the pin clamps can translate on the external fixator rail in a proximal and distal direction to reduce the difficulty of the reapplication of the device.*

- *If translation in the sagittal plane appears at the osteotomy site, a specialized pin clamp (sandwich clamp) is used that allows the pins to be placed more anteriorly.*

  - *Bulky pin wrap dressings allow for mild compression of the soft tissues around the pin sites that stabilizes the soft tissues and reduces external fixator–to-bone distance.*

PITFALLS

- *If concurrent angular deformity correction is performed and residual translation at the osteotomy is present, the angular correction needs to be reversed and the translation needs to be corrected. After translational correction, then the angular correction can be performed.*

  - *If the distracting device is not pretensioned, then several days of distraction will be wasted in order to tension the system. During this time, the osteotomy will not distract and this will increase the risk of preconsolidation.*

STEP 7

- The external fixator is placed back onto the pins through the same pin clamp holes utilized to place the half-pins.
  - Gentle manipulation should be performed to reduce the amount of translation and trauma that occurs at the osteotomy site.
  - Ensure that the pin clamps and rail connecting the bolts are loose to give all degrees of freedom to facilitate the reapplication of the external fixator.
  - The osteotomy is reduced by bringing the pins into a collinear position in the pin clamps on the external fixator rail.
- The osteotomy is now visualized under fluoroscopy and any residual translation is corrected by pulling or pushing the pins through a loose clamp.
- The pin clamps are tightened, leaving 1 fingerbreadth of distance between the external fixator and the skin.
- The pins are cut, leaving approximately 1–2 cm residual length outside of the clamp, and sterile dressings are applied to pin sites and incision sites.
- The distractor/lengthening device is placed between the clamps and distracted approximately two to three turns (2–3 mm) to pre-tension the system.
- A Sawbones model of a completed femoral lengthening external fixator with hinged bridging of the knee joint is shown in Figure 12A. The distal osteotomy can be utilized for concurrent deformity correction or lengthening in congenital femoral deficiency patients. (Note that only two-pin fixation was used for model construction; however, in clinical practice all segments must have at least three points of fixation.)
- A typical femoral external fixator with bridging across the knee joint is shown in a clinical picture (Fig. 12B) and radiograph (Fig. 12C) of a 9-year-old patient with congenital femoral deficiency after 8-cm femoral lengthening.

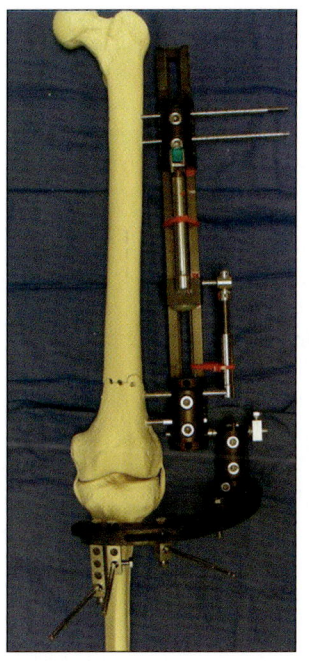

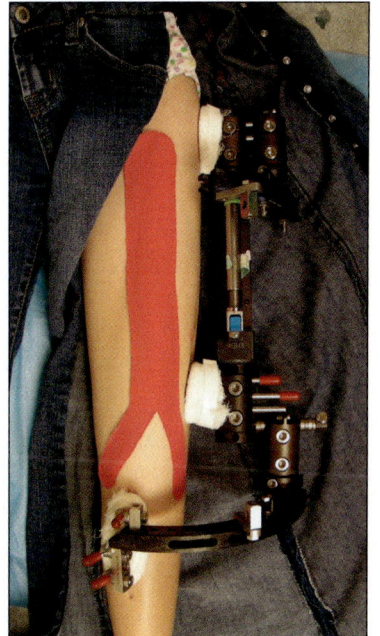

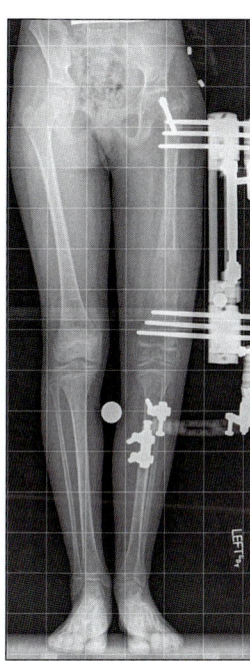

A

B

C

FIGURE 12

POSTOPERATIVE CARE AND EXPECTED OUTCOMES

PAIN MANAGEMENT AND ANTIBIOTICS

- Postoperative epidural analgesia is used for the first 48 hours, with gradual conversion to oral pain medications.
  - Muscle spasms are controlled with diazepam (0.4–0.8 mg/kg/day).
    - Intraoperative Botox injection into the quadriceps muscle is utilized to reduce postoperative muscle spasms (10 units/kg; maximum 200 units per muscle group).
- Prophylactic antibiotics are given for 24 hours.
  - Intravenous (IV) antibiotics continue after the initial 24 hours for as long as the epidural catheter is present.

DISTRACTION STRATEGY

- Distraction begins 5–7 days after the osteotomy, which is termed the latency period.
  - The latency period allows the bone to recover from the insult of the osteotomy, enabling early bone formation before distraction.
  - Increased latency periods of 10–14 days are beneficial for overtly traumatic osteotomies or conditions with poor regenerate bone formation.
- Distraction rate
  - 0.75 mm/day for children less than 6 years of age (three $\frac{1}{4}$-turns)
  - 1.0 mm/day for children greater than 6 years of age (four $\frac{1}{4}$-turns)
- The distraction rate is adjusted during the lengthening period depending on regenerate bone formation and joint range of motion.
  - Distraction rates are decreased:
    - If the regenerate bone becomes narrow or hypotrophic
    - If the fibrous interzone is greater than 5–6 mm in width
    - If there is a significant decrease in the hip or knee joint range of motion
  - Distraction rates are increased:
    - If the regenerate bone becomes hypertrophic with a width greater than the normal bone diameter
    - If early preconsolidation of the osteotomy is apparent on radiographs

POSTOPERATIVE PHYSICAL THERAPY

- Physical therapy is essential for a successful femoral lengthening.
- Physical therapy is required:
  - 5 days per week (1–2 hr/day) during the distraction period of the lengthening treatment
  - 2–3 days per week (1 hr/day) during the consolidation period of the lengthening treatment
- Physical therapy can include both land and hydrotherapy.
- Weight bearing:
  - Patients less than 6 years of age are allowed weight bearing as tolerated.
  - Patients greater than 6 years of age are allowed 50% weight bearing.
- Range-of-motion requirements:
  - Patients must maintain a certain amount of motion in the involved joints to be able to continue the distraction process.
    - ◆ < 20° of hip flexion contracture
    - ◆ > 20° of hip abduction
    - ◆ > 45° of knee flexion
    - ◆ Maintenance of full knee extension
  - **Continued distraction despite inadequate range of motion will result in joint contractures requiring extensive surgical and physiotherapeutic intervention.**

FRAME MAINTENANCE AND PIN CARE

- Preoperative and perioperative education is essential for the family.
- An external fixation manual is provided for each family.
- A patient education nurse performs an education session with the family about the specific external fixator and its adjustment schedule while the operation is being performed.
  - Daily reinforcement of external fixator specifics and care is performed during the hospital stay.
- Pin care
  - The initial pin dressing change is performed 24 hours after surgery by nursing staff with instructions to the parents.
  - Pin care is performed daily by the family.
    - ◆ For the first week, the pin sites are cleaned with sterile normal saline daily and wrapped with rolled gauze.
    - ◆ After the first week, the pins are cleaned using a simple antibacterial soap and water when the patient performs the daily bath.
    - ◆ Most patients keep the pin sites wrapped with rolled gauze to reduce skin motion and protect the sites from the environment.

PIN SITE INFECTIONS

- Infections are very common, with an average of one pin site infection per month of frame wear.
- The vast majority of pin site infections are superficial skin infections easily treated with oral antibiotics.
- The earliest sign of pin site infection is increasing pain at the pin site.
  - This pain rapidly increases over the ensuing 6–12 hours.
  - Other pin site qualities such as drainage, erythema, and skin changes can be misleading for parents and are not indicative of infection unless pain is also present.
- Oral antibiotic treatment is initiated at the earliest sign of pin infection.
  - Primary antibiotic tier
    - Keflex (50–100 mg/kg/day) qid for 10 days
    - Bactrim DS (penicillin-allergic patients) bid for 10 days
  - Secondary antibiotic tier (patients who fail with the primary antibiotic tier)
    - Bactrim DS bid for 10 days
    - Clindamycin (10–25 mg/kg/day) tid for 10 days
  - Tertiary antibiotic tier
    - Ciprofloxacin (10–20 mg/kg/dose) bid, not to exceed 750 mg/dose no matter the child's size.
    - Tailor antibiotics according to sensitivities from pin swab culture taken for difficult pin sites.
- Organism identification
  - The vast majority of pin site infections are treated empirically.
  - Difficult pin sites that are resistant to routine oral antibiotic treatment may undergo swab culture.
    - Culture results must be analyzed with the correct perspective of the routine skin flora.
    - Swab results are helpful to identify unusual organisms such as *Pseudomonas* or resistant organisms such as methicillin-resistant *Staphylococcus aureus.*
    - Swab results are used to tailor antibiotic treatment.
- Severe pin site infections are rare and usually deeper.
  - Severe infections begin as a typical pin site infection with pain and eventual progressive erythema.
  - They cause constitutional symptoms such as fever, lethargy/malaise, and nausea.
  - Symptoms must not be ignored, and the patient must be treated immediately.
  - The patient is admitted to the hospital for IV antibiotics.
  - If the infected pin site does not respond within 24 hours to the IV antibiotics, the pin is removed and the site is débrided and curetted in the OR.

CLINICAL FOLLOW-UP STRATEGY

- The patient is seen within 2 weeks from hospital discharge.
- Clinical follow-up visits occur every 2 weeks during the distraction or lengthening phase of the treatment for clinical and radiographic examination.
- Clinical examination and review of physical therapy notes:
  - Normal neurovascular status of the limb is ensured.
  - Overall clinical alignment in the coronal and sagittal plane is checked.
  - Joint motion measurements recorded during physical therapy are reviewed.
  - The frame and distraction device are checked for stability and position (i.e., overall mechanical check of frame and connections).
  - Pin sites and pin stability are checked.
- Radiographic examination
  - Anteroposterior and lateral radiographs of the femur are obtained; these must include the hip and the knee.
    - Radiographs are checked to ensure that the hip and knee are in normal position with no contracture or subluxation.
    - The length of distraction and quality of the regenerate bone are evaluated.
    - The joint orientation measurements for both the hip and the knee are evaluated to ensure that malalignment is not occurring.
  - A bilateral standing AP radiograph of the legs, to include hips to ankles, is obtained.
    - An overall measurement of LLD and extremity alignment is performed.
- Clinical follow-up does not occur during the consolidation/ healing phase of the treatment.
- The family obtains radiographs (AP and lateral) of the femur in their home town and mails the films to the office every 4 weeks.
- When the intermittent radiographs demonstrate complete consolidation, the patient is notified and a surgical removal of the external fixator is scheduled.

PROCEDURE: EXTERNAL FIXATOR REMOVAL AND IM NAIL INSERTION

- Determine the timing of external fixation removal.
  - The consolidation phase is completed when three of four cortices have healed on radiographs.
  - The estimated total frame time equals 1 month for every centimeter gained in bone length.
- The external fixator is removed under general anesthesia.

STEP 1: EXTERNAL FIXATOR REMOVAL

- The pin sites are cleaned and external fixator pin clamps loosened.
- The half-pins are removed through the pin clamp to reduce torque on the femur.
- The frame is removed from the last half-pin; the femur is supported while this pin is removed.
- Anteroposterior and lateral radiographs are obtained.
  - The quality of regenerate bone and the half-pin sites are checked radiographically.
  - If radiographs demonstrate adequate healing, then bulky sterile dressings are applied with mild compression. Dressings are removed 48 hours after surgery.
  - If the regenerate bone is narrowed or the half-pin sites are at risk for a post-lengthening fracture, then intramedullary (IM) nail support is applied (see Step 2).
    - Figure 13 presents a case example of an 8-year-old female with an LLD secondary to polio demonstrated in preoperative standing long-leg radiographs (Fig. 13A and 13B). A post-lengthening radiograph (Fig. 13C) demonstrated a narrow regenerate bone formation at risk for fracture, resulting in placement of a prophylactic IM rod in the femur after external fixation removal (Fig. 13D).

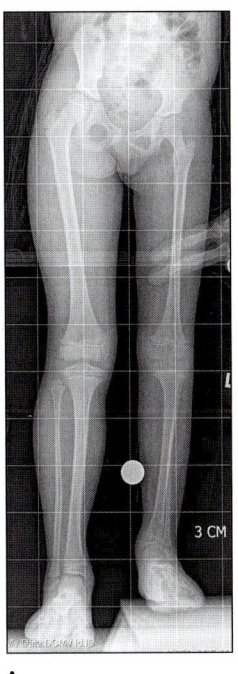

A

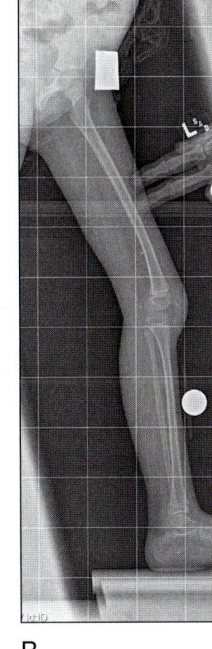

B

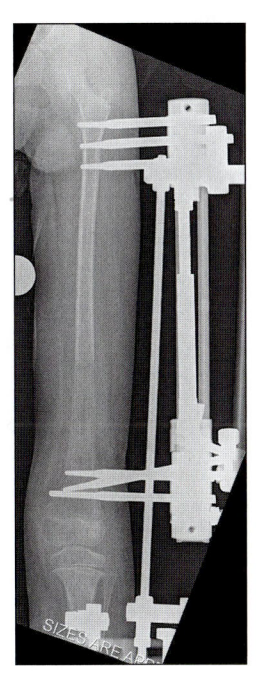

C

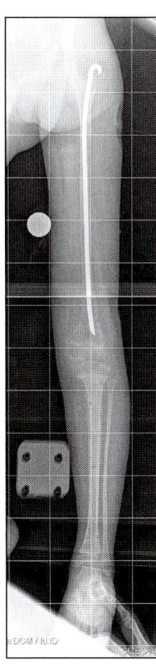

D

FIGURE 13

◆ Figure 14 presents a case example of an achondroplastic male undergoing bilateral lower extremity lengthening. A preoperative standing long-leg film demonstrated a normal mechanical axis bilaterally (Fig. 14A). Interval radiographs (Fig. 14B and 14C) during the lengthening process demonstrated good regenerate bone formation and maintenance of overall alignment. Radiographs obtained after the completion of lengthening show a 15-cm (6-inch) lengthening of the bilateral lower extremities and an 8-cm lengthening of each femur (Fig. 14D and 14E). A postremoval standing long-leg film demonstrates excellent healing and alignment with a total of 15 cm lengthening (Fig. 14F). Note the postremoval prophylactic IM rods in the femur to protect against post-lengthening fracture.

STEP 2: IM NAIL INSERTION

- After the external fixator is removed, the pin sites are prepared with a Betadine solution.
- The pin sites are isolated with Tegaderm dressings.
- The entire lower limb, to include the iliac crest, groin, and gluteal region, is prepared and draped in the typical fashion.
  • The Tegaderm dressings are prepared the same as the rest of the skin surface.
- Under fluoroscopy, a 1.8-mm wire is inserted into the greater trochanter and checked in both the AP and lateral views.
- A small stab incision is created around the guidewire and a 4.8-mm cannulated drill is used to create a starting hole in the greater trochanter.
- T-handled reamers are used to sequentially ream the canal from a 4.5-mm diameter to a 5.5- or 6.0-mm diameter canal.
  • The reamers are passed by hand under careful biplanar fluoroscopy.
- The appropriate size and length of Rush rod are determined.
  • A small bend is placed on the end of the Rush rod with the apex of the bend on the same side as the bevel of the tip.
- The rod is inserted into the start hole and carefully driven down the prepared canal under fluoroscopic guidance.
- The rod is driven into its final position and checked radiographically.
- The insertion site is sutured in the typical fashion and the pin sites are covered as previously described.
  • The pin sites are not curetted or released if an IM rod is inserted; this will increase the risk of infection.
  • Recent study indicates infection rates of less than 6% when inserting IM rods after long-term external fixation.
  • Personal experience demonstrates infection rates of less than 1% with IM rod insertion after femoral lengthening.

POSTOPERATIVE CARE AND EXPECTED OUTCOMES

- The patient is admitted postoperatively for 24 hours of IV antibiotics.
- Oral antibiotics are continued for an additional 10 days after IM rod insertion.
- The patient is allowed partial weight bearing and continues with gentle range of motion for 4 weeks after external fixator removal.
- Postremoval protocols for weight bearing and physical therapy are the same with or without IM rod insertion.

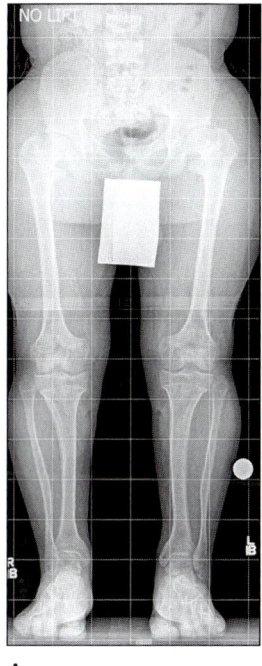

A

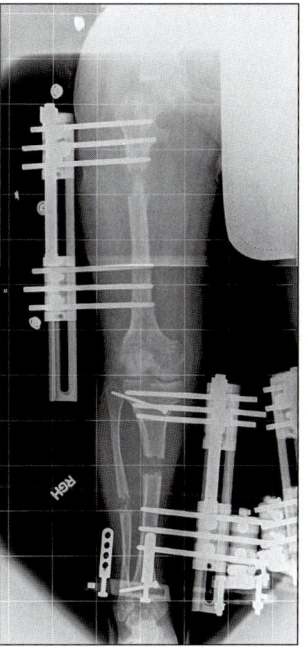

B

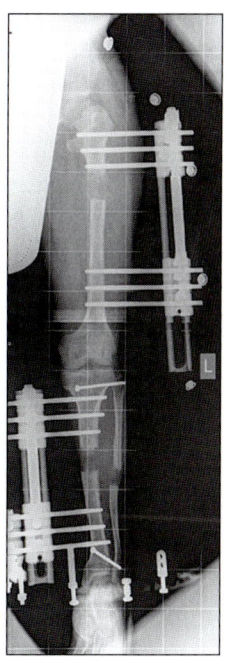

C

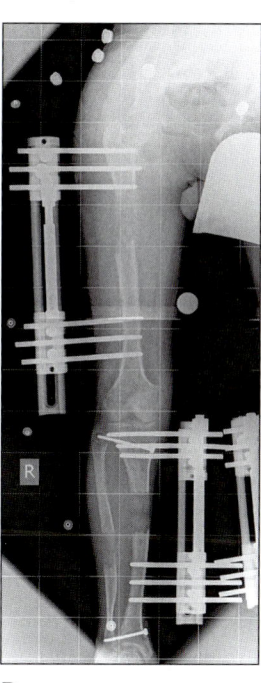

D

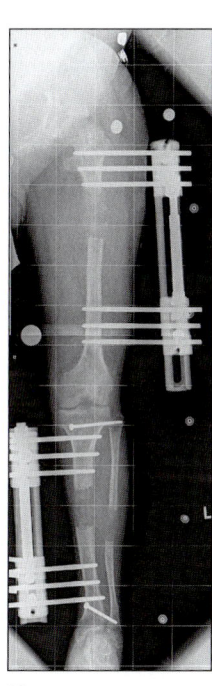

E

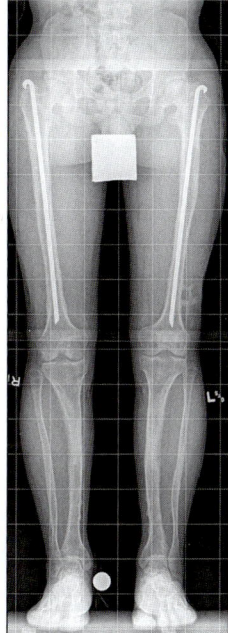

F

FIGURE 14

EVIDENCE

Chotel F, Braillon P, Sailhan F, Gadeyne S, Panczer G, Pedrini C, Berard J. Bone stiffness in children: part I. In vivo assessment of the stiffness of femur and tibia in children. J Pediatr Orthop. 2008;28:534–7.

Chotel F, Braillon P, Sailhan F, Gadeyne S, Gellon JO, Panczer G, Pedrini C, Berard J. Bone stiffness in children: part II. Objectives criteria for children to assess healing during leg lengthening. J Pediatr Orthop. 2008;28:538–43.

De Bastiani G, Aldegheri R, Renzi-Brivio L, et al. Limb lengthening by callus distraction (callostasis). J Pediatr Orthop. 1987;7:128–34.

Glorion C, Pouliquen JC, Langlais J, Ceolin JL, Kassis B. Femoral lengthening using the callotasis method: study of the complications in a series of 70 cases in children and adolescents. J Pediatr Orthop. 1996;16:161–7.

Guidera K, Hess W, Highhouse K, et al. Extremity lengthening: Results and complications with the Orthofix system. J Pediatr Orthop. 1991;11:90–4.

Herzenberg JE, Branfoot T, Paley D, Violante FH. Femoral nailing to treat fractures after lengthening for congenital femoral deficiency in young children. J Pediatr Orthop [Br]. 2010;19:150–4.

Min WK, Min BG, Oh CW, Song HR, Oh JK, Ahn HS, Park BC, Kim PT. Biomechanical advantage of lengthening of the femur with an external fixator over an intramedullary nail. J Pediatr Orthop [Br]. 2007;16:39–43.

Viehweger E, Pouliquen JC, Kassis B, Glorion C, Langlais J. Bone growth after lengthening of the lower limb in children. J Pediatr Orthop [Br]. 1998;7:154–7.

Greater Trochanteric Transfer/ Relative Femoral Neck Lengthening

Benjamin J. Shore and Michael B. Millis

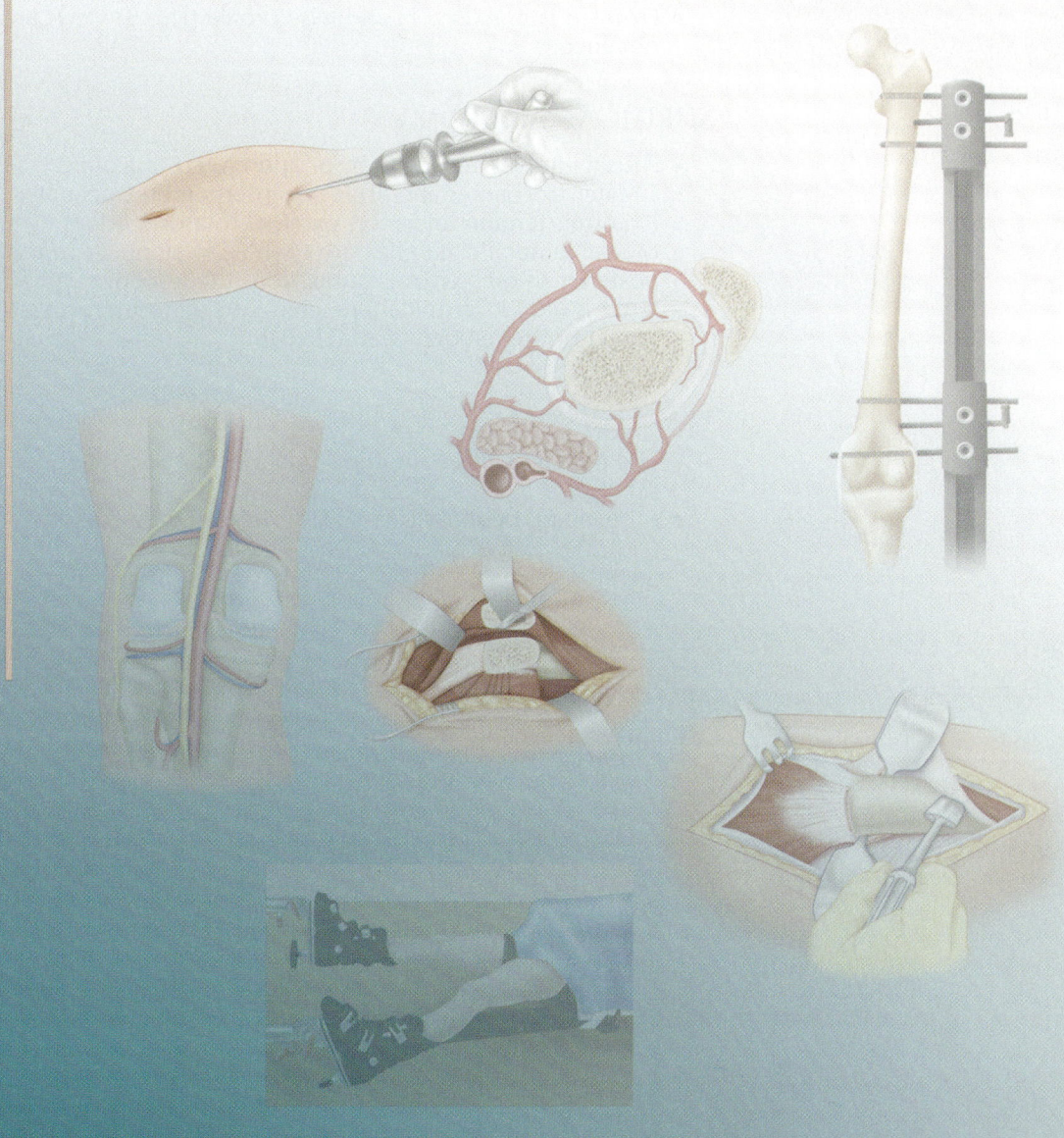

Controversies

• If the intra-articular malalignment is an indication for valgus intertrochanteric osteotomy, the valgus realignment may make unnecessary an otherwise-indicated trochanteric transfer.

Treatment Options

• "Simple" distal/lateral transfer of the greater trochanter

• Valgus intertrochanteric osteotomy (occasionally)

Equipment

• Pegboard or beanbag

Controversies

• The supine or "sloppy lateral" position is a poor alternative.

INDICATIONS

■ Extra-articular hip impingement associated with short femoral neck/high greater trochanter
  • Often done in conjunction with intra-articular surgery to address concomitant impingement via the surgical dislocation approach
  • Abductor insufficiency associated with short femoral neck/high greater trochanter

EXAMINATION/IMAGING

■ Supine and standing anteroposterior (AP) radiographs of both hips are obtained (Fig. 1).
■ Frog-leg lateral (Fig. 2) and false profile (Fig. 3) views are also obtained.

SURGICAL ANATOMY

■ Fascial interval between tensor and gluteus maximus
■ Greater trochanter and abductor insertion on trochanter
■ Piriformis tendon and short external rotator tendons
■ Medial femoral circumflex artery (MFCA) along its course posterior to greater trochanter, from the level of quadratus femoris until its terminal branches into the posterolateral/lateral aspect of the femoral head (Fig. 4)

POSITIONING

■ The patient is placed in the lateral decubitus position, operative side up.
■ A beanbag, pegboard, or similar stabilizing device is favored (Fig. 5).

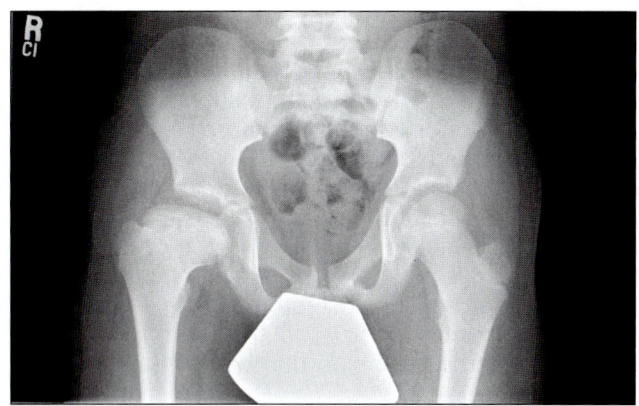

FIGURE 1

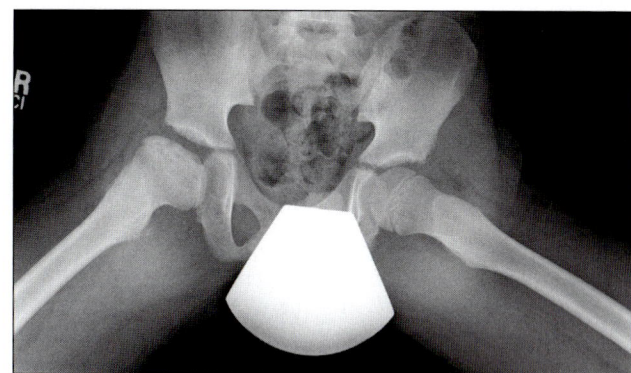

FIGURE 2

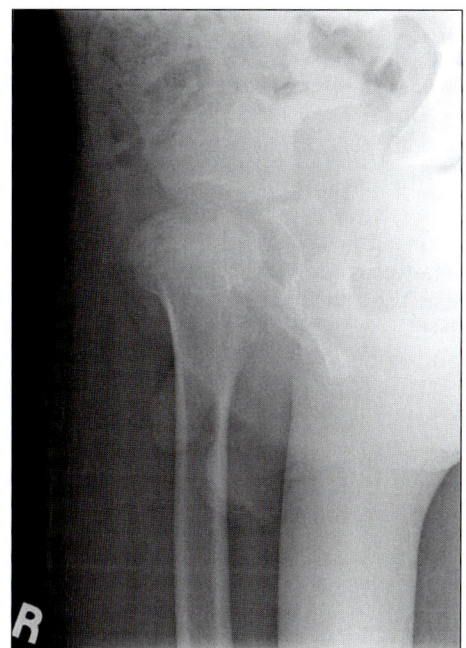

FIGURE 3

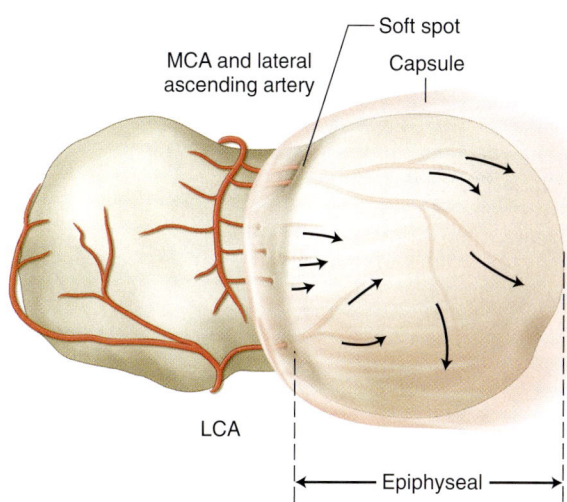

FIGURE 4

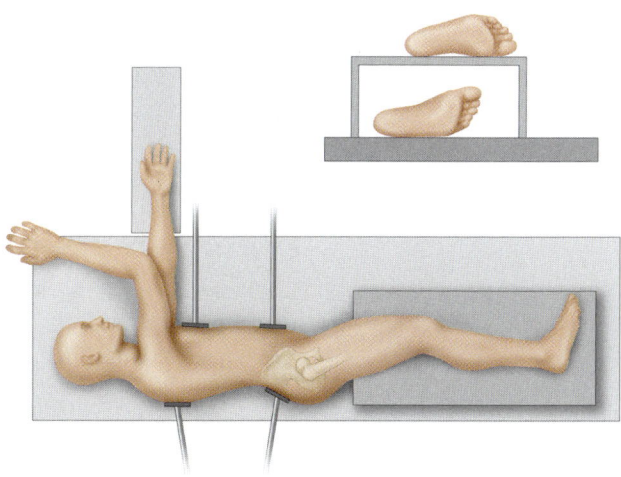

FIGURE 5

PORTALS/EXPOSURES

- A direct lateral skin incision is made; fasciotomy by the Gibson approach is preferred. The incision is continued in the proximal interval between the posterior edge of the tensor fasciae latae (TFL) and the anterior edge of the gluteus maximus (Fig. 6).
- Proximal to the tip of the greater trochanter, elevation of the abductors in an anterior direction occurs in the interval between the anterior edge of the piriformis tendon and the posterior edge of the gluteus medius muscle.
- The plane for the posteroanterior osteotomy of the greater trochanter is at a level just superficial to the piriformis tendon insertion onto the posterosuperior portion of the base of the trochanter (Fig. 7).
- The proximal plane lies between the posterolateral capsule and the tip of the greater trochanter (this dissection is most safely done subperiosteally, hugging the bone of the posterosuperior edge of the greater trochanter) (Fig. 8).

PROCEDURE

STEP 1

- A longitudinal incision is made through the TFL, extending distally at least to the level of the gluteus maximus tendon insertion on the femur and proximally at least 3 cm proximal to the tip of the greater trochanter (Fig. 9).
- The obturator externus tendon insertion on the posterior aspect of the trochanter is identified, and the course of the piriformis tendon, from the sciatic notch to its insertion onto the posterolateral base of the greater trochanter, is traced (Fig. 10).
- The level and angle of the trochanteric osteotomy, just superficial to the level of the piriformis tendon, is determined.
- The vastus lateralis is elevated subperiosteally in an anterior direction off the lateral intermuscular septum, leaving intact its attachment to the distal aspect of the greater trochanter (Fig. 11).

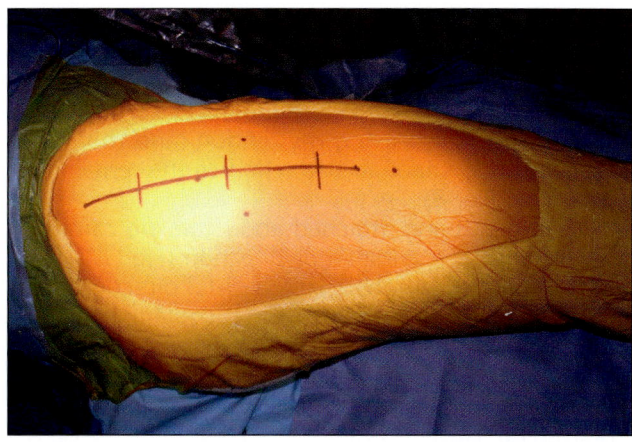

FIGURE 6

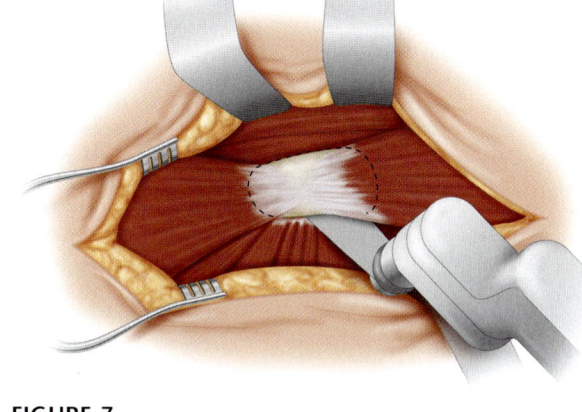

FIGURE 7

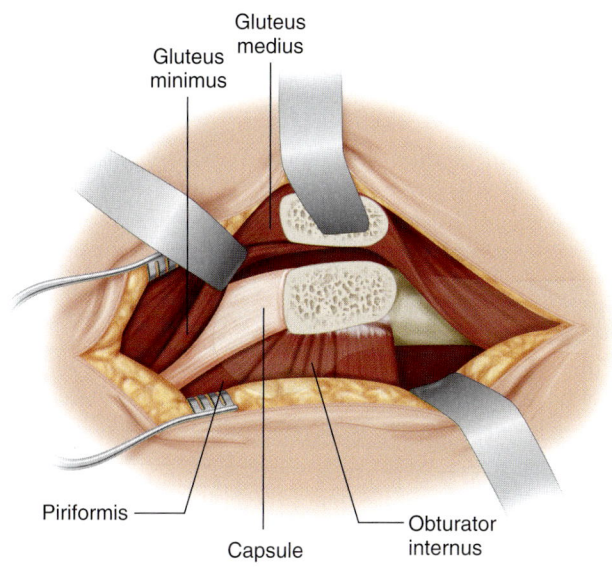

Gluteus
medius

Gluteus
minimus

Piriformis

Capsule

Obturator
internus

FIGURE 8

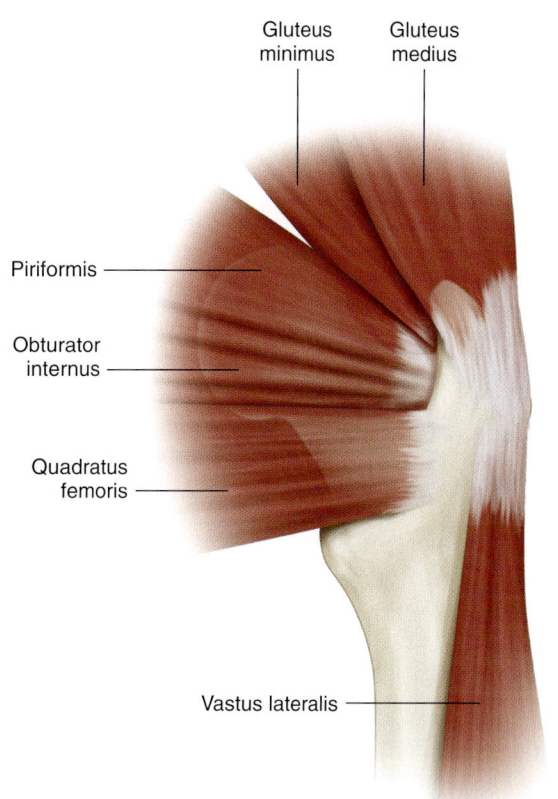

Gluteus
minimus

Gluteus
medius

Piriformis

Obturator
internus

Quadratus
femoris

Vastus lateralis

FIGURE 10

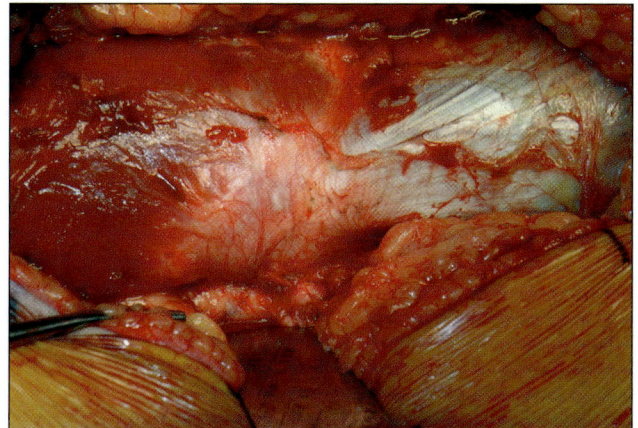

FIGURE 9

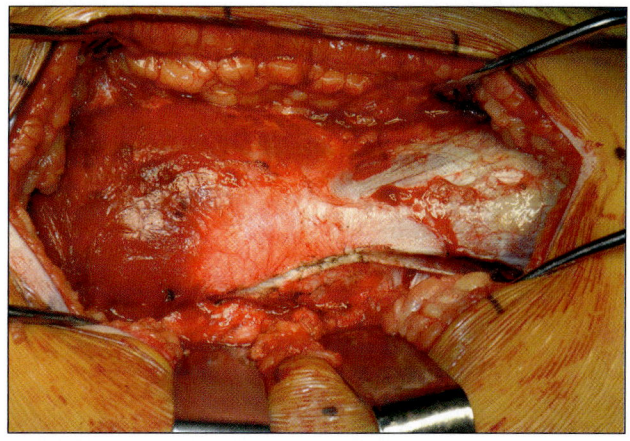

FIGURE 11

Step 2

- Osteotomy of the greater trochanter is performed with an oscillating saw or chisel, beginning posteriorly and directing the cut anteriorly. The level of the cut is just superficial to the piriformis tendon proximally, leaving the tendon (and the nearby important vessels) intact and attached to the remaining trochanteric base (see Fig. 8).
- The trochanteric fragment and attached abductors are carefully elevated from the capsule in an anterior direction (Fig. 12).
- The trochanteric fragment is mobilized in a distal direction by sharply dividing any adhesions between the capsule and the trochanter. The surgeon must stay as close as possible to the proximal tip of the trochanter to avoid damaging either the femoral head blood supply traversing the capsule or the abductor muscles (Fig. 13).

Controversies

- A deeper osteotomy of the trochanter, taking the piriformis tendon along with the trochanteric fragment, is simple but very risky to the femoral circumflex vessels and should be avoided.

PEARLS

- *Internal rotation and extension facilitates the trochanteric ostreotomy by relaxing the TFL and gluteus maximus.*

- *Abduction and external rotation facilitates safe dissection and mobilization of the proximal end of the trochanter and abductors from the hip joint capsule and adjacent vessels.*

- *Mobilization of the trochanteric fragment usually is sufficient when gentle distal traction on the fragment yields an elastic feel, rather that a tight, "check-rein" feeling.*

PITFALLS

- *In most patients requiring distal transfer of the greater trochanter, the MFCA is at risk as it enters the hip capsule because the femoral neck is short. This necessitates great care in freeing the trochanteric fragment from the capsule and is an important reason for the subperiosteal resection of bone from the proximal portion of the trochanteric base in Step 2.*

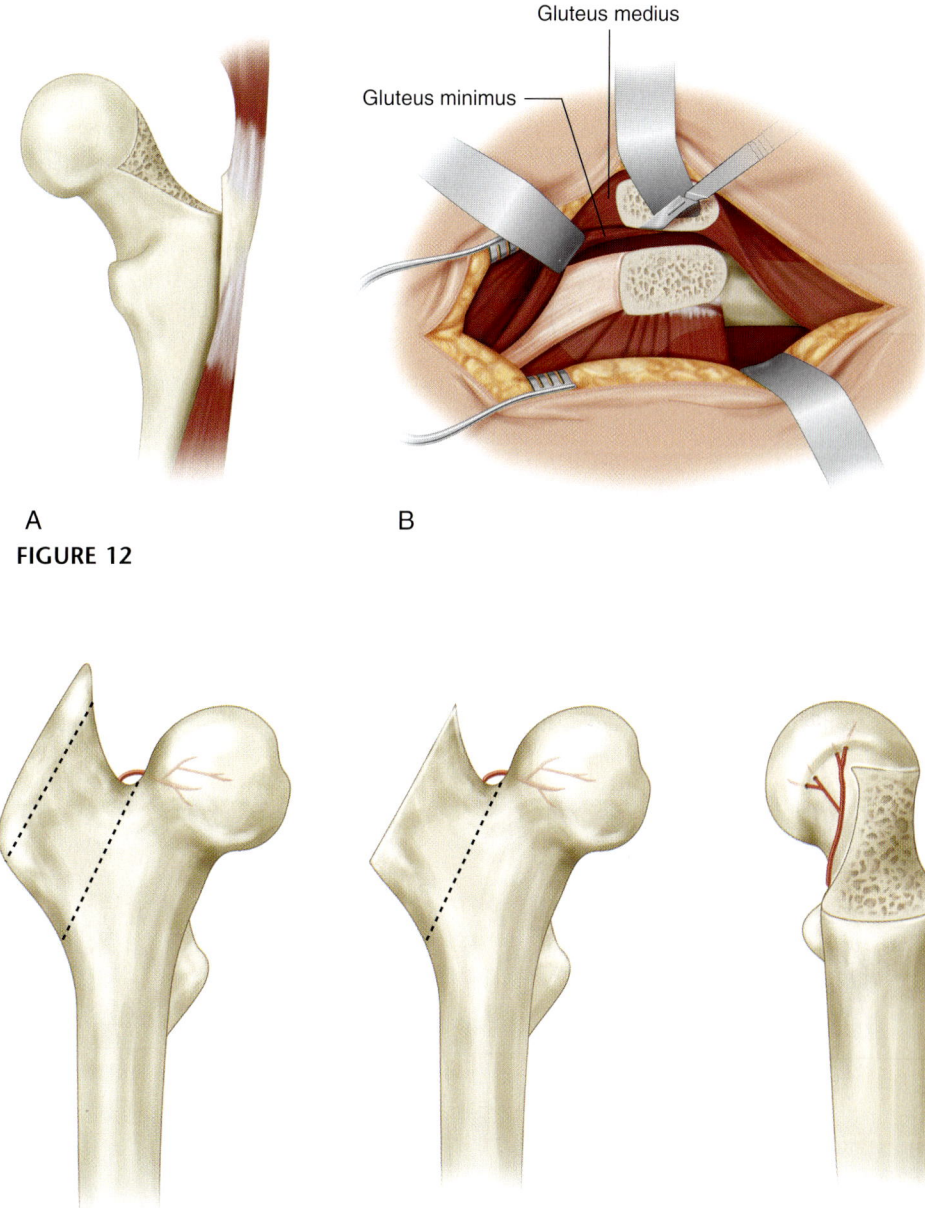

A

B

Gluteus medius

Gluteus minimus

FIGURE 12

A   B   C

FIGURE 13

STEP 3

■ A careful subperiosteal dissection exposes the bone of the portion of the "stable" trochanter that lies proximal to the femoral neck. This allows subsequent safe removal of this bone to remodel the femoral neck without risk to the vessels supplying the femoral head (Fig. 14).

■ The proximal trochanteric bone resection is performed from inside the periosteum, carefully using a knife, rongeur, and osteotome as indicated.

■ The trochanteric base is remodeled until it is the desired shape to receive the distally transferred trochanteric fragment.

STEP 4

■ The trochanteric fragment is transferred to its desired position, usually both distal and lateral to its former location.

■ Provisional fixation is done with Kirschner wires.

■ Hip motion is checked to confirm freedom from impingement in abduction and flexion. If motion adequate, then an AP image intensifier image is made to confirm that position is optimal (Figs. 15 and 16).

■ Definitive fixation is done with screws (Figs. 17 and 18).

■ The hip is carried through a careful range of motion, to confirm both stability of fixation and the limits of passive motion as determined by ligaments and the shape of the femoral head and acetabulum.

■ Soft tissue closure is carried out.

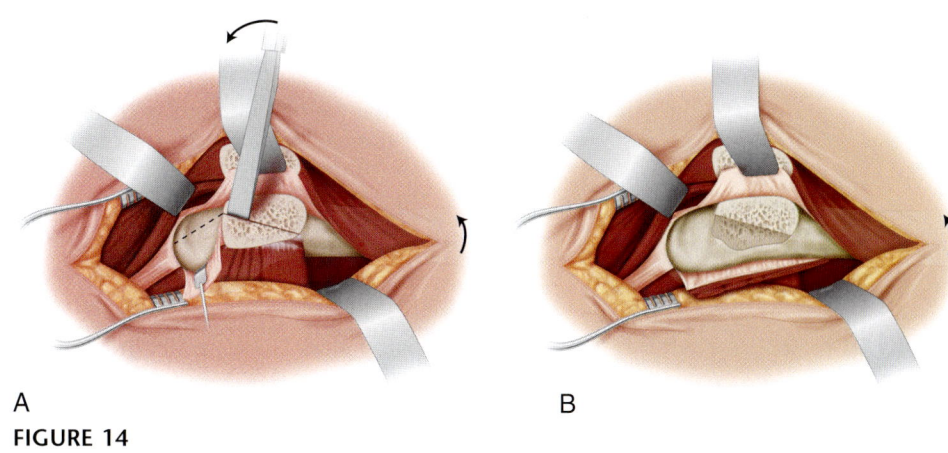

A   B

FIGURE 14

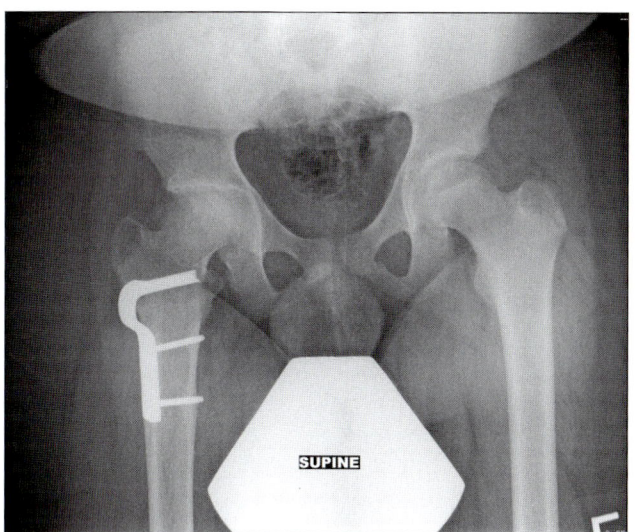

FIGURE 15

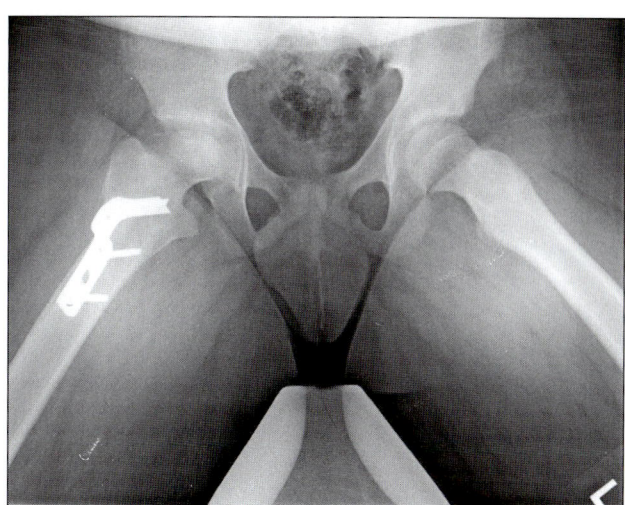

FIGURE 16

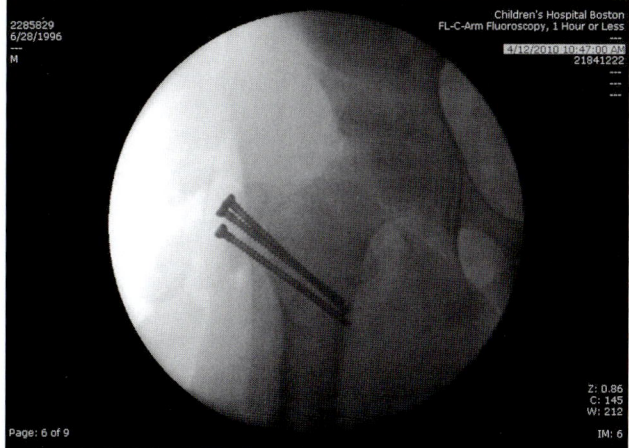

FIGURE 17

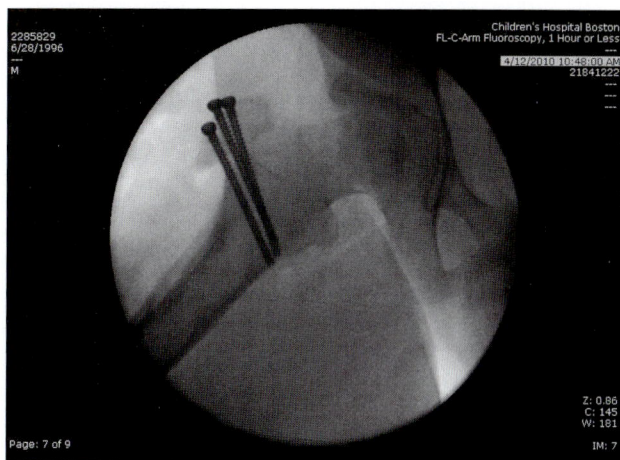

FIGURE 18

POSTOPERATIVE CARE AND EXPECTED OUTCOMES

- Partial weight bearing with one-sixth body weight (the weight of the ipsilateral limb) is permitted until bony healing of the transferred fragment is confirmed by radiographs (Figs. 19 through 22).

PEARLS

- *Do not go beyond the range of passive motion determined intraoperatively.*

PITFALLS

- *Inappropriate weight bearing—either too little or too much—must be avoided. Ambulation with less than one-sixth body weight will stress the osteosythesis, as will more than one-sixth body weight.*

- *Changing positions from lying to sitting or from sitting to standing involves high stress to the trochanteric osteosynthesis. Care must be used in such postion changes for the first few postoperative weeks.*

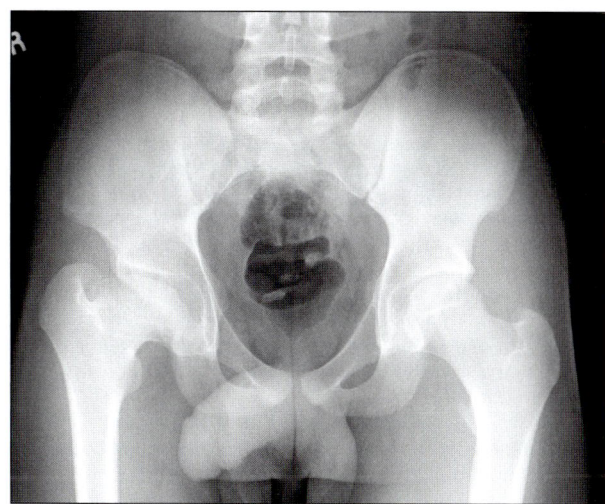

FIGURE 19

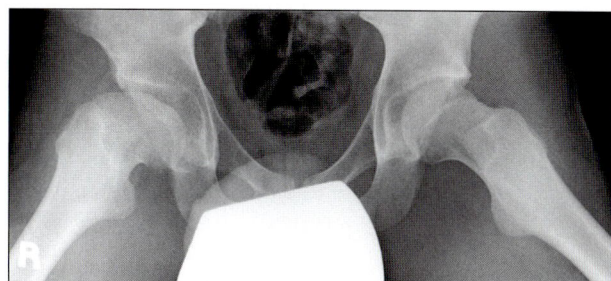

FIGURE 20

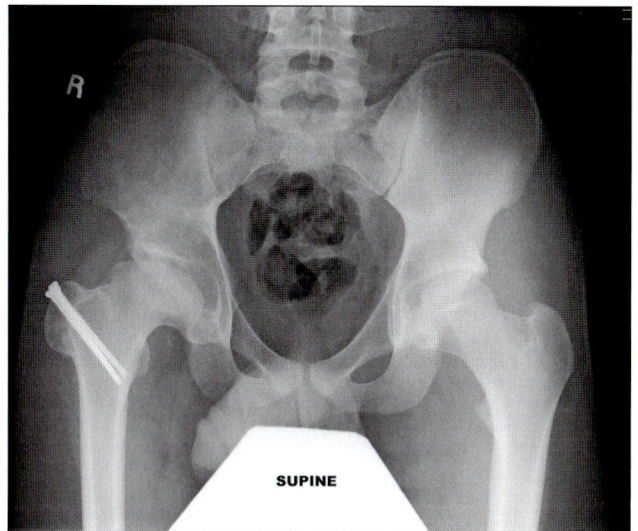

FIGURE 21

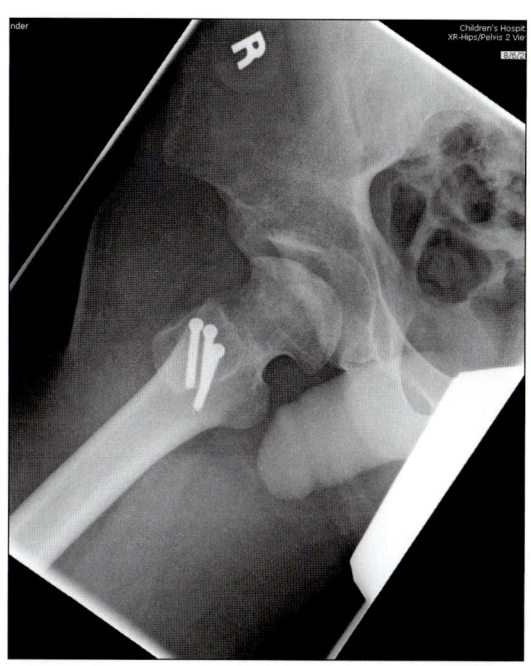

FIGURE 22

EVIDENCE

Hasler CC, Morscher EW. Femoral neck lengthening after growth disturbance of the proximal femur. J Pediatr Orthop B. 1999;8:271–5.

The authors achieved absolute neck lengthening by two parallel osteotomies at the level of the upper and lower neck, plus a third osteotomy at the base of the greater trochanter. This procedure allowed actual lengthening of both the neck and the femur, but with the disadvantage of multiple osteotomies and complex fixation issues. (Level IV evidence)

Holder G, Wagner H. Osteotomy of the greater trochanter. In Schatzker J (ed). The Intertrochanteric Osteotomy. Berlin/Heidelberg: Springer Verlag, 1984.

This classic publication detailed the indications and technique for traditional distal transfer of the greater trochanter. No details were provided for protecting the at-risk vessels in the trochanteric sulcus. (Level V evidence)

Ganz R, Huff T, Leunig M. Extended retinacular soft-tissue flap for intraarticular hip surgery: surgical technique, indications, and results of application. Instr Course Lect. 2009;58:241–55.

This superb article described the general techniques for developing an extended retinacular soft tissue flap to protect the blood supply to the femoral head during intra-articular hip surgery. It also described specific details of relative femoral neck lengthening. (Level V evidence)

Ganz R, Gill T, Gautier E, Ganz K, Krugel N, Berlemann U. Surgical dislocation of the adult hip: a technique with full access to the femoral head and acetabulum without the risk of avascular necrosis. J Bone Joint Surg [Br]. 2001;83:1119–24.

This classic article described an extensile, safe, and open surgical technique for the treatment of intra-articular hip impingement through a lateral trans-trochanteric approach. (Level IV evidence)

Femur Fracture: Lateral Trochanteric Entry Rigid Nailing

Kathryn A. Keeler and J. Eric Gordon

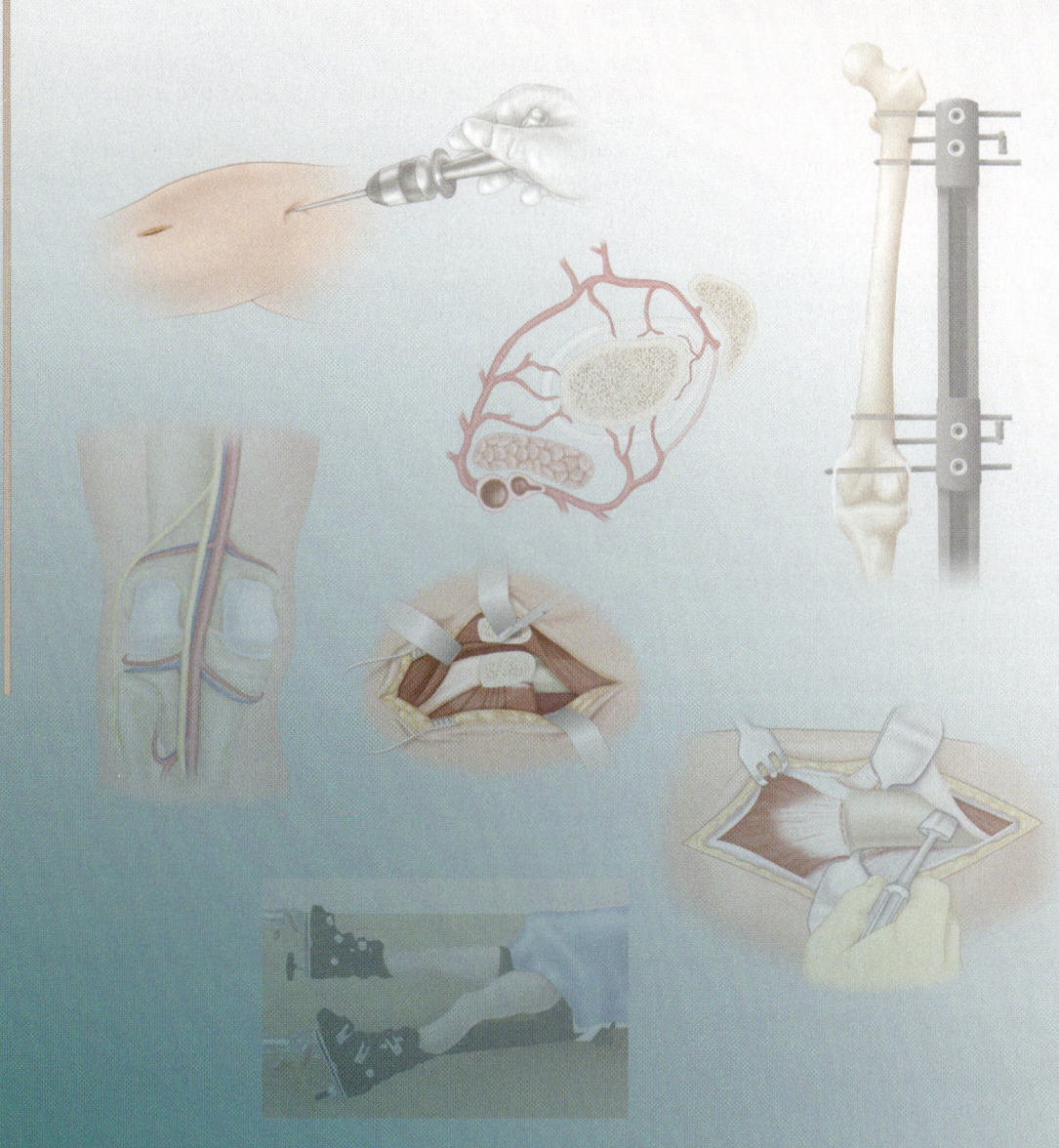

Controversies

- Avascular necrosis of the femoral head has been reported after IM nailing through the piriformis fossa, with an incidence of 0 to 5%.

- Avascular necrosis of the femoral head has also been reported after IM nailing through the tip of the greater trochanter.

- Femoral neck narrowing and proximal femoral valgus have been reported in children after IM nailing through the piriformis fossa and the tip of the greater trochanter.

INDICATIONS

- Rigid intramedullary (IM) nail fixation for femoral diaphyseal fractures in children and adolescents over the age of 8 years until skeletal maturity.
- All fracture patterns, including transverse, spiral, oblique, and comminuted fractures, can be successfully managed with this technique.
- This technique is particularly useful in unstable fracture patterns.
- The technique can also be used for stabilization of femoral diaphyseal osteotomies in patients age 8 years to skeletal maturity.

EXAMINATION/IMAGING

- Standard anteroposterior (AP) (Fig. 1A) and lateral (Fig. 1B) radiographs of the femur as well as of the ipsilateral hip and knee should be obtained.
- In patients with comminuted fractures, radiographs of the contralateral femur can be used to determine the length of the injured femur.

Treatment Options

- Submuscular bridge plating
- Titanium elastic nails
- Antegrade nailing through the tip of the greater trochanter
- Open reduction and plate fixation
- External fixation
- Traction with subsequent spica cast application

SURGICAL ANATOMY

- Vasculature about the proximal femur is at risk (Fig. 2).

POSITIONING

- The patient may be positioned in the hemilithotomy position on a fracture table. Traction is applied through a boot (Fig. 3). The post should be well padded where it contacts the perineum.
- As an alternative, the patient may be positioned supine on a radiolucent table. This is the preferred table for performing osteotomies. If this is used for fractures, an assistant will be needed to apply traction to the lower extremity to bring the fracture out to length.
- An image intensifier should be draped for visualization of the femur. Figure 4 shows draping of the extremity.

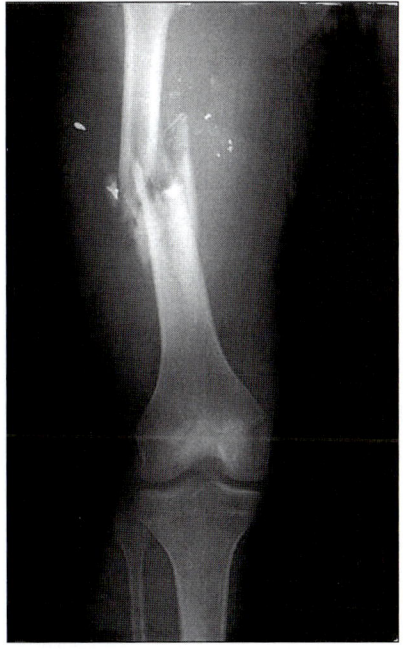

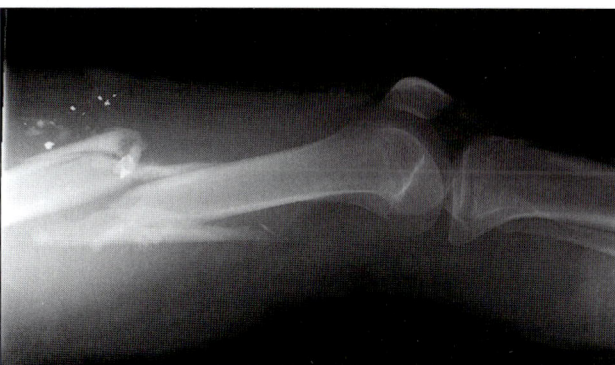

A

B

FIGURE 1

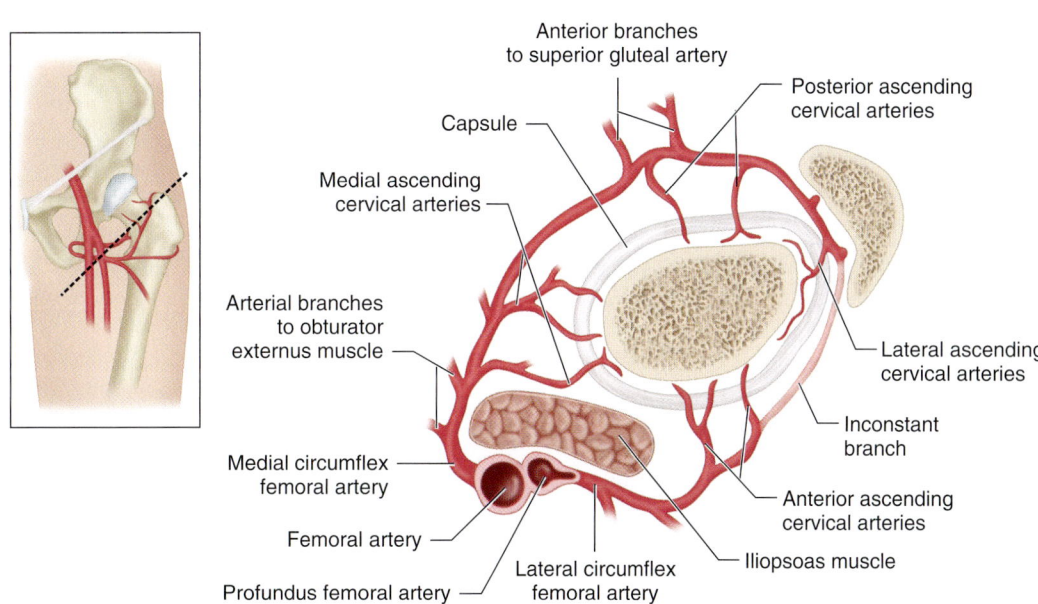

Anterior branches
to superior gluteal artery

Posterior ascending
cervical arteries

Capsule

Medial ascending
cervical arteries

Arterial branches
to obturator
externus muscle

Lateral ascending
cervical arteries

Inconstant
branch

Medial circumflex
femoral artery

Anterior ascending
cervical arteries

Femoral artery

Profundus femoral artery

Lateral circumflex
femoral artery

Iliopsoas muscle

FIGURE 2

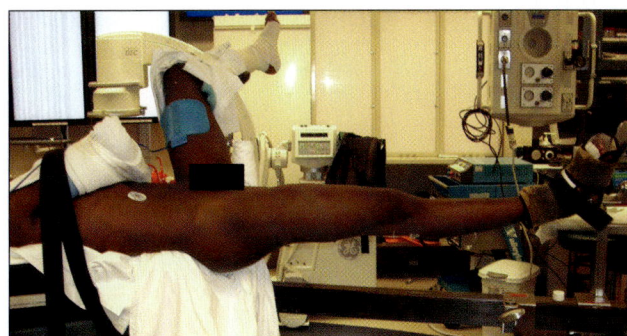

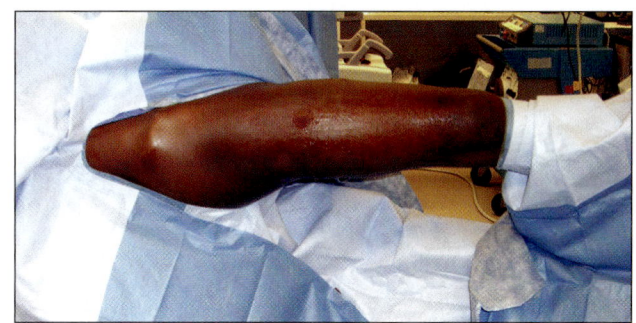

FIGURE 3

FIGURE 4

PORTALS/EXPOSURES

- The image intensifier is used to assess the entry point. Because the proximal fragment tends to externally rotate on the fracture table, it is helpful to arc the image intensifier over the patient's hip to visualize the lateral aspect of the greater trochanter.
- A 3.2-mm guidewire is placed via percutaneous entry (Fig. 5). Using fluoroscopic guidance, the tip of the guidewire is placed into the lateral aspect of the greater trochanter.
- The guidewire is advanced into the medullary canal aimed slightly medially.
- Placement of the guidewire is confirmed by fluoroscopy in both the AP (Fig. 6A) and lateral (Fig. 6B) planes.
- A small incision (approximately 1.5 cm) is made extending proximal from the insertion site of the guidewire to allow for passage of the entry reamer.

Instrumentation

- A 3.2-mm threaded-tip guidewire

Controversies

- Some authors have advocated a tip-of-the-trochanter entry point for antegrade rigid femoral nailing. This is probably associated with a lower incidence of avascular necrosis, although nailing through the tip of the trochanter has been associated with avascular necrosis in at least one report. This likely is due to the entry point slipping medially and damaging the medial femoral circumflex vessels.

PEARLS

- *Often, when the patient is placed onto the fracture table, the proximal fragment is externally rotated. To better visualize the lateral aspect of the trochanter, the image intensifier should be arced over the field so that the posteroanterior beam is directed from medial and posterior to lateral and anterior (Fig. 7).*

- *Because the proximal fragment is flexed, particularly in more proximal fractures, the guidewire should be angled anteriorly to stay in alignment with the femoral shaft.*

PITFALLS

- *Care should be taken to ensure that the guidewire is not placed into the region of the femoral neck as this could potentially injure the vessels.*

- *Dissection posterior to the greater trochanter or in the area of the femoral neck should be avoided to avoid injury to the medial femoral circumflex vessels.*

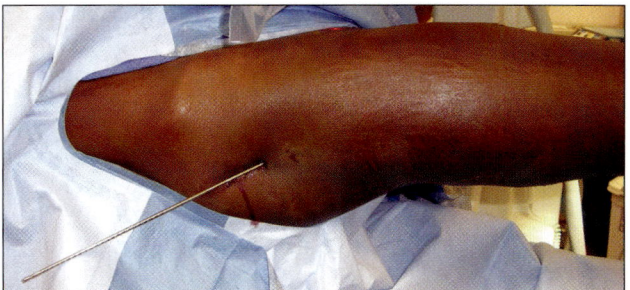

FIGURE 5

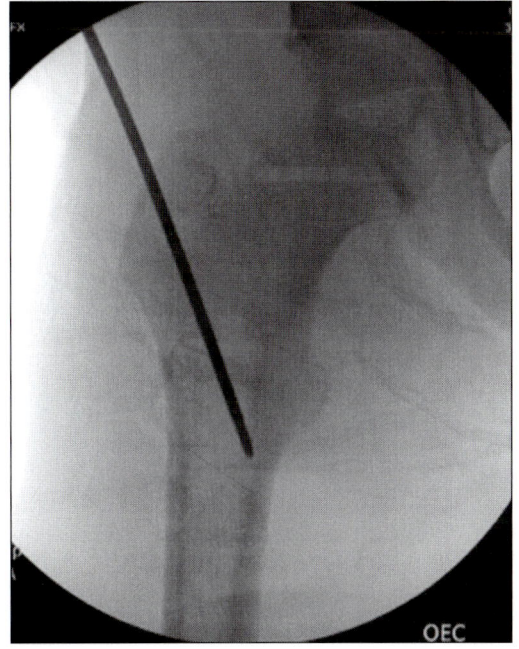

A

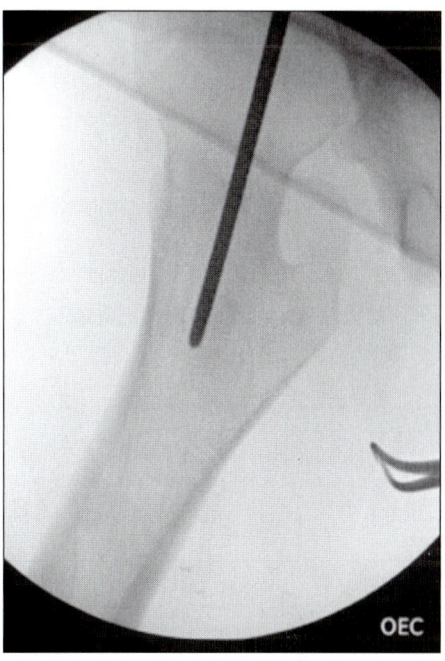

B

FIGURE 6

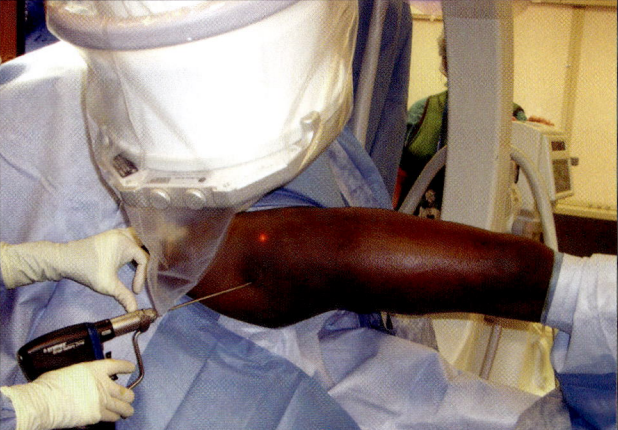

FIGURE 7

PROCEDURE

STEP 1

- A rigid 8-mm reamer is advanced over the guidewire into the medullary canal (Fig. 8).
- The reamer is then removed, leaving the guidewire in place, and a short exchange tube is placed over the guidewire and advanced into the medullary canal.
- The guidewire is then removed.
- A 3.0-mm ball-tipped guidewire is then advanced through the exchange tube and down into the medullary canal.
- The exchange tube is then withdrawn.
- The nail length should then be measured either by using a measuring device placed over the guidewire or by placing a radiolucent ruler on the anterior thigh (Fig. 9A) and placing the distal end slightly proximal to the distal femoral physis (Fig. 9B) and measuring up to the greater trochanteric apophysis (Fig. 9C).

Instrumentation/ Implantation

- 8-mm cannulated rigid reamer
- Ball-tipped guidewire (1 m long, 3.0-mm diameter)

PEARLS

- *Bend the ball-tipped guidewire at a 20° angle approximately 1 cm from the tip of the guidewire. This allows passage of the guidewire into the canal and allows it to be directed down the medullary canal after it strikes the medial calcar region of the proximal femur.*

- *When measuring the nail length, make sure that the fracture site is at the appropriate length. If shortened or overlengthened, the measured nail length will be incorrect.*

- *Plan to leave the proximal end of the nail buried just below the trochanteric apophysis but proximal to the physis.*

- *Plan to leave the distal end of the nail 1–2 cm proximal to the distal femoral physis.*

PITFALLS

- *If the guidewire is passed without bending the tip or at an angle too great to allow this to bounce off of the medial calcar and slide down the canal, there is a potential of pushing the guidewire through the medial femoral cortex.*

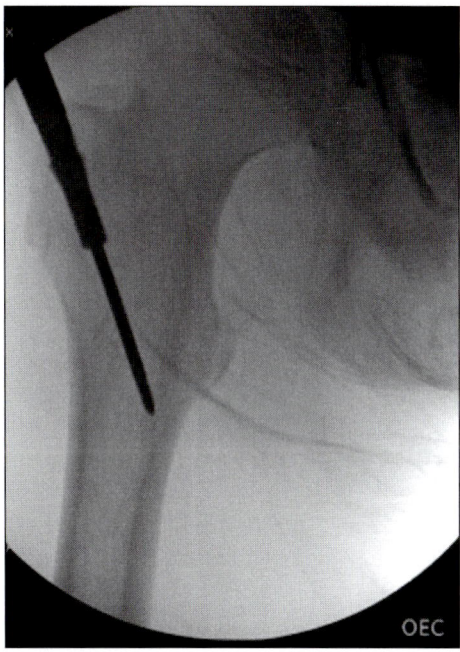

FIGURE 8

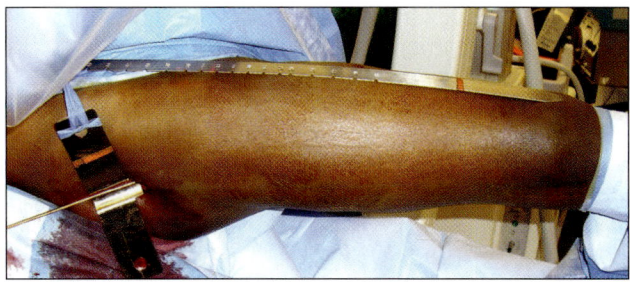

A

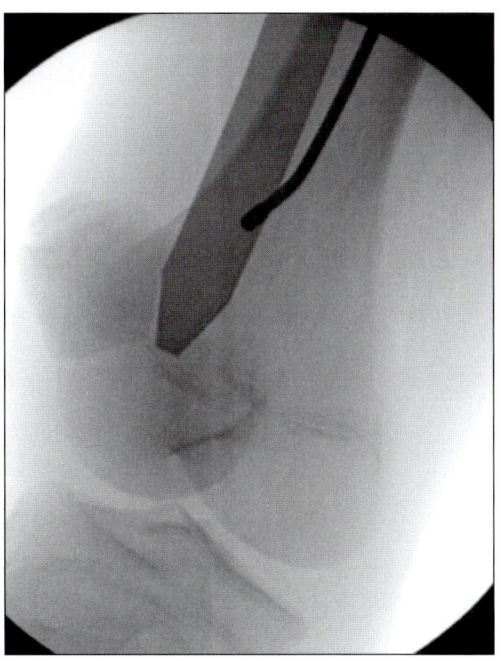

B

FIGURE 9

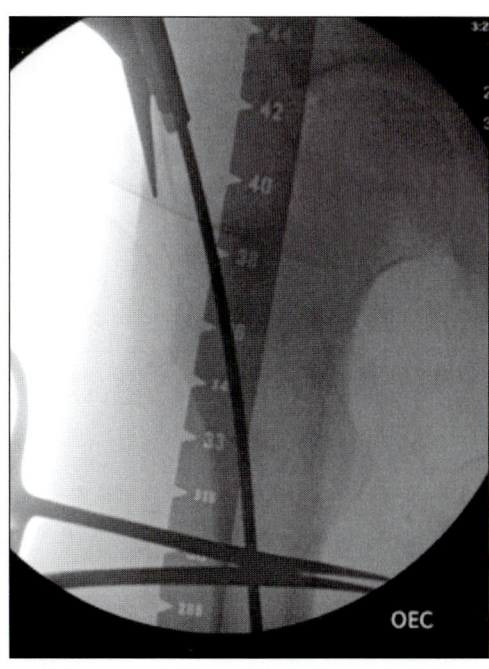

C

STEP 2

- The guidewire is driven down to the fracture site (Fig. 10), and the fracture is manually reduced.
- The guidewire is then driven across the fracture site and passed down into the lateral femoral metaphysis, where it is impacted into the cancellous bone in the metaphysis.

PEARLS

- *Preparing and draping the patient's limb circumferentially allows the surgeon to reduced the fracture manually rather than relying on crutches or other nonsterile implements wielded by a nonsterile assistant, as would be used if the patient were draped out with an impervious vertical curtain.*

- *If the fracture cannot be reduced manually, a 3-mm Steinman pin can be used percutaneously from the anterolateral aspect of the thigh to push one of the fragments into alignment and allow passage of the guidewire.*

- *Alternatively, irreducible fractures can often be reduced through a small, 2-cm lateral incision, with a Cobb elevator used to clear the fracture site and reduce the fracture.*

STEP 3

- Under power, a cannulated flexible reamer (Fig. 11A) is passed over the guidewire beginning with an 8-mm end-cutting reamer.
- The reamer is advanced upward in the femoral canal by 0.5-mm increments until resistance is noted (Fig. 11B).

Instrumentation/ Implantation

- Flexible reamer system

PEARLS

- *If difficulty is encountered when passing the reamer across the bend in the guidewire proximally just distal to the greater trochanter, the reamer should be withdrawn and the flutes cleaned of impacted bone.*

- *If difficulty is encountered when passing the reamer beyond the bend in the guidewire in the intertrochanteric area, the guidewire should be grasped with a large needle holder and withdrawn 1–2 cm while the reamer is advanced under power in order to avoid cutting the guidewire.*

- *When reaming, keep in mind that "filling the canal" is not necessary in pediatric patients. Look at the nail diameters available in the desired nail length and plan to ream 1.5–2.0 mm larger than the selected nail diameter.*

PITFALLS

- *When reaming the canal in younger children, the flutes of the reamer often become clogged with impacted bone. If the reamer is not advancing as expected, remove the reamer and inspect the flutes. If they are clogged with bone, clean the flutes with a small hemostat.*

STEP 4

- When reaming is completed, an exchange tube is passed down the femur beyond the fracture site (Fig. 12) and the 3.0-mm guidewire is withdrawn.

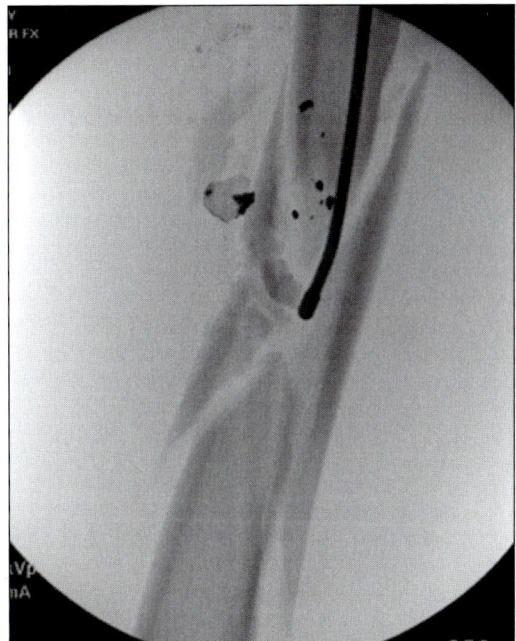

FIGURE 10

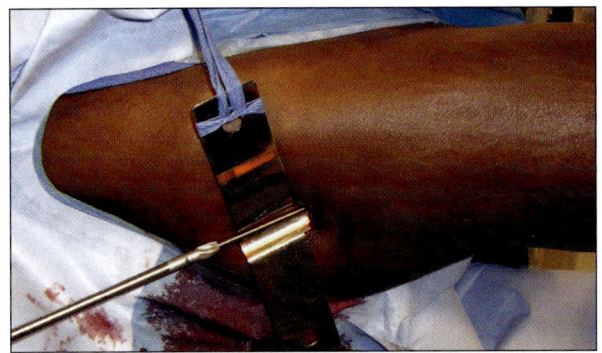

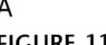

A

FIGURE 11

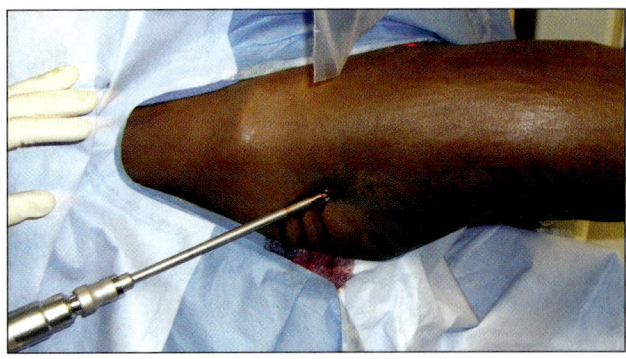

B

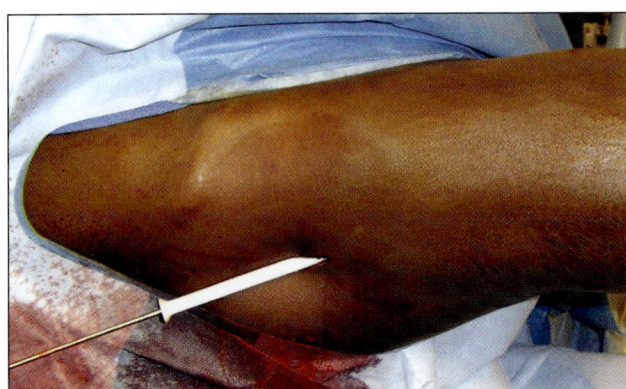

FIGURE 12

- A 2.0-mm smooth guidewire is then passed down the canal into the distal femur (Fig. 13) and the exchange tube is withdrawn (Fig. 14).
- After the selected IM nail has been mounted on the insertion jig, this should be passed by hand down over the guidewire into the femur (Fig. 15). Typically this can be passed down to an area 3–5 cm distal to the lesser trochanter relatively easily.
- After this point, the nail should be driven using a slotted mallet down to the level of the fracture site (Figs. 16 and 17). Any residual fracture angulation should be corrected, and the nail driven across the fracture and into the distal femur.
- After the nail is well down in the distal femoral medullary canal, the 2.0-mm guidewire should be removed.
- The nail is then impacted into place, just below the surface of the greater trochanter (Fig. 18).

Instrumentation/ Implantation

- Insertion jig for the pediatric trochanteric entry nail
- Smooth 2.0-mm guidewire

PEARLS

- *When impacting the nail into its final position, the traction applied through the boot should be relaxed, allowing the fracture ends to impact.*

PITFALLS

- *As the nail is passed down to the fracture site, it must bend slightly to pass down the canal. If the nail is driven forcefully, comminution of the medial cortex can occur. To avoid this, drive the nail firmly but slowly up to the fracture site.*

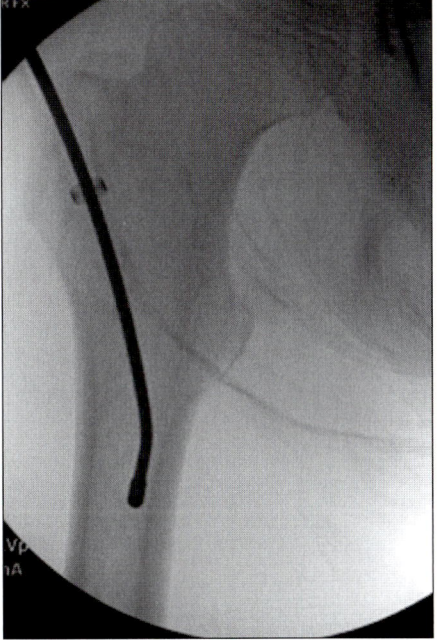

FIGURE 13

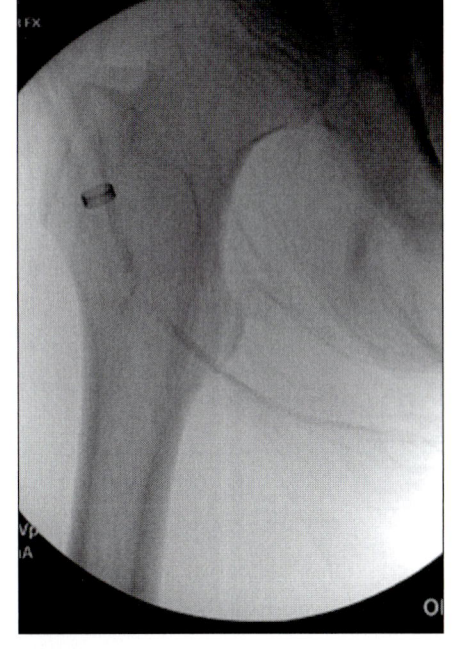

FIGURE 14

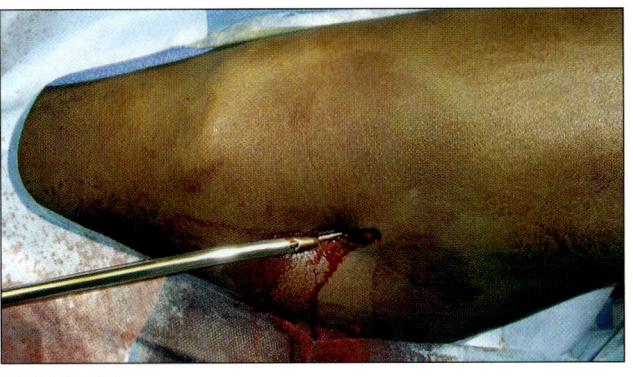

FIGURE 15

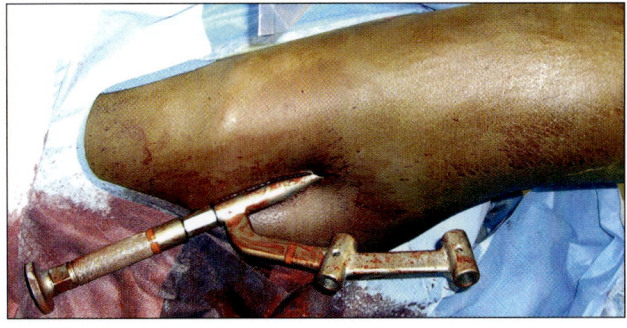

FIGURE 16

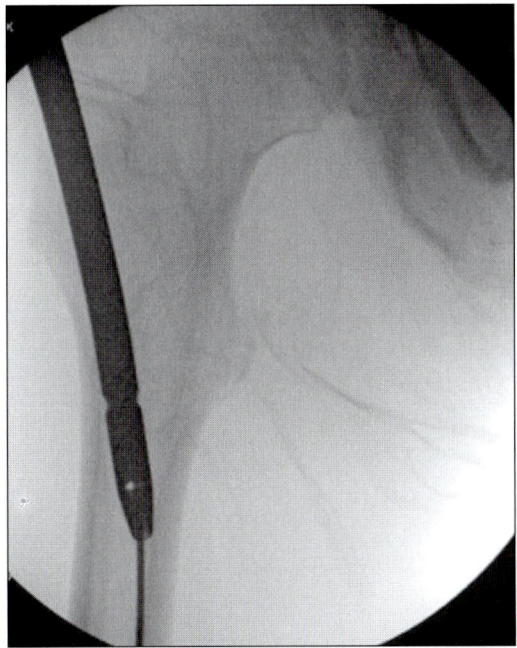

FIGURE 17

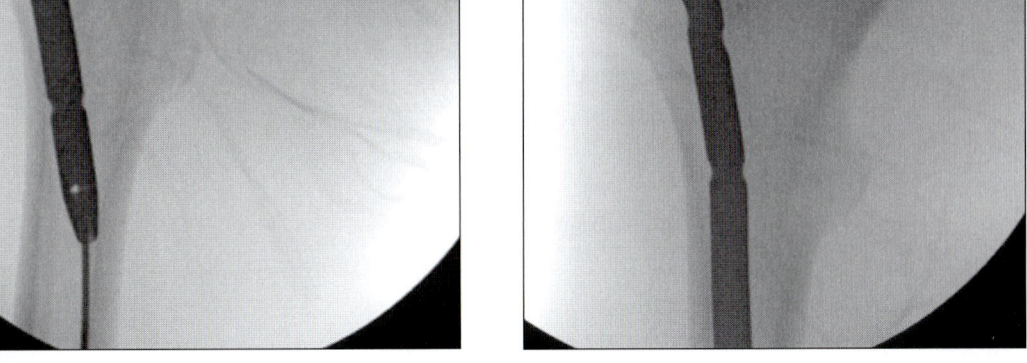

FIGURE 18

Instrumentation/ Implantation

- Guide tube and trochar for proximal interlocking screw
- 2.7-mm drill bit with drill

STEP 5

- Proximal interlocking should be performed using the guide. The guide tube with the trochar should be placed through the guide in the insertion jig and the skin marked for incision.
- A 1-cm incision is then made in the proximal lateral thigh and carried down sharply through the tensor fascia lata.
- The guide tube and trochar are driven down through the vastus lateralis down to the lateral femur as confirmed by image intensifier. The guide tube is then locked into the insertion jig.
- The trochar is then removed and an interlocking drill used to drill the hole for the proximal interlocking screw (Fig. 19). The screw length should be read off of the scale on the side of the drill bit. The drill is then withdrawn.
- The screw is then inserted and tightened into place (Fig. 20).

STEP 6

- Limb rotation should be confirmed clinically and by examining the fracture site under image intensification.
- The distal interlocking hole should be visualized under image intensification and the angle of the intensifier adjusted so that a completely round hole is visible.
- The projected insertion site is visualized by marking the spot on the skin overlying the interlocking hole.
- A 1-cm incision is made (Fig. 21) and blunt dissection is performed down to the bone.

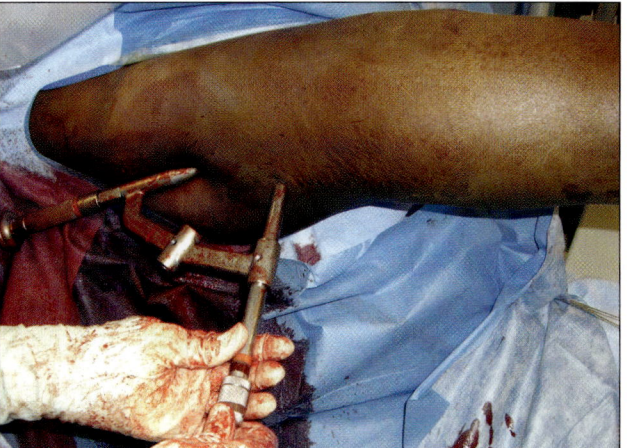

FIGURE 19

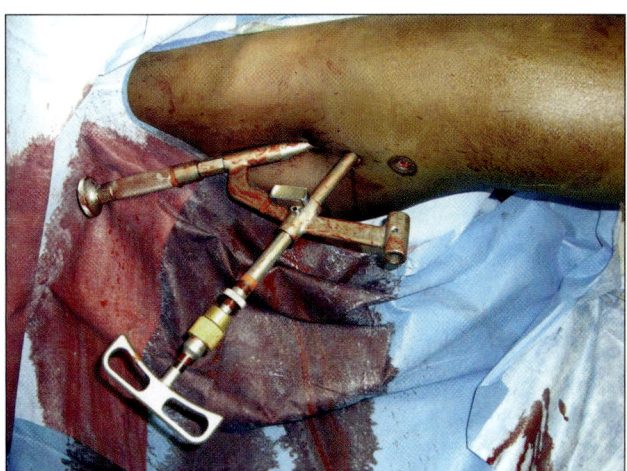

FIGURE 20

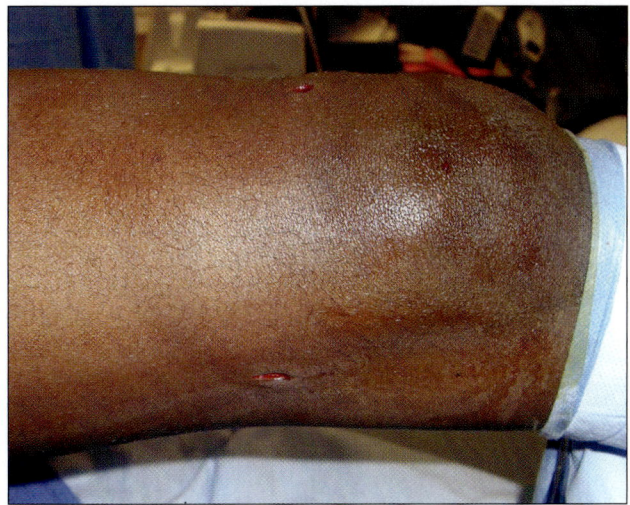

FIGURE 21

Instrumentation/Implantation

- 2.7-mm drill bit with drill.

- A 2.7-cm drill is then used to drill through the interlocking hole through both cortices.
- The screw length is assessed by depth gauge or by measurement of the preoperative radiographs.
- The screw is placed, and a second interlocking screw is then placed if necessary. Intraoperative radiographs are used to confirm proximal (Fig. 22A) and distal (Fig. 22B) screw placement through the interlocking hole.
- Final intraoperative radiographs are obtained to confirm screw placement. Figure 23 shows AP radiographs of the distal (Fig. 23A) and proximal (Fig. 23B) femur and a lateral view of the distal femur (Fig. 23C).

POSTOPERATIVE CARE AND EXPECTED OUTCOMES

- Patients are not immobilized postoperatively.
- Patients are allowed to bear weight as tolerated on crutches or a walker immediately postoperatively.

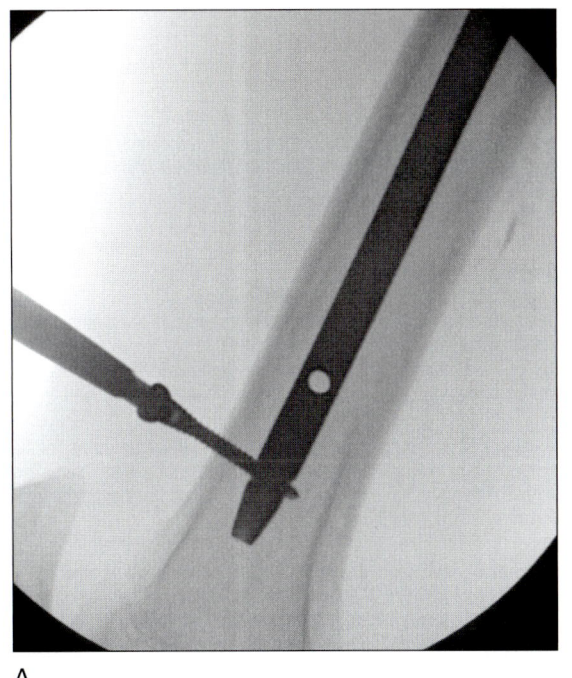
A

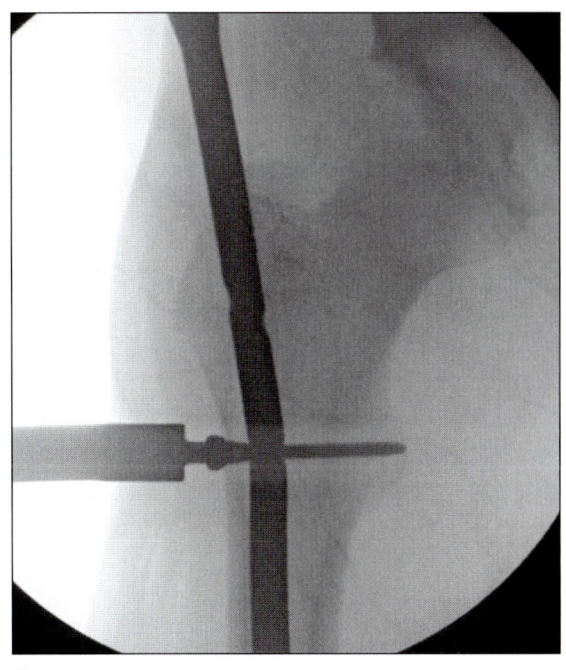
B

FIGURE 22

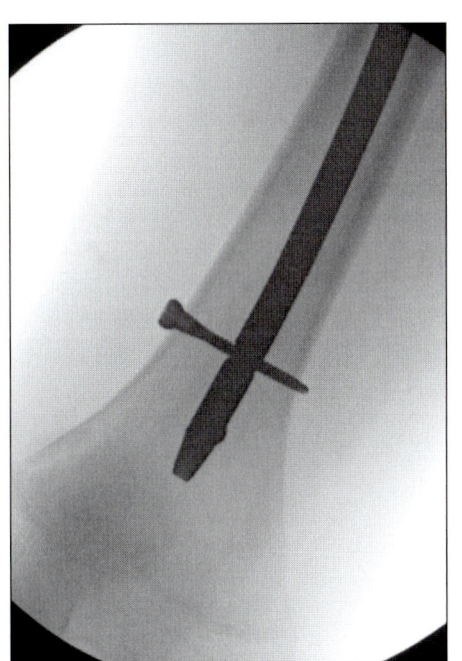
A

FIGURE 23

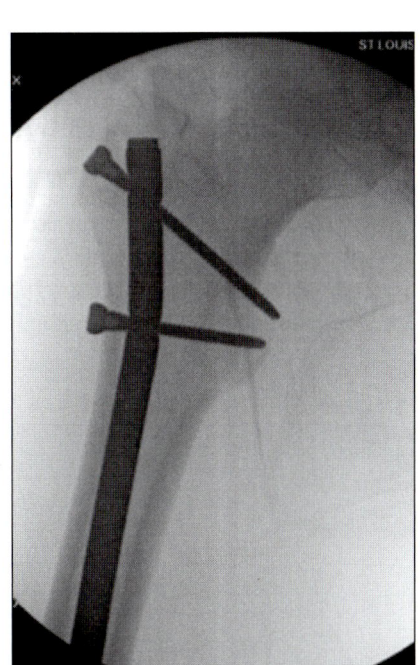
B

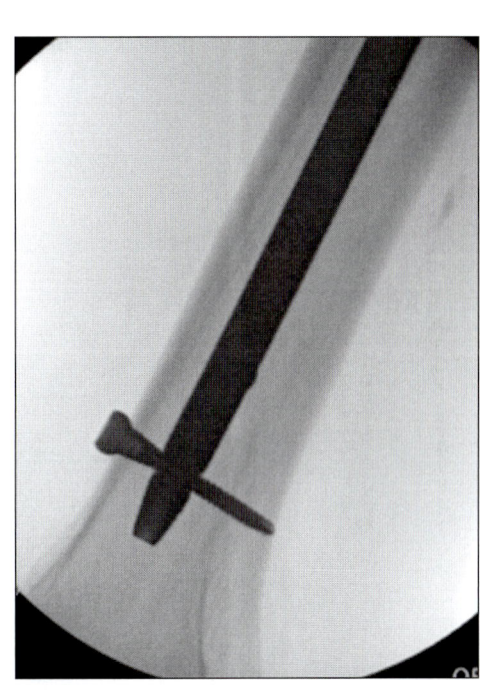
C

EVIDENCE

Anglen JO, Choi L. Treatment options in pediatric femoral shaft fractures. J Orthop Trauma. 2005;19:724–33.

The authors recommended surgical treatment of femoral shaft fractures in older or larger children and adolescents. Rigid antegrade nailing was noted to carry a risk of avascular necrosis.

Chung SMK. The arterial supply of the developing proximal end of the femur. J Bone Joint Surg [Am]. 1976;58:961–70.

The author reported the results of a cadaveric study of the arterial supply to the proximal femur. Two anastomotic rings were found: an extracapsular ring formed by the medial and lateral femoral circumflex arteries, and a subsynovial intra-articular ring at the junction of the articular cartilage and femoral neck.

Gordon JE, Khanna N, Luhmann SJ, et al. Intramedullary nailing of femoral fractures in children through the lateral aspect of the greater trochanter using a modified rigid humeral intramedullary nail: preliminary results of a new technique in 15 children. J Orthop Trauma. 2004;18:416–22.

In this retrospective study, skeletally immature patients with femoral shaft fractures were treated using a rigid IM nail placed through the lateral aspect of the greater trochanter. All fractures healed at a mean of 7 weeks. No patients developed avascular necrosis, femoral neck valgus, femoral neck narrowing, or other complications.

Gordon JE, Swenning TA, Burd TA, Szymanski DA, Schoenecker PL. Proximal femoral changes after lateral transtrochanteric intramedullary nail placement in children: a radiographic analysis. J Bone Joint Surg [Am]. 2003;85:1295–301.

This retrospective study examined proximal femoral changes after IM nailing through the lateral aspect of the trochanter, indicating the lack of avascular necrosis or femoral neck narrowing in patients 8 years and older.

O'Malley DE, Mazur JM, Cummings RJ. Femoral head avascular necrosis associated with intramedullary nailing in an adolescent. J Pediatr Orthop. 1995;15:21–3.

This case report described development of avascular necrosis of the femoral head after IM nail treatment of a femoral shaft fracture. The authors attributed the process to injury to the posterior superior ascending branch of the medial femoral circumflex artery in the piriformis fossa at the time of nail insertion.

Stevens PM, Anderson D. Correction of anteversion in skeletally immature patients: percutaneous osteotomy and transtrochanteric intramedullary rod. J Pediatr Orthop. 2008;28:277–83.

The authors reported their experience using a lateral trochanteric entry nail in performing derotational osteotomies in pediatric patients with increased femoral anteversion.

Submuscular Plating for Pediatric Femur Fractures

Ernest L. Sink

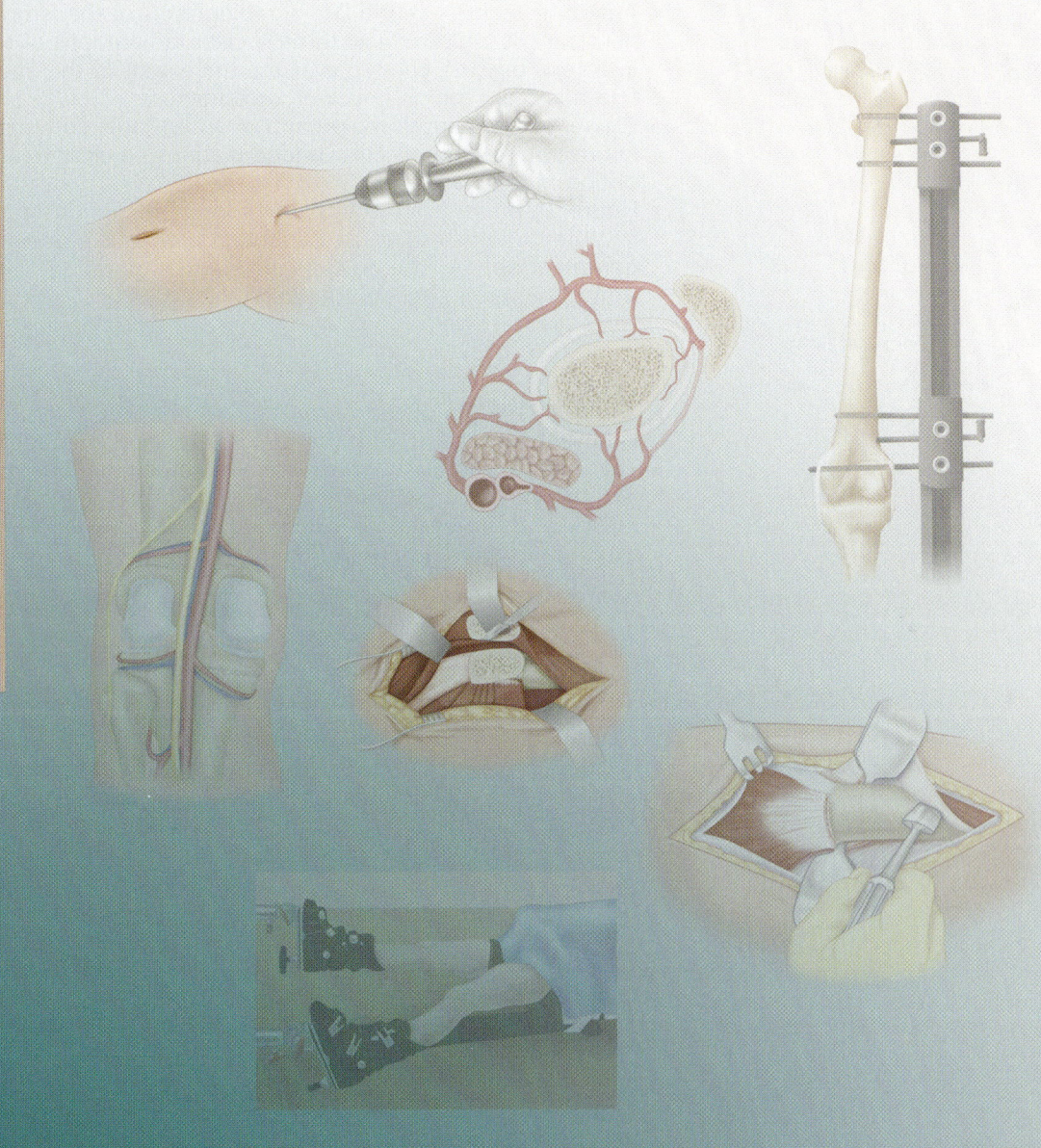

Controversies

- There is no consensus for submuscular bridge plating in stable transverse femur fractures. We prefer flexible intramedullary nailing in the stable transverse or short-oblique fractures.

Treatment Options

- Other options for unstable femur fractures in older patients are rigid trochanteric intramedullary nails. Elastic intramedullary nails (stainless and titanium) are less appealing in unstable fratures but can be used if technical details are strictly followed.

- Traction and external fixation are also options for treatment but are less appealing due to the complications of external fixation and prolonged immobilization in traction.

INDICATIONS

- This procedure is indicated for patients ≥ 5 years until skeletal maturity.
- Submuscular plating is ideally suited for comminuted or long-oblique unstable femur fractures.
- Submuscular plating is also a good option for proximal-third or distal-third femur fractures. In the proximal-third and distal-third fractures, there needs to be enough room for two to three screws in the proximal or distal diaphysis.

EXAMINATION/IMAGING

- Anteroposterior (AP) and lateral radiographs of the femur are necessary. It is also critical to have clear radiographs of the ipsilateral hip and knee to evaluate the extent of the fracture and rule out a femoral neck or knee fracture.
- Figure 1 shows an AP radiograph of an unstable comminuted femur frature. Submuscular bridge plating is a clear treatment option in this fracture.
- Figure 2A presents an example of a long-oblique unstable femur fracture for which submuscular bridge plating is a good treatment option. The postoperative AP radiograph in Figure 2B shows the result after submuscular plating.

SURGICAL ANATOMY

- The distal margin of the vastus lateralis muscle is deep to the iliotibial fascia in line with the proximal pole of the patella.
- The fibers of the distal vastus lateralis are oblique. The muscle is not attached to the bone, and there is a plane between the muscle and the lateral periosteum of the femur that is easily explored for plate insertion (Fig. 3).

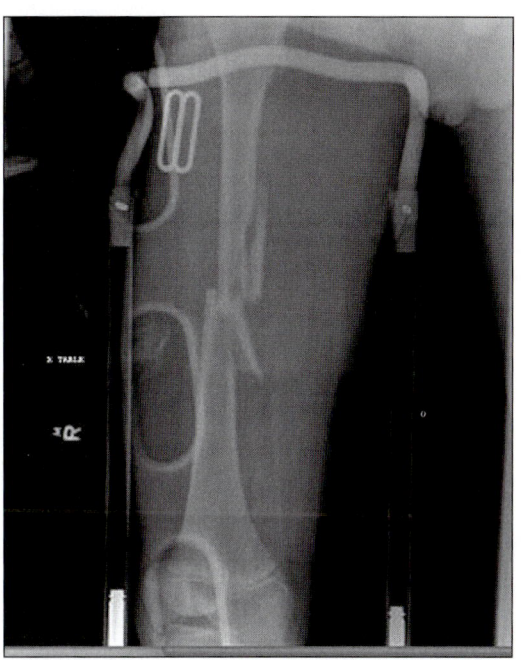

FIGURE 1

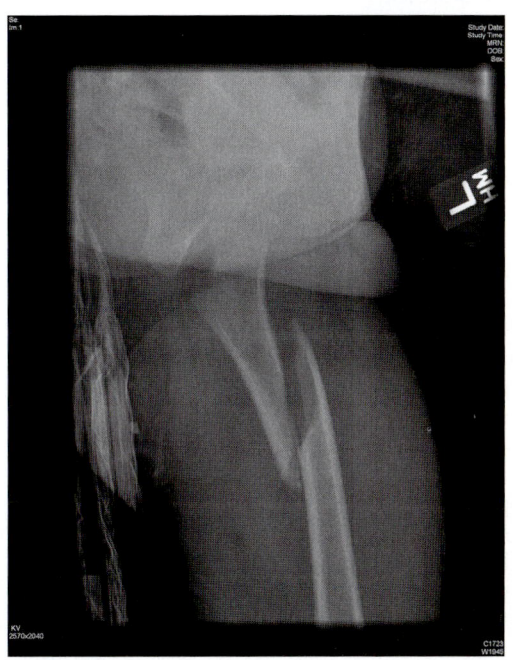

FIGURE 2 A

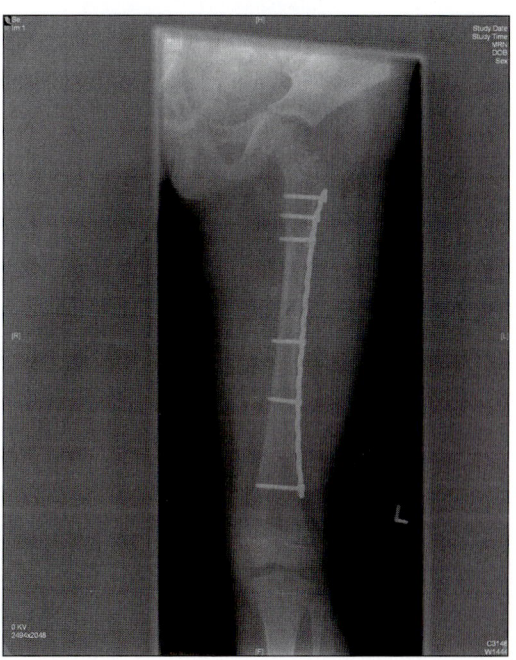

B

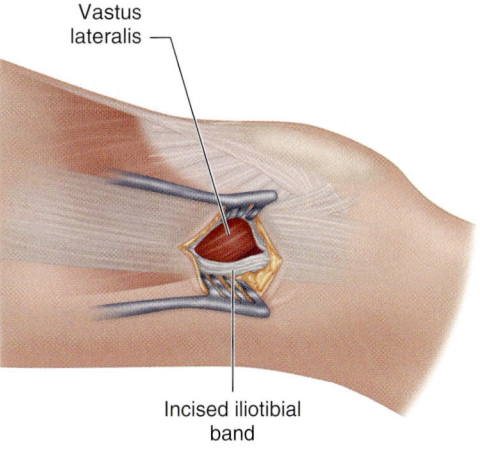

Vastus
lateralis

Incised iliotibial
band

FIGURE 3

PEARLS

- *Make sure patients are positioned to allow a good fluoroscopic lateral view to facilitate the placement of percutaneous screws.*

PITFALLS

- *In communuted fractures, be aware of malrotation of the distal leg.*

Equipment

- A traction bed that accommodates the pediatric patient will facilitate treatment.

Controversies

- We prefer a distal incision with retrograde plate insertion over a proximal incision. The vastus lateralis does not insert into the femur distally; thus developing the subvastus plane for plate insertion is easier than with a proximal incision where the vastus lateralis inserts into the proximal femur. Retrograde plate insertion has been successful in proximal fractures.

POSITIONING

- Patients are positioned supine on a fracture table. The well leg is extended and slightly abducted to allow a true lateral fluoroscopic image of the fractured femur. Alternatively, a "well-leg" holder may also be used.
- Provisional reduction restoring femoral length and rotation is obtained with boot traction and verified fluoroscopically. Figure 4 shows patient positioning on the traction table with boot traction. In this case, the legs are scissored in the anterior-posterior direction to give the C-arm access to obtain clear AP and lateral images.
- In comminuted fractures, special attention should be given to rotation. Final alignment is performed with plate fixation as described later.

PORTALS/EXPOSURES

- A small (4- to 7-mm) incision is made at the distal lateral thigh. The incision is midway anterior-posterior and as distal as the proximal pole of the patella. The incision is similar to the lateral incision for retrograde insertion of elastic nails.
- As the dissection is advanced through the tensor fascia lata, the distal oblique fibers of the vastus lateralis muscle will be exposed (Fig. 5). Blunt dissection is performed deep to the distal muscle fibers to enter the plane between the vastus lateralis and lateral femur periosteum. This plane is easily entered and allows proximal plate advancement with minimal force.

PROCEDURE

STEP 1: CHOOSING AND PRECONTOURING A PLATE

- After the patient has had length and rotation provisionally restored with boot traction and confirmed with C-arm fluoroscopy, the surgical field is routinely prepped and draped. Prior to making the incision, the appropriate-length plate is chosen.
- A long, narrow 4.5-mm plate with no staggering of screw holes is most often used. This plate is easy to contour and is readily available in many different lengths, and percutaneous screw fixation is forgiving. In smaller patients, a 3.5-mm plate may be used, although a 4.5-mm plate fits most femurs in children. Having 4.5-mm self-tapping screws allows easier percutaneous screw insertion and implant removal as the larger screw head is easier to engage with the screwdriver in a percutaneous manner.
- Historically, a nonlocking stainless steel plate has been used. Our experience is that the nonlocking plate achieves enough stability in this age group. Also percutaneous screw insertion and fracture reduction to the plate is easier with a nonlocking plate. In the pediatric age group, there have been no plate failures or nonunions to our knowledge with a nonlocking stainless plate.
  - A locking plate may also be used depending on surgeon preference, in osteopenic patients, or for very proximal or distal fractures where there is little available room for screws.

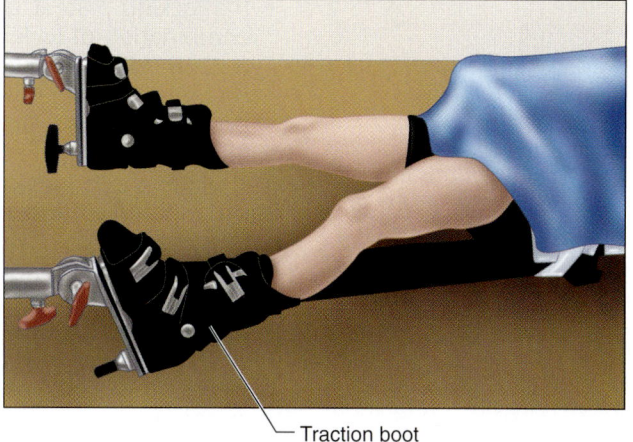

Traction boot

FIGURE 4

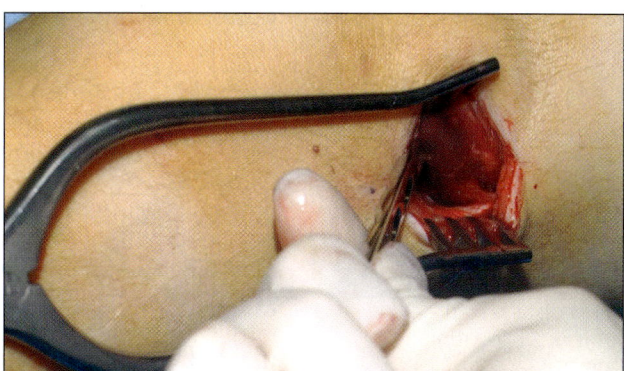

FIGURE 5

PEARLS

- *Use a long, narrow plate that spans from the trochanteric apophysis to the distal femur. Precontour the plate to accommodate to proximal and distal metaphyses and check the contour by using an AP image with the plate on the anterior thigh shadowing the lateral femur.*

PITFALLS

- *Do not overcontour. Contour the plate as close to anatomic as possible as the final aligment will be that of the plate.*

Instrumentation/ Implantation

- We prefer a 4.5-mm narrow plate and screws as percutaneous screw insertion and eventual removal are easier.

Controversies

- In our experience, a nonlocking plate has been successful in all cases. Locking plate technology is increasing in utilization. A locking plate can be used based on surgeon preference, osteopenic bone, or more proximal and distal fractures. If a locking plate is used, we would recommend using nonlocking screws as well.

PEARLS

- *Use a combination of C-arm views and "feel" to guide the plate past the fracture. Make sure the plate is in a good position in anterior-posterior planes with the C-arm prior to securing the plate on the femur.*

- *Use K-wires in the most proximal and distal screw holes to hold the plate in position prior to screw placement. The K-wire can be used to manipulate the plate into position.*

- If a locking plate is used, the surgeon should use a combination of locking and nonlocking screws to reduce the fracture to the precountoured plate. Also, with a distal metaphyseal bend in the plate, the surgeon should avoid the possibility of a locking screw trajectory crossing the distal femoral physis.

■ The plate length chosen is normally 10–16 holes. The plate should span from just below the greater trochanteric apophysis to the metaphysis of the distal femur. If possible, the plate should allow for six holes above and/or below the fracture margins to allow a large screw spread. Frequently the fracture location allows for only three screw holes, which is adequate as long as a long plate is chosen. A key determinate to stability is plate length. A long plate is more important to stability than the number of screws.

■ Once the appropriate length is chosen, it is necessary to use a table plate bender to contour the plate to accommdate the proimal and distal metaphyseal flare. Since the screws "pull" the femur to the pecountoured plate, the final varus/valgus alignment will be that of the precontoured plate. Therefore, it is important to contour the plate as close to anatomic as possible. Once the plate is contoured, we place it on the anterior thigh (Fig. 6A) and use an AP C-arm image to shadow the lateral aspect of the femur to check the contour and length (Fig. 6B). In our experience, we have not had any significant postoperative malalignment due to poor contouring.

STEP 2: PLATE ADVANCEMENT

■ A small (4- to 7-mm) incision is made at the distal lateral thigh. The exposure is advanced through the tensor fascia lata to expose the distal oblique fibers of the vastus lateralis muscle. Blunt dissection is performed deep to the distal muscle fibers to enter the plane between the vastus lateralis and lateral femur periosteum. This plane is easily entered and allows proximal plate advancement with minimal force.

■ The plate is then slowly tunneled proximally along the lateral femur in this plane (Fig. 7A). A Kocher clamp may be used to grasp the distal aspect of the plate for guidance.

- Care is taken to keep the plate on the lateral femur as it is advanced proximally past the fracture to the region of the greater trochanteric apophysis.

- The plate may be more difficult to pass along the lateral femur as it passes the fracture. The surgeon may facilitate plate advancement by pulling the plate back and redirecting it using C-arm guidance (Fig. 7B).

■ Once the plate is fully advanced, it sits "comfortably" on the lateral femur. Anteroposterior and lateral images are obtained to make sure the plate is in a good position in both planes and the femoral length is restored.

■ The plate is provisionally fixed to the femur with Kirshner wires (K-wires) placed in the most proximal and distal screw holes (Fig. 8A and 8B). In proximal fractures, where screw holes are limited, the surgeon will have to make sure the plate is positioned as proximal as possible while performing the temporary K-wire fixation. If the fracture is "sagging" posterior, the femur can be lifted in an anterior direction while a K-wire is placed through the plate to engage the femur in this region. The K-wire may also be used to manipulate the plate.

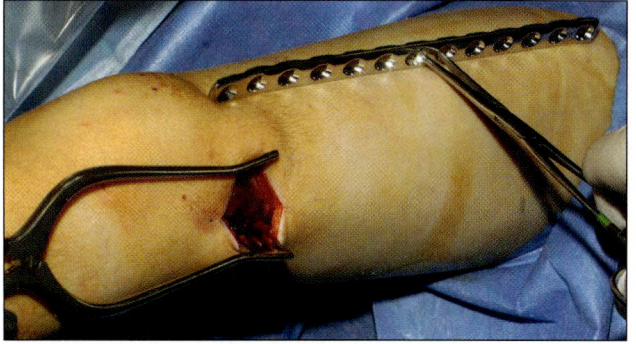
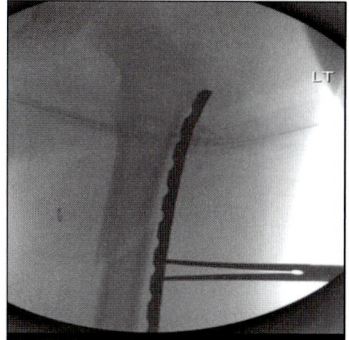

A

B

FIGURE 6

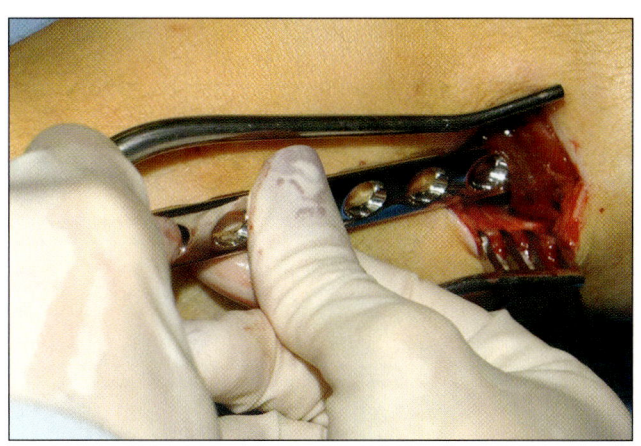
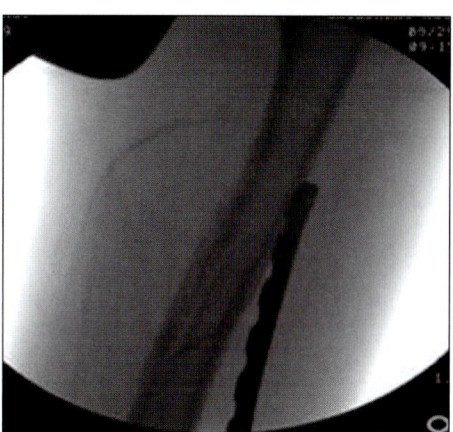

A

B

FIGURE 7

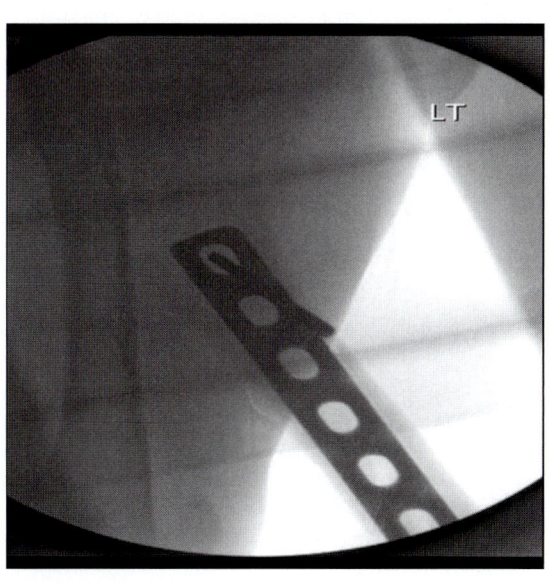
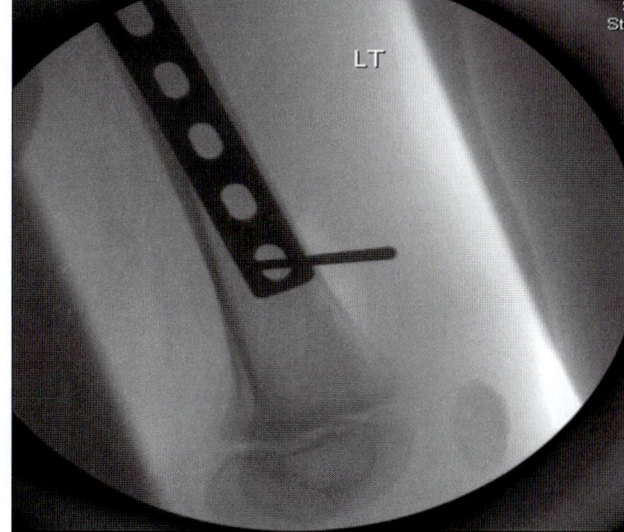

A

B

FIGURE 8

Instrumentation/ Implantation

- Self-tapping screws are critical for percutaneous incisions.

STEP 3: PERCUTANEOUS SCREW PLACEMENT

- Obtaining maximal screw spread with a long plate (long working length of the plate) is important for construct stability. It is important that a screw be placed just proximal and another just distal to the proximal and distal extents of the fracture.
  - The first screw placed should be near the proximal or distal extent of the fracture where the femur is furthest from the plate. This screw will reduce the femur to the precontoured plate and act as a "reduction screw." As the screw engages the far cortex, the femur will be reduced to the precontoured plate (Fig. 9A). The fracture is "bridged" and no attempt is made to place a screw to lag the fracture fragments.
  - The second screw is placed in the opposite margin of the fracture (Fig. 9B).
  - The remaining screws are placed as far apart as possible (Fig. 9C). Three screws proximal and three screws distal to the fracture are optimal.

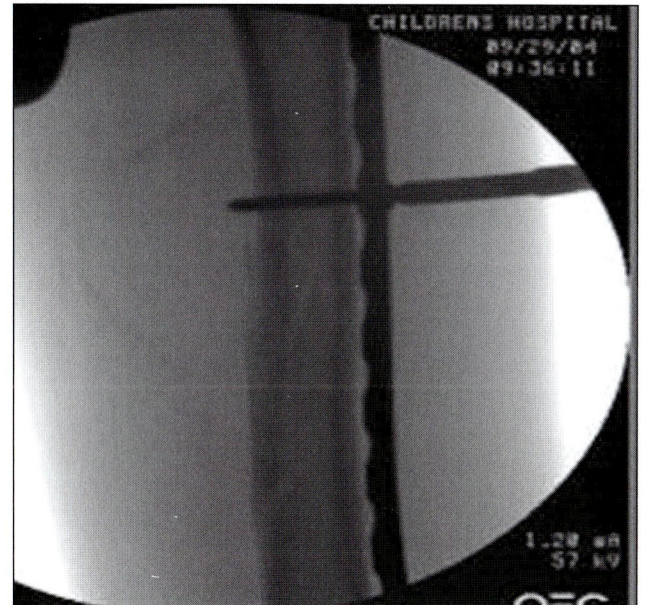

A

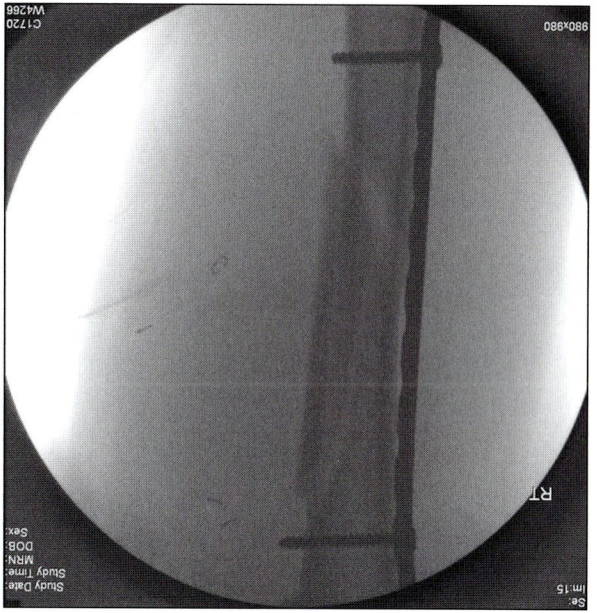

B

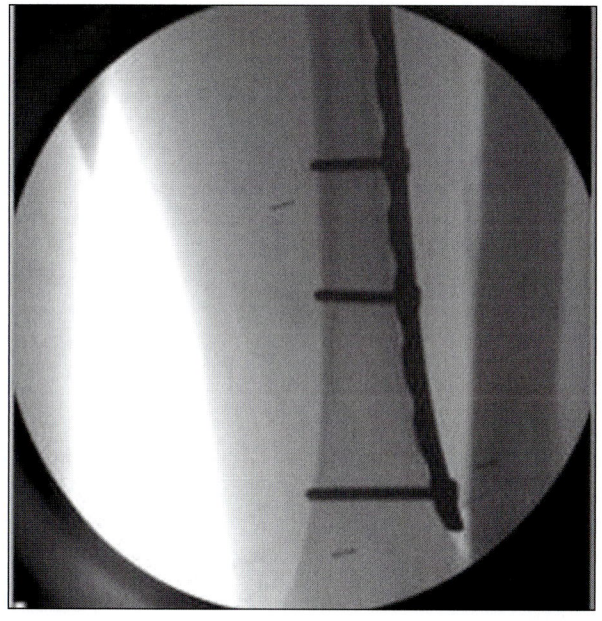

C

FIGURE 9

- Screws are placed using a "perfect circle" technique. The technical aspects of percutaneous screw placement are as follows:
  - Using the fluoroscopic image in the lateral plane, a #15 blade scalpel is placed on the skin over the desired hole and then rotated horizontal to the beam through the skin, tensor fascia, and vastus fascia (Fig. 10A).
  - Using freehand technique, a 3.2-mm drill is placed in this small incision and its location in the desired hole is confirmed with fluoroscopy (Fig. 10B). The hole is then drilled through both cortices.
  - The length of the screw is approximated by placing the depth gauge on the anterior thigh as the C-arm is used in the anterior-posterior position (Fig. 10C).
  - It is important to tie a #0 Vicryl suture around the 4.5-mm fully threaded cortical screw head so it will not be lost in the soft tissue if the screw inadvertently disengages from the screwdriver (Fig. 10D).
  - The screw is then placed though the plate and across the femur (Fig. 10E). The first screw placed is placed just proximal to the fracture where the femur is furthest from the plate (Fig. 10F).
  - The Vicryl ties are cut and the incisions are closed with absorbable subcuticular sutures after all screws are placed.

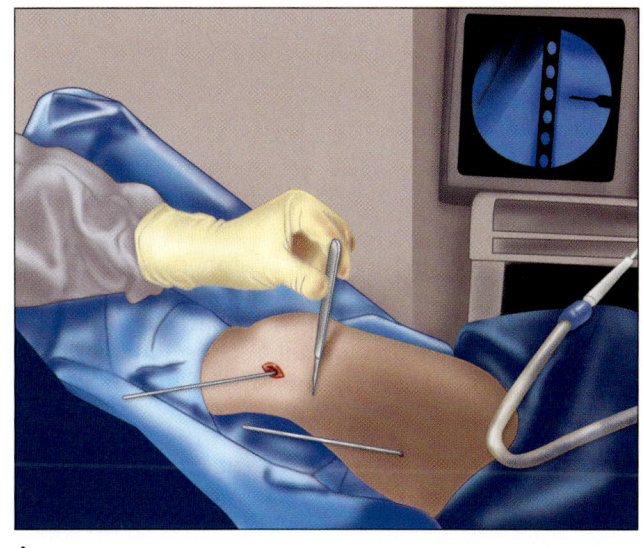

A

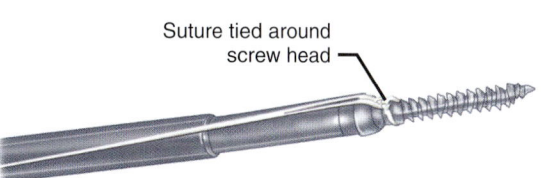

Suture tied around
screw head

D

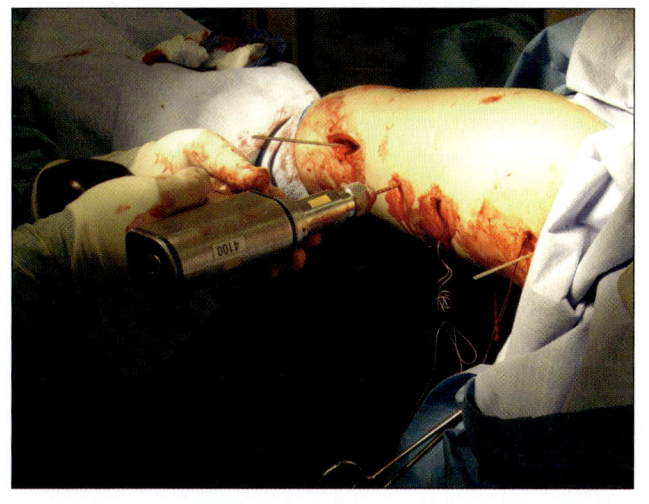

B

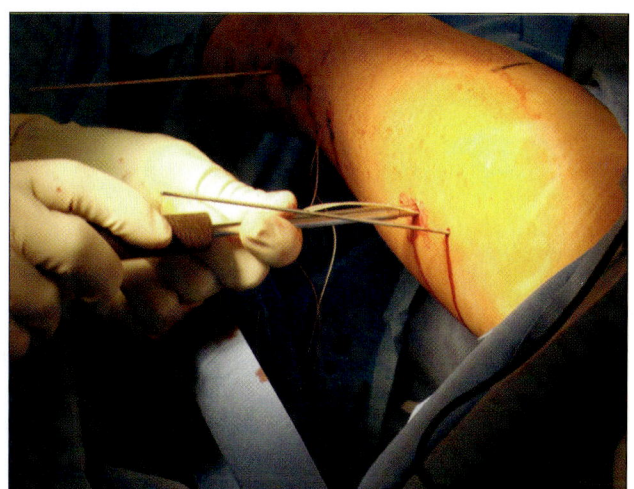

E

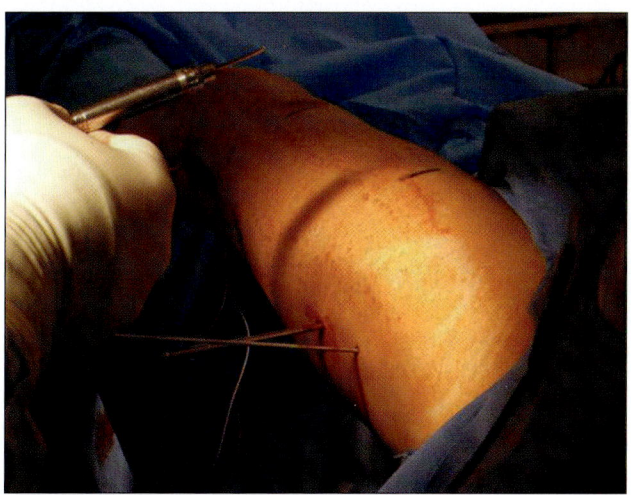

C

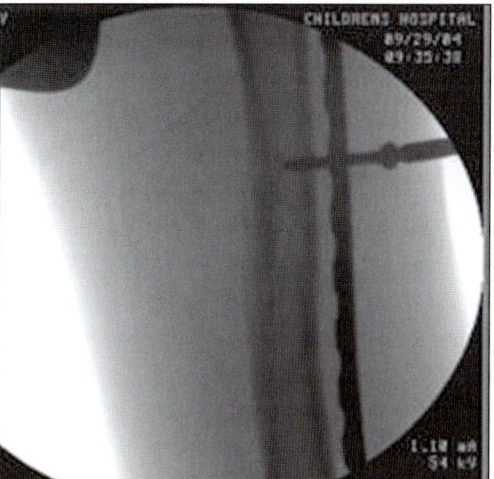

F

FIGURE 10

■ Figure 11 shows a comminuted fracture in a 7-year-old patient from the AP (Fig. 11A) and lateral (Fig. 11B) views before submuscular plating and the AP (Fig. 11C) and lateral (Fig. 11D) views after submuscular plating.

POSTOPERATIVE CARE AND EXPECTED OUTCOMES

■ A soft dressing is applied postoperatively. Postoperative spica casting is not necessary.
■ A knee immobilizer can be used for patient comfort.
■ Patients are restricted to toe-touch weight bearing until early callus is visualized on postoperative radiographs. The usual time to advance weight bearing is 6–8 weeks.
■ Hip and knee range of motion is encouraged as tolerated. Patients can usually return to full activity in 10–12 weeks.

PEARLS

• *Make sure to check for any rotational malalignment in comminuted fractures prior to the patient leaving the operating room.*

PITFALLS

• *Overgrowth of the operative side (up to 1–2 cm) is not uncommon after anatomic reduction in pediatric femur fractures. Overgrowth in most cases has no clinical relevance.*

Controversies

• Plate removal is dependent on surgeon and family preference. There are no data on the benefits of plate removal. In the author's experience, plate removal is performed on an outpatient basis and the plate is removed in a percutaneous manner. We have not had any cases of refracture after plate removal. The recommendation after plate removal is weight bearing as tolerated but limiting athletic activities for 6 weeks.

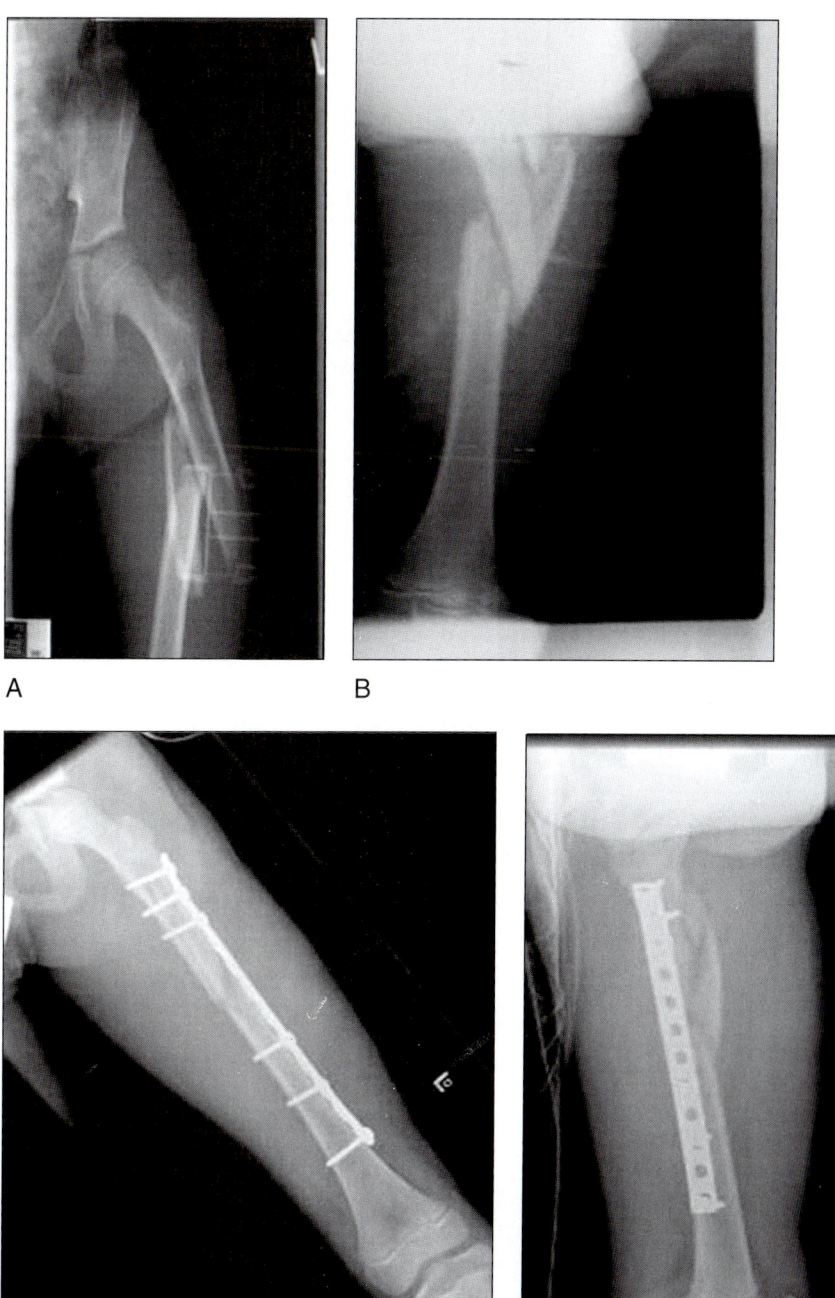

A

B

C

D

FIGURE 11

EVIDENCE

All of the papers in the literature regarding submuscular plating in pediatric femur fractures are retrospective case series and descriptive technical articles.

Angus H, Kalenderer O, Eranilmaz G, et al. Biologic internal fixation of comminuted femur shaft fractures by bridge plating in children. J Pediatr Orthop. 2003;23: 184–9.

Hedequest DJ, Bishop J, Hresko T. Locking plate fixation for pediatric femur fractures. J Pediatr Orthop. 2008;28:6–9.

Hedequist DJ, Sink EL. Technical aspects of bridge plating for pediatric femur fractures. J Orthop Trauma. 2004;19:276–79.

Kanlic EM, Anglen JO, Smith DG. Advantages of submuscular plating for complex femur fractures. Clin Orthop Relat Res. 2004;(426):244–51.

Sink EL, Hedequist DJ, Morgan SJ, et al. Results and technique of pediatric femur fractures treated with submuscular bridge plating. J Pediatr Orthop. 2006;26:177–81.

Flexion Osteotomy for Slipped Capital Femoral Epiphysis

Paul R.T. Kuzyk

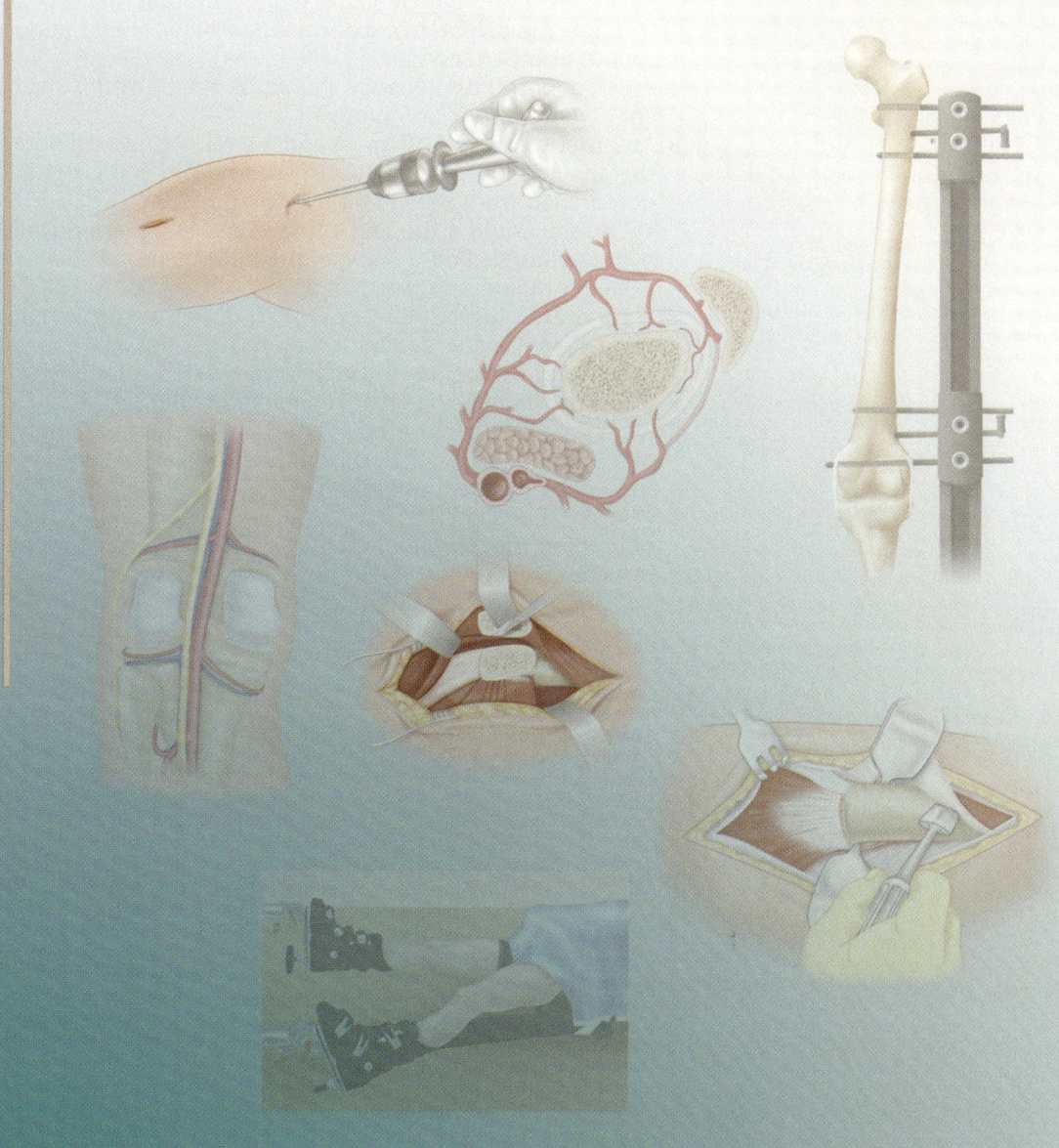

Controversies

- Slipped capital femoral epiphysis with a slip angle less than 30° may be treated with femoral neck osteoplasty performed with hip arthroscopy, anterior arthrotomy, or surgical hip dislocation.

- Slipped capital femoral epiphysis with a slip angle greater than 60° may be treated with subcapital osteotomy.

INDICATIONS

- Chronic and subacute slipped capital femoral epiphysis with slip angles of 30–60° on a lateral radiograph.
- Avascular necrosis affecting a focal segment of the femoral head. The goal of a intertrochanteric osteotomy in this clinical scenario is to move an unaffected portion of the femoral head into the weight-bearing area.

EXAMINATION/IMAGING

- The hip is examined for range of motion. It is especially important to document deficiency of internal rotation and flexion as these may be corrected with rotation and flexion through the osteotomy. Extension, abduction, and adduction should also be recorded.
- Any leg length discrepancy should be noted as this may be corrected with the osteotomy.
- Anteroposterior (AP) (Fig. 1) and lateral (Fig. 2) radiographs of the affected hip must be obtained. The slip angle should be determined from the lateral radiograph.
  - The slip angle is the angle between a line perpendicular to the epiphysis and a line parallel to the femoral shaft on the lateral radiograph (see Fig. 2).
- A computed tomography (CT) scan of the proximal femur with three-dimensional rendering may provide the surgeon with a better understanding of the deformity (Fig. 3A and 3B).
- Contrast magnetic resonance imaging (MRI) of the hip may be used to identify intra-articular pathology, such as labral tears and chondral flaps, arising from mechanical damage due the presence of the chronic slip.
- MRI or CT may be used to assess overall femoral version and determine the degree of internal rotation of the distal fragment required to correct the external rotation deformity.

Treatment Options

- Nonoperative management may be considered for small slips (< 30°) that do not cause symptomatic restriction of range of motion.
- Some authors advocate the use of osteoplasty through surgical hip dislocation for slips between 30° and 60°.
- Severe slips (> 60°) may be managed with subcapital osteotomy.

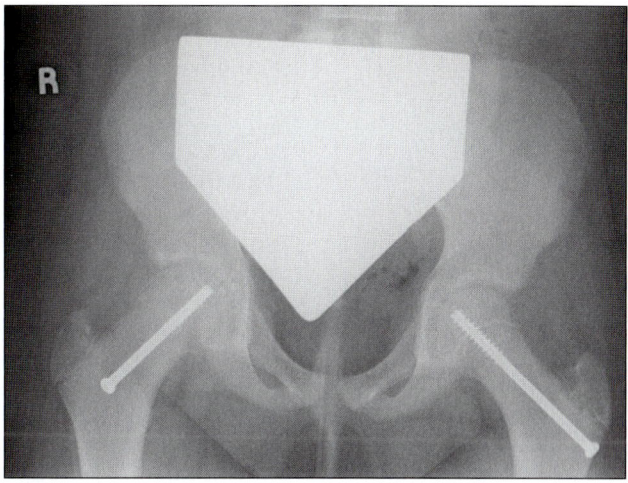

FIGURE 1

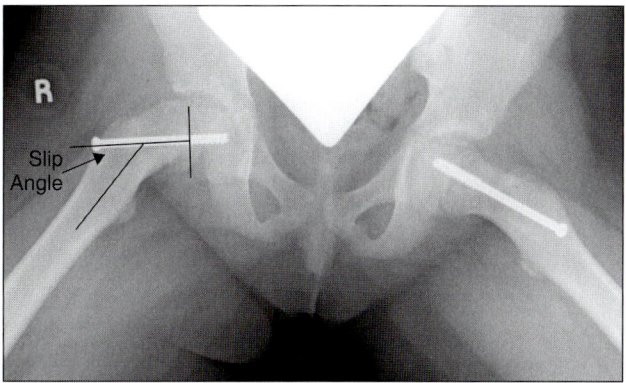

Slip
Angle

FIGURE 2

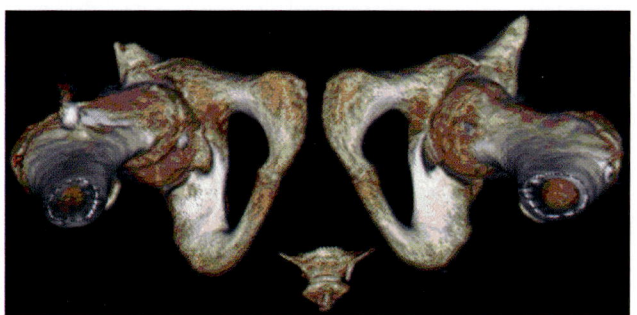

A

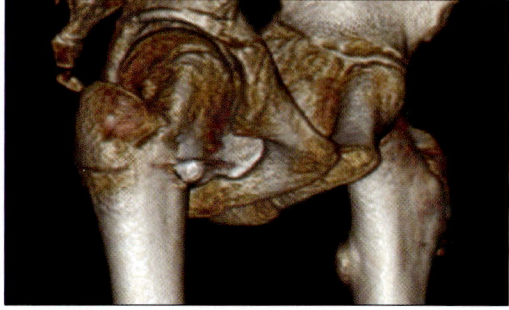

B

FIGURE 3

SURGICAL ANATOMY

- Superficial anatomy includes the gluteus maximus muscle, tensor fascia lata muscle, and iliotibial band (Fig. 4).
- Deep anatomy includes the gluteus medius and vastus lateralis muscles.
- Perforating vessels may be found entering the vastus lateralis through the intermuscular septum (see Fig. 4). These vessels should be identified and coagulated as the vastus lateralis is reflected off the intermuscular septum and lateral aspect of the femur.
- The vastus ridge is the site of insertion of both the gluteus medius and vastus lateralis muscles (Fig. 5). This bony landmark is useful for planning the osteotomy.
- It is important to understand the blood supply to the femoral head.
  - The deep branch of the medial femoral circumflex artery constitutes the main blood supply to the femoral head (see Fig. 5). This artery lies anterior to the obturator externus tendon and may be damaged by vigorous retraction in this area.
  - The trochanteric branch is visible on the lateral-posterior aspect of the trochanter during the surgical approach. The trochanteric branch is at the level of the obturator externus tendon and therefore serves as a rough landmark for the medial femoral circumflex artery.

POSITIONING

- The patient should be positioned supine on a radiolucent table. A radiolucent support may be placed under the ipsilateral hip (Fig. 6).
- The ipsilateral arm should be draped over the chest to allow room for the surgeon and assistants. The contralateral arm may be left free for intravenous access.
- The operative leg should be prepped and draped free to allow for manipulation during surgery. A leg bag should be placed over the foot.
- The groin should be draped out of the sterile field. The sterile field should extend proximally to the anterior superior iliac spine and medially to the umbilicus. A padded Mayo stand may be used to help position the leg during surgery.
- The fluoroscope should be draped and brought in from the contralateral side of the operating table.

PEARLS

- *The fluoroscope should be used to image the area of interest on the femur prior to prepping and draping the patient. This is to ensure that adequate AP and lateral fluoroscopic images may be obtained prior to beginning the operation.*

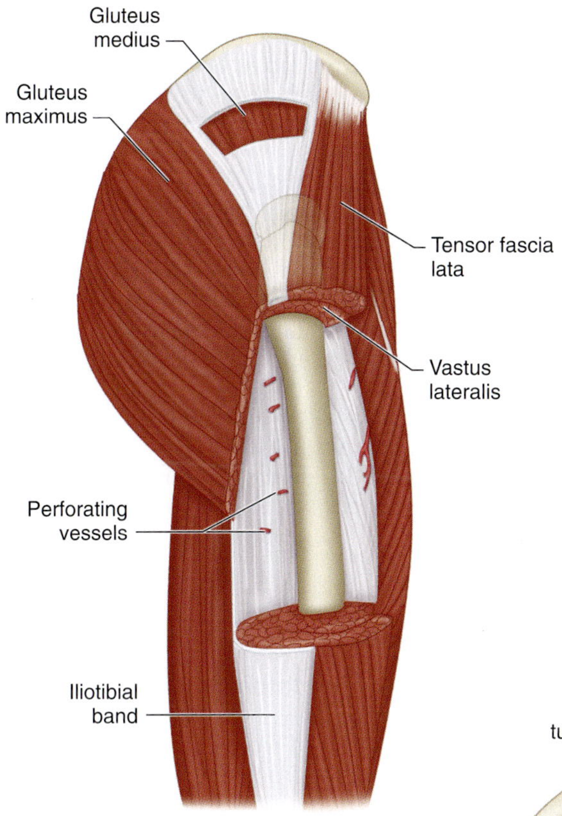

Gluteus
medius

Gluteus
maximus

Tensor fascia
lata

Vastus
lateralis

Perforating
vessels

Iliotibial
band

FIGURE 4

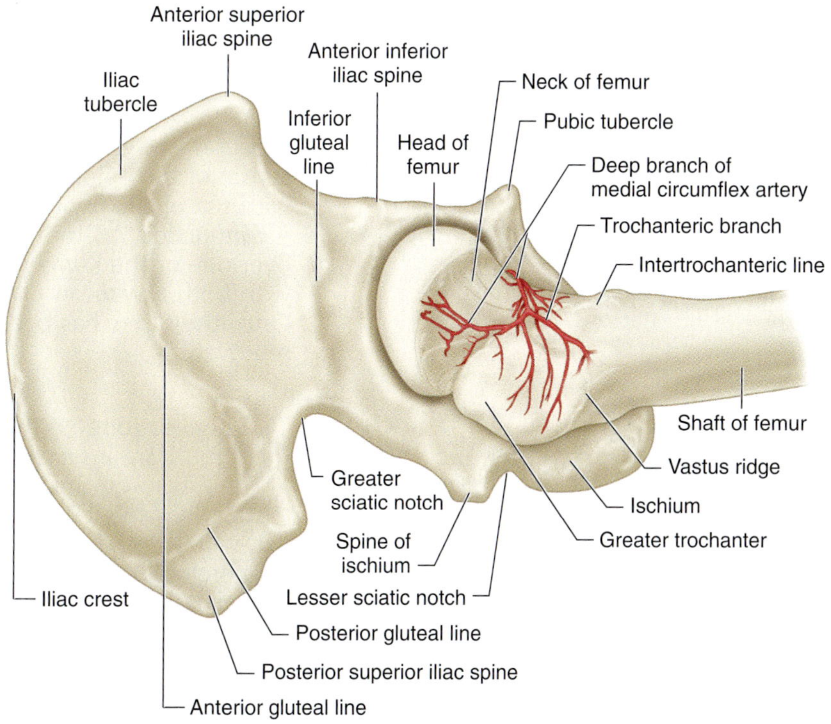

Anterior superior
iliac spine

Anterior inferior
iliac spine

Iliac
tubercle

Inferior
gluteal
line

Head of
femur

Neck of femur

Pubic tubercle

Deep branch of
medial circumflex artery

Trochanteric branch

Intertrochanteric line

Shaft of femur

Vastus ridge

Greater
sciatic notch

Spine of
ischium

Lesser sciatic notch

Ischium

Greater trochanter

Iliac crest

Posterior gluteal line

Posterior superior iliac spine

Anterior gluteal line

FIGURE 5

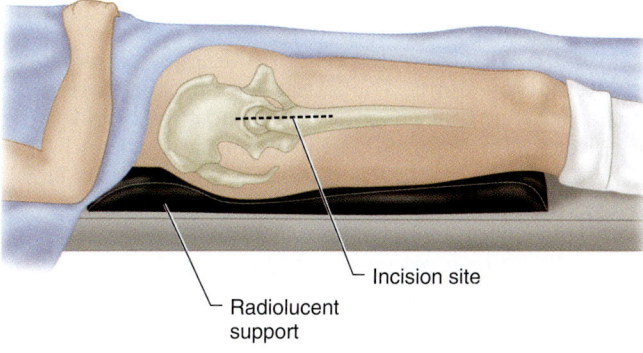

Incision site

Radiolucent
support

FIGURE 6

Instrumentation

• Self-retaining retractors and Hohmann retractors may be used to aid exposure.

Instrumentation/ Implantation

• 3.0-mm K-wires and fully threaded 7.3-mm cannulated screws

Controversies

• Some authors recommend fixing the epiphysis with two screws. However, this may increase the risk of avascular necrosis.

Instrumentation/ Implantation

• K-wires

• Blade plate chisel, handle for chisel

• Slotted hammer, mallet

PORTALS/EXPOSURES

■ The lateral skin incision extends from a point 6 cm proximal to the tip of the greater trochanter to 6 cm distal to the vastus ridge. The incision is centered over the greater trochanter and femoral shaft (see Fig. 6).

■ The iliotibial band is incised longitudinally in the interval between the tensor fascia lata and iliotibial band (Fig. 7). The incision in the iliotibial band should be carried distal to expose the vastus ridge and the upper portion of the vastus lateralis.

■ The origin of the vastus lateralis is reflected off the vastus ridge using an L-shaped incision. The vastus lateralis muscle is reflected off the lateral intermuscular septum and retracted anteriorly (see Fig. 7). Care is taken to coagulate or ligate the perforating branches of the profunda femoris that pierce the septum and supply the vastus lateralis muscle.

■ A longitudinal incision is made in the periosteum and a Cobb elevator is used to free the periosteum both anteriorly and posteriorly off the lateral aspect of the femur.

PROCEDURE

STEP 1

■ Two Kirschner wires (K-wires) are used to provisionally stabilize the femoral epiphysis. Since the epiphysis has slipped posteriorly, the K-wires must be inserted from the anterior aspect of the femoral neck and directed posteriorly to enter the center of the epiphysis (Fig. 8A). The K-wires should be placed with use of the fluoroscope.

■ A cannulated 7.3-mm fully threaded screw may then be inserted over one of the K-wires (Fig. 8B). This screw should be placed with both K-wires in place to prevent rotation of the epiphysis. Once the screw has been inserted, both K-wires may be removed.

STEP 2

■ Two K-wires (one on the greater trochanter and one distal on the femur) are inserted to help plan fixation of the osteotomy.
  • The K-wire on the greater trochanter should be placed slightly superior (about 1 cm) to the insertion site for the blade. This K-wire is intended to be a guide for insertion of the blade. Therefore, care should be taken to ensure that the K-wire lies in the appropriate direction on the AP and lateral projections. The K-wire should be roughly in the center of the femur on the lateral projection and at an angle of 90° to the femur to ensure maintenance of the normal neck-shaft angle.
  • The distal K-wire should be placed 2–3 cm distal to the anticipated distal end of the blade plate. This K-wire is intended to mark rotation and should be placed parallel to to the K-wire in the greater trochanter to ensure neutral rotation of the femur after the osteotomy (Fig. 9).

■ The blade should be placed central within the femoral neck on the AP and lateral projections. The lateral femoral cortex is scored using a 3.2-mm drill bit prior to seating the chisel for the blade. The chisel should be at 90° to the femoral shaft and parallel to the K-wire placed in the greater trochanter (see Fig. 9). The handle for the chisel should be rotated 30° to the femoral shaft, so that the blade plate will sit on the femoral shaft when the 30° flexion osteotomy is completed.

■ The blade plate chisel should be advanced to the length of the chosen blade plate. An adolescent blade plate may be used for small femurs.

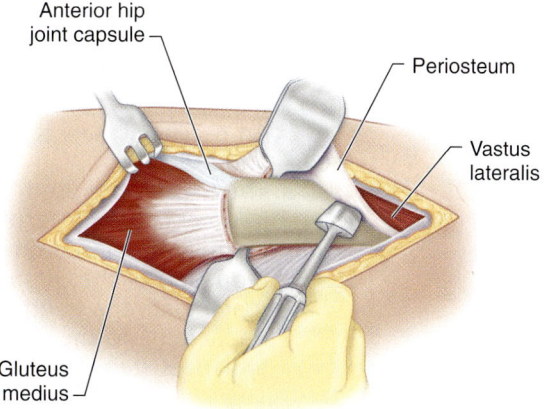

Anterior hip joint capsule

Periosteum

Vastus lateralis

Gluteus medius

FIGURE 7

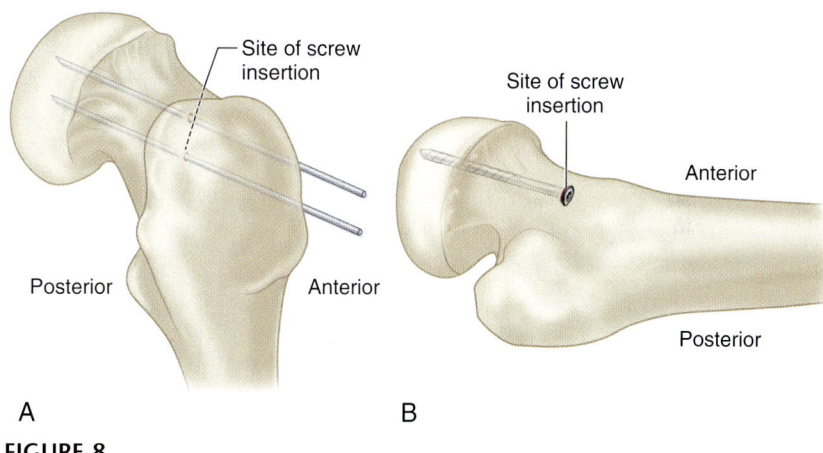

Site of screw insertion

Posterior

Anterior

Site of screw insertion

Anterior

Posterior

A

B

FIGURE 8

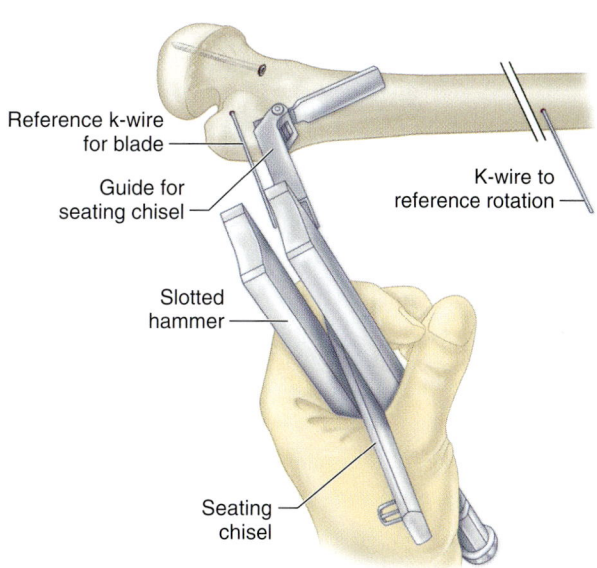

Reference k-wire for blade

Guide for seating chisel

Slotted hammer

Seating chisel

K-wire to reference rotation

FIGURE 9

STEP 3

- The intertrochanteric osteotomy should be performed just proximal to the lesser trochanter. Two Hohmann retractors are placed at the site of the osteotomy to protect the soft tissues. An oscillating saw is used to perform the osteotomy (Fig. 10A and 10B)

- The K-wires are used to assess rotation of the fragments. The fragments are distracted using laminar spreaders (Fig. 11). The leg may be placed on a padded Mayo stand (Fig. 12A) to aid in reduction of the osteotomy. Large reduction forceps are used to manipulate the fragments. The edge of the proximal fragment is impacted into the shaft (Fig. 12B). This produces flexion and enhances stability of the osteotomy.

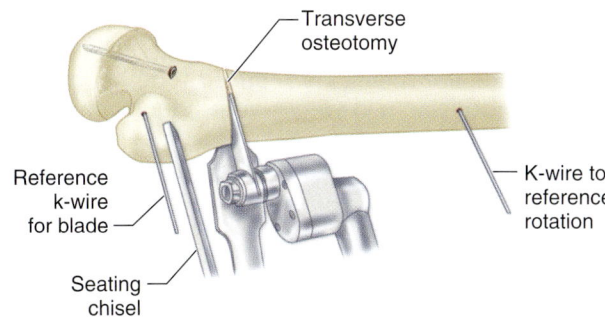

Transverse
osteotomy

Reference
k-wire
for blade

K-wire to
reference
rotation

Seating
chisel

A

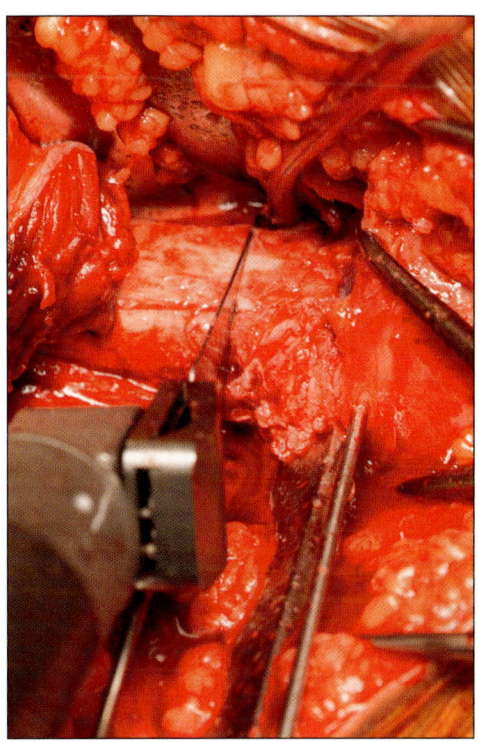

B
FIGURE 10

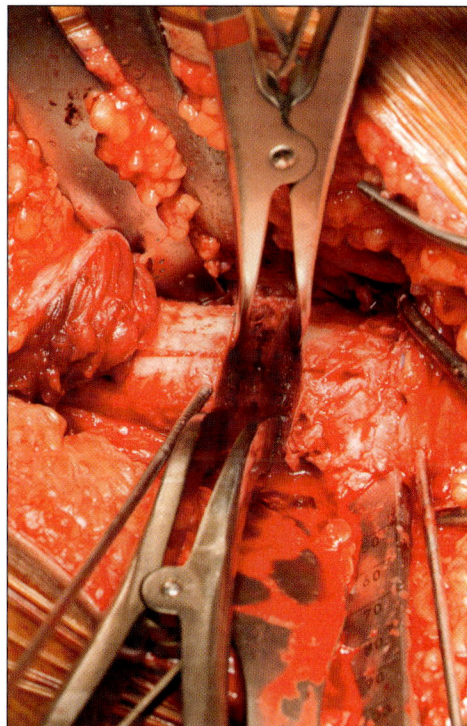

FIGURE 11

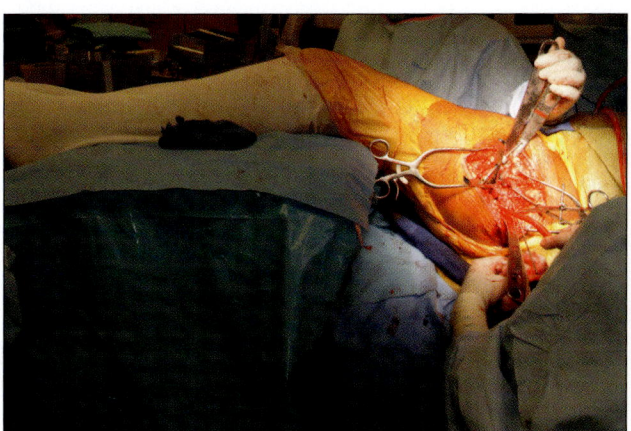

A
FIGURE 12

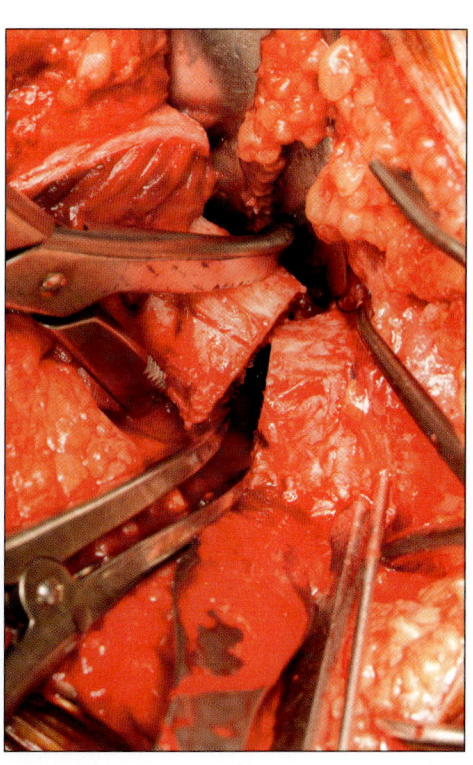

B

STEP 4

- The blade plate chisel is removed and the blade plate is placed (Fig. 13A). The two bone fragments are reduced together and the blade plate is provisionally held with a Verbrugge clamp (Fig. 13B and 13C).

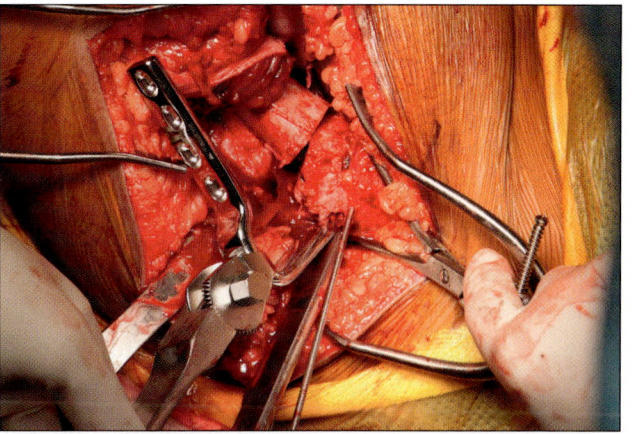

A

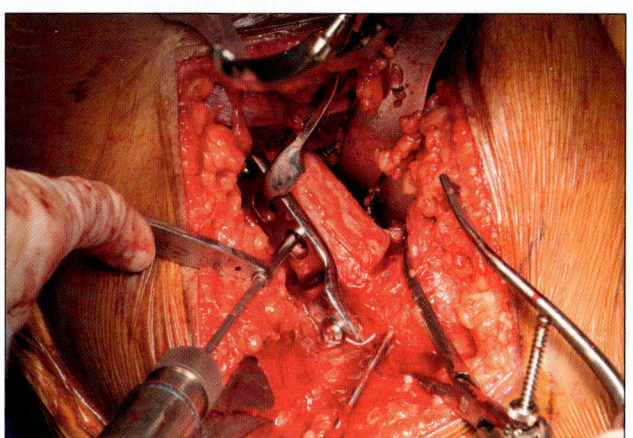

B

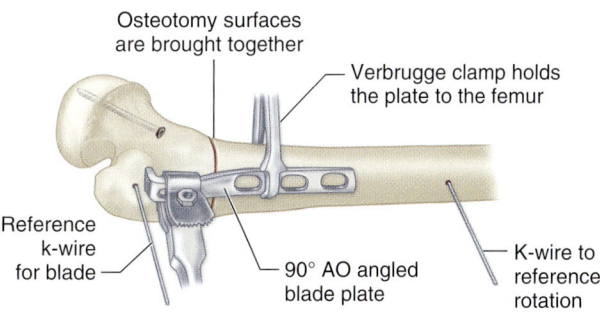

Osteotomy surfaces
are brought together

Verbrugge clamp holds
the plate to the femur

Reference
k-wire
for blade

90° AO angled
blade plate

K-wire to
reference
rotation

C

FIGURE 13

- Screws are used to fix the blade plate to the femur. Screws should be placed to create compression across the osteotomy site (Fig. 14A and 14B), as verified on AP (Fig. 15A) and lateral (Fig. 15B) radiographs.
- The vastus lateralis fascia is repaired using 2-0 Vicryl, the fascia lata is repaired using #1 Vicryl, and a subcuticular suture is used to close the skin.

POSTOPERATIVE CARE AND EXPECTED OUTCOMES

- Patients should be restricted to partial weight bearing for 6 weeks. Weight bearing may be gradually increased with evidence of bone healing on radiographic follow-up. Generally full weight bearing is permitted at 3–4 months.
- Hardware may be removed at 1 year.

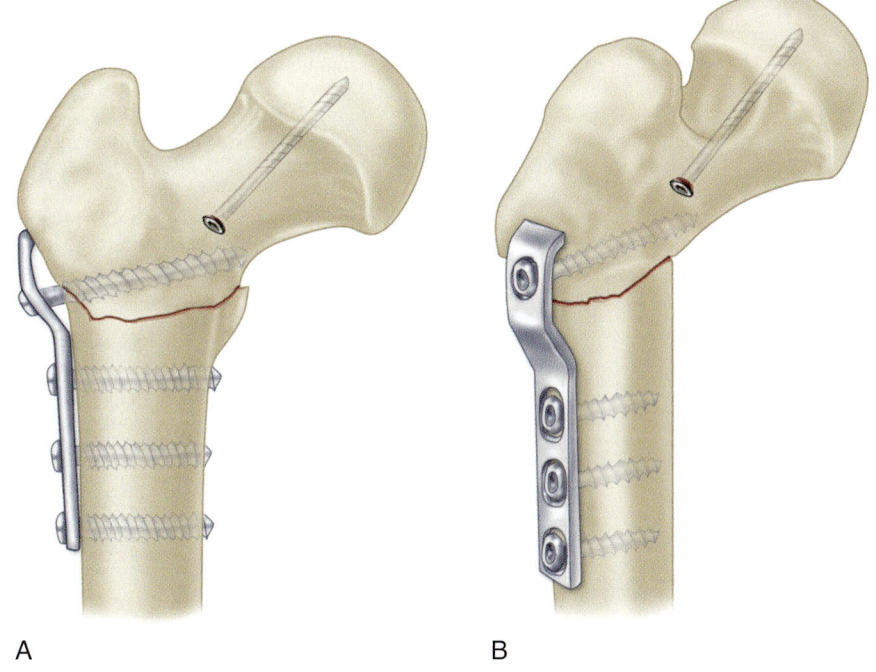

A   B

FIGURE 14

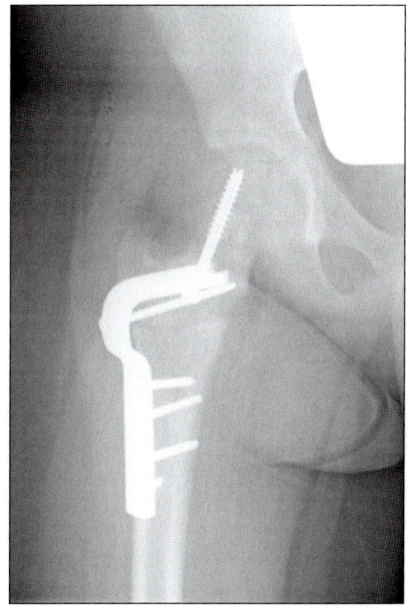

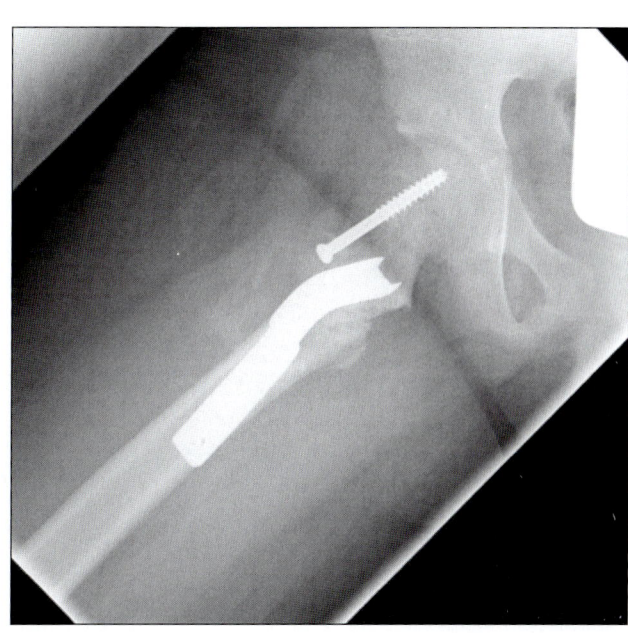

A   B

FIGURE 15

EVIDENCE

Diab M, Hresko MT, Millis MB. Intertrochanteric versus subcapital osteotomy in slipped capital femoral epiphysis. Clin Orthop Relat Res. 2004;(427):204–12.

Flexion intertrochanteric osteotomy was found to be an effective, safe, and reproducible realignment osteotomy for treatment of chronic, severe, stable slipped capital femoral epiphysis. (Level IV evidence [case series])

Schai PA, Exner GU, Hänsch O. Prevention of secondary coxarthrosis in slipped capital femoral epiphysis: a long-term follow-up study after corrective intertrochanteric oste-otomy. J Pediatr Orthop B. 1996;5:135–43.

Imhauser intertrochanteric osteotomy prevented osteoarthritis of the hip as compared to natural history. (Level IV evidence [case series])

Witbreuk MM, Bolkenbaas M, Mullender MG, Sierevelt IN, Besselaar PP. The results of downgrading moderate and severe slipped capital femoral epiphysis by an early Imhauser femur osteotomy. J Child Orthop. 2009;3:405–10.

Imhauser intertrochanteric osteotomy of the femur combined with epiphysiodesis per-formed on patients with moderate and severe slipped capital femoral epiphysis gave sat-isfactory results. (Level IV evidence [case series])

Femur Fracture: Closed Reduction and Spica Cast

Matthew Diltz and Mininder S. Kocher

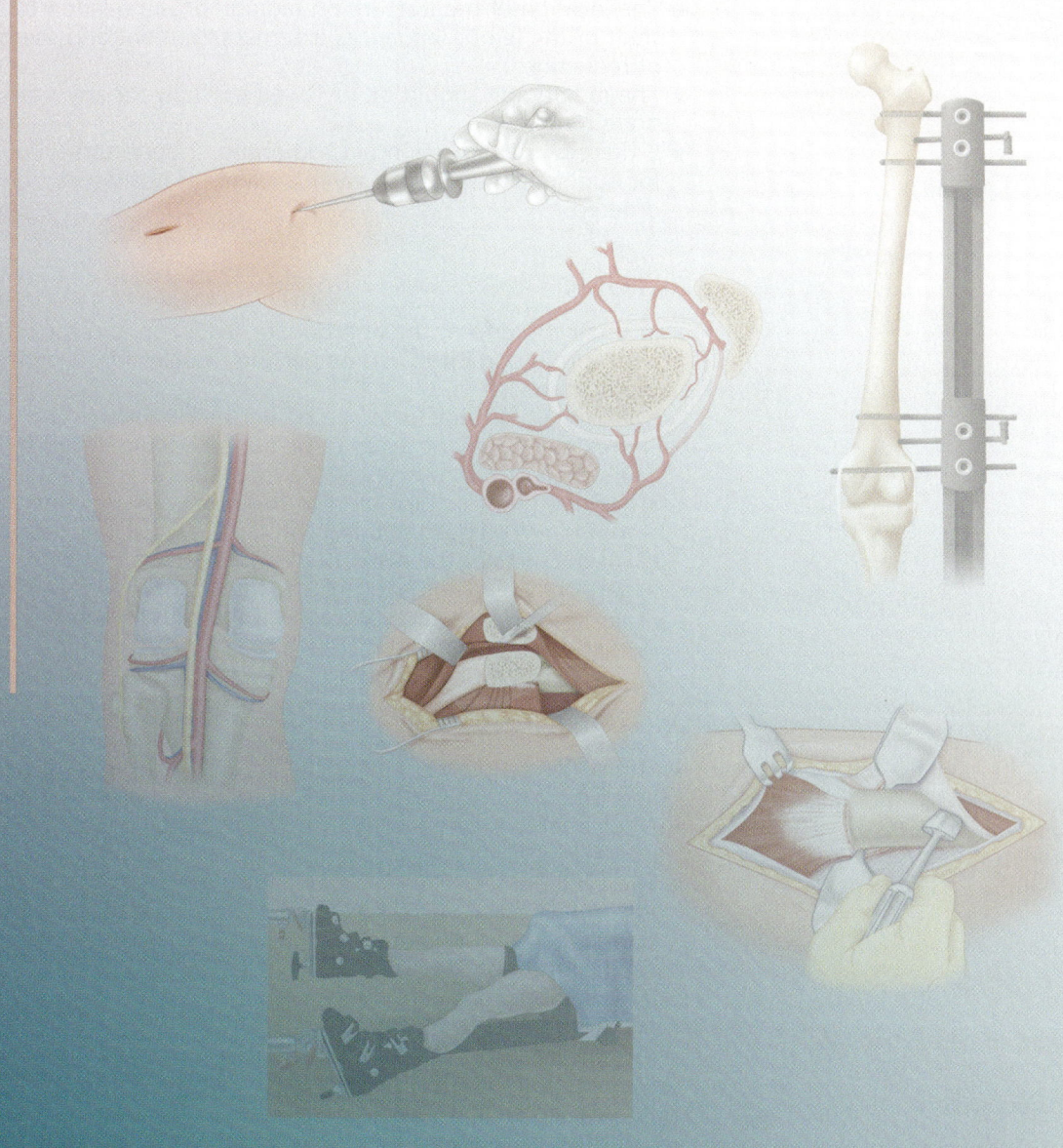

Treatment Options

- Pavlik harness in children less than 6 months
- Flexible nails
- External fixation
- Submuscular plating
- Intramedullary nail

Equipment

- Radiographs demonstrating the fracture
- Pediatric spica table
- Fluoroscopy

INDICATIONS

- Closed fracture of the femoral shaft
- Children less than 6 years old

EXAMINATION/IMAGING

- As with any case of trauma, it is important to evaluate the entire patient.
- The neurovascular status of the extremity should be documented
  - Vascular injuries are not uncommon with femur fractures in children
- The location of the fracture on radiographs in relation to the shaft of the femur influences external treatment and the method of reduction.
- The radiograph should be reviewed carefully for any signs of bone tumor.
- If there is any indication of child abuse, a bone survey looking for additional fractures in various stages of healing can be ordered.

ANATOMY

- In order to perform the appropriate reduction and mold the cast, it is important to remember the muscles forces acting on the fracture.
  - Proximal-third fractures can be hard to maintain. The proximal fragment tends to be abducted and flexed by the insertion of the muscles at the trochanters.
  - Middle-third fractures tend to fall into varus and external rotation. A valgus mold is important to resist this deformity.
  - For fractures of the distal third of the femur, the gastrocnemius tends to pull the fracture into recurvatum. Flexing the knee takes tension off the muscle and helps to maintain the reduction.

POSITIONING

- The patient is placed supine on a radiolucent table (Fig. 1A and 1B).
- A spica table is prepared with padding of the central perineal post (Fig. 2).
- The position of the leg is dependent on the location of the fracture. General guidelines for leg positioning are as follows:
  - Proximal-third fractures
    - Hip flexion: 45°
    - Hip abduction: 30°
    - External rotation: 20°
  - Midshaft fractures
    - Hip flexion: 30°
    - Hip abduction: 20°
    - External rotation: 15°
  - Distal-third fractures
    - Hip flexion: 20°
    - Hip abduction: 20°
    - External rotation: 15°

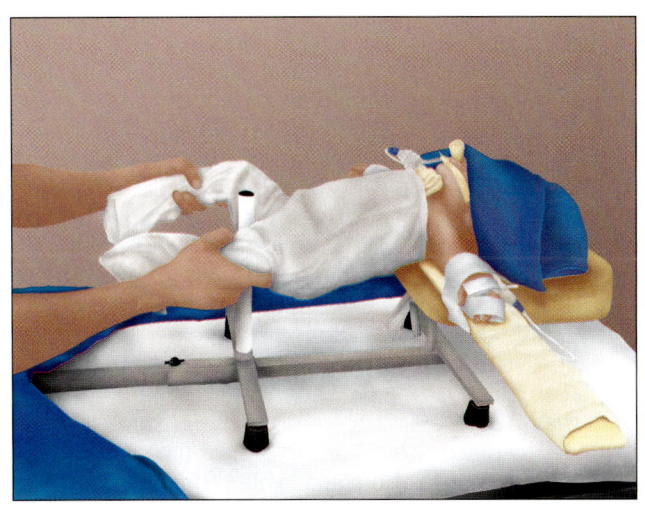
A
FIGURE 1

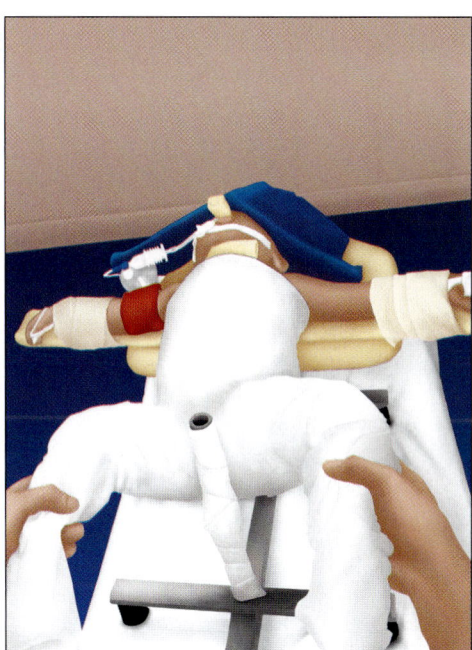
B

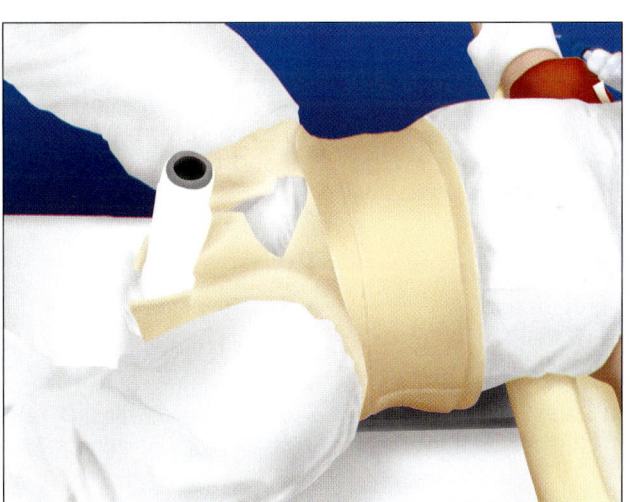
FIGURE 2

PEARLS

- *Two cuts are made in the lower portion of the torso stockinette. The anterior and posterior limbs are loosely tied together. This helps the stockinette stay in the appropriate position, and the limbs can be folded back during the application of the fiberglass cast.*

- *Bony prominences to inspect include the ribs, anterior superior iliac crest, posterior superior iliac crest, femoral condyles, patella, malleoli, Achilles tendon, and calcaneus.*

- *The word spica is derived from the Latin for "grain of wheat." The way the padding is placed resembles a grain of wheat with a V pattern at the perineum. Start on inner aspect of one thigh, wrap around completely one time, then wrap over/under the abdomen, and down onto the other thigh (see Fig. 4).*

PROCEDURE

STEP 1

- The first step is to appropriately prepare the patient for the application of the cast.

- After the induction of anesthesia, the patient is placed on the radiolucent table. Conscious sedation with ketamine is possible. General anesthesia with paralysis may be necessary.

- The patient's skin should be thoroughly examined for any signs of child abuse, such as bruises and burns. If these are noted, they should be documented in the medical record. Pictures of these lesions should be taken if possible.

- Two sizes of stockinette are placed based on the patient's proportions, one for the torso and one for each leg. These should extend to the toes, knee, and nipple line so they can be folded back. Figure 3 demonstrates a folded stockinette placed over the chest and abdomen to create space in order to prevent excessive chest or abdominal compression during spica placement.

- It may be necessary to remove the cushions from the table in order to place the spica table on a firm support. The patient is transferred onto the spica table. The stockinette goes around the back support. The peroneal post is well padded with Webril.

- Additional felt padding is applied to bony prominences.

- A small towel roll is placed at the abdomen extending to the chest.

- Fluoroscopy is now utilized. The optimal position for fracture reduction with patient comfort is determined. Gentle manipulation is used to align the fracture. Assistance is necessary to maintain this position throughout the remainder of the procedure.

- The cast padding is now applied. Either Webril or Gore-Tex is applied from just below the nipple line to the metatarsal heads and the contralateral thigh (Fig. 4).

Controversies

- Some pediatric orthopaedic surgeons recommend applying a short-leg cast, then applying traction with the knee at 90° to maintain the reduction. This can lead to increased pressure in the popliteal fossa and risk of compartment syndrome.

Instrumentation/Implantation

- Stockinette: one size for the torso and another for the leg (see Fig. 3).

- Towel roll to place at chest/abdomen

- Large amount of cast padding (Gore-Tex soft wrap provides easier maintenance of hygiene, but Webril will suffice) (see Fig. 4)

- Foam padding

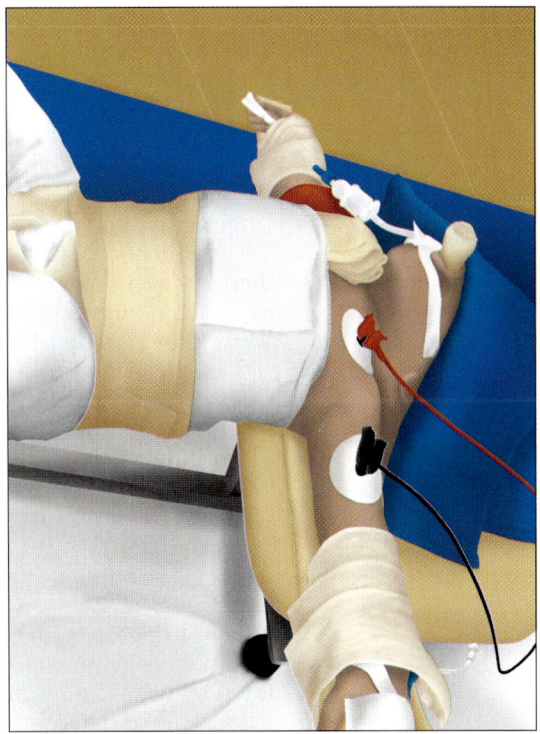

FIGURE 3

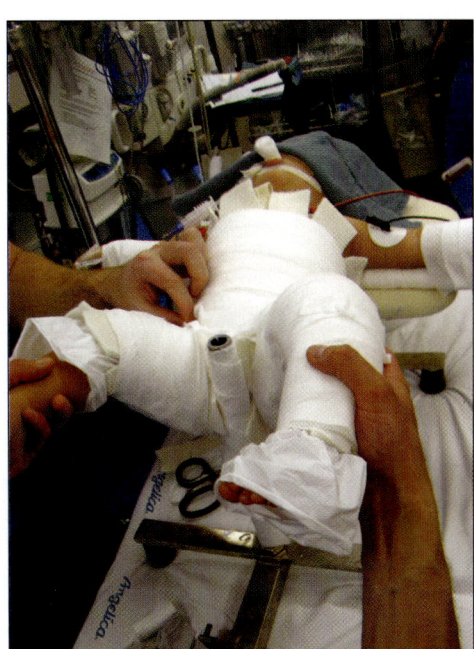

FIGURE 4

Instrumentation/ Implantation

• Multiple widths of fiberglass (reinforcing strips are useful as well)
• Basin with "baby bath" warm water
• Cast saw
• Cast wedges should be available
• Felt (moleskin)

STEP 2

■ The second portion of the procedure involves maintaining the reduction as the fiberglass cast is applied.
  • If two assistants are available, one holds the injured limb and the other holds the contralateral leg. Position of the fractured leg is matched on the other side.
  • Both legs are placed in sufficient abduction to aid in perineal care.
■ After verification of fracture reduction, five to six layers of fiberglass are now applied. The cast should extend from the level of the xiphoid process to the foot and opposite thigh. The stockinette is folded back at the perineum, chest, toes, and thigh (Figs. 5 and 6).
  • Reinforcing fiberglass strips can be utilized at the groin and lateral torso to below the fracture
■ For midshaft femur fracture, overcorrection with a valgus flexion mold is useful to maintain the reduction.
■ Fluoroscopy is used again to check the alignment of the fracture.
■ If necessary, some correction can be made by wedging the cast (see Pearls).
■ Once satisfactory reduction has been determined, the cast saw is used to trim the cast. The anterior aspect should be trimmed down to near the umbilicus to allow for chest and abdominal expansion. An alternative is to cut a hole at the abdomen. Sufficient room for placement of a diaper is necessary in the perineum.
■ The sharp edges of fiberglass are trimmed with a scalpel.
■ Moleskin is then applied to provide soft edges (Fig. 7).

POSTOPERATIVE CARE AND EXPECTED OUTCOMES

■ The patient is followed closely after the application of the spica cast. At 1 week, repeat films are obtained and the skin is inspected for any signs of ulceration.
■ Depending on the age of the patient and the stability of the fracture, weekly or biweekly appointments are made for follow-up.

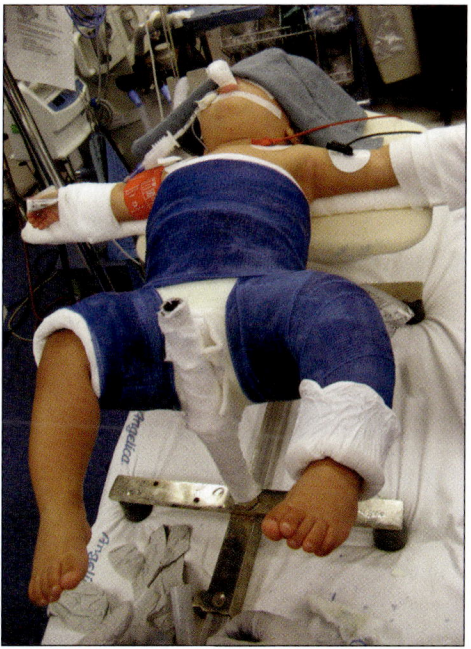

FIGURE 5

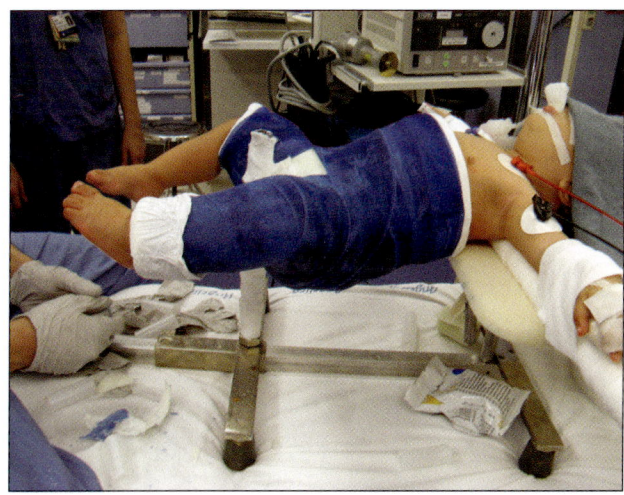

FIGURE 6

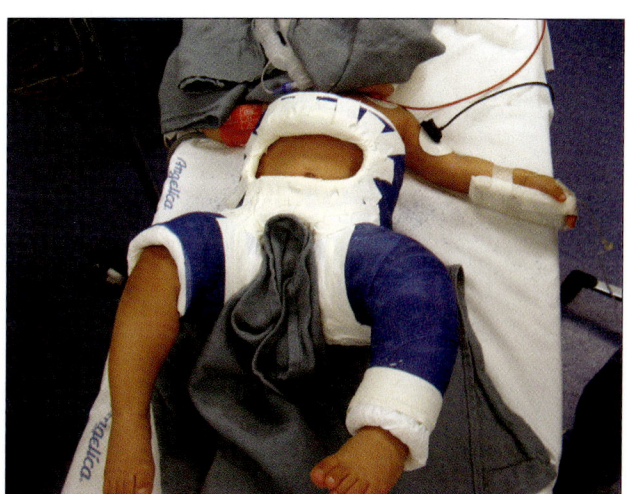

FIGURE 7

EVIDENCE

Ferguson J, Nicol RO. Early spica treatment of pediatric femoral shaft fractures. J Pediatr Orthop. 2000;20:189–92.

This prospective study followed early spica treatment of 101 femur fractures in patients less than 10 years of age. An age older than 7–8 years was the only variable that might be used to predict the need for a change in treatment at 7–10 days.

Illgen R 2nd, Rodgers WB, Hresko MT, Waters PM, Zurakowski D, Kasser JR. Femur fractures in children: treatment with early sitting spica casting. J Pediatr Orthop. 1998;18:481–7.

This paper reviewed the treatment of 114 children with early spica cast for fractures of the femur. The authors found a spica knee flexion angle of less than 50° to be predictive of eventual loss of reduction. Initial shortening of greater than 2 cm was not a contraindication to early spica casting.

Large TM, Frick SL. Compartment syndrome of the leg after treatment of a femoral fracture with an early sitting spica cast: a report of two cases. J Bone Joint Surg [Am]. 2003;85:2207–10.

The author describes two cases in which the treatment of a pediatric femur fracture with a spica cast resulted in the development of a compartment syndrome. In each of the cases, a three step technique was used in the application of the spica cast. The author felt that the use of a short leg cast to assist with traction and reduction of the fracture contributed to the complication. (Level IV evidence)

Mubarak SJ, Frick S, Sink E, Rathjen K, Noonan KJ. Volkmann contracture and compartment syndromes after femur fractures in children treated with 90/90 spica casts. J Pediatr Orthop. 2006;26:567–72.

Nine pediatric patients with low-energy femur fractures were treated with 90/90 spica casts and developed leg compartment syndromes, Volkmann contracture, and ankle skin loss. The authors believed the technique of an initial below-the-knee cast, and then use of that cast for applying traction while immobilizing the child in the 90/90 spica cast, was potentially dangerous. Alternative spica application methods were advocated. (Level IV evidence)

Epiphysiodesis of the Distal Femur/Proximal Tibia-Fibula

Samantha A. Spencer

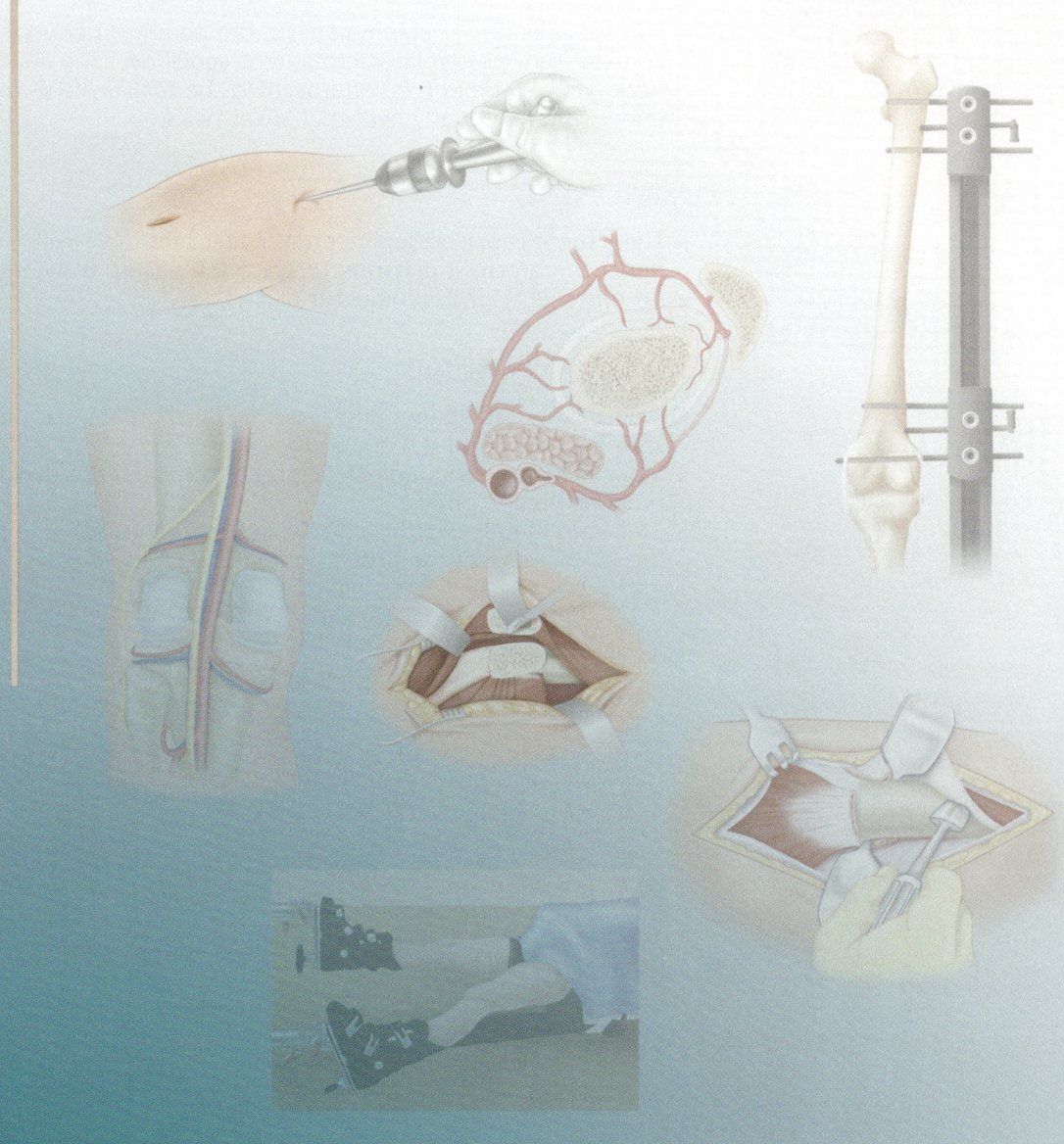

Treatment Options

- Observation with a shoe lift or with later lengthening of the contralateral side or ipsilateral femoral shortening when mature

Equipment

- Radiolucent table (flat Jackson table or fluoroscopy foot extension)
- Intraoperative fluoroscopy

INDICATIONS

- Leg length discrepancy (LLD) projected to be greater than 2.5 cm at the end of growth

EXAMINATION/IMAGING

- An anteroposterior (AP) hips-to-ankles radiograph (Fig. 1) and/or scanograms should be obtained, as well as AP and lateral views of the knee.
- Bone age of the wrist should be determined.

SURGICAL ANATOMY

- For proximal fibular epiphysiodesis, the peroneal nerve is coming from posterolateral to anteromedial over the fibular neck (Fig. 2). Avoid it by approaching the fibular physis under direct vision anteriorly over the fibular head.

POSITIONING

- The patient is placed supine on a radiolucent table with a bump under the greater trochanter to place the patella anteriorly.
- An unsterile thigh tourniquet is placed.

PORTALS/EXPOSURES

- Identify the distal femur and proximal tibial and fibular physes with fluoroscopy and mark on the skin.
- Make a 2.0-cm longitudinal incision directly anterior over the proximal fibular physis.
- Spread longitudinally through the subcutaneous tissue and open the lateral edge of the tibialis anterior fascia.

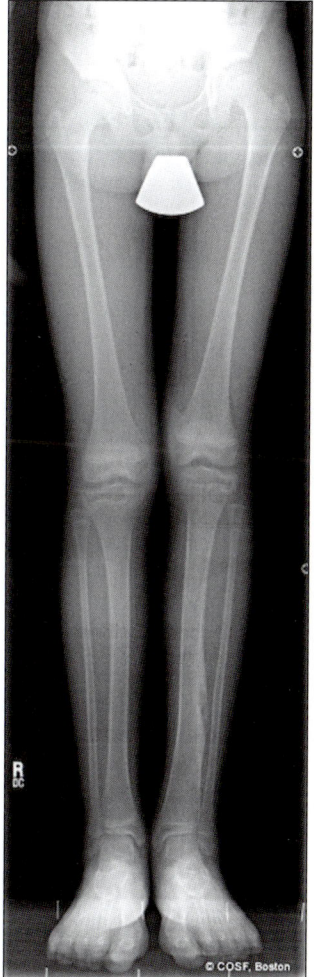

FIGURE 1

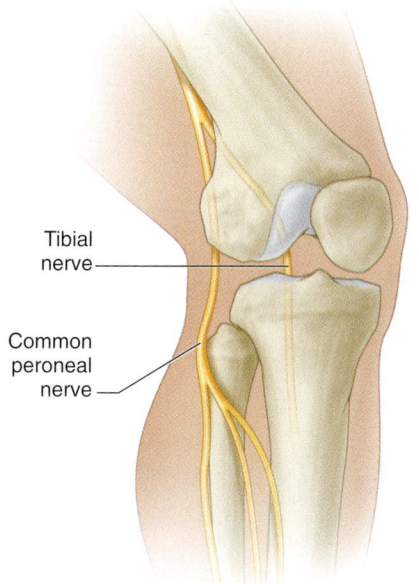

Tibial nerve

Common peroneal nerve

FIGURE 2

Instrumentation/Implantation

- Small angled curettes

Controversies

- If the patient has under 2 years of growth remaining and/or the proximal fibula is inferior to the proximal tibia, a proximal fibular epiphysiodesis is unnecessary.

PROCEDURE

STEP 1

- The muscle is bluntly cleared off the overlying periosteum. Position over the physis is verified with fluoroscopy.
- An H-shaped periosteal incision is made with a knife anteriorly and medial and lateral periosteal flaps are elevated (Fig. 3).
- The proximal fibular physis is visualized directly (Fig. 4A) and curetted out under direct vision (Fig. 4B).

STEP 2

- Tissues are bluntly spread anterior to the proximal tibial lateral physis.
- This position is localized with fluoroscopy and a 3.5- to 4.5-mm drill bit is drilled into the physis (Fig. 5).

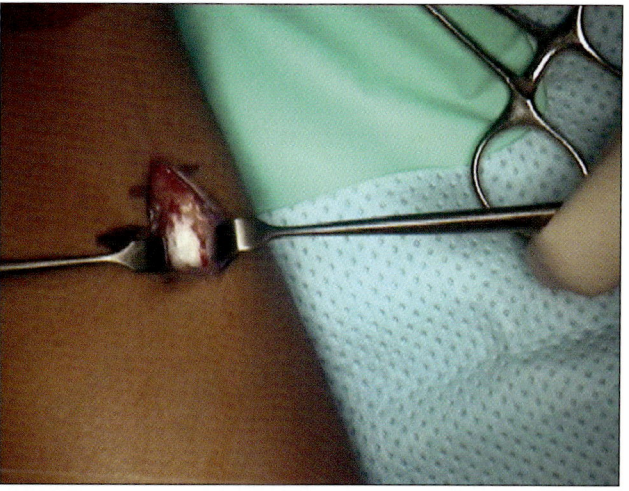

FIGURE 3

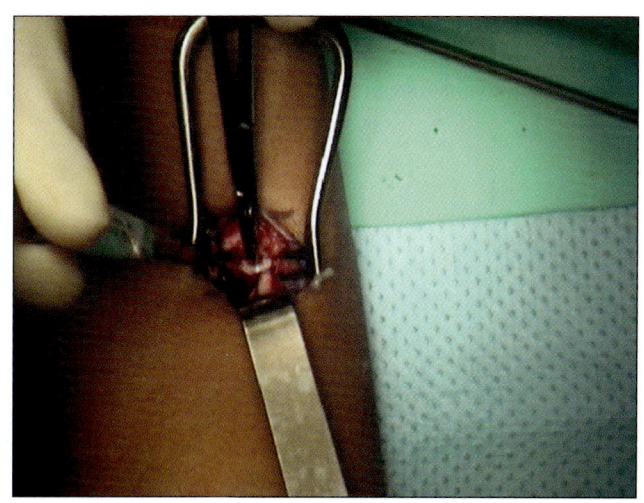

A
FIGURE 4

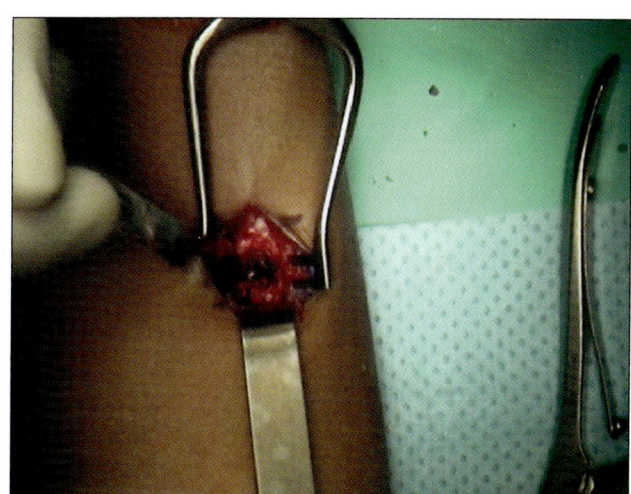

B

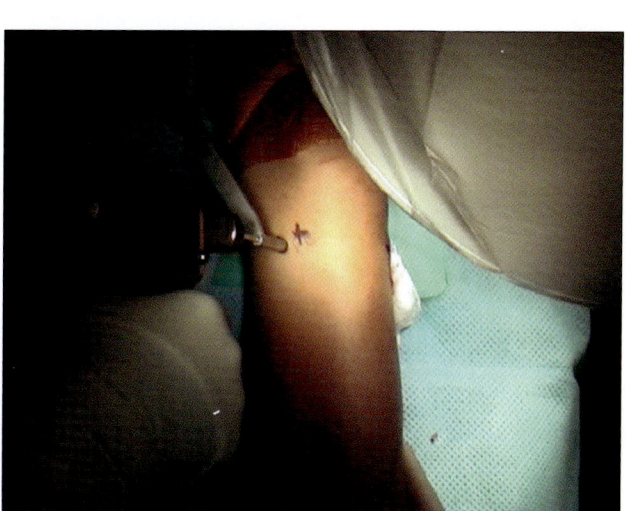

FIGURE 5

Instrumentation/ Implantation

- Solid drill bits sized 3.5–4.5 mm, depending on the size of the patient

- Small straight and angled curettes

- The drill is withdrawn to the edge of the cortex and fanned in 5° increments anteriorly and posteriorly (Fig. 6A), taking care not to violate the far cortex and checking fluoroscopic images as needed (Fig. 6B).
- When a free path exists from drilling, the drill is withdrawn and angled curettes are inserted, scraping any remaining physis (Fig. 7).
- This procedure is repeated on the medial side: the medial proximal tibial physis site is localized with a radiopaque instrument, a stab incisionis made, tissues are spread to bone, and drilling and curetting are done as above.
- The surgeon must check in the AP plane that the curette can cross the physis superiorly into the epiphysis (Fig. 8A) and inferiorly into the metaphysis (Fig. 8B), and in the lateral plane that it reaches anteriorly and posteriorly.

STEP 3

- The medial and lateral distal femoral physes are identified as in Step 2
- Percutaneous stab incisions are made, tissues are spread to bone, and a drill bit with guide is placed at the edge of each physis.
- The position is verified with fluoroscopy, then drilling is done as above, fanning in 5° increments anteriorly and posteriorly.
- Curetting is done as above in Step 2.

POSTOPERATIVE CARE AND EXPECTED OUTCOMES

- A knee immobilizer is placed for 2 weeks, and partial weight bearing with crutches is recommended for a month postoperatively to protect against fracture.
- Anteroposterior and lateral radiographs of the knee should show evidence of physeal closure by 3 months postoperatively.
- Correction expected is the amount of growth remaining on the contralateral side.
  - In general, the distal femur grows $\frac{3}{8}$ inch (1.0 cm) per year and the proximal tibia $\frac{1}{4}$ inch (0.6 cm) per year; thus $\frac{5}{8}$ inch (1.6 cm) of correction can be expected for each year of growth remaining if both these physes successfully close.
  - In general, there is 1 inch (2.5 cm) of growth remaining in the proximal tibial physis at age $10\frac{1}{2}$ in a girl and age $11\frac{1}{2}$ in a boy. There is 1 inch (2.5 cm) of growth remaining in the distal femoral physis at age $12\frac{1}{2}$ in a girl and age $13\frac{1}{2}$ in a boy.

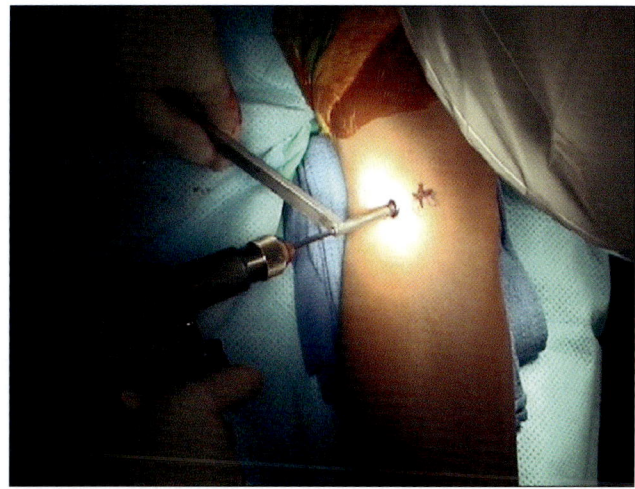

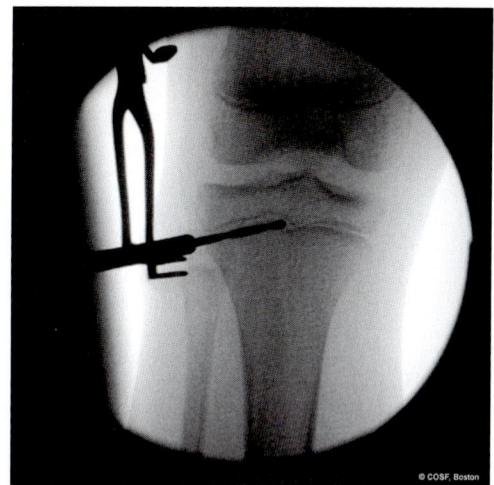

A

B

FIGURE 6

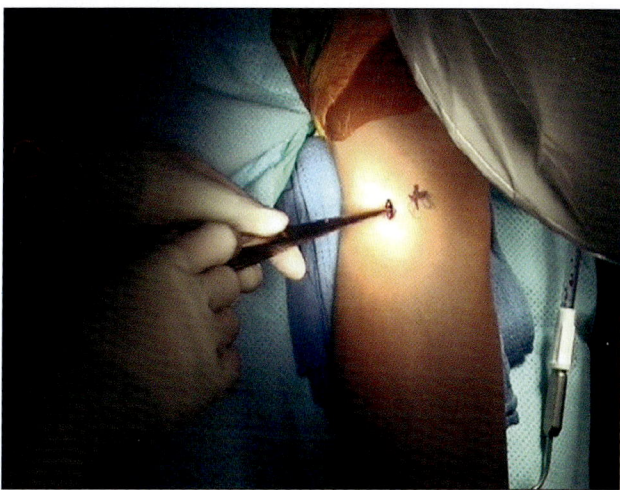

FIGURE 7

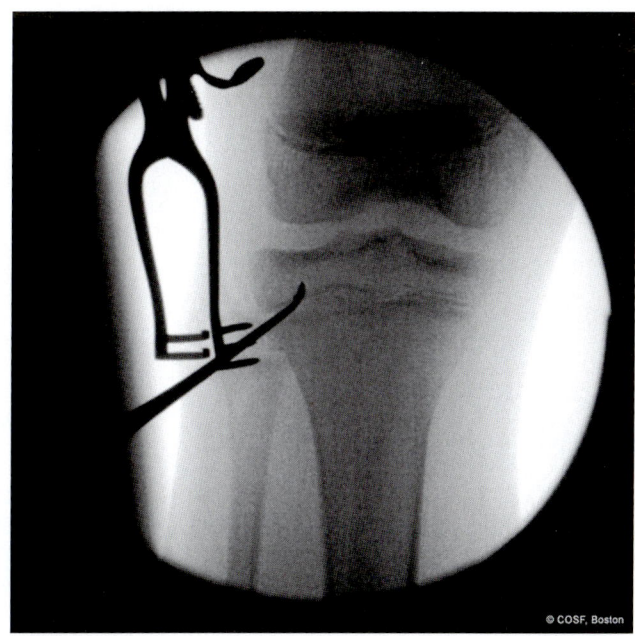

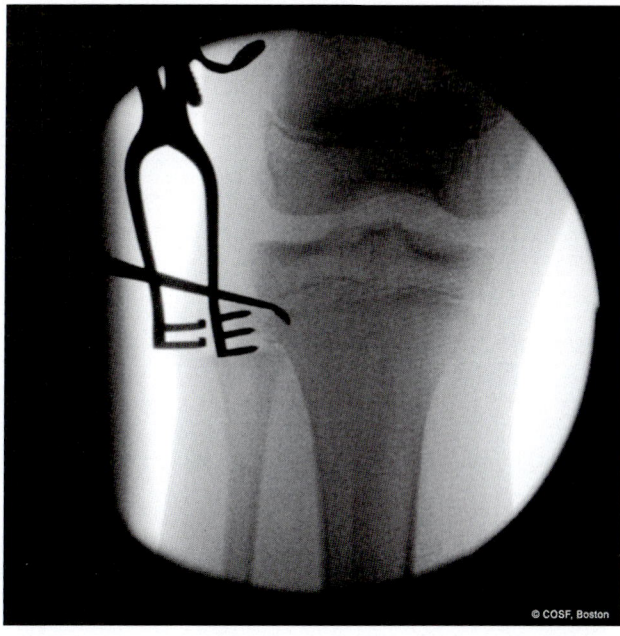

A

B

FIGURE 8

EVIDENCE

Aguilar JA, Paley D, Paley J, Santpure S, Patel M, Herzenberg JE, Bhave A. Clinical validation of the multiplier method for predicting limb length discrepancy and outcome of epiphysiodesis, part II. J Pediatr Orthop. 2005;25:192–6.

The authors validate the multiplier method for residual limb length discrepancy after epiphysiodesis by applying it retrospectively to a previously published series of patients. It performed statistically significantly better than the Moseley method. (Grade A recommendation; Level IV evidence)

Inan M, Chan G, Littleton AG, Kubiak P, Bowen JR. Efficacy and safety of percutaneous epiphysiodesis. J Pediatr Orthop. 2008;6:648–51.

In this retrospective review, 97 patients were followed to skeletal maturity after percutaneous epiphysiodesis. Three had failure of the epiphysiodesis; 88 had correction of the leg length discrepancy to an average of 1.3 cm. The procedure was found to be safe and efficacious. (Grade A recommendation; Level IV evidence)

Paley D, Bhave A, Herzenberg JE, Bowen JR. Multiplier method for predicting limb-length discrepancy. J Bone Joint Surg [Am]. 2000;82:1432–46.

The authors published a description of the multiplier method for calculating limb length difference.

Sofield Osteotomy with Intramedullary Rod Fixation of the Long Bones of the Femur/Tibia

Samantha A. Spencer

PITFALLS

- *Be certain the bone is large enough for the rod chosen.*

- *Counsel the patient and family regarding the risks of this surgery: complication rates are 55% in OI, regardless of rod type; 51% rate of re-rodding for simple rods and 27% rate of re-rodding for telescoping rods.*

- *For severe OI patients, be sure the cervical spine has been imaged appropriately and that an experienced anesthesia team is available; fiberoptic intubation is often needed.*

Controversies

- Sofield osteotomy and rodding for deformity alone may not improve function.

Treatment Options

- Bracing for deformity
- Cast immobilization for fracture
- Observation

INDICATIONS

- Severe long-bone deformity such as in osteogenesis imperfecta (OI) or rickets
- Long-bone fracture with deformity
- Recurrent fracture

EXAMINATION/IMAGING

- Anteroposterior (AP) and lateral radiographs of the entire bone are obtained (Fig. 1).

SURGICAL ANATOMY

- In the relevant long bone, neurovascular injury may be avoided by making the incision over the apex of the deformity, spreading longitudinally through muscle, and then doing careful subperiosteal dissection around the bone at the osteotomy site.

POSITIONING

- The patient is placed supine on a radiolucent table.
- Intraoperative fluoroscopy is utilized.
- The entire gluteal area must be draped free to access the greater trochanter for rodding; the entire lower extremity is prepped out.
- For surgery on one lower extremity, a trochanter roll is appropriate (Fig. 2), with the ipsilateral arm across the chest.
- For surgery on bilateral lower extremities, access to both gluteal areas is ensured using a stack of blankets to elevate the patient if needed (Fig. 3).

PEARLS

- *A stack of blankets for a small patient allows good access to the legs and works for bilateral procedures. This will allow access to the greater trochanters and will allow enough knee flexion for concomitant tibial rodding if needed.*

PITFALLS

- *To place an intramedullary device down the femur, the patient needs to be at the side of the table or elevated enough to allow room to access the entry point to the femoral canal.*

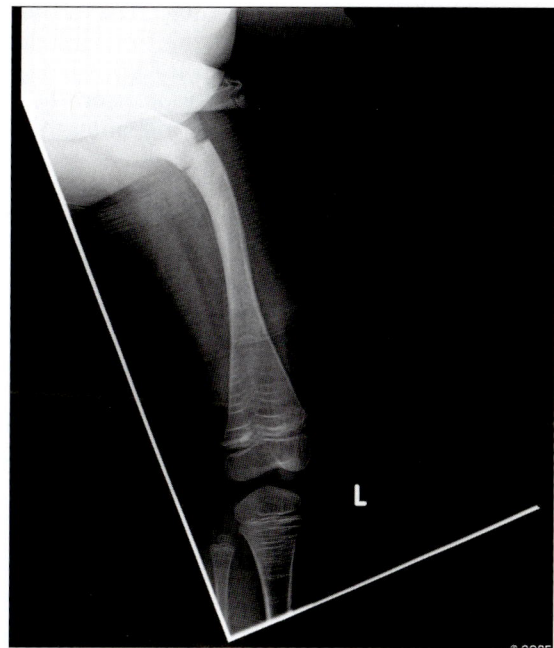

FIGURE 1

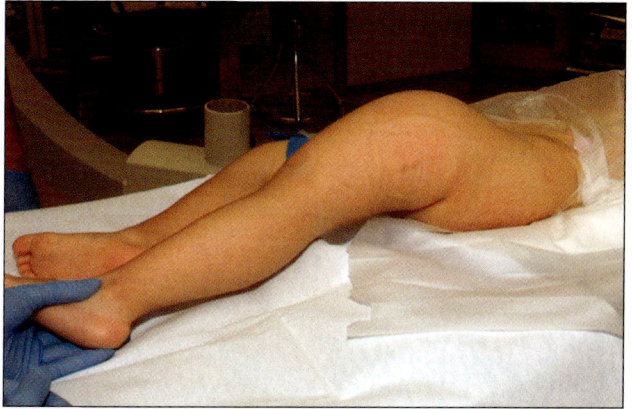

FIGURE 2

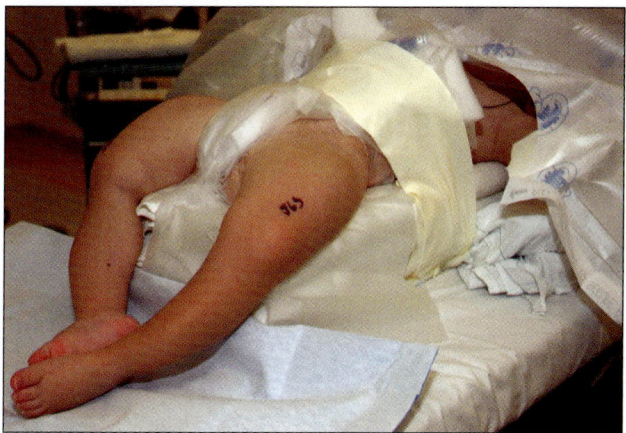

FIGURE 3

PORTALS/EXPOSURES

STEP 1 (APPROACH A)

- The entry point to the greater trochanter is identified. Figure 4 shows the trochanteric entry point for a femoral rodding with a Schnidt forceps marking the first osteotomy.
- The incision needs to be posterior and inferior to the tip of the greater trochanter. A 2-cm incision is sufficient.
- Dissection is performed bluntly and longitudinally, spreading through the gluteus maximus until the tip of the greater trochanter can be accessed.

PROCEDURE

STEP 1 (APPROACH B)

- The fracture site is accessed first, and a guidewire is passed retrograde through the greater trochanter (Fig. 5). The guidewire is drilled into the greater trochanter and down the canal, and AP and lateral radiographs are checked for position.
- Drilling stops when the wire is at a cortex; this will be the apex of the deformity and the appropriate position for the first osteotomy.
- If using a simple rod (Rush rod or large Kirschner wire), the guidewire may now be overdrilled with a cannulated drill, and the larger implant placed. For a Rush rod, this will require precutting the rod based on x-ray measurements at this stage.
- For the tibia, the starting point is as for an adult nail: extra-articular medial to the patellar tendon and anterior.

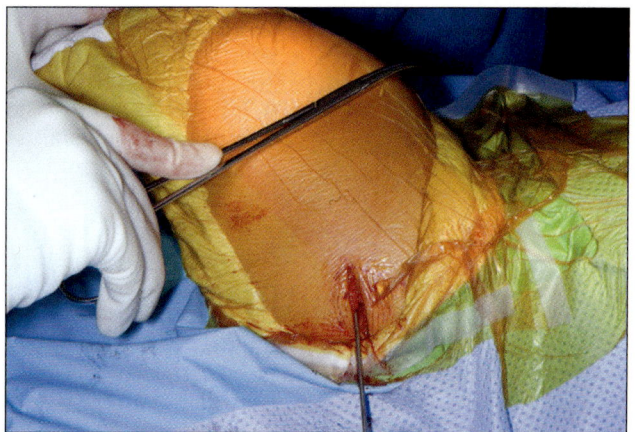

FIGURE 4

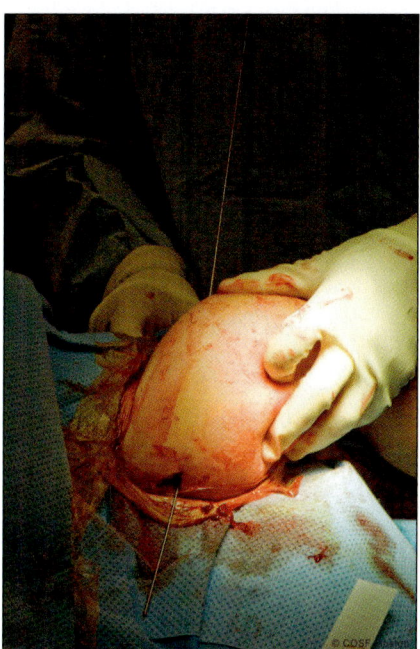

FIGURE 5

STEP 2

- Using fluoroscopy, the point where the wire stops is marked and the wire left in place with the wire driver removed (Fig. 6).
- A 1.5- to 2.0-cm incision is made over the apex of the deformity (usually anterolateral for the femur and tibia) (Fig. 7). Dissection is performed bluntly through muscle, spreading longitudinally.
- The periosteum is opened longitudinally and careful dissection is done subperiosteally (see Fig. 7).
- Retractors are placed.
- Using a drill a small (0.5-cm) anterior wedge of bone , is marked out to be removed.
- The osteotomy is gently completed with osteotomes (Fig. 8), preserving the posterior periosteum and using gentle osteocleisis to complete the posterior cortex.
- The small wedge of bone is removed with a rongeur and saved (Fig. 9).

PEARLS

- *Baby Bennett retractors are ideal for subperiosteal retraction.*
- *For soft bone, a drill and osteotomes are safer than a saw.*

PITFALLS

- *Do not take a big wedge of bone to start; this will destabilize the osteotomy.*
- *Be sure you are subperiosteal before starting the osteotomy; the periosteum protects adjacent structures, and it is easy to place a sharp pointed retractor through soft bone rather than around it.*

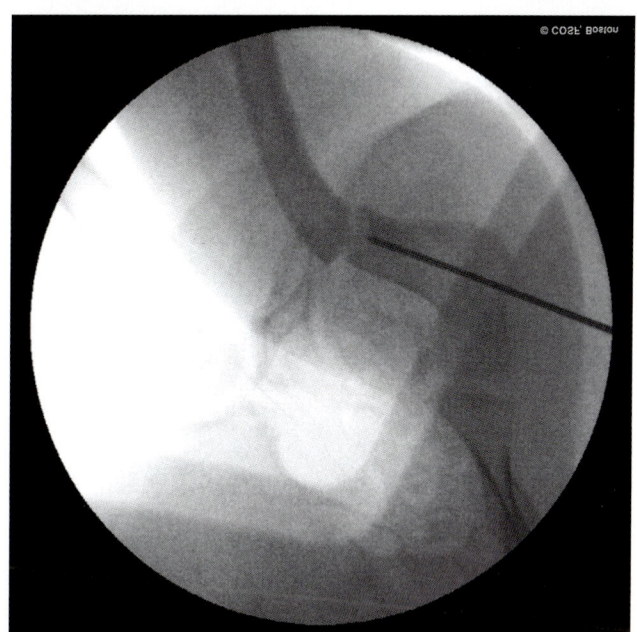

FIGURE 6

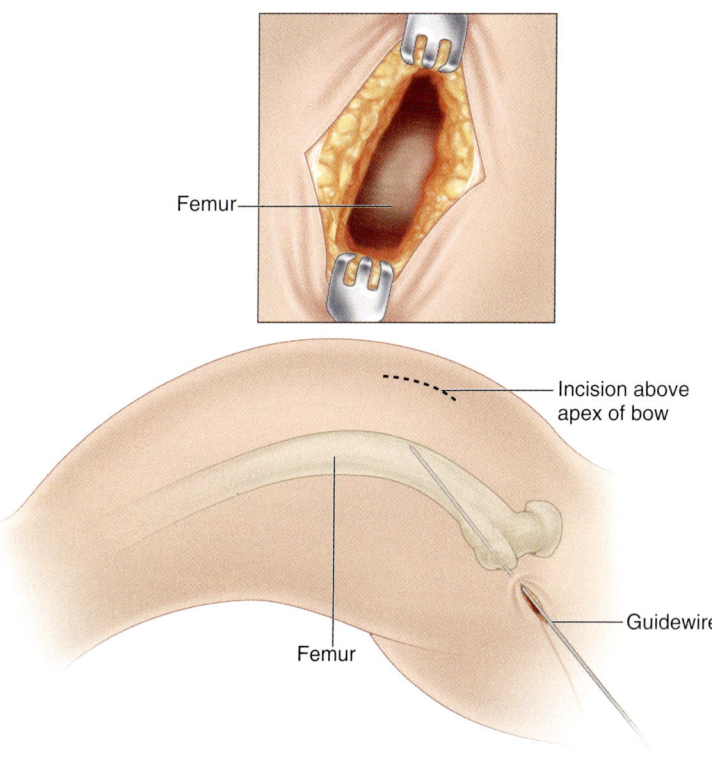

Femur

Incision above
apex of bow

Femur

Guidewire

FIGURE 7

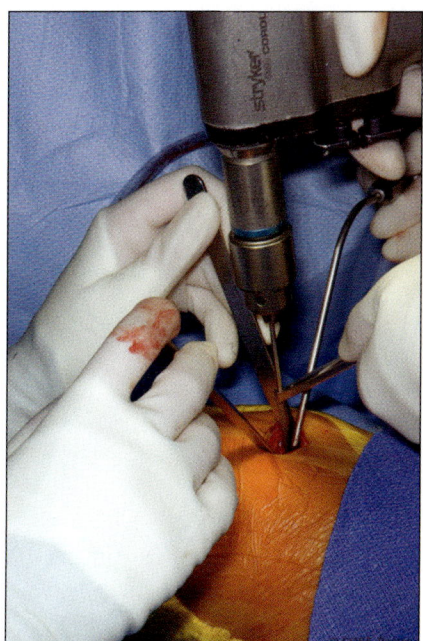

FIGURE 8

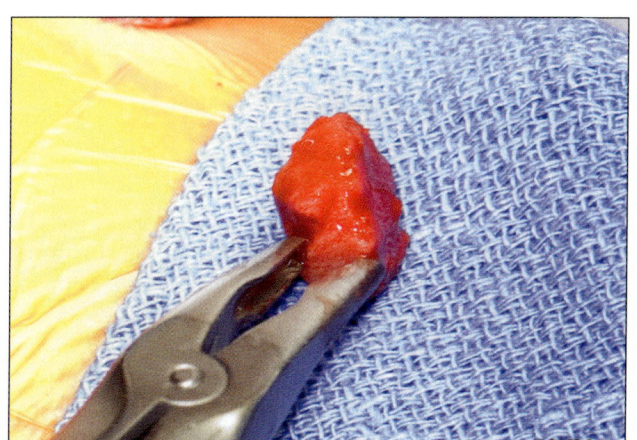

FIGURE 9

PEARLS

- *It is better to perform an extra osteotomy than to have a malpositioned rod that will cut out.*

- *For telescoping rods, the guidewire must be as central as possible in the physis; if it is eccentric, it is better to perform another osteotomy.*

- *To aid guiding the wire, the cannulated drill/reamer can be advanced over the wire to help guide it distally.*

PEARLS

- *With deformity, it is very difficult to template rod length off radiographs; thus the above wire measurement method may be easier. It is better to cut the final rod too long and have to shorten it than to have it be too short and leave part of the bone unprotected.*

- *To cut a telescoping rod, a diamond-wheel burr is essential or the female rod will deform and will not fit over the male rod.*

- *Be sure the cut end of the female rod is smooth and will telescope by checking that the male nail still fits through it easily.*

STEP 3

- The guidewire is advanced across the osteotomy down the canal. If it hits another cortex before arriving distally (Fig. 10), a second osteotomy is performed as in Step 2.
- The wire can be put into the distal canal under direct vision if needed, using blunt fracture reduction clamps; if the canal is obscured, the surgeon should consider drilling it with a Kirschner wire or small drill.

STEP 4

- The canal is over-reamed to the desired amount. This can be done easily by hand using a cannulated drill and T-handled chuck for soft fragile bone (Fig. 11).
- The rod length is measured off the guidewire by placing a similar wire to the tip of the trochanter and subtracting the difference.
- The simple rod or the female part of the telescoping rod is cut to this length with a burr (Fig. 12).

STEP 5

- While the assistant holds the leg with the osteotomies reduced, the guidewire is carefully withdrawn.
- Either the simple rod or the male part of the telescoping rod is placed down the long bone. Gentle traction or manual manipulation is used to realign the osteotomies during this step.
- For a telescoping (e.g., Fassier-Duval) rod, the surgeon must be certain the rod is central at the physis in the AP and lateral planes, then carefully twist it across until the threads are buried in the epiphysis.

PEARLS

- *For simple rod placement, a larger cannulated drill might be placed over the smaller guidewire across the osteotomy/osteotomies; then the guidewire may be withdrawn and the simple rod placed.*

PITFALLS

- *For the telescoping Fassier-Duval rods, there is no cannulated rod so it is easy to lose the reduction after withdrawing the guidewire and pass the male nail falsely. Avoid this by rechecking AP/lateral radiographs as each osteotomy is crossed.*

- *Multiple passes across the physis will risk growth disturbance and destabilize the purchase of the male nail in the physis; be sure the male nail tip is in the central desired position before passing it.*

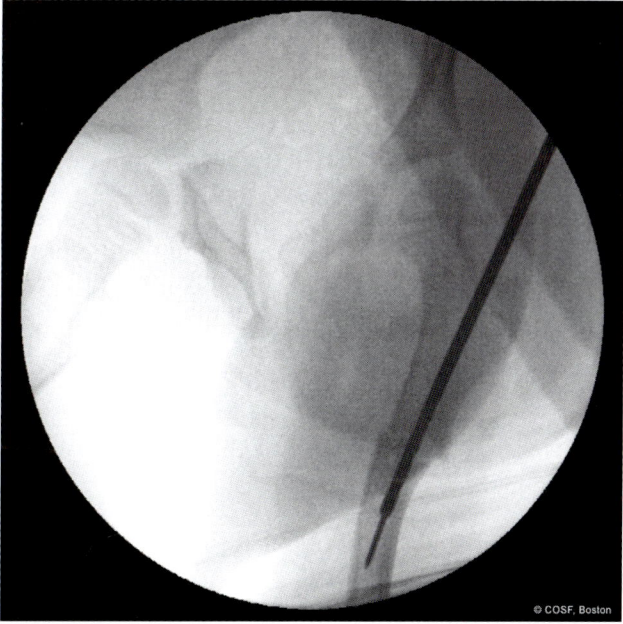

FIGURE 10

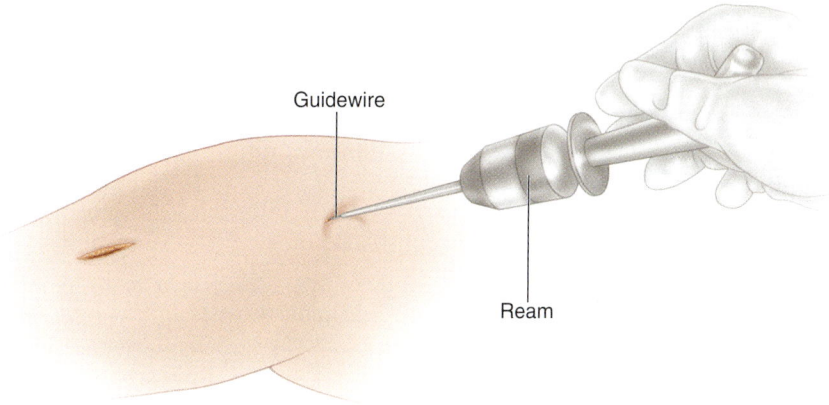

Guidewire

Ream

FIGURE 11

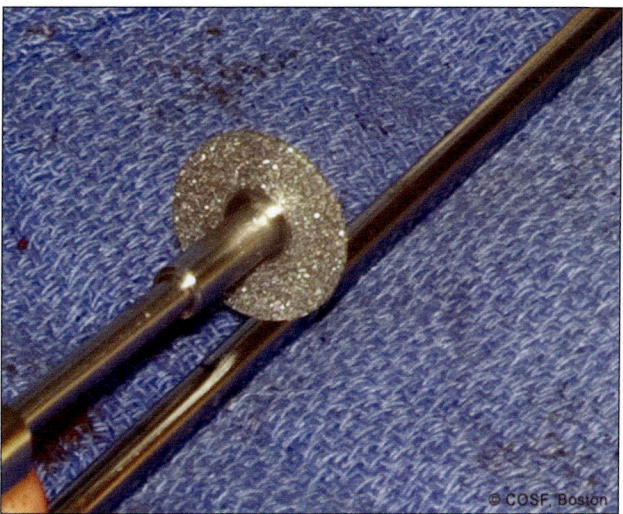

FIGURE 12

PEARLS

- *If it is necessary to withdraw the female rod and recut it, be sure to use counterpressure against the male nail to prevent backout.*

- *It is desirable to leave up to 2–3 cm of male nail protruding at the proximal femur; less than 1 cm should be left at the proximal tibia to allow maximal telescoping.*

- *Check that the cut male nail does not block hip abduction or knee extension clinically.*

- *Be sure the tip of the male nail is smooth enough to telescope after cutting. For the Fassier-Duval system, the rod cutter in the kit is quite large and difficult to use with small patients. The author has found careful use of gold-tipped wire cutters to be adequate.*

STEP 6

- The precut female rod is placed over the male nail and carefully twisted down with the driver.
- Radiographs are checked as the female rod advances, particularly across the osteotomies to be sure it is not driving the male nail intra-articularly. If this is happening, the mail nail is untwisted with a heavy needle driver.
- The nail should screw into either the greater trochanteric apophysis or the proximal tibial physis with several threads, but the threads should not cross the physis.
- The male nail is cut and checked to ensure that it is not bent.
- The saved bone graft is applied as desired, and the wounds are closed (Fig. 13).

POSTOPERATIVE CARE AND EXPECTED OUTCOMES

- Light posterior splints are applied for older, cooperative patients. For younger patients, long-leg A-frame casts versus spicas (if the osteotomies are unstable) are better.
- At 3 weeks postoperative, gentle motion with a brace or a bivalved and lined cast may begin after verifying rod position by radiography.
  - The 4-month postoperative radiographs in Figure 14 show a telescoping rod in the femur in lateral (Fig. 14A) and AP (Fig. 14B) views.
- Rod backout, refracture, and need for surgical revision are common: approximately 50% in simple roddings and 30% in telescoping rod systems.

PEARLS

- *While brief light immobilization is desirable for OI patients, for toddler patients casts are easier for the parents and patients than splints.*

PITFALLS

- *Be sure to obtain flat-plate AP and lateral radiographs before leaving the operating room and deal with any malpositioned rods at that time. Particularly in combined femoral/tibial rodding, the first rod placed may dislodge after the subsequent rod is placed.*

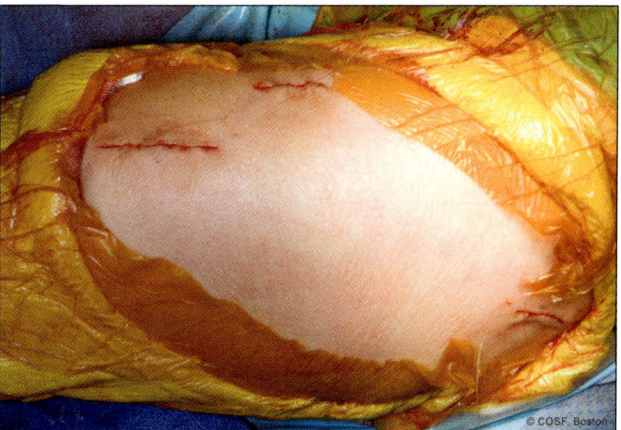

FIGURE 13

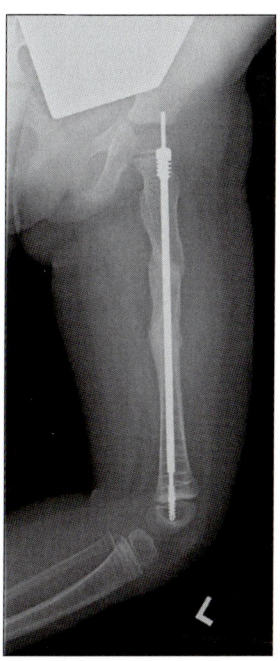

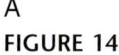

A

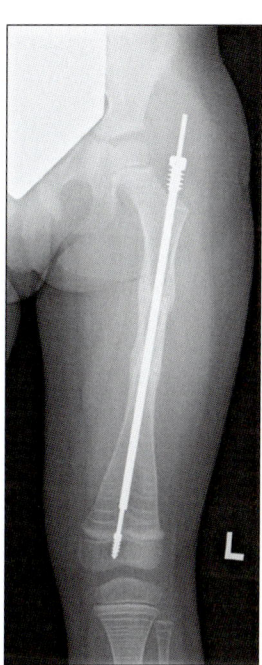

B

FIGURE 14

EVIDENCE

Bailey RW, Dubow HI. Evolution of the concept of an extensible nail accommodating to normal longitudinal bone growth: clinical considerations and implications. Clin Orthop Relat Res. 1981;00(159):157–70.

This paper detailed the evolution to a telescoping rod system. (Note that this rod system is no longer available and required distal osteotomy for insertion of the male nail.) (Level IV evidence)

Sofield HA, Millar EA. Fragmentation, realignment and intramedullary rod fixation of deformities of the long bones in children: a ten year appraisal. J Bone Joint Surg [Am]. 1959;41:1371–91.

This is the classic article describing this technique. (Level IV evidence)

Wilkinson JM, Scott BW, Clarke AM, Bell MJ. Surgical stabilization of the lower limb in osteogenesis imperfecta using the Sheffield Telescopic Intramedullary Rod System. J Bone Joint Surg [Br]. 1998;80:999–1004.

The authors reviewed the Sheffield type of rodding. (Level IV evidence)

Zeitlin L, Fassier F, Glorieux FH. Modern approach to children with osteogenesis imperfecta. J Pediatr Orthop. 2003;12:77–87.

This comprehensive review article documented the overall complication rates of various types of rodding for OI as well as reviewing types and current classification. (Level IV evidence)

KNEE

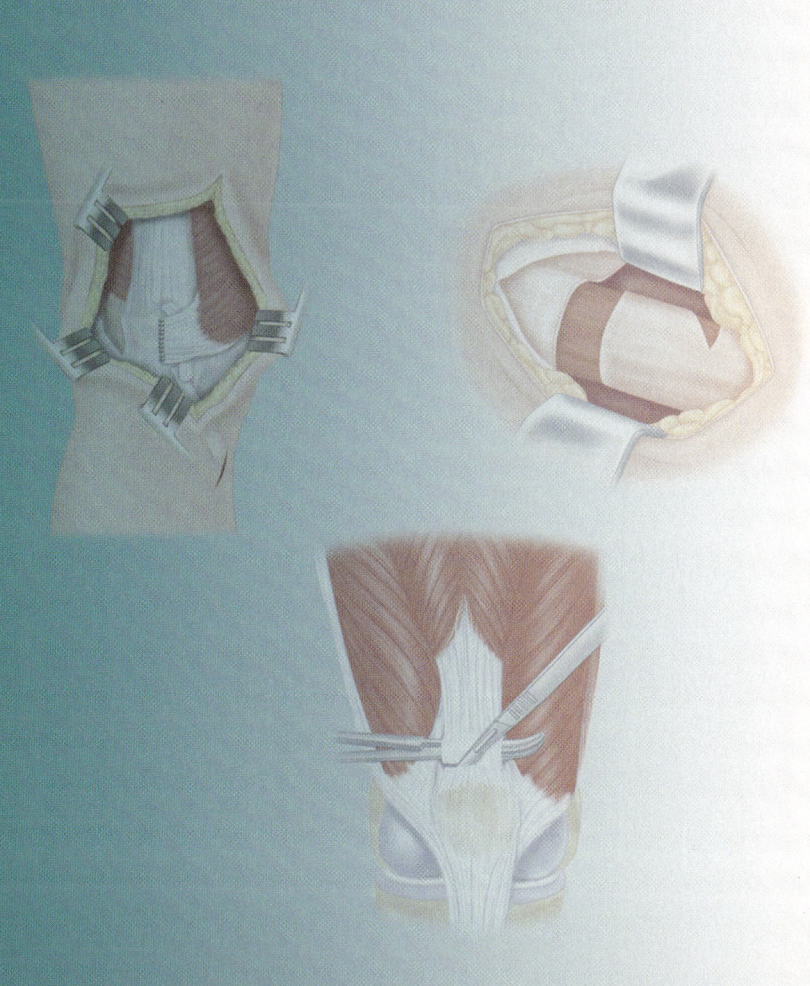

Discoid Lateral Meniscus

Hua Ming Siow and Theodore J. Ganley

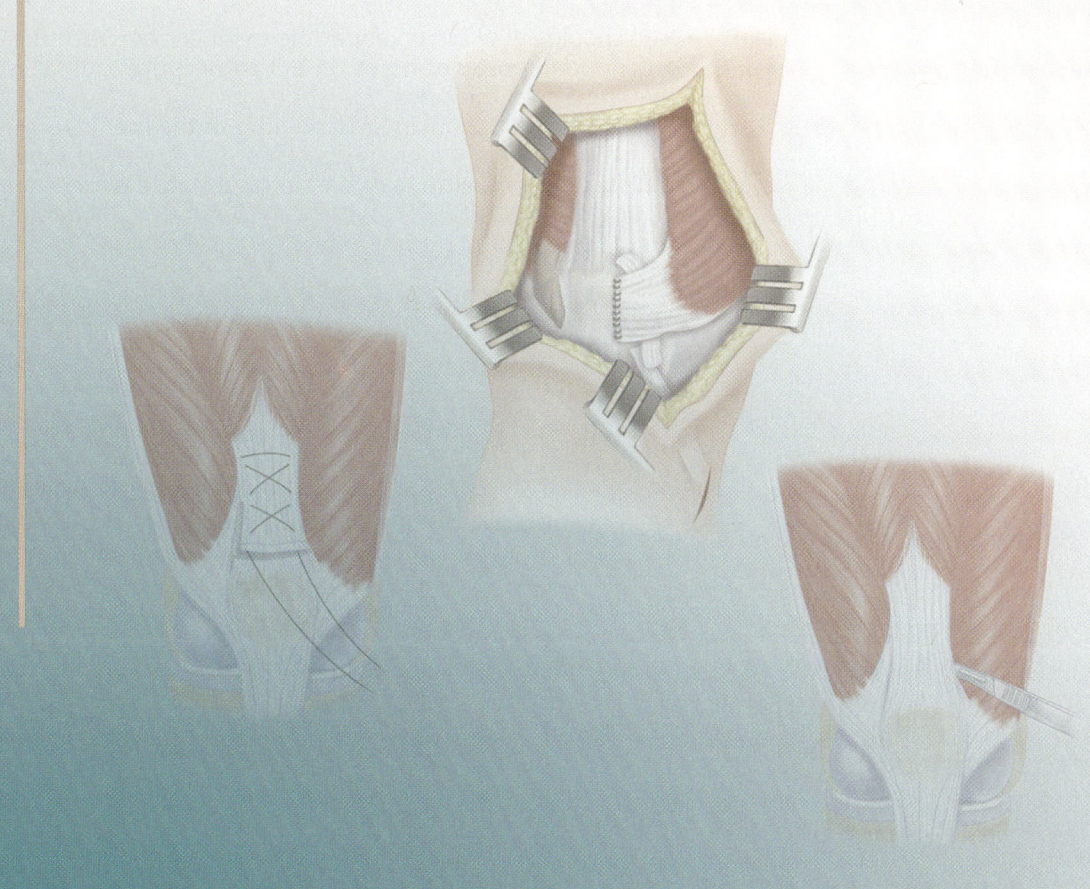

INDICATIONS

- The presence of a discoid lateral meniscus on magnetic resonance imaging (MRI) associated with symptoms or a tear.
- Symptoms include pain, swelling, locking, instability, and extension block.

EXAMINATION/IMAGING

- Examination may show joint line tenderness, effusion, decreased range of motion, quadriceps atrophy, bulge at the anterolateral joint line in full flexion, click and shift of the meniscus on extension, and a positive McMurray's sign.
- Radiographs may show widening of the lateral joint space, cupping of the lateral tibial plateau, flattening of the lateral femoral condyle, tibial spine hypoplasia, and elevation of the fibular head.
- MRI should show continuity of the meniscus between the anterior and posterior horns on ≥ 3 consecutive sagittal sections that are 5 mm thick (Fig. 1).
- MRI should also show increased width of the meniscus at the midpoint of the anterior and posterior horns on a coronal view.
- MRI will help visualize tears and intrasubstance degeneration.

SURGICAL ANATOMY

- Watanabe classification
  - Type I: complete (Fig. 2A)
  - Type II: incomplete (Fig. 2B)
  - Type III: Wrisberg variant (Fig. 2C)

POSITIONING

- The patient is placed in the supine position.
- The hip is flexed and abducted, with external rotation when applying varus stress in the figure-of-4 position.
- A bolster is placed behind the knee to allow for 70–90° of flexion at rest.
- A tourniquet is applied and inflated after Esmarch bandaging.

PORTALS/EXPOSURES

- Standard anterior medial and lateral portals are used (Fig. 3).
- Midpatellar medial and lateral portals are added as required (see Fig. 3).
- A posterolateral incision is made as necessary for inside-out meniscal repairs.
- An anterolateral incision is made as necessary for outside-in meniscal repairs.

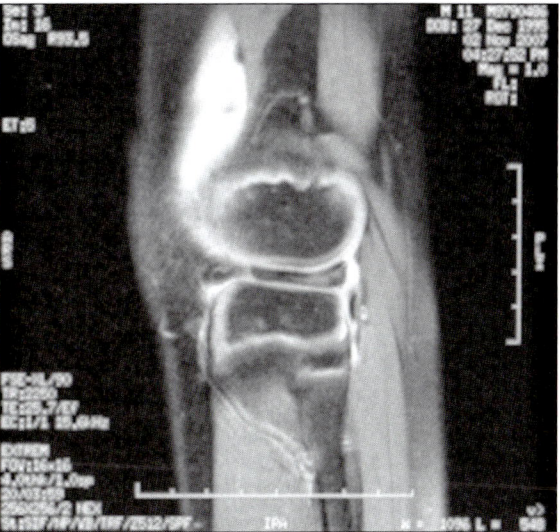

FIGURE 1

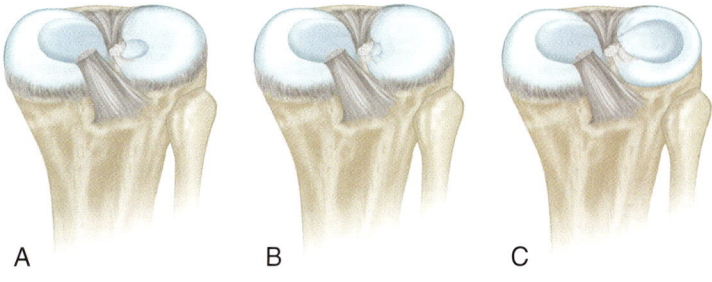

A   B   C

FIGURE 2

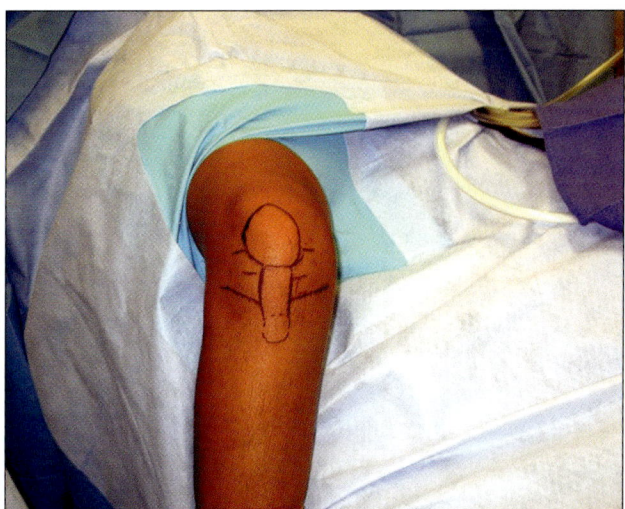

FIGURE 3

Instrumentation/ Implantation

- Standard 30° oblique 4-mm arthroscope
- Probe

Instrumentation/ Implantation

- Punches—straight, angled 45° or 90°, and reverse
- Curved scissors
- Motorized meniscal shaver
- Graspers
- Probe

Controversies

- Total meniscectomy may be preferred if extensive irreparable tears compromise the peripheral rim.

PROCEDURE

STEP 1: ARTHROSCOPIC ASSESSMENT

- The surgeon must visualize the discoid meniscus and determine its extent. Figure 4 shows an incomplete discoid meniscus.
- An assessment is made for tears and instability of the discoid meniscus.
- The surgeon should assess for chondral damage, osteochondritis dissecans lesions, and loose bodies.

STEP 2: PARTIAL MENISCECTOMY

- Scissors, punches, and a shaver are used to resect the central portion of the meniscus (Fig. 5), leaving ≥ 8 mm of peripheral rim.
- Resection is started from the medial free edge, progressing sequentially to the peripheral rim. A probe is used to determine the extent of resection.
  - Figure 6A shows resection of a discoid meniscus anterior horn.
  - Figure 6B shows the completed resection.
- Contouring of the rim is done with punches angled at 45° to the horizontal and a shaver. Contouring will help to distribute contact pressure of the remnant meniscal rim, resulting in decreased incidence of further chondral injury, osteochondritis dissecans, and meniscal tears.

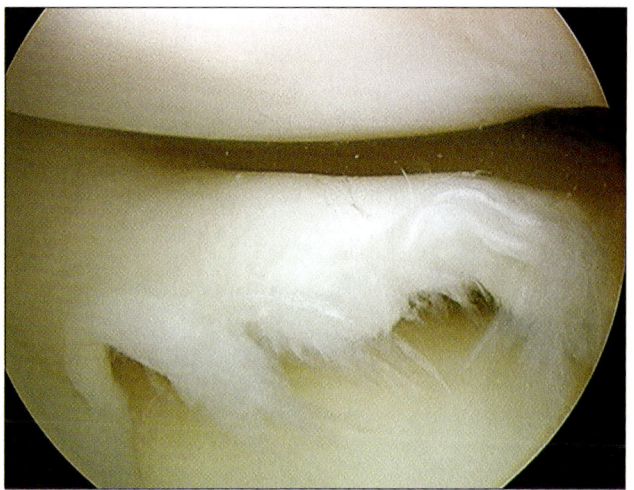

FIGURE 4

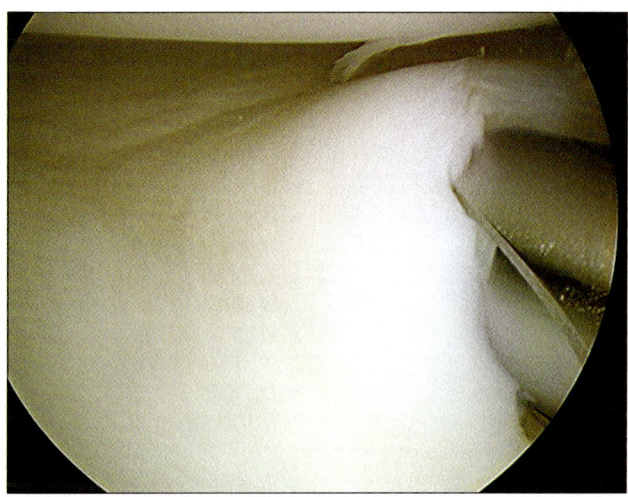

FIGURE 5

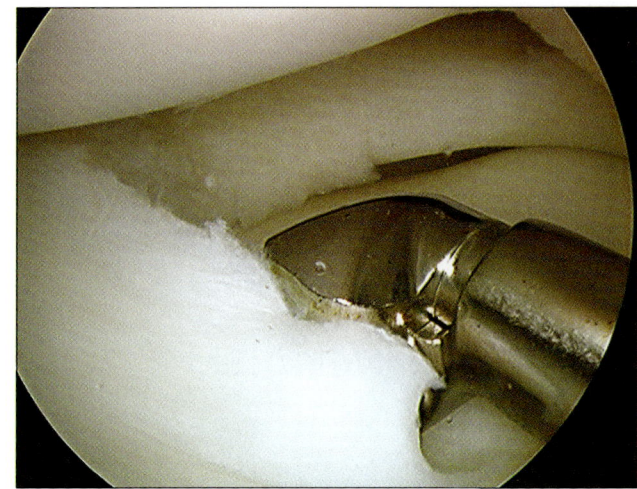

A

FIGURE 6

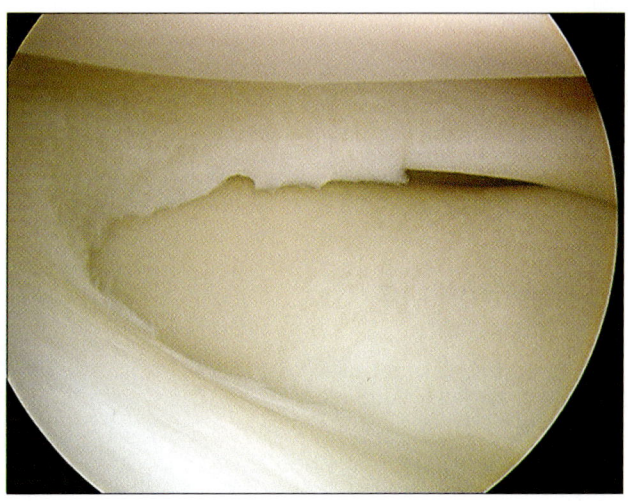

B

Instrumentation/ Implantation

- Bioresorbable arrow all-inside suture implants with integrated delivery system

- Straight or curved suture needles for outside-in and inside-out repairs

- Suture cutter

Controversies

- Some bioresorbable implants are more prominent and risk scuffing of chondral surfaces.

- Adverse reactions to implant or suture may occur.

- Implants may lose fixation.

Instrumentation/ Implantation

- Bioresorbable arrow all-inside suture implants with integrated delivery system

- Straight or curved suture needles

- Suture cutter

- Probe

STEP 3: REPAIR OF REMNANT MENISCAL TEARS

- After resection of the central portion of the meniscus, remnant tears are addressed, commonly with an all-inside repair using a bioresorbable arrow allowing for tensioning across the repair (Fig. 7).
- Outside-in or inside-out meniscal suture repair is performed as necessary.
- Intrasubstance degeneration is repaired to prevent tear propagation.

STEP 4: STABILIZATION OF UNSTABLE RIM

- Stabilization of an unstable rim is concurrently achieved with meniscal repair if using all-inside bioresorbable arrows with meniscocapsular anchoring.
- All-inside implants can also be used independent of meniscal repair.
- Otherwise suture stabilization is used with techniques similar to outside-in and inside-out meniscal repairs.
- A probe used to assess stability after repair.

POSTOPERATIVE CARE AND EXPECTED OUTCOMES

- A hinged knee brace is used for 6 weeks. It is locked in extension for 4 weeks, but unlocked for range-of-motion exercises.
- Flexion during exercises is limited to 90° for 4 weeks.
- Partial weight bearing is permitted for 1 week, then progressive full weight bearing.
- Walking, swimming, and cycling exercises are started at 6 weeks; running and jumping are allowed at 3 months.
- Return to sports is permitted after 4 months of rehabilitation with an asymptomatic knee while doing exercises.
- Longer term results, ranging from 3 to 17 years, have shown good or excellent results in 55–100% of patients. Results are improved with pediatric patients.
- A small risk of degenerative change has been noted.

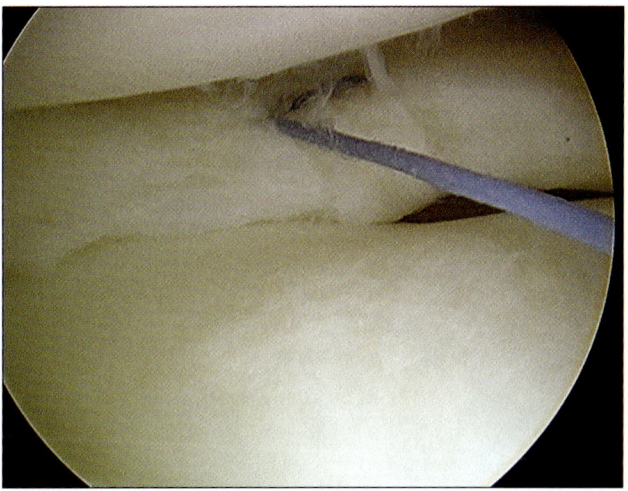

FIGURE 7

PEARLS

- *Avoid deep squats for 3 months to protect the repair.*

PITFALLS

- *Myositis ossificans has been observed with aggressive early rehabilitation after operation.*
- *Complete resection is associated with increased degenerative changes.*

POTENTIAL COMPLICATIONS

- Degenerative changes to the chondral surfaces
- Osteochondritis dissecans
- Further tears
- Risk of lateral instability if complete meniscectomy performed
- Complete resection associated with increased degenerative changes
- Quadriceps atrophy and weakness
- Persistent pain or effusion
- Decreased range of motion
- Radiologic degenerative changes:
  - Lateral joint space narrowing
  - Lateral femoral condyle flattening
  - Ridge formation along the lateral femoral condyle
  - Spurring and sclerosis of the tibial plateau

EVIDENCE

Aichroth PM, Patel DV, Marx CL. Congenital discoid lateral meniscus in children: a follow-up study and evolution of management. J Bone Joint Surg [Br]. 1991;73:932–6.

The authors presented a retrospective review of 62 knees with an average follow-up of 5.5 years. Average age was 10.5 years and osteochondritis dissecans was seen in seven knees. Of the 62 knees, 48 had total meniscectomy, 6 had partial meniscectomy, and 8 knees were observed. There were 84% good or excellent results on the Ikeuchi scale. (Level III evidence)

Atay OA, Doral MN, Leblebicio lu G, Tetik O, Aydingöz U. Management of discoid lateral meniscus tears: observations in 34 knees. Arthroscopy. 2003;19:346–52.

In this retrospective study, 34 knees were followed up for an average of 5.6 years after partial meniscectomy. The patients had an average age of 19.8 years; 85% had good or excellent results on the Ikeuchi scale. (Level III evidence)

Davidson D, Letts M, Glasgow R. Discoid meniscus in children: treatment and outcome. Can J Surg. 2003;46:350–8.

In this retrospective study of 36 knees, partial resection was performed in 19, complete resection in 13, and 4 knees were observed, with an average 3-year follow-up. Outcome was graded good or excellent in 74% of the knees on the Ikeuchi scale. The authors noted that 65% of the cases were female. (Level III evidence)

Good CR, Green DW, Griffith MH, Valen AW, Widmann RF, Rodeo SA. Arthroscopic treatment of symptomatic discoid meniscus in children: classification, technique, and results. Arthroscopy. 2007;23:157–63.

This was a retrospective review of 23 knees with a 37.4-month follow-up. Meniscal instability was noted in 77% of knees, most commonly in the anterior horn. The authors noted slow return of range of motion postoperatively in children under 6 years of age. (Level III evidence)

Hayashi LK, Yamaga H, Ida K, Miura T. Arthroscopic meniscectomy for discoid lateral meniscus in children. J Bone Joint Surg [Am]. 1988;70:1495–500.

The authors presented a retrospective study of 53 knees followed up for an average of 31.2 months. They recommended a remnant rim width of 6 mm for complete discoid menisci and 8 mm for incomplete discoid menisci, in order to reduce the incidence of further tears. (Level III evidence)

Ikeuchi H. Arthroscopic treatment of the discoid lateral meniscus: technique and long-term results. Clin Orthop Relat Res. 1982;(167):19–28.

In this retrospective review of 24 knees followed up for an average of 4.3 years, there were 71% good or excellent results on the author's grading. (Level III evidence)

Klingele KE, Kocher MS, Hresko MT, Gerbino P, Micheli LJ. Discoid lateral meniscus: prevalence of peripheral rim instability. J Pediatr Orthop. 2004;24:79–82.

In this retrospective review of 128 knees, meniscal tear was noted in 69.5% of knees. The authors noted peripheral rim instability in 28.1% of cases, which was significantly more common in complete discoid menisci and younger patients. (Level III evidence)

Räber DA, Friederich NF, Hefti F. Discoid lateral meniscus in children: long-term follow-up after total meniscectomy. J Bone Joint Surg [Am]. 1998;80:1579–86.

The authors presented a retrospective review of 17 knees followed up for an average of 19.8 years after total meniscectomy. In 10 of 17 knees there were clinical symptoms of osteoarthritis, and 10 of 11 knees had radiologic osteoarthritic changes. Osteochondritis dissecans developed in two knees. (Level III evidence)

Vandermeer RD, Cunningham FK. Arthroscopic treatment of the discoid lateral meniscus: results of long-term follow-up. Arthroscopy. 1989;5:101–9.

This was a retrospective review of 25 knees evaluated at an average of 54 months. The average patient age was 31.9 years. Of the symptomatic torn lesions, 55% were graded good or excellent on the Ikeuchi scale. Moderate to severe degenerative changes noted at operation were associated with a 66% rate of unsatisfactory outcome; 66% of patients less than 20 years of age at operation were graded good or excellent on follow-up. (Level III evidence)

Washington ER, Root L, Liener UC. Discoid lateral meniscus in children: long-term follow-up after excision. J Bone Joint Surg [Am]. 1995;77:1357–61.

In this retrospective review, 18 knees treated with complete meniscectomy were followed up for an average of 17 years. Average age at operation was 10.5 years; 72% had a good or excellent result on the Ikeuchi scale. Six of 14 knees had mild lateral instability and 3 of 8 knees had slight narrowing of the joint space and flattening of the femoral condyle. (Level III evidence)

Patellar Instability: Lateral Release and Medial Plication

John Hunt Udall and Dennis E. Kramer

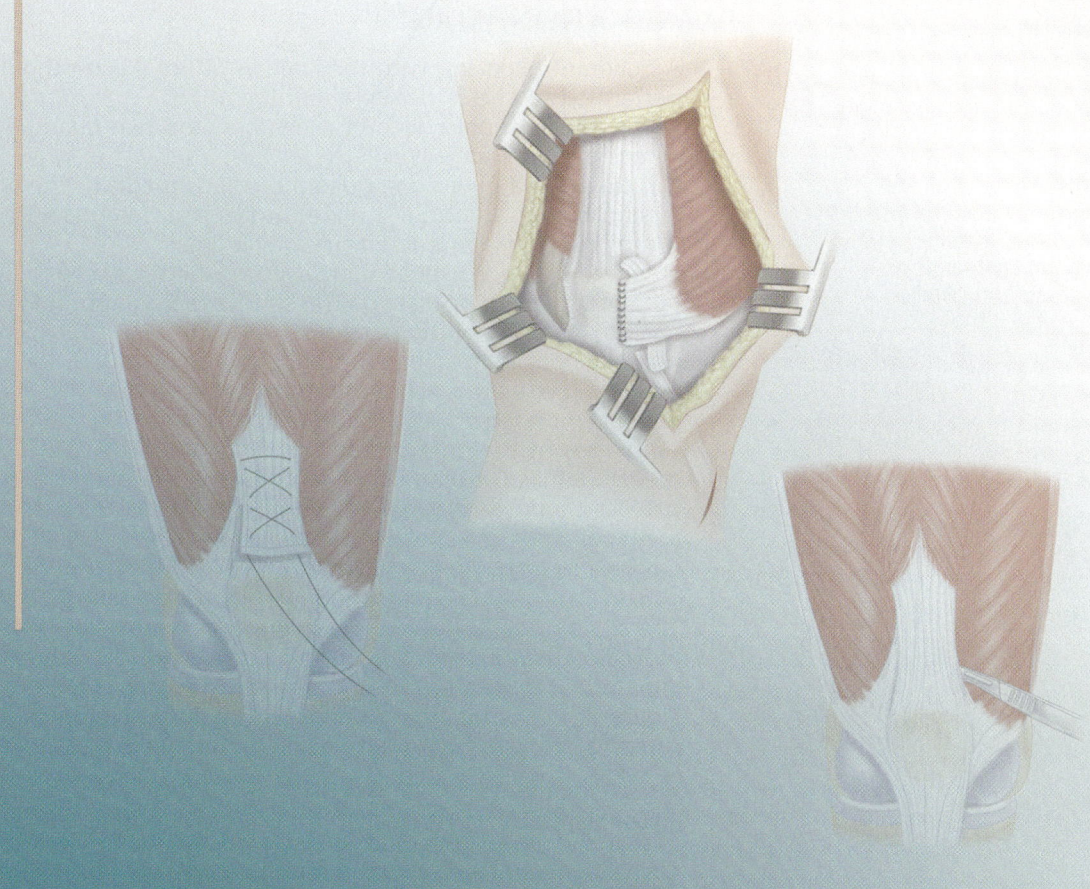

Controversies

• Patients with chondromalacia of the patella have a poorer prognosis following all types of treatment.

Treatment Options

• Depending on patient anatomy, severity of patellar malalignment, injured structures, previous failed procedures, age of the patient, and status of the physes, surgical options include lateral release with medial plication, medial patellofemoral ligament reconstruction, and patellar realignment tibial tubercle osteotomy.

INDICATIONS

- Lateral release is indicated in patients with patellar tilt and/or a tight lateral retinaculum with patellofemoral pain.
- Medial plication can be added if the patient has recurrent patellar subluxations or dislocations or for patellar maltracking following lateral release.
- Medial plication is typically done in conjunction with a lateral release but can be done alone if there is no patellar tilt or tight lateral retinaculum.
- For patellofemoral pain without instability, extensive nonoperative treatment, including physical therapy for quadriceps strengthening and stretching of the lateral structures, should be done in all patients for at least 6 months prior to surgical treatment.

EXAMINATION/IMAGING

- A quadrant glide test with the knee in 30° of flexion should be performed to check for lateral tightness.
  - The patella should glide between one and two quadrants medially and laterally.
  - If the patella glides one quadrant or less medially, the lateral retinaculum is tight. If it glides more than two quadrants medially, the lateral retinaculum is loose.
- Standard views as well as sunrise views of both knees should be obtained prior to operating. The sunrise radiograph in Figure 1A reveals lateral tilt of the patella.
- Magnetic resonance imaging (MRI) can be helpful in determining whether chondral injury is present in the patellofemoral joint. An axial MRI after patellar dislocation (Fig. 1B) shows hemarthrosis, lateral subluxation of the patella, medial retinacular tear, lateral femoral condyle bone bruise, and patellar chondromalacia.

SURGICAL ANATOMY

- The superior genicular vessels are near the vastus lateralis musculotendinous junction and must be coagulated thoroughly after lateral release to prevent hemarthrosis.
- Figure 2 shows the arterial supply to the knee. Note where the superolateral genicular artery nears the vastus lateralis.

POSITIONING

- The patient is placed in supine position with a nonsterile, well-padded thigh tourniquet.

PORTALS/EXPOSURES

- A standard anterolateral portal should be made next to the patellar tendon and at the level of the inferior pole of the patella.
- An anteromedial portal is made in the standard position.
- Medial plication requires a 4-cm incision placed 1 cm medial to the medial border of the patella.
- Figure 3 shows the standard positions for arthroscopic portals, and the potential incision for a medial plication is marked.

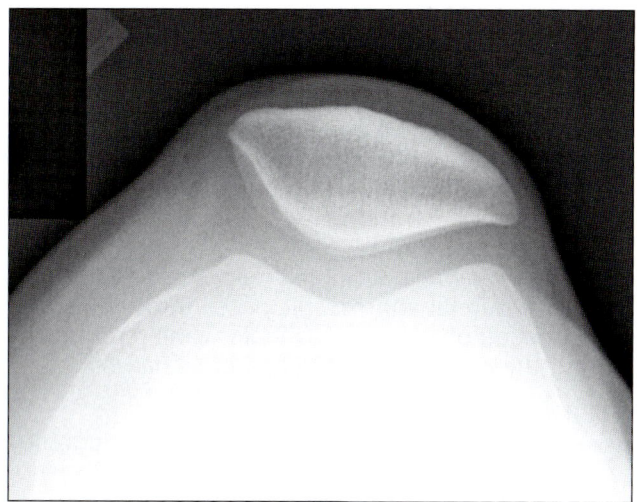
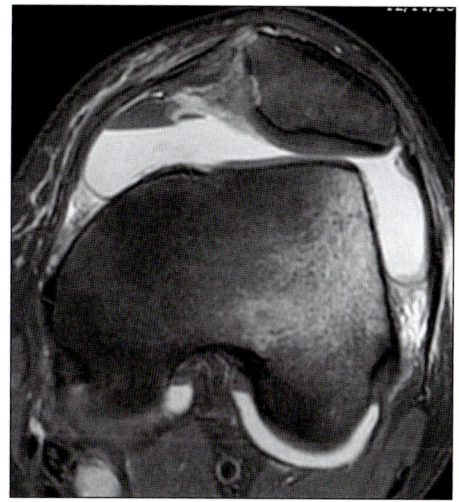

A
B

FIGURE 1

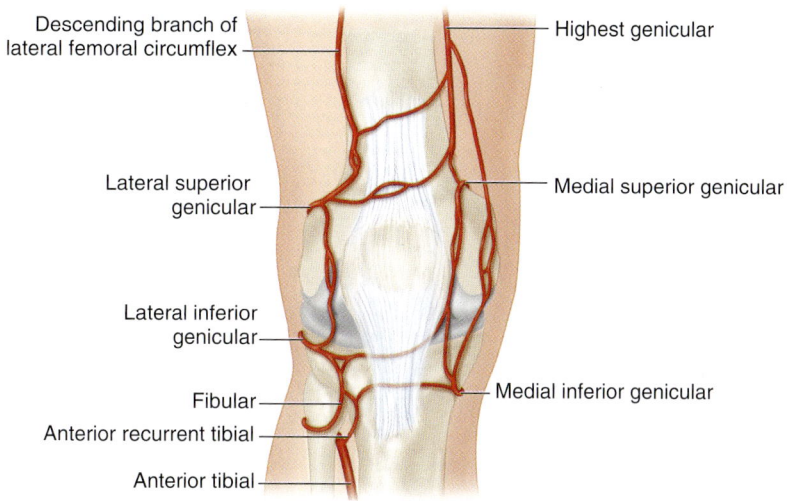

Descending branch of
lateral femoral circumflex —

— Highest genicular

Lateral superior
genicular —

— Medial superior genicular

Lateral inferior
genicular —

Fibular —

Anterior recurrent tibial —

Anterior tibial —

— Medial inferior genicular

FIGURE 2

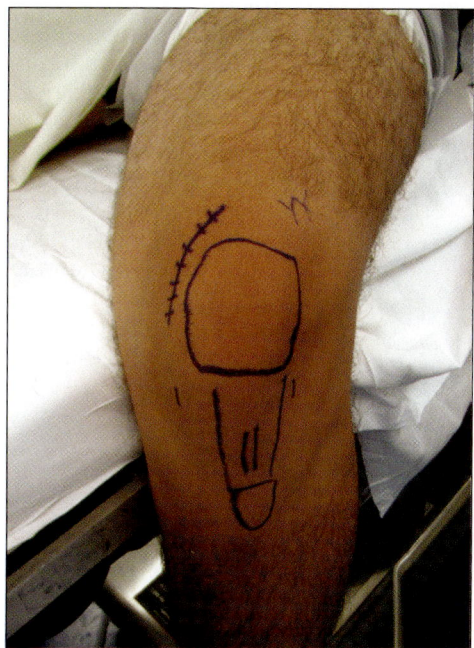

FIGURE 3

PROCEDURE: ARTHROSCOPIC LATERAL RELEASE

STEP 1

- The anterolateral portal is made first, and a standard diagnostic arthroscopy proceeds. Patellar tilt and tracking should be observed in relation to the trochlear groove.
- The lateral release can be performed with either electrocautery or Metzenbaum scissors.
- The lateral release should be performed from the level of the anterolateral arthroscopic portal to the musculotendinous junction of the vastus lateralis, aiming approximately 20° lateral to the patella while heading proximally.

STEP 2

- For scissor release of the lateral retinaculum, first the lateral portal is made slightly larger, then the Metzenbaum scissors are placed through the portal into the knee joint, sliding up the lateral gutter.
  - The Metzenbaum scissors are then withdrawn superficially and used like a Cobb elevator to define the plane between the lateral retinaculum and the overlying soft tissue approximately 1 cm lateral to the lateral border of the patella.
  - The scissors are then partially replaced into the knee joint so that the lower shear blade is in the knee joint and the upper shear blade is in the layer between the lateral retinaculum and the superficial soft tissues.
  - The patella is then held everted while the scissors are used to cut the retinaculum to the level of the vastus lateralis (just proximal to the superior pole of the patella) (Fig. 4).
- Alternatively, the lateral release can be performed with an electrocautery device under direct visualization (Fig. 5).
  - In these cases, first using the Metzenbaum scissors to define the plane between the lateral retinaculum and superficial soft tissues aids in the electrocautery release.
- The path of the lateral release heads proximally at a 20° angle lateral to the patella.

STEP 3

- After the lateral release has been performed, check the orientation of the patella in the trochlear groove to determine if tracking is adequate. If the patella is still maltracking, or subluxed in a lateral position, medial plication is indicated.
- The lateral overhang of the patella over the lateral femoral condyle with the knee in full extension can be measured before and after the release to judge improvement in alignment.
  - Figure 6 shows the patellar tilt (*top*) and lateral overhang (*bottom*) prior to a lateral release.
  - Figure 7 shows the patellar tilt (*top*) and overhang (*bottom*) after the lateral release.
- Prior to doing the medial plication, meticulous hemostasis must be achieved at the lateral release site with an arthroscopic electrocautery device (particular attention should be paid at the proximal aspect of the release).

PEARLS

- *Make sure that the patella can be everted at least 60° after the release; if not, there are likely some bands of retinaculum that need to be cut.*

PITFALLS

- *The patella is often normally laterally subluxed with the knee in full extension. Patellar tracking relative to the trochlear groove is better assessed at 30° of knee flexion.*

- *Meticulous hemostasis must be achieved following the lateral release to prevent a hemarthrosis.*

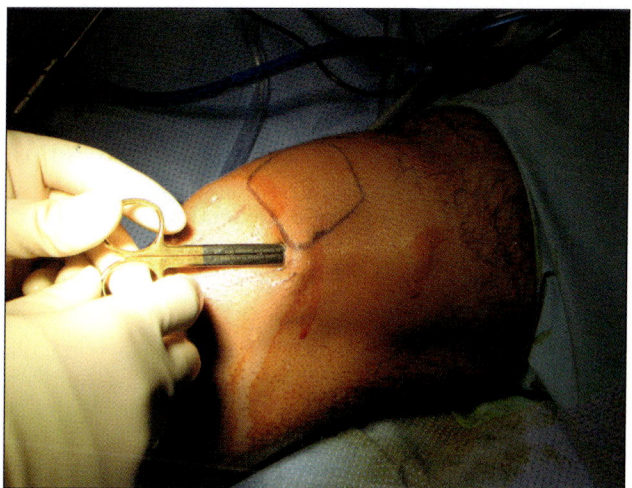

FIGURE 4

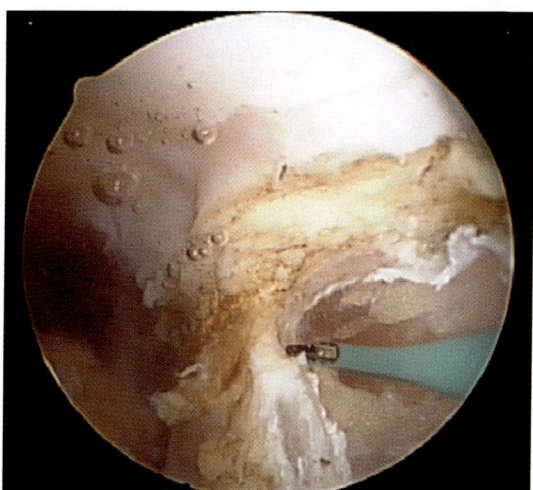

FIGURE 5

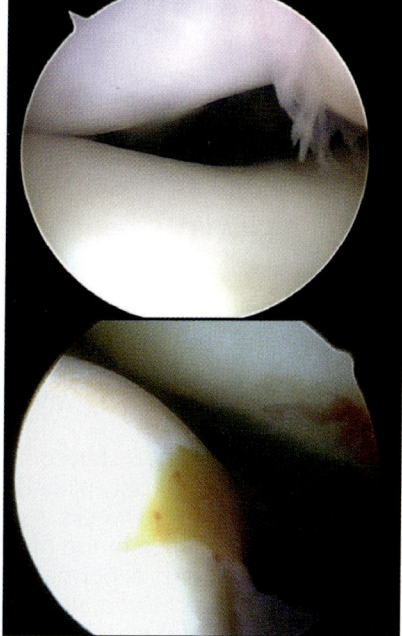

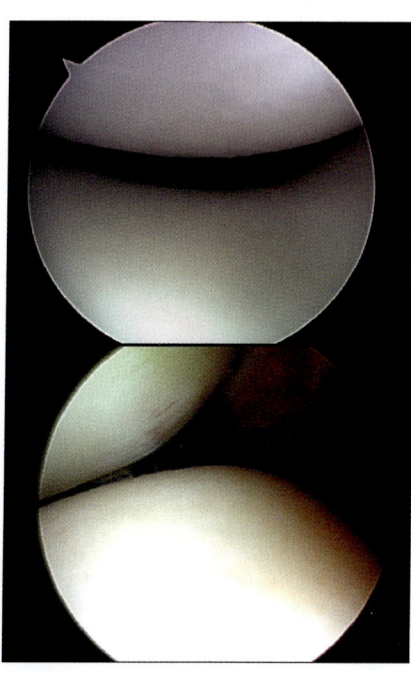

FIGURE 6   **FIGURE 7**

PROCEDURE: OPEN MEDIAL PLICATION

STEP 1

- The medial plication incision should be about 4 cm in length, positioned 1 cm medial to the medial border of the patella and extending from just proximal to the superior pole of the patella to near the level of the inferior pole of the patella (Fig. 8).
- Dissection is carried down to the medial retinaculum.
- If a defect in the medial patellofemoral ligament (MPFL) is visible or palpable, this can be repaired with suture imbrication.

STEP 2

- If no obvious retinacular defect is present (more common), an arthrotomy incision is made positioned 1 cm medial to the medial border of the patella down to but not through the synovium of the knee.
  - The arthrotomy incision should go from the superior pole to the inferior pole of the patella.
- A "pants-over-vest" imbrication is then performed over the arthrotomy incision by suturing the vastus lateralis and the medial retinacular flap onto the periosteum of the patella at its midportion (Fig. 9).
- Three horizontal mattress sutures placed 1 cm apart (from superior to inferior) are utilized for the imbrication.
  - The most proximal suture grabs tissue from the vastus lateralis and advances it to the midportion of the superior pole of the patella.
  - The middle and inferior sutures are used to imbricate the MPFL and medial retinaculum to the midportion of the middle and inferior pole of the patella.
  - Each suture grabs approximately 1 cm of tissue on the medial side of the arthrotomy incision and sutures it to the periosteum of the patella.
- The number of sutures and amount of plication varies depending on the patient's anatomy.

STEP 3

- All sutures are placed and secured first before any knots are tied. The arthroscope is then placed back in the knee joint and the patellofemoral articulation is observed with knee flexion.
- If the plication is deemed adequate, the knots are then tied with the knee in 30° of flexion.
- Following knot-tying, the knee is flexed from 0 to 90° to ensure the knots are secure and the knee has not been overtightened. Patellofemoral articulation is assessed during this maneuver with the surgeon's thumb and index finger on the patella.

POSTOPERATIVE CARE AND EXPECTED OUTCOMES

- Protocols vary; our preference is presented here.
- A hinged knee brace is used, with range of motion progressing from 0 to 90° over 6 weeks.
- Partial weight bearing with crutches is permitted during this time.
- Physical therapy is started at 4–6 weeks postoperatively, focusing on quadriceps and vastus medialis strengthening.
- The brace after 6 weeks is discontinued and physical therapy aims for full knee range of motion.
- Return to sports is permitted at 3 months postoperatively if the patient has achieved all full motion and strength.
- An elastic patellar stabilization brace is utilized if necessary.

PEARLS

- *The plication sutures should be tied only after visualization of satisfactory patellofemoral tracking with the sutures secured.*
- *Square knots are necessary to secure the plication and prevent knot loosening or breakage.*

PITFALLS

- *Overtightening the medial structures or over-release of the lateral structures can cause medial patellar subluxation-dislocation or loss of flexion postoperatively.*

Instrumentation/Implantation

- Either absorbable or nonabsorbable suture (#1 or #2) can be utilized for the plication.

PEARLS

- *Flexing the knee intraoperatively from 0 to 90° after the plication ensures that the repair can tolerate this amount of knee motion.*

PITFALLS

- *Hemarthrosis from inadequate cauterization following lateral release can slow rehabilitation and cause stiffness.*

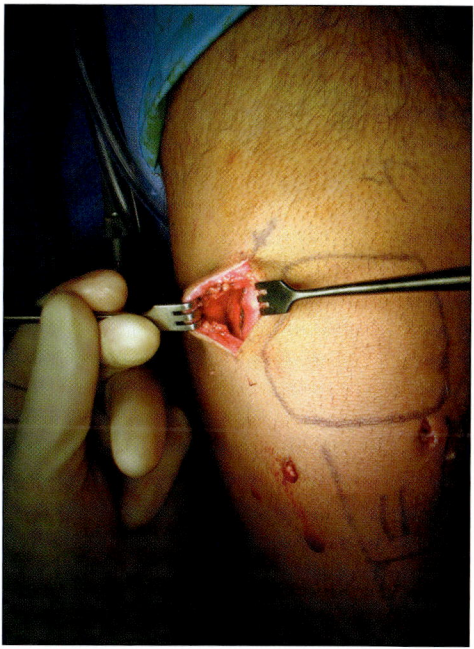

FIGURE 8

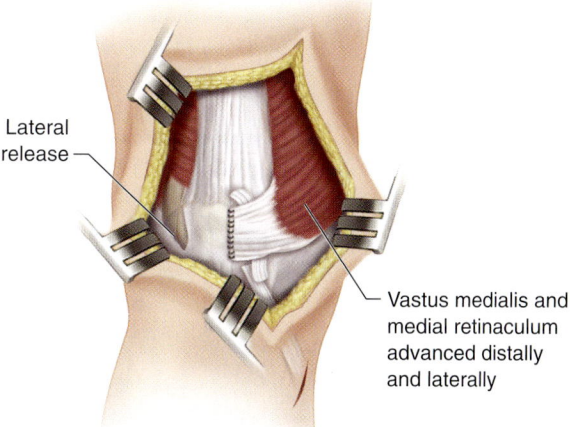

Lateral release

Vastus medialis and medial retinaculum advanced distally and laterally

FIGURE 9

EVIDENCE

Colvin AC, West RV. Patellar instability. J Bone Joint Surg [Am]. 2008;90:2751–62.

The authors review the various soft tissue and bony pathologies which contribute to patellar instability and discuss both nonoperative and operative management options. Indications and contraindications for various surgical procedures are described. A literature review is included.

Gerbino PG, Zurakowski D, Soto R, Griffen E, Reig TS, Micheli LJ. Long-term functional outcome after lateral patellar retinacular release in adolescents: an observational cohort study with minimum 5-year follow-up. J Pediatr Orthop. 2008;28:118–23.

The authors perform a retrospective cohort study evaluating the mid-term results of lateral patellar retinacular release in adolescents. Most patients demonstrated improvement in knee scores at latest follow-up and overall satisfaction improved as time from operating increased. Twenty five of 140 patients required reoperation although no differences were found in this subgroup. (Level IV evidence)

Miller JR, Adamson GJ, Pink MM, Fraipont MJ, Durand P Jr. Arthroscopically assisted medial reefing without routine lateral release for patellar instability. Am J Sports Med. 2007;35:622–9.

The authors present a case series of 24 patients with patellofemoral instability who underwent arthroscopically assisted medial reefing without lateral release. Significant improvement was noted in postoperative knee scores and radiographic parameters of patellar tilt were improved as well. No patients experienced a recurrent dislocation or subluxation at short term follow-up. (Level IV evidence)

Ricchetti ET, Mehta S, Sennett BJ, Huffman GR. Comparison of lateral release versus lateral release with medial soft-tissue realignment for the treatment of recurrent patellar instability: a systematic review. Arthroscopy. 2007;23:463–8.

The authors perform a systemic review of 14 level 3 and level 4 studies that reported on the surgical success of lateral retinacular release vs. lateral retinacular release with medial soft tissue realignment for recurrent lateral patellar instability. This systematic review found that isolated lateral release yields significantly inferior long-term results with respect to symptoms of recurrent lateral patellar instability compared with lateral release with medial soft tissue realignment. (Level III evidence)

Knee Surgery for Children with Cerebral Palsy I: Hamstring Lengthening

Benjamin J. Shore and Brian Snyder

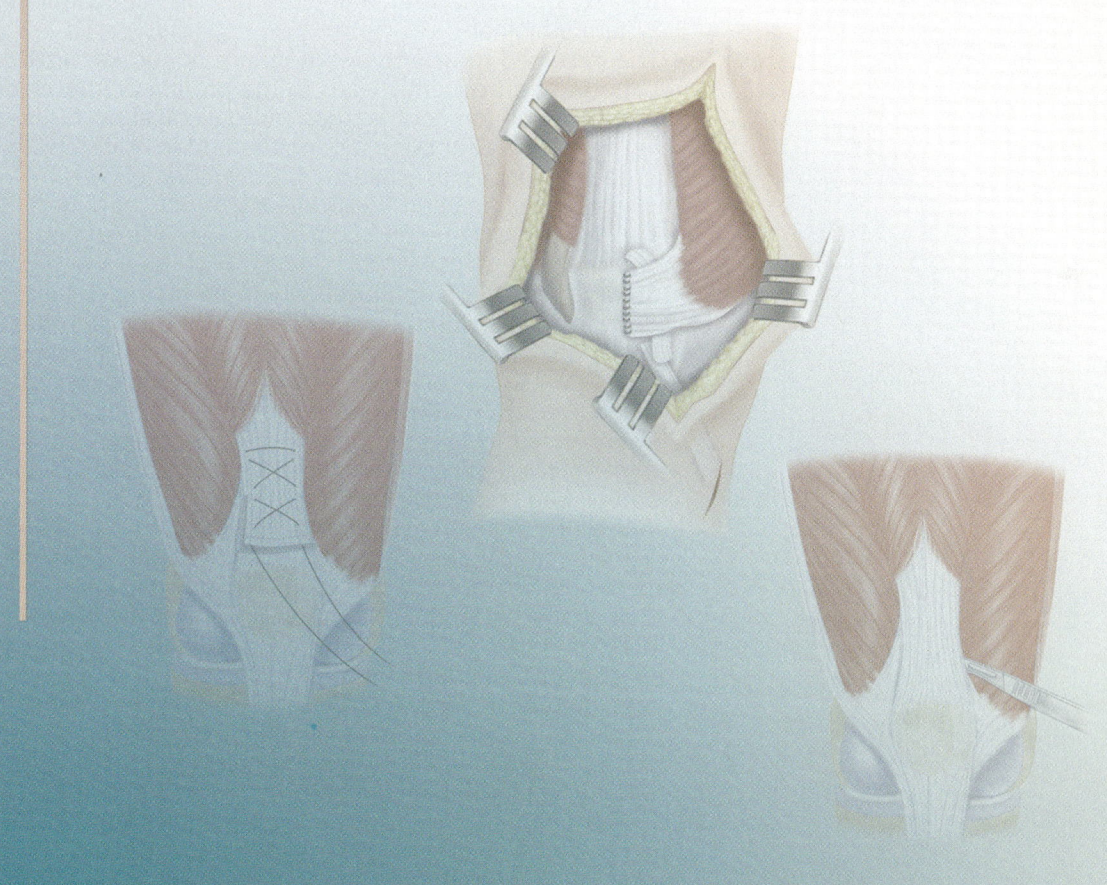

INTRODUCTION

- Children with cerebral palsy demonstrate three primary abnormalities of gait: (1) loss of selective motor control, (2) impaired balance, and (3) abnormal muscle tone.
  - As a child with cerebral palsy matures, incongruous growth between the muscle and bone occurs so that the muscle is relatively shorter than the bone it subtends. Biarticular muscles tend to be more affected than monoarticular muscles; this pattern appears to be more profound distally than proximally, resulting in contractures of the gastrocnemius-soleus, hamstrings, rectus femoris, and psoas muscles.
  - Spasticity is the most common abnormality of muscle seen in patients with cerebral palsy. The hallmark feature of spasticity is velocity-dependent stiffness of the muscle in proportion to the rate of muscle stretch, indicating a loss of central nervous system inhibition.
  - The increased muscle tone can induce abnormal movement patterns and frequently leads to the progressive development of muscle-tendon contractures and skeletal abnormalities, including torsional bone deformities and joint instability.
- The goal of surgery for children with cerebral palsy is to improve overall function by addressing structural bone deformities, muscle-tendon contractures, and lever arm dysfunction.
  - Surgical results are optimized when the timing of surgery is delayed until children have reached a functional "plateau." At this point, the child has exhausted nonsurgical measures (physical therapy, orthoses, and pharmacologic spasticity management), has failed to demonstrate significant improvement over a 6-month follow-up period, and experiences significant functional impairments affecting ambulation and activities of daily living.
- In our clinic, preoperative analysis includes physical examination, observational gait analysis, and frequently quantitative three-dimensional computerized motion analysis.
  - Gait analysis is an important component of the surgical decision-making algorithm for children with cerebral palsy. Quantitative gait analysis can provide objective information regarding deviations in three-dimensional joint kinematics involving multiple joints simultaneously and often provides additional information to the surgeon beyond that ascertained by physical examination alone.
- Different gait patterns involving the knee have been described in ambulatory children with cerebral palsy. Most recently, Rhodda et al. (2004) identified four gait patterns in children with spastic diplegia and outlined surgical and nonsurgical treatment for each pattern (Fig. 1).
  - **True equinus gait** occurs when the ankle is fixed in equinus but the knee, hip, and pelvis demonstrate a normal dynamic range of motion.
  - **Jump gait** occurs when the ankle is fixed in equinus, and the hip and knee demonstrate a flexed posture in early stance and extend to a variable degree in late stance, yet never reach full extension.

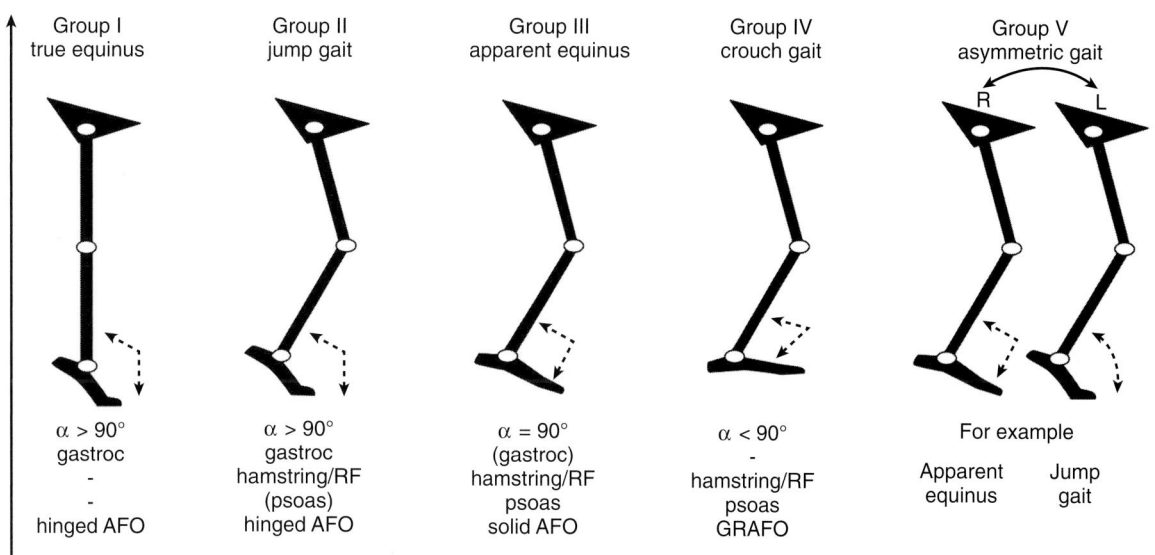

Sagittal gait patterns: spastic diplegia

Group I
true equinus

$\alpha > 90°$
gastroc
-
-
hinged AFO

Group II
jump gait

$\alpha > 90°$
gastroc
hamstring/RF
(psoas)
hinged AFO

Group III
apparent equinus

$\alpha = 90°$
(gastroc)
hamstring/RF
psoas
solid AFO

Group IV
crouch gait

$\alpha < 90°$
-
hamstring/RF
psoas
GRAFO

Group V
asymmetric gait

R   L

For example

Apparent   Jump
equinus   gait

FIGURE 1

- **Apparent equinus gait** occurs when the ankle has a normal dynamic range of motion but the hip and knee demonstrate increased flexion throughout the stance phase so that the patient appears to be up on his or her toes; often the pelvis may be tilted anteriorly (contracted psoas muscle).
- **Crouch gait** is defined as calcaneus or hyperdorsiflexion of the ankle with increased flexion at the hip and knee throughout stance; the pelvis may be tilted posteriorly (hamstring contracture).
- **Stiff-knee gait,** which was previously described by Sutherland and Davids (1993) and represents the delayed and decreased dynamic knee flexion amplitude during the swing phase of the gait cycle, was seen across three of the four gait patterns described by Rhodda et al. (2004). As a result, it was considered to be a specific knee pattern but not a specific gait pattern.
- In light of these specific gait patterns and their implications for treatment affecting functional outcomes, it is important for the treating orthopedic surgeon to carefully examine the hip and ankle when considered knee surgery in children with cerebral palsy.
- Surgical treatment of knee pathology in children with cerebral palsy rarely involves isolated muscle-tendon lengthening. This procedure highlights two of the surgical techniques commonly employed to treat knee pathology relative to the observed gait disturbances in children with cerebral palsy: hamstring lengthening and distal rectus femoris transfer (see Knee Surgery in Children with Cerebral Palsy II).

INDICATIONS

- Inability to fully extend the knee during midstance phase and at terminal swing
- Knee popliteal angle greater than 50°
- Fixed knee flexion contracture greater than 20°

EXAMINATION/IMAGING

- Observational gait analysis is important in assessing which of the four gait patterns is present.
- The hip is examined for the presence of hip flexion contracture with the Thomas test.
  - The patient is placed in supine, with the pelvis positioned such that the anterior superior iliac spine (ASIS) is vertically aligned with the posterior superior iliac spine (PSIS), and lumbar lordosis is reduced.
  - One hip is flexed to 90° and the contralateral leg is assessed in full extension.
  - Any flexion of the contralateral leg indicates the presence of a hip flexion contracture.
  - If there is a concomitant knee flexion contracture, the patient is positioned so that the leg extends beyond the end of the examination table to accommodate the knee flexion contracture.
- The knee is examined for hamstring tightness and the presence of fixed knee flexion contracture.
- The knee-popliteal angle (KPA) is an effective tool to assess hamstring length (Fig. 2).
  - The patient is positioned in supine with one hip flexed to 90° and the contralateral leg extended.

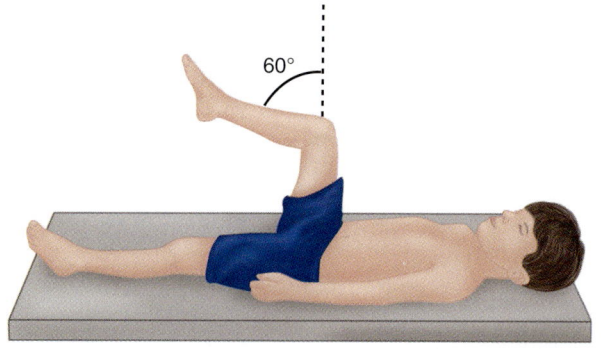

FIGURE 2

Treatment Options

- The semitendinosus and gracilis can be treated by tenotomy at the muscle-tendon junction.

- The tendinous portion of the gracilis and semitendinosus can be used as an anchor for concomitant rectus femoris transfer.

- Semitendinosus transfer around the adductor magnus tendon can also be used in concert with medial hamstring lengthening to act as a "tether" to prevent excessive anterior pelvic tilt and lumbar lordosis, which can be seen after overlengthening the medial and lateral hamstring muscles.

- Fractional aponeurotic lengthening of the semimembranosus (occasionally with the biceps femoris) helps preserve muscle function without overlengthening.

- Initially the ipsilateral knee is flexed to greater than 90° and then slowly the knee is extended until the first endpoint of resistance is felt and the pelvis begins to "rock"; the measurement (in degrees) lacking full extension is the KPA (Fig. 3).
- The unilateral KPA is a measure of "functional hamstring contracture." Functional KPA ranges from 0 to 49° (Katz et al., 1992); angles greater than 50° require surgical intervention.
- The bilateral KPA is determined with the contralateral hip flexed until the ASIS and PSIS are in a vertical line, decreasing lumbar lordosis and pelvic tilt. The bilateral KPA gives a measure of "true hamstring contracture."
- The difference between the unilateral and the bilateral KPA is the "hamstring shift." Hamstring shift greater than 20° indicates significant anterior pelvic tilt from (Delp et al., 2006):
  - ◆ Tight hip flexor musculature
  - ◆ Weak abdominals
  - ◆ Weak pelvic/hip extensors
- Examination for fixed knee flexion contracture is preformed with the patient prone, feet overhanging the edge of the examination table. Any lack of full knee extension indicates persistent knee flexion contracture.
- A straight leg raise examination is performed.

SURGICAL ANATOMY

- The semitendinosus, gracilis, and semimembranosus make up the medial-side hamstring muscles that commonly insert onto the pes anserinus of the proximal medial tibia (Fig. 4).
- Superficially and medial to the midline lies the semitendinosus, which is palpable as a tight tendon just proximal to the popliteal crease. At this level, the semitendinosus is purely tendinous with no visible muscle belly.
- Deep and medial to semitendinosus lie the semimembranosus and gracilis. The gracilis is the most medial of the three muscles and can be tightened with abduction of the hip and extension at the knee. At this level, the tendon of the gracilis is intramuscular, lying on the anteromedial aspect of the muscle belly.
- The semimembranosus lies deep to the semitendinosus and gracilis and demonstrates a broad muscular attachment with five separate insertions on the back of the knee.
- The medial intermuscular septum lies deep between the interval of the semimembranosus and gracilis. A 10-cm window through this septum is opened longitudinally to facilitate transfer of the rectus femoris to the semitendinosus/gracilis or semitendinosus transfer around the adductor magnus tendon.
- The adductor magnus muscle forms a discrete tendon that inserts on the adductor tubercle on the medial femoral condyle and lies anterior to the medial intermuscular septum.
- The biceps femoris lies on the lateral border of the popliteal fossa. This tendon can be palpated proximal to the popliteal crease. Medial to the biceps femoris (lateral to medial) lie the common peroneal nerve, tibial nerve, popliteal vein, and popliteal artery (see Fig. 4).
- The common peroneal nerve lies along the posterior/medial border of the biceps femoris and can be difficult to isolate from the muscle-tendon junction of the biceps femoris in very contracted knees (see Fig. 4).

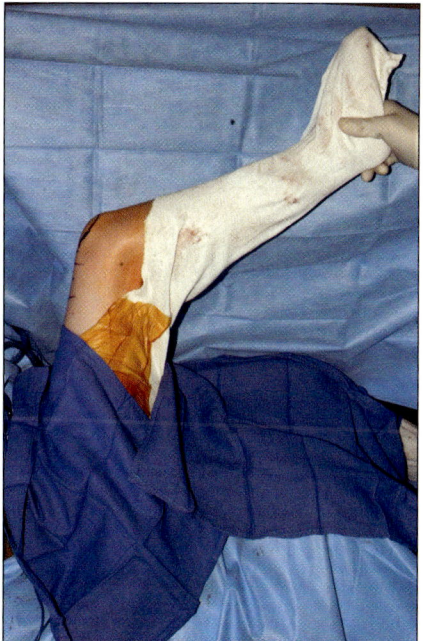

FIGURE 3

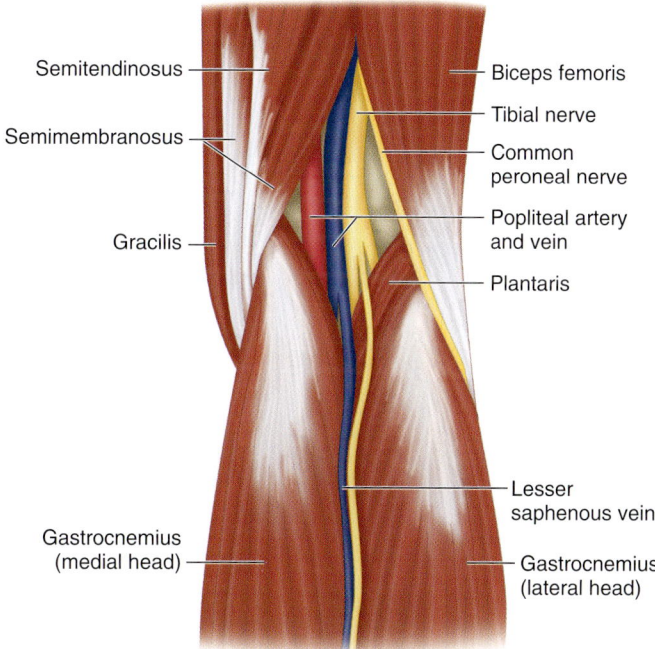

Semitendinosus

Semimembranosus

Gracilis

Biceps femoris

Tibial nerve

Common
peroneal nerve

Popliteal artery
and vein

Plantaris

Lesser
saphenous vein

Gastrocnemius
(medial head)

Gastrocnemius
(lateral head)

FIGURE 4

Equipment

- A tourniquet is not needed for hamstring lengthening.

POSITIONING

- The patient is examined under general anesthesia and physical examination findings are compared to those when awake. The differences may be attributed to spasticity that requires pharmacologic tone management.
- When considering positioning, the surgeon should always assess for the presence of hip flexion contracture.
- If no concurrent lengthening of the psoas is to be performed, surgery may be performed supine or prone. However, if the psoas is to be lengthened, then supine positioning is preferred.
- In the prone position, the patient is positioned on the chest and iliac crest bolsters are placed transversely to decompress the abdomen.
- In the supine position, each leg is free draped to allow for intraoperative examination of the hip, knee, and ankle.

PORTALS/EXPOSURES

- A single incision, 3–6 cm in length, just medial or lateral to the palpable semitendinosus tendon at the mid- to distal third of the posterior thigh can be used to access all the hamstring tendons (Fig. 5).
- Sharp dissection through skin and electrocautery through subcutaneous tissue minimize blood loss.

PROCEDURE

STEP 1

- The muscle-tendon junction of the semitendinosus is palpated. The sheath of the tendon is incised using a #15 blade or electrocautery.
- A right-angle clamp is placed around the tendon from *lateral to medial* to prevent inadvertent injury to the neurovascular bundle (Fig. 6A and 6B).
- Electrocautery is used to amputate the semitendinosus at the level of the musculotendinous junction.
- If the semitendinosus is being used for rectus femoris transfer, then amputation occurs slightly more proximal to ensure sufficient length to facilitate the transfer.
- If the semitendinosus is being used for adductor magnus transfer, then the knee is flexed up and tenotomy scissors are used to dissect the semitendinosus tendon distally free to the insertion on the tibia at the pes anserinus. The tendon is amputated distally so as to preserve as much length as possible for later transfer around the adductor magnus tendon.

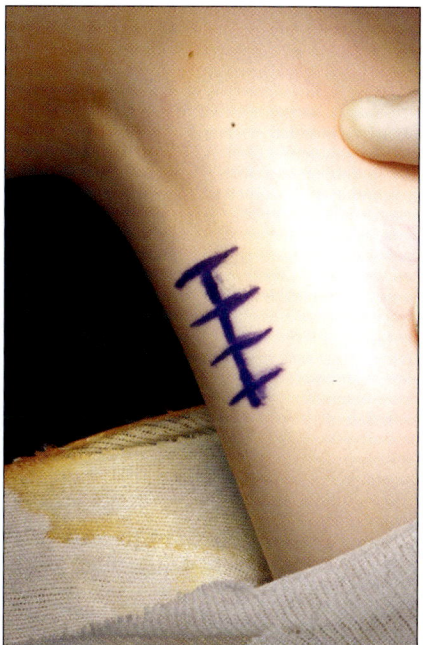

FIGURE 5

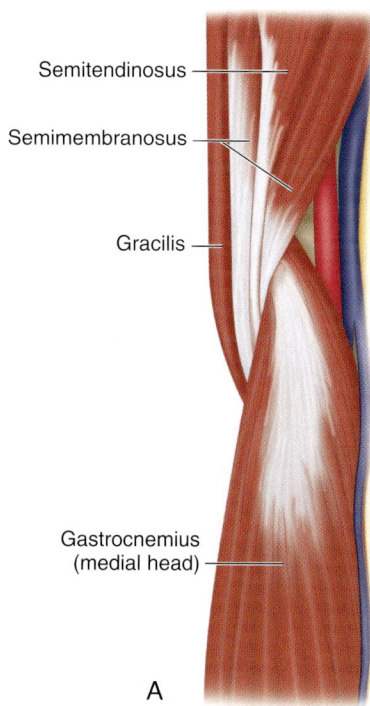

Semitendinosus

Semimembranosus

Gracilis

Gastrocnemius
(medial head)

A

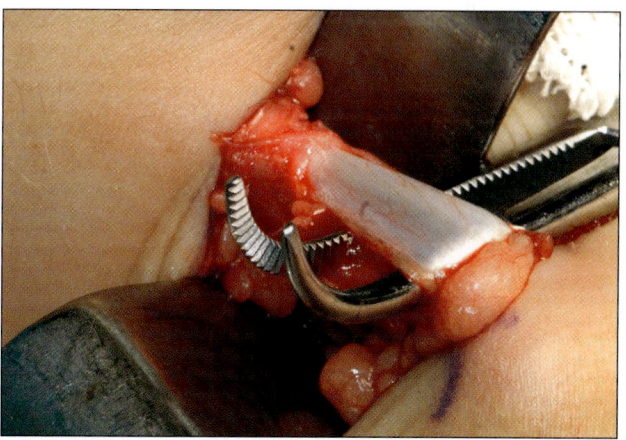

B

FIGURE 6

STEP 2

- The muscle-tendon junction of the gracilis, which lies medial and slightly deeper than the semitendinosus, is palpated; it is smaller in size than the semitendinosus.
- At this level, the tendon of the gracilis is intramuscular. The electrocautery or tenotomy scissors are used to incise the sheath of the gracilis muscle. The tendon lies anteriorly and medially within the muscle. A right-angle clamp is used to mobilize the tendon and it is bisected with the electrocautery.

STEP 3

- The semimembranosus muscle lies deep to the semitendinosus and slightly lateral to the gracilis muscle. The medial and lateral borders of the muscle are identified with the help of a rake or Senn retractor. The fat layer surrounding the aponeurosis of the semimembranosus is incised longitudinally. A Cobb elevator is used to circumferentially expose the aponeurosis. A #15 blade or electrocautery is used to make one or two transverse cuts (spaced 1 cm apart) through the aponeurosis of the semimembranosus at its muscle-tendon junction, preserving the underlying muscle (Fig. 7).
- Incisions in the aponeurotic fascia of the semimembranosus are begun proximally. If with careful stretching more extension is needed, further transverse incisions in the aponeurotic fascia are made distally (Fig. 8).
- The muscle fibers of the incised semimembranosus will stretch approximately 1–1.5 cm with each aponeurotic incision (Fig. 9).
- The wound is irrigated, and closure is done in layers with absorbable sutures.

STEP 4

- If there is a significant contracture of the lateral hamstring still restricting adequate knee extension, the biceps femoris can be fractionally lengthened through the same incision.
- Tenotomy scissors are used to dissect through the superficial fat laterally to the muscle-tendon junction of the biceps femoris.
- The surgeon must be mindful of the neurovascular structures that lie medially. A Senn or Army-Navy retractor is used to facilitate the exposure.
- The fat enveloping the biceps femoris aponeurosis is incised longitudinally.
- The muscle-tendon junction is exposed using a Cobb elevator.
- The biceps femoris is fractionally lengthened by transversely incising the fascia of the aponeurosis, preserving the underlying muscle.
- The knee is extended so that the muscle fibers stretch 1–1.5 cm; the popliteal angle should be reduced to approximately 20°.
- When lengthening both the medial and lateral hamstrings, the surgeon must use **extreme caution** to avoid overlengthening the neurovascular structures.

POSTOPERATIVE CARE AND EXPECTED OUTCOMES

- A well-padded long-leg cast with the knee in maximal safe extension that does not unduly stretch the sciatic nerve is applied.
- Adequate padding is applied anteriorly on the knees as well as posteriorly over the heels. The surgeon must ensure that there is no compression at the popliteal fossa as this may also lead to injury to neurovascular structures.

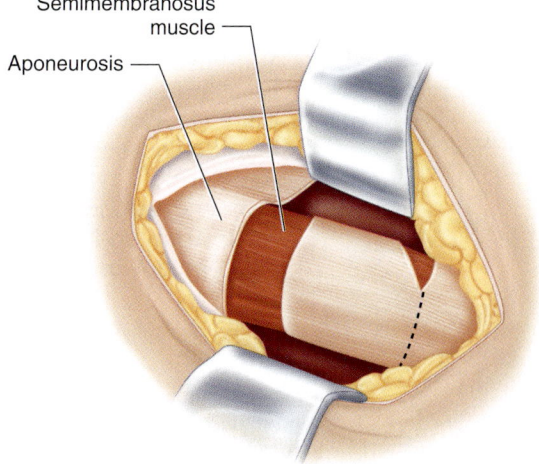

Semimembranosus
muscle

Aponeurosis

FIGURE 7

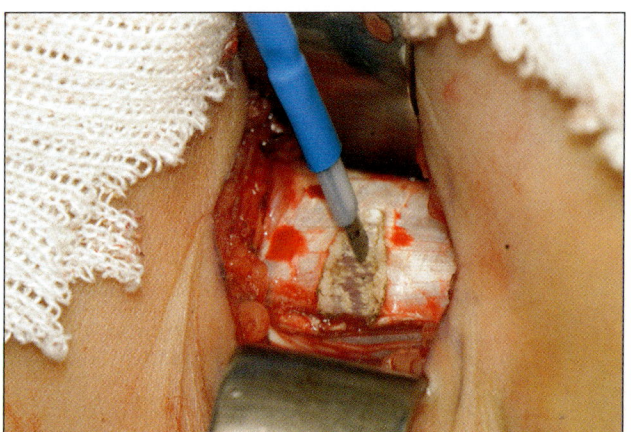

FIGURE 8

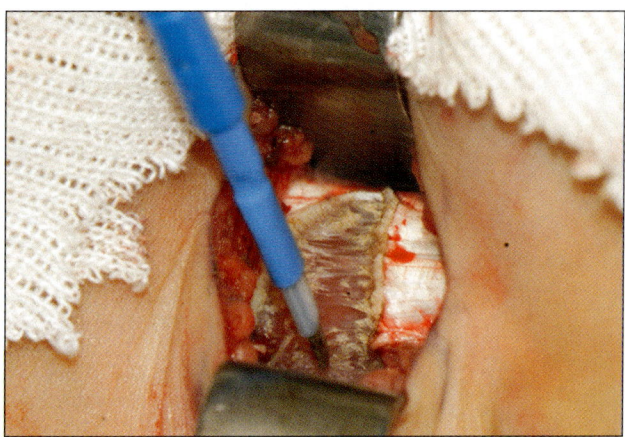

FIGURE 9

Controversies

• Passive stretching using long-leg casts, knee immobilizers, or a dynamic extension orthosis may be considered.

■ Casts are worn for 3 weeks, and then patients are transitioned to nighttime three-point splints or knee immobilizers.
■ Stiff-knee gait caused by spastic rectus femoris can develop after isolated hamstring lengthening.
■ Knee recurvatum can also develop if overaggressive hamstring lengthening occurs in the setting of tight gastrocnemius muscles.
■ Overlengthening of the hamstring muscles can generate knee recurvatum and increased anterior pelvic tilt if there is concomitant psoas contracture.

EVIDENCE

Delp SL, Arnold AS, Speers RA, Moore CA. Hamstring and psoas lengths during normal and crouch gait: implications for muscle-tendon surgery. J Orthop Res. 2006; 14:144–51.

A graphics based model of the lower extremity was used in conjunction with 3-D kinematic data obtained from gait analysis to estimate the lengths of the hamstrings and psoas during normal and crouch gaits. Eighty percent of subjects in crouch had hamstrings of normal length or longer despite persistent knee flexion during stance. All patients had psoas muscles that were shorter than normal by greater than 1 standard deviation. (Level IV evidence)

Katz K, Rosenthal A, Yosipovitch Z. Normal ranges of popliteal angle in children. J Pediatr Orthop. 1992;12:229–31.

The popliteal angle in 482 normal children, 1–10 years of age, was measured. Between the ages of 1 and 3 years, the mean angle was 6° (range, 0–15). At age 4, the angle rose to 17° in girls and 27° in boys (range, 5–45). At greater than or equal to 5 years the mean angle was 26° with little change (range, 0–50). A popliteal angle of greater than 50° in the above age groups indicates abnormal hamstring tightness. (Level IV evidence)

Rhodda JM, Graham HK, Carson L, Galea MP, Wolfe R. Sagittal gait patterns in spastic diplegia. J Bone Joint Surg [Br]. 2004;88:251–8.

This was a cross-sectional study of 187 children with spastic diplegia who attended gait analysis. A simple classification of sagittal gait patterns based on a combination of pattern recognition and kinematic data was developed. Then the evolution of gait patterns in a longitudinal study of 34 children who were followed for more than one year demonstrated the reliability of the classification. (Level IV evidence)

Schutte LM, Hayden SW, Gage JR. Lengths of hamstring and psoas muscles during crouch gait: effects of femoral anterversion. J Orthop Res. 2007;15:615–21.

In this study, normal adult musculoskeletal models were used to calculate hamstring and psoas lengths for children with cerebral palsy. A group of subjects with cerebral palsy who walk with a crouch gait were investigated to assess the changes in muscle lengths that arise when a patient-specific representation of clinically measured femoral anteversion was added to a model of normal musculoskeletal geometry. The calculation of psoas muscle length was found to be very sensitive to femoral anteversion whereas the calculation of hamstrings length was found to be relatively insensitive to this osseous deformity. (Level IV evidence)

Sutherland DH, Davids DR. Common abnormalities of the knee in cerebral palsy. Clin Orthop Relat Res. 1993;(288):139–47.

A retrospective review of 588 patients with cerebral palsy who underwent gait analysis. Four primary gait abnormalities of the knee were identified: jump knee, crouch knee, stiff knee, and recurvatum knee. In this review, each abnormality is described by its motion analysis laboratory profile (physical examination, motion parameters, electromyography [EMG] data, and force plate data). The most common etiologies and the consequences for gait of each disorder are also considered. (Level IV evidence)

Knee Surgery for Children with Cerebral Palsy II: Distal Rectus Femoris Transfer

Benjamin J. Shore and Brian Snyder

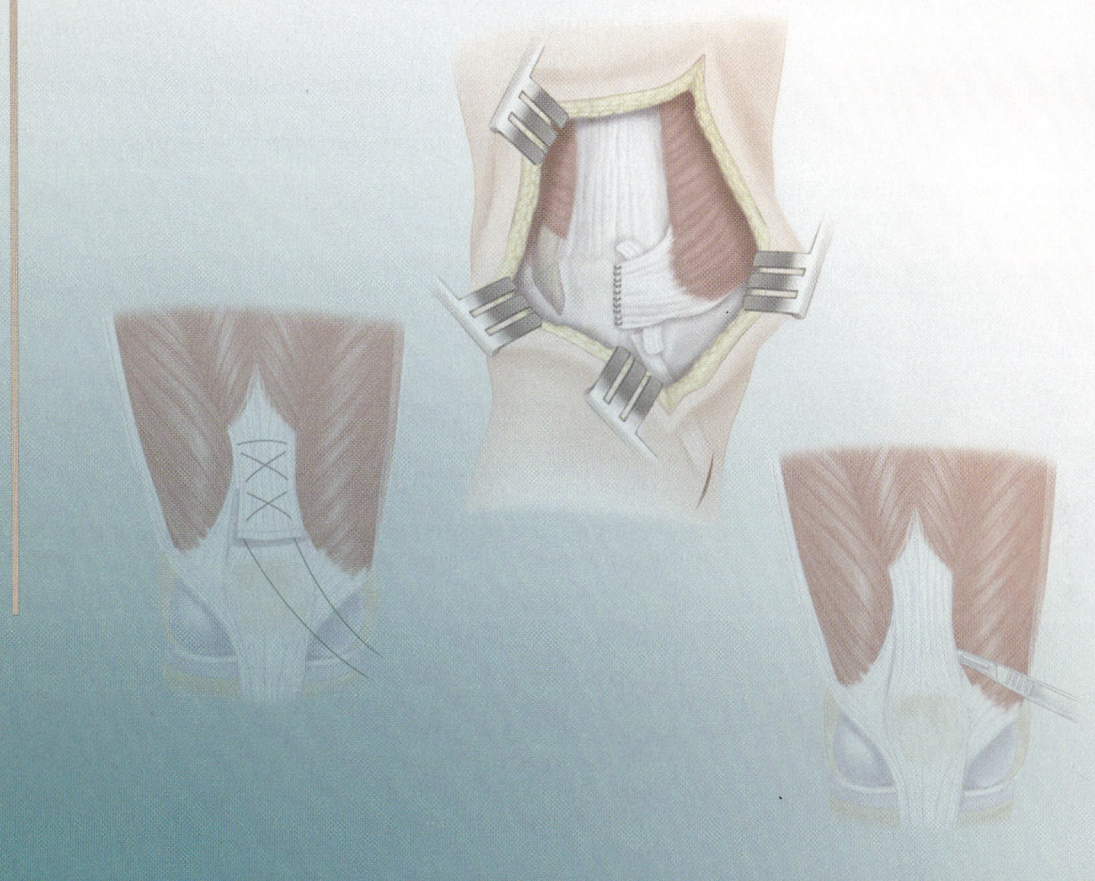

PITFALLS

- *Not all patients with rectus femoris transfers improve their knee range of motion, and transfers should be avoided in GMFCS IV children or those who are minimal ambulators with significant crouch gait (Gage et al., 1987; Kay et al., 2004).*

- *Consider other causes of stiff-knee gait, including spastic or contracted gastrocnemius (altered plantar flexion, knee extension moment), weak quadriceps or gastrocnemius, and previously overlengthened hamstring muscles (Ounpuu et al., 1993a).*

Controversies

- Rectus femoris transfer has been performed to medial and lateral insertion points, including the sartorius, gracilis, semitendinosus, and iliotibial band, with comparable results (Ounpuu et al., 1993b). Most authors now favor transfor to a medial insertion point, finding little significant difference in rotational alignment of the leg during gait.

- If preoperative knee range of motion is greater than 80% of normal, rectus femoris transfer provides results similar to distal rectus release. If preoperative knee range of motion is less than 80% of normal, rectus femoris transfer provides results superior to distal release (Marks et al., 2003).

- At the time of surgery, coexistent fixed flexion contractures of the hip (iliopsoas) and knee (hamstring) are addressed.

PITFALLS

- *Caution should be exercised when using the Duncan-Ely test alone to assess rectus spasticity.*

- *Gait analysis and fine-wire dynamic electromyographic testing of the rectus femoris are helpful and reliable investigations to perform to determine if rectus activity is prolonged or firing out of phase.*

INDICATIONS

- Decreased and delayed peak knee flexion in the swing phase of gait (< 45°) combined with overactivity of the rectus femoris during swing phase.
- Patients with "stiff-knee" gait and increased difficulty in clearance of foot during the swing phase, resulting in tripping or dragging of toes and inefficient gait.
- The goal is to convert the rectus femoris tendon from a hip flexor/knee extender to a hip flexor/knee flexor.

EXAMINATION/IMAGING

- Complete lower extremity examination is important.
- Associated lever arm dysfunction must be identifed.
- Associated flexion contracture of the hip (iliopsoas) and knee (hamstring) must be identifed.
- The rectus femoris acts proximally as a hip flexor and distally as a knee extender.
- The Duncan-Ely test is commonly used to assess rectus spasiticity.
  - With the patient prone, the knee is flexed rapidly to 90° (Fig. 1).
  - A spastic rectus femoris will cause the ipsilateral pelvis to rise up with knee flexion.
  - However, this test does not differentiate between a spastic rectus femoris or iliopsoas muscle (Rethlefsen et al., 2009).
- Rectus spasticity may also be tested in the supine position through rapid knee flexion.
  - Resistance in velocity-dependent knee flexion will also indicate rectus femoris spasticity.

SURGICAL ANATOMY

- The confluence of the vastus muscles must be appreciated. The rectus femoris is the most superficial and midline muscle of the complex, and care must be taken to separate this muscle from the underlying vastus intermedius, medialis, and lateralis (Fig. 2).
  - Separation between the muscles is best appreciated at the most proximal extent of the incision.
  - Once a surgical plane is developed between the rectus femoris tendon and underlying vastus intermedius, blunt dissection should facilitate dissection.
  - If dissection is not progressing with blunt dissection, careful re-evaluation of the surgical dissection should take place.
- The femoral artery and vein lie superficial to the adductor longus muscle on the medial aspect of the femur.
  - The vessels lie in a depression known as the subsartorial canal of Hunter. The canal lies between the extensor and adductor compartments of the thigh. The roof is formed by a fascial layer from the sartorius muscle, the posterior wall is from the adductor muscles (adductor longus superiorly and adductor magnus inferiorly), and the anterior wall is formed by the vastus medialis (see Fig. 2).
  - Running with the artery and vein at this level is the saphenous nerve.
- The femoral artery and vein pierce the adductor magnus muscle approximately 5–7 cm proximal to the insertion of the adductor magnus tendon on the adductor tubercle of the medial femoral condyle.

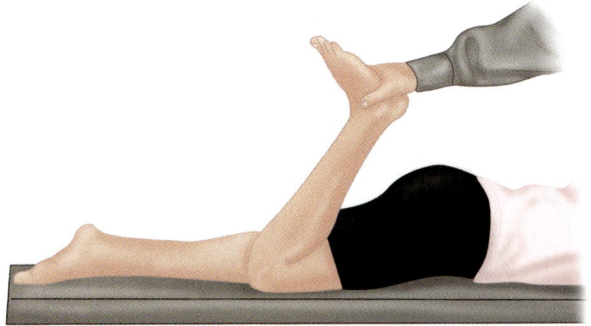

FIGURE 1

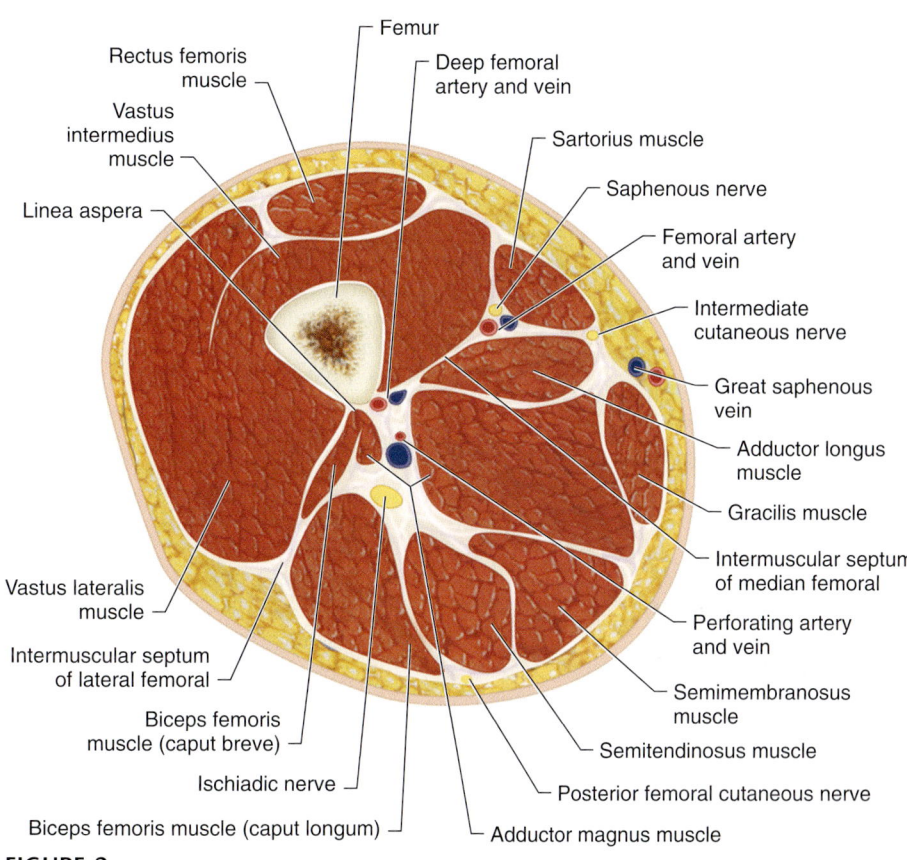

Rectus femoris muscle

Femur

Deep femoral artery and vein

Vastus intermedius muscle

Sartorius muscle

Linea aspera

Saphenous nerve

Femoral artery and vein

Intermediate cutaneous nerve

Great saphenous vein

Adductor longus muscle

Gracilis muscle

Intermuscular septum of median femoral

Perforating artery and vein

Vastus lateralis muscle

Semimembranosus muscle

Intermuscular septum of lateral femoral

Semitendinosus muscle

Biceps femoris muscle (caput breve)

Ischiadic nerve

Posterior femoral cutaneous nerve

Biceps femoris muscle (caput longum)

Adductor magnus muscle

FIGURE 2

Equipment

• Avoid tourniquet control as it tends to bind the rectus muscle and decrease the overall excursion that is vital for a successful transfer.

■ The anterior and medial compartments of the upper leg are divided by a medial intermuscular septum that connects the medial aspect of the vastus medialis with the lateral border of the adductor magnus tendon. It is this intermuscular septum that must be pierced to facilitate the transfer of the rectus femoris tendon into the medial compartment to join with either the semitendinosus or the gracilis (Fig. 3).

POSITIONING

■ The patient is placed supine with a bump placed under the knee to allow 30° of flexion of the knee.
■ The posterior preparation of the hamstring tendons can be accomplished medially by abducting and externally rotating the leg while the patient is supine.

PORTALS/EXPOSURES

■ A longitudinal midline incision from the superior pole of the patella 6–10 cm proximally is preferred (Fig. 4); however, several different incisions have been described in the literature, including a transverse incision.
■ Sharp dissection is carried down to the deep fasica of the thigh.
■ Proximally, the rectus femoris tendon is isolated from the underlying vastus intermedius and adjacent vastus medialis and lateralis.
  • Proximally, small longitudinal incisions (1–2 cm) are made along the medial and lateral borders of the rectus femoris.
  • A septal or Freer elevator is inserted to bluntly establish the plane between the rectus femoris and vastus intermedius (Fig. 5). Once the plane has been established, further blunt dissection with an index finger can help facilitate the dissection distally.
  • A combination of sharp and blunt dissection using a scissors and/or knife (beaver blade) to free up the remaining soft tissue attachments is acceptable (Fig. 6).
  • The surgeon must take care to ensure that the joint is not violated distally near the patella and that the insertion of the vastus intermedius is not violated.
■ Next a full-thickness medial skin flap is developed bluntly to the posterior border of the vastus medialis (a knee retractor can help facilitate the exposure).
  • The deep fascia over the vastus medialis is opened. A plane of dissection is developed deep to the vastus medialis fascia and carried to the posterior border of the vastus medialis. Here the medial intermuscular septum is visualized (Fig. 7).

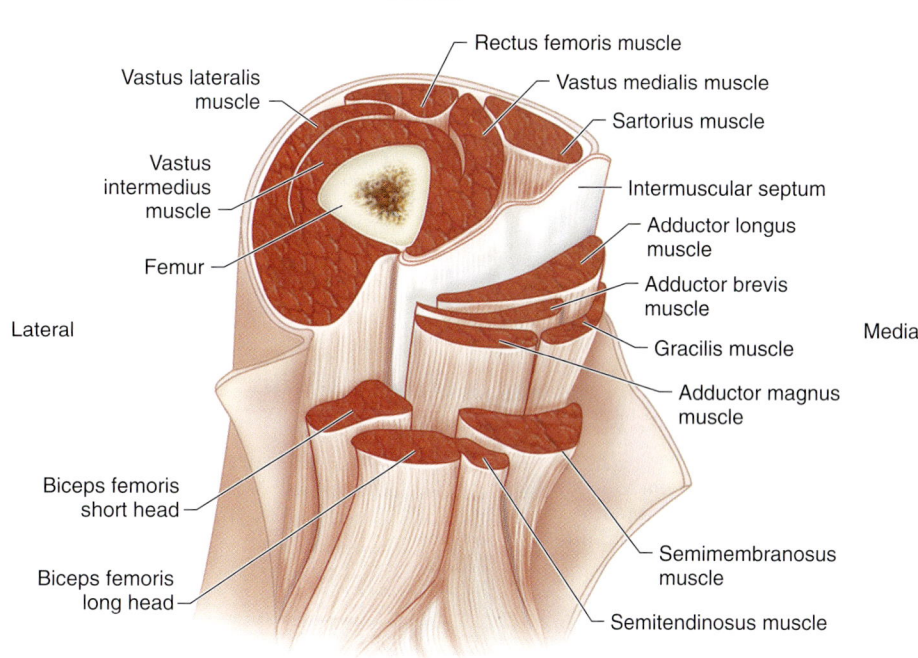

Anterior

Rectus femoris muscle

Vastus lateralis muscle

Vastus medialis muscle

Sartorius muscle

Vastus intermedius muscle

Intermuscular septum

Adductor longus muscle

Femur

Adductor brevis muscle

Lateral

Gracilis muscle

Medial

Adductor magnus muscle

Biceps femoris short head

Semimembranosus muscle

Biceps femoris long head

Semitendinosus muscle

Posterior

FIGURE 3

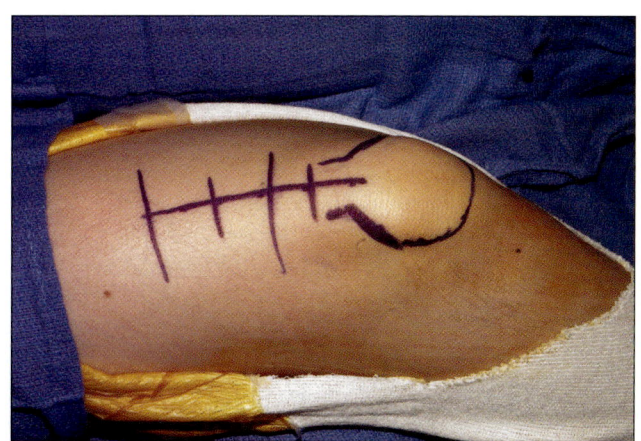

FIGURE 4

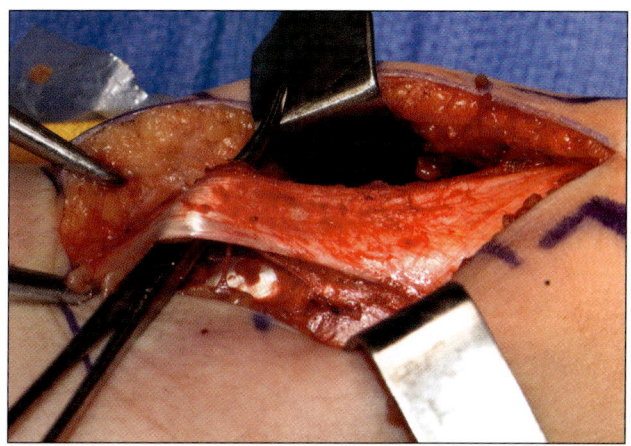

FIGURE 5

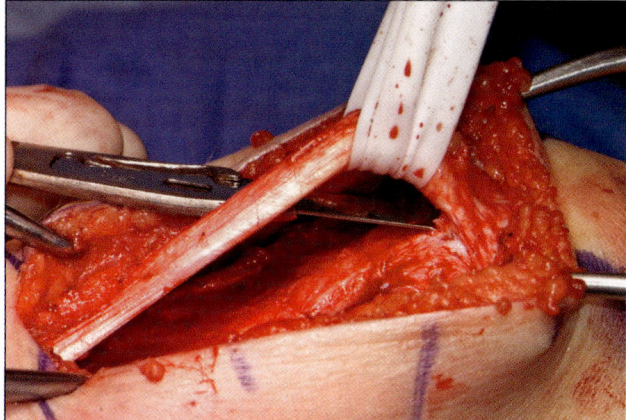

FIGURE 6

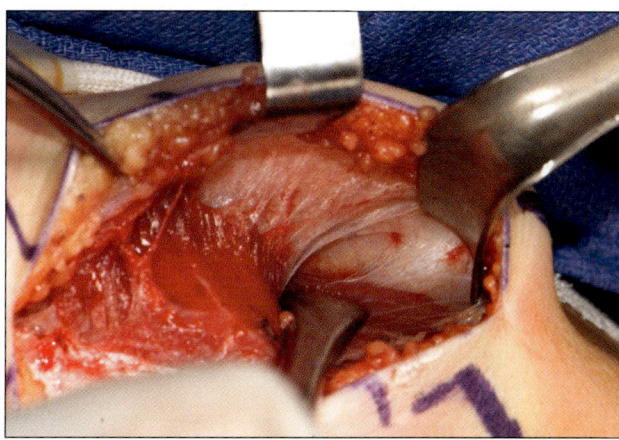

FIGURE 7

PEARLS

- *The rectus femoris can be adherent to the vastus intermedius distally at the patella; therefore, dissection of the rectus femoris off the vastus intermedius is easiest in the proximal extent of the inicision.*

PITFALLS

- *If dissection of the rectus femoris is difficult with blunt dissection, this can be a clue that the surgical plane is incorrect, and careful re-evaluation of surgical planes should follow.*

- *For the transfer to be successful, the rectus tendon must have a gradual curve medially in the anterior thigh; acute angles will compromise the function of the transfer.*

- A posterior incision for isolated hamstring lengthening is made at this point to identify and prepare the semitendinosus or gracilis tendon for transfer (see Portals/Exposure in Knee Surgery for Children with Cerebral Palsy I).
- The medial intermuscular septum is palpated from the anterior and posterior compartments of the thigh simultaneously prior to creating a window in the septum (Fig. 8).
  - The window in the septum is created through a combination of sharp and blunt dissection (6 cm in length) (Fig. 9).
  - The track created should be sufficiently large to prevent tethering of the rectus femoris as it is reorientated from the anterior to the posterior compartment.

PROCEDURE

STEP 1

- Once the rectus femoris is clearly dissected free from the remaining vastus structures, the tendon is amputated 1 cm proximal to the superior pole of the patella (Figs. 10 and 11).

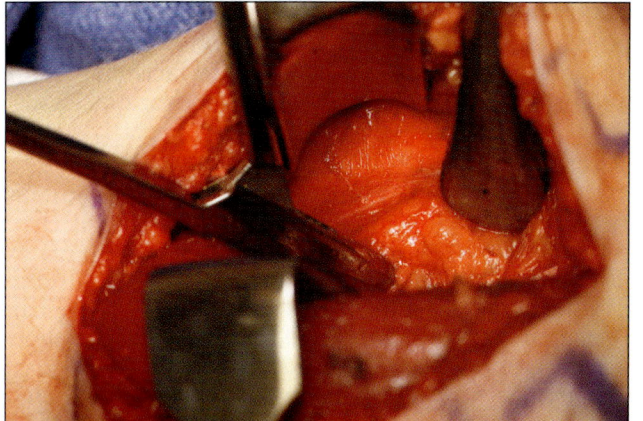

FIGURE 8

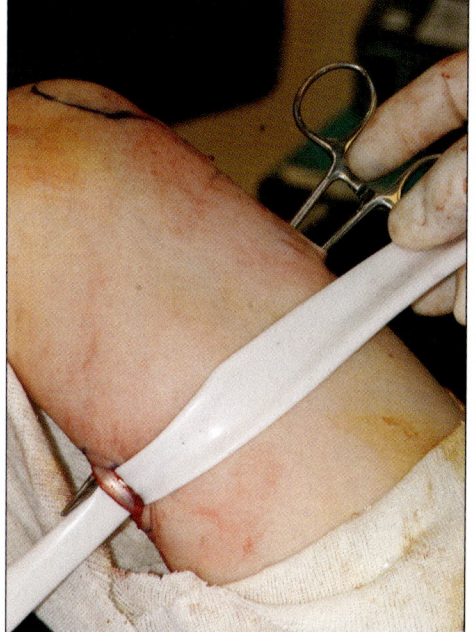

FIGURE 9

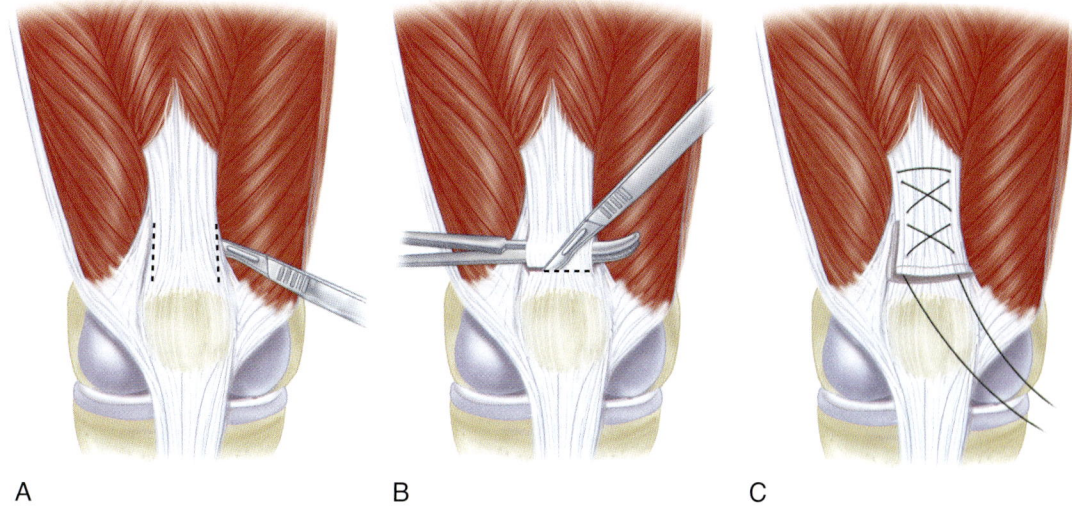

A   B   C

FIGURE 10

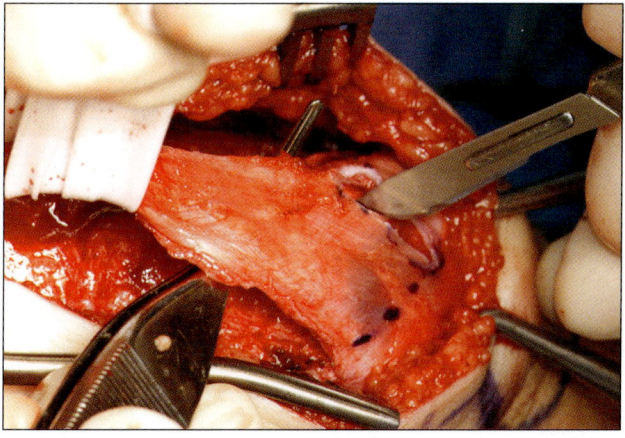

FIGURE 11

PEARLS

- *Wide exposure of the window in the medial intermuscular septum facilitates the transfer of the rectus femoris from the anterior to the posterior compartment and decreases the risk of scarring.*

- *Simultaneous palpation of the medial intermuscular septum from the anterior and posterior compartments minimizes the risk of injury to the femoral artery and vein and the saphenous nerve, which runs along the posterior border of the sartorius.*

- A locking whipstitch is placed using size 0 or 2-0 Ethibond (nonabsorbable braided suture) in the distal stump of the tendon (5 cm), and the tendon is tubularized to facilitate tenodesis to the stump of the semitendinosus and/or gracilis (Fig. 12).

- Once the rectus femoris tendon is prepared, care is taken to bluntly dissect the muscle belly proximally well beyond the extent of the skin incision. It is important to free the rectus femoris proximally from its surrounding attachments as much as possible so that a gradual transition of the tendon occurs from the anterior to the posterior compartment of the thigh (Fig. 13).

- Once the whipstitch is placed within the tendon, in-line traction can be applied to ensure that there is adequate tendon excursion and all underlying soft tissue attachments have been addressed.

- Gracilis is the tendon of choice for our transfer (Fig. 14). The gracilis tendon is identified at its musculotendinosus junction and sharply transected. Proximally, the gracilis can also be tenodesed to the tendinous stump of the semitendinosus to reinforce the distal point of attachment.

- The tendon of the gracilis is prepared distally with a locking stitch for easier recognition at the time of transfer (Fig. 15).

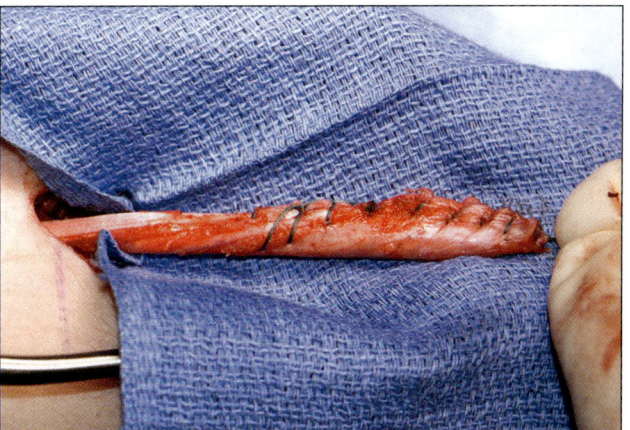

FIGURE 12

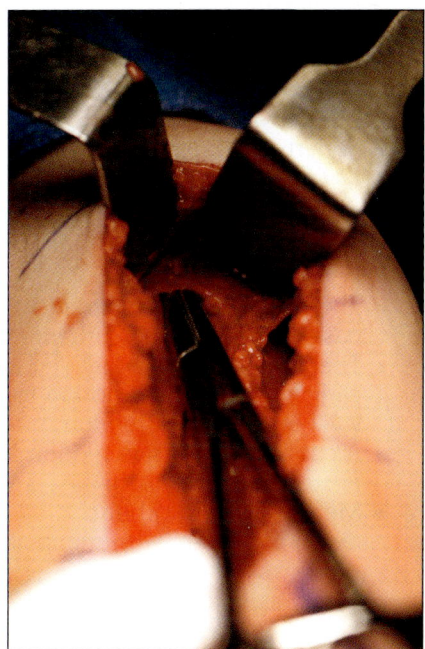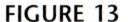

FIGURE 13

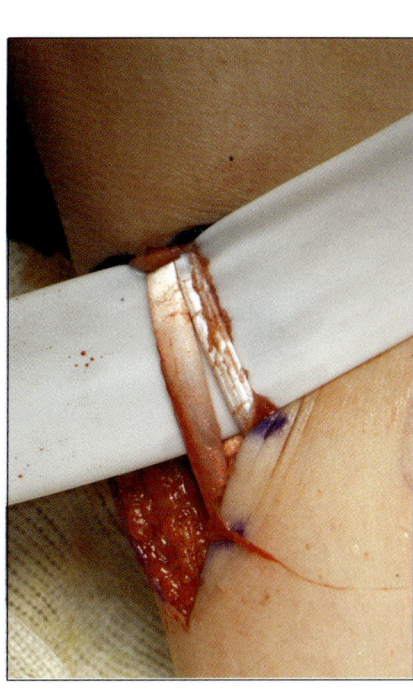

FIGURE 14

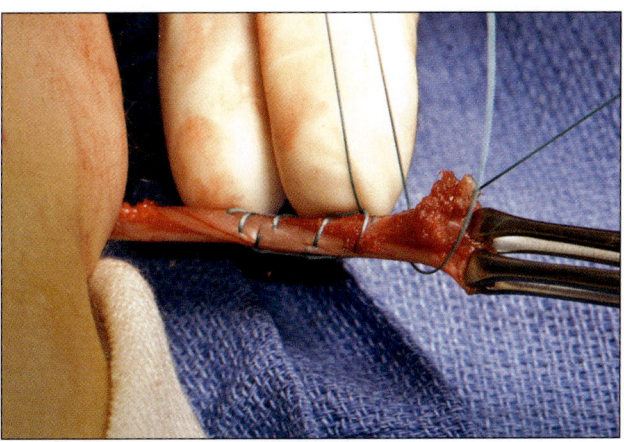

FIGURE 15

Controversies

• Early mobilization of the knee is believed by some to create wound problems; however, the authors believe that a vertical midline incision and careful soft tissue handling permit early safe postoperative passive range of motion with minimal risk for wound breakdown.

• If a transverse incision is utilized, wound breakdown risk with early range of motion becomes a greater concern.

• Avoid rectus tendon transfers in GMFCS IV or V patients, as minimal ambulators tend to benefit least from this procedure.

STEP 2

■ The rectus femoris tendon is brought through the intermuscular septum and sutured to the gracilis in a side-to-side fashion (Fig. 16).

■ The transfer is fixed with the knee at 20–30° of flexion to generate the appropriate degree of tension with the rectus femoris tendon being brought into the posterior compartment for fixation.

■ The knee should be able to reach full extension after the transfer, and care should be taken to ensure that there are no soft tissue attachments impeding smooth excursion of either muscle.

■ The two tendons are sutured in a series of side-to-side repair using a series of horizontal mattress stitches with nonabsorbable suture (Ethibond) (Fig. 17).

■ Some surgeons advocate a Pulvertaft-type weave of the two tendons. However, in children with small-diameter tendons, this is often quite challengeing and runs the risk of damaging the integrity and quality of the recipient gracilis tendon.

STEP 3

■ The wounds are closed in layers.

■ The partial-thickness defect in the quadriceps is repaired with 2-0 Vicryl suture (Fig. 18).

■ Robert-Jones dressings are applied with knee immobilizers.

POSTOPERATIVE CARE AND EXPECTED OUTCOMES

■ The postoperative regimen and weight-bearing status will vary based on associated surgeries.

■ The authors believe that key to success for this procedure is early knee range of motion to prevent scar formation at the level of the rectus tendon.

■ A continuous passive motion knee machine is used postoperatively for the first 3 weeks.

■ Meticulous surgical dissection and closure facilitates early passive range of motion with minimal postoperative skin complications.

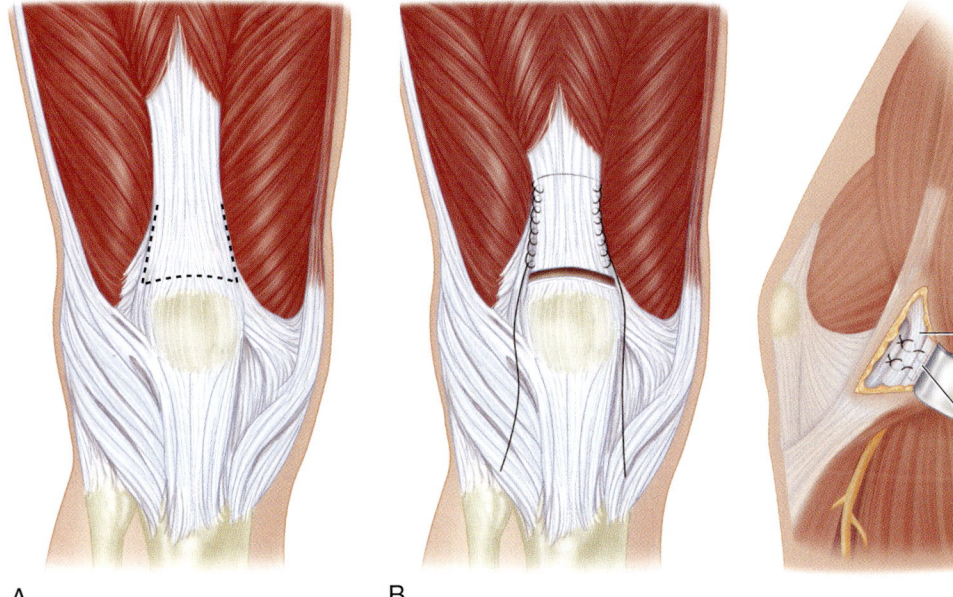

A   B

FIGURE 16

Rectus
femoris
tendon

Semitendinosus
tendon

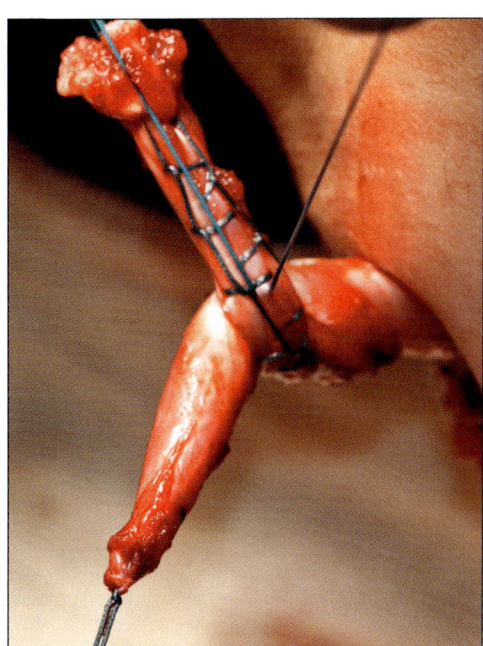

FIGURE 17

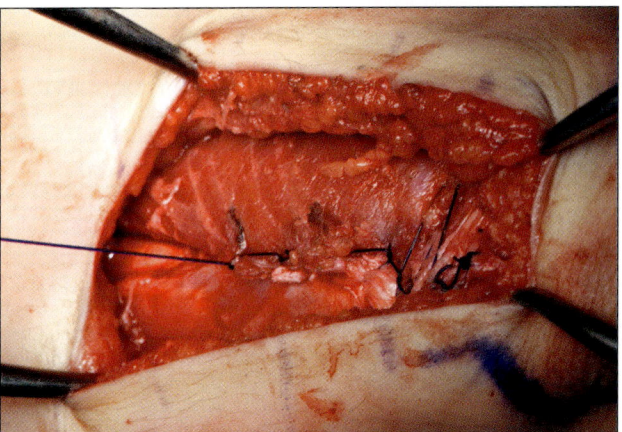

FIGURE 18

EVIDENCE

Gage JR, Perry J, Jicks RR, Koop S, Werntz JR. Rectus femoris transfer to improve knee function of children with cerebral palsy. Dev Med Child Neurol. 1987;29:159–66.

This paper presents the outcome of transfer of the distal end of the rectus femoris in conjunction with hamstrings lengthening in 37 knees, and compares it with a control group of 24 knees in which only hamstrings lengthening was done. In the first group swing-phase knee flexion was improved by $16.0 \pm 14.4°$, compared to $9.5 \pm 7.5°$ in the control group, and residual knee flexion in stance was reduced to $8.9 \pm 8.1°$, compared to $15.1 \pm 13.8°$ in the controls. Poor outcome in the transfer-plus-lengthening group was associated mainly with foot rotation in excess of 8° internally or externally, or postoperative knee flexion in stance. (Level IV evidence)

Kay RM, Rethlefsen SA, Kelly JP, Wren TA. Predictive value of the Duncan-Ely test in distal rectus femoris transfer. J Pediatr Orthop. 2004;24:59–62.

A retrospective review of 56 patients who underwent 94 distal rectus femoris transfers with pre- and postoperative gait analyses. Patients were divided into three groups based on pre- and postoperative Duncan-Ely tests. Group A (34 limbs) had positive tests both before and after surgery. Group B (46 limbs) had positive tests before surgery and negative tests after surgery. Group C (13 limbs) had negative tests both before and after surgery. Knee arc increased significantly in both groups with positive preoperative Duncan-Ely tests (groups A and B), but not in the group with negative preoperative tests (group C). The timing of peak knee flexion in swing improved in all groups, but the change was smaller and not statistically significant in the group with negative preoperative tests (group C). The findings of the current study indicate that the Duncan-Ely test may be a helpful predictor of outcome in children for whom distal rectus femoris transfer is being considered. (Level IV evidence)

Marks MC, Alexander J, Sutherland DH, Chambers HG. Clinical utility of the Duncan-Ely test for rectus femoris dysfunction during the swing phase of gait. Dev Med Child Neurol. 2003;45:763–8.

In this retrospective review, patients' dynamic knee range of motion (ROM) during gait and an electromyogram (EMG) were compared with the results of the Ely test. Data for 70 patients (44 males, 26 females; 104 limbs) were included. All patients were diagnosed with cerebral palsy and ambulatory (spastic diplegia, n = 42; spastic quadriplegia, n =15, and hemiplegia, n = 13). For the gait variables examined (decreased dynamic knee ROM, timing of peak knee flexion, and abnormal EMG in swing) the sensitivity of the Ely test ranged from 56 to 59% and the specificity ranged from 64 to 85%. For the same variables the positive predictive value ranged from 91 to 98% and the negative predictive value ranged from 4 to 19%. (Level IV evidence)

Ounpuu S, Muik E, Davis III RB, Gage JR, DeLuca PA. Rectus femoris surgery in children with cerebral palsy. Part I: The effect of rectus femoris transfer location on knee motion. J Pediatr Orthop. 1993a;13:325–30.

This was a retrospective review of rectus femoris muscle (RF) surgery on 98 children (136 sides) with cerebral palsy (CP). Gait analysis was performed just before and approximately 1 year after surgery. When preoperative knee range of motion (ROM) was > 80% of normal, there were no significant changes in knee motion in either the RF transfer or distal release groups. In patients with < 80% of normal knee ROM preoperatively, RF transfer was followed by maintained knee flexion in swing; patients who underwent distal RF release or no RF procedure showed a decrease (10° and 6°, respectively) in knee flexion postoperatively. These results suggest that the RF should be transferred and not released when knee ROM is < 80%. (Level IV evidence)

Ounpuu S, Muik E, Davis III RB, Gage JR, DeLuca PA. Rectus femoris surgery in children with cerebral palsy. Part II: A comparison between the effect of transfer and release of the distal rectus femoris on knee motion. J Pediatr Orthop. 1993b;13:331–5.

This was a retrospective review of 78 children (105 sides) with cerebral palsy (CP) who underwent rectus femoris transfer. The transfer was either medial to the sartorius (62 sides), semitendinosus (19 sides), or the gracilis (14 sides) muscles, or laterally to the iliotibial band (10 sides). Gait analysis performed before and 1 year after operation demonstrated increased knee range of motion (ROM) with increased extension at initial contact and in midstance and maintained knee flexion in swing. There were no statistically significant differences between the four transfer sites in the effect on those variables. There was no consistent change in transverse plane motion of the hip or foot progression angles between the two gait analyses, suggesting that rectus femoris transfer does not affect gait abnormalities observed in the transverse plane. (Level IV evidence)

Rethlefsen SA, Kam G, Wren TA, Kay RM. Predictors of outcome of distal rectus femoris transfer surgery in ambulatory children with cerebral palsy. J Pediatr Orthop B. 2009;18:58–62.

This retrospective review examined pre- and postoperative gait data for 81 patients, focusing on knee flexion/extension range. Outcome was 'good' for 46 patient and 'poor' for 35. The poor outcome group had no improvement in knee range because of increased crouch postoperatively. Outcome was unrelated to quadriceps strength, crouch, velocity, or type of cerebral palsy. Gross Motor Function Classification System was predictive of outcome, with poor results in all level IV patients (P ≤ 0.008). In conclusion, Gross Motor Function Classification System IV patients may not benefit from distal rectus femoris transfer because of increased postoperative crouch. (Level IV evidence)

TIBIA AND ANKLE

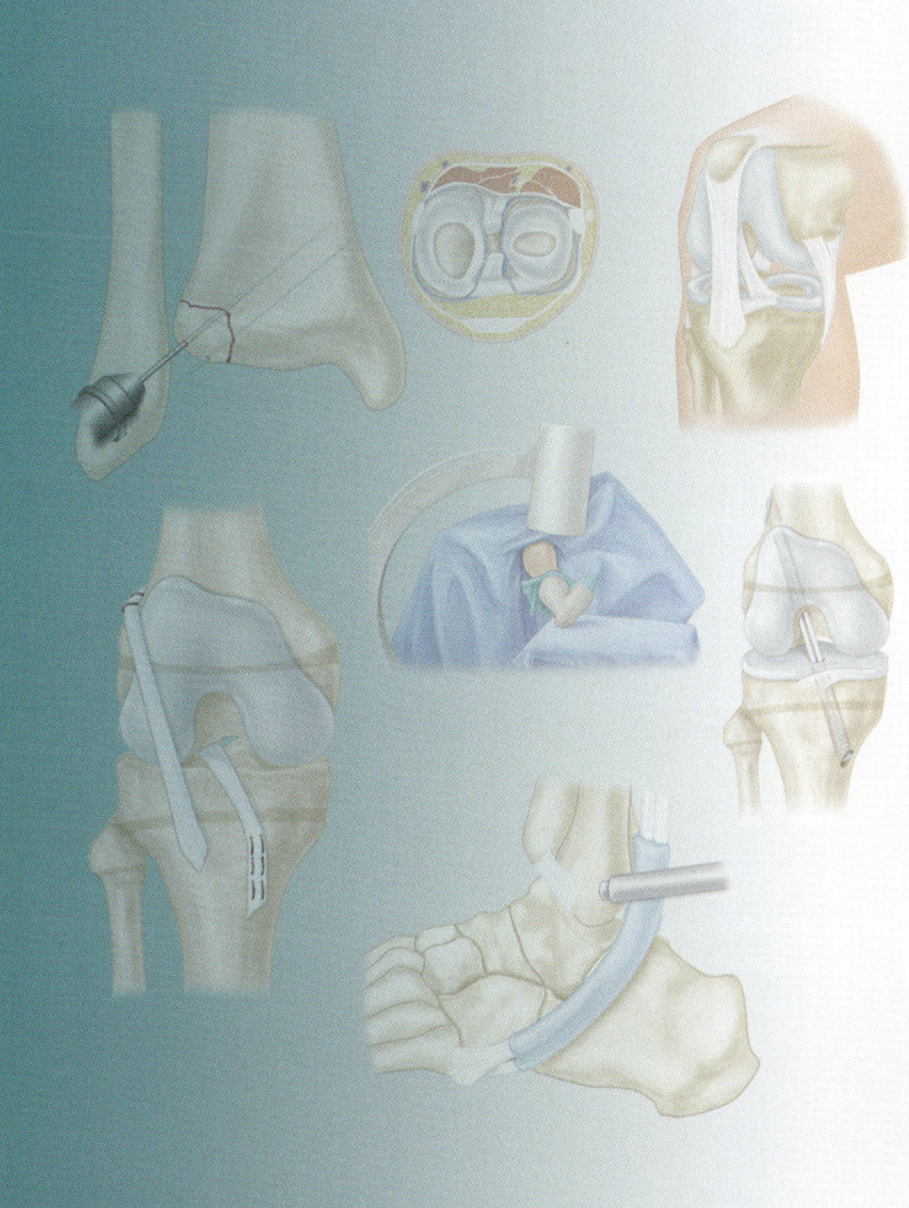

Tibial Spine Fracture: Arthroscopic and Open Reduction and Internal Fixation

Dennis E. Kramer

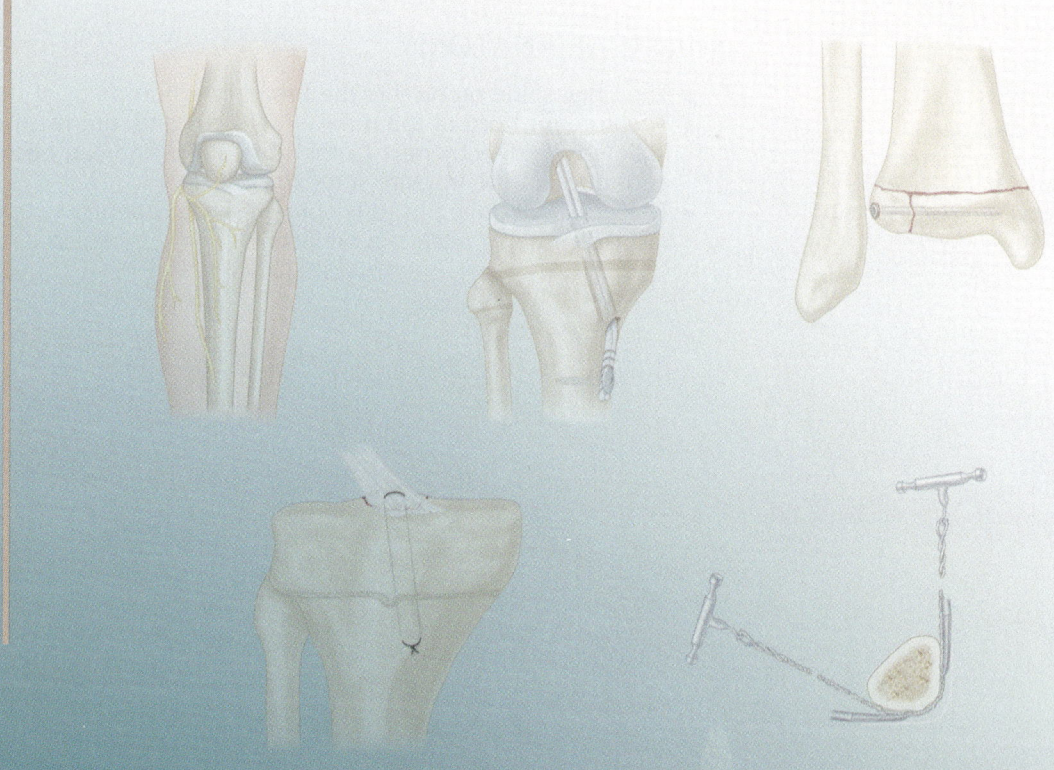

PITFALLS

- *Displacement may be difficult to determine on radiographs. If uncertain, a computed tomography scan can be obtained to accurately measure displacement.*
- *Proximal displacement of the anteriormost portion of the tibial spine may not be clinically relevant. If the majority of the anterior cruciate ligament (ACL) insertion on the tibia is reduced, the fracture can be treated conservatively.*

Controversies

- If Lachman's sign is positive, it may be indicative of concurrent plastic deformation of the ACL. Some feel this is a relative surgical indication as the fracture can be over-reduced to re-tension the ACL.

Treatment Options

- Arthroscopic versus open reduction of fragment
- Fixation with metal or bioabsorbable screws or sutures

INDICATIONS

- Displaced type 2 tibial spine fractures that do not reduce in extension
- All type 3 tibial spine fractures

EXAMINATION/IMAGING

- Anteroposterior and lateral (Fig. 1A) radiographs are mandatory.
- Computed tomography (CT) or magnetic resonance imaging (MRI) may be obtained depending on surgeon preference.
  - CT (Fig. 1B) is most useful for determining fragment size and accurately measuring displacement.
  - MRI (Fig. 1C) assesses integrity of the ACL and helps to identify concurrent meniscal pathology.

SURGICAL ANATOMY

- The tibial spine represents the broad insertion point of the ACL.
- The anterior horn of the medial meniscus and intermeniscal ligament lie directly next to the tibial spine and can become entrapped in the fracture site (Fig. 2).
- The proximal tibial physis is open in most patients, as fracture most commonly occurs in skeletally immature adolescents.

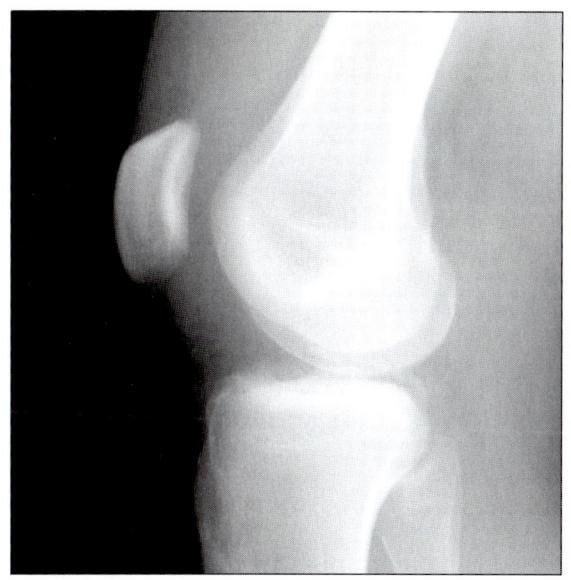

A

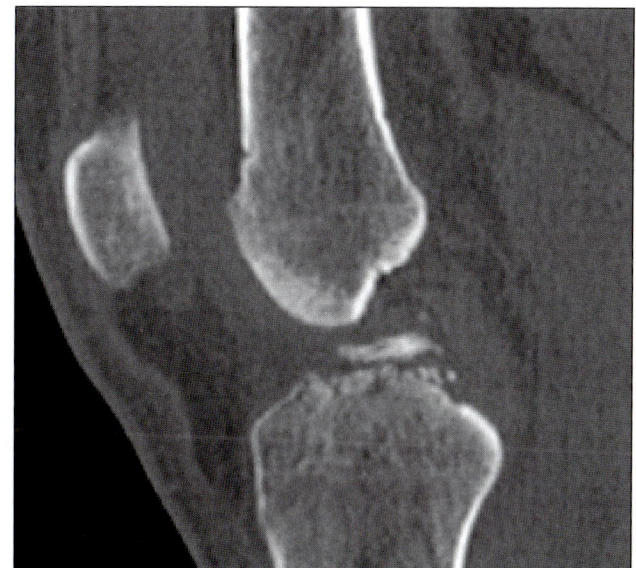

B

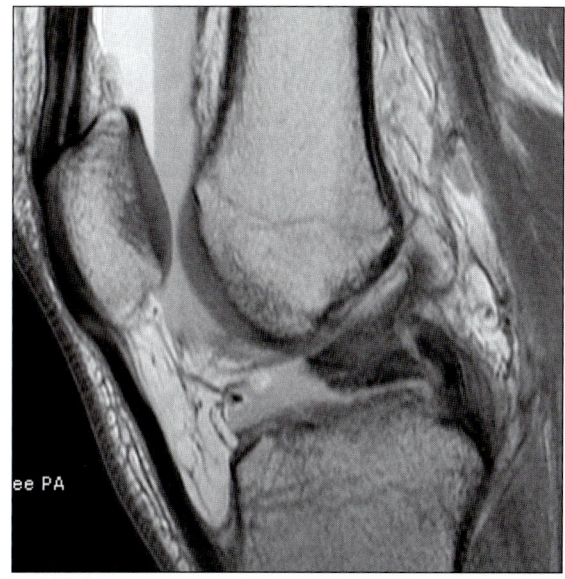

C

FIGURE 1

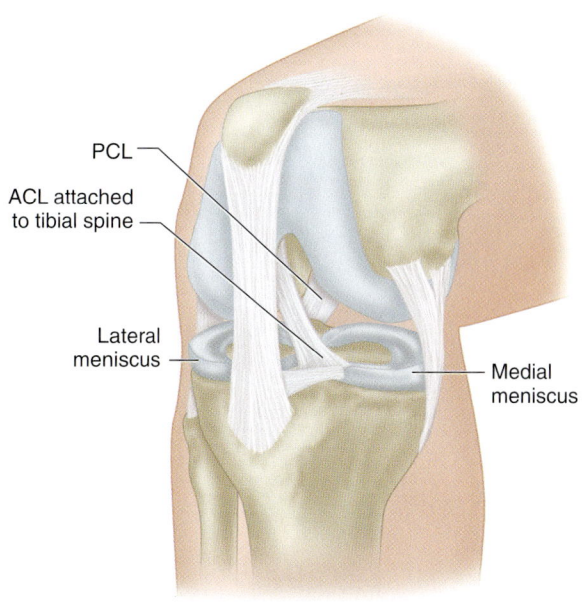

FIGURE 2

PEARLS

- *Ensure proper positioning of the fluoroscopy unit to limit the amount of knee manipulation necessary to obtain a lateral image following fragment reduction.*

PITFALLS

- *A low-positioned tourniquet can interfere with proximal portals used for screw placement.*

Equipment

- In our experience, a mini C-arm is preferable to a larger fluoroscopy unit.

PEARLS

- *A superomedial portal positioned at the proximal medial border of the patella will provide the best access for fragment fixation. This should be utilized for the first fixation device. Use a superolateral portal for supplementary fixation if necessary.*

Controversies

- The inferomedial incision site for the suture lasso technique may be placed proximal or distal to the tibial physis. Both techniques have been described. A distal incision site allows for easier tunnel placement but the suture crosses the physis.

POSITIONING

- The patient is placed supine with the leg hanging over the side of the bed.
- A tourniquet is positioned proximally on the thigh.
- A standard fluoroscopy unit or mini C-arm is positioned so that it can easily be brought in to obtain a lateral fluoroscopic image of the reduction and fixation (Fig. 3). This can be accomplished with the leg in the figure-of-4 position.

PORTALS/EXPOSURES

- Figure 4 illustrates potential portals used in arthroscopic reduction and internal fixation of tibial spine fractures.
  - Standard anteromedial and anterolateral arthroscopy portals
  - Superomedial portal for placement of first cannulated screw or Kirschner wire (K-wire)
  - Alternate superolateral portal for placement of second screw or K-wire
  - Inferomedial incision for suture lasso technique

PROCEDURE

STEP 1: EXPOSURE OF THE FRAGMENT

- The arthroscope is placed in the anterolateral portal.
- The knee is lavaged immediately to clear hemarthrosis.
- An oscillating shaver is used to perform extensive fat pad débridement.
- Diagnostic arthroscopy is performed to identify and treat concurrent meniscal pathology.
  - The tibial spine fracture site is identified.
  - The surgeon should look for an entrapped anterior horn of the medial meniscus or intermeniscal ligament.
  - An arthroscopic probe is used to pull out the meniscus or intermeniscal ligament from the fracture site.
- A spinal needle is used through the anteromedial portal to place a temporary outside-in suture (0 Prolene works well) around the anterior horn of the medial meniscus or intermeniscal ligament (Fig. 5). This suture is used to retract the anterior horn and keep it out of the fracture site during reduction and fixation.

PEARLS

- *Place a heavy Kelly clamp around the Prolene suture coming out of the anteromedial portal to allow gravity to retract the anterior horn of the medial meniscus.*

PITFALLS

- *Insufficient fat pad débridement will impede visualization during the key steps of reduction and fixation.*

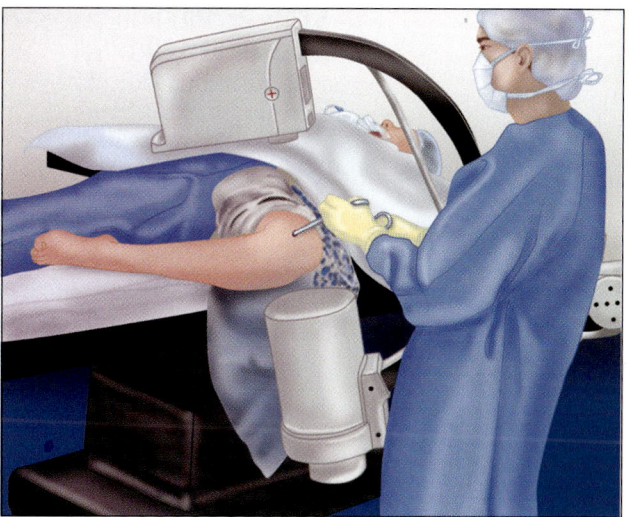

FIGURE 3

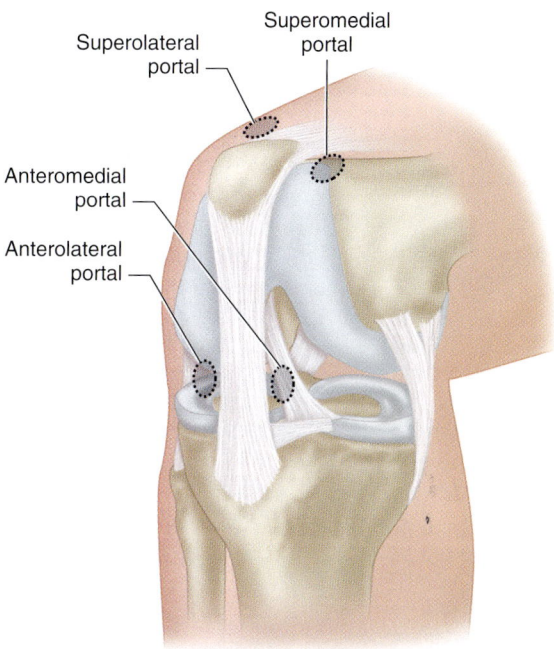

Superolateral portal

Superomedial portal

Anteromedial portal

Anterolateral portal

FIGURE 4

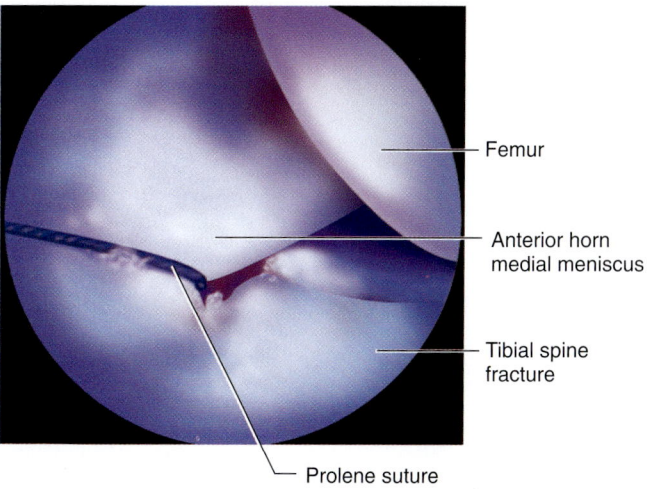

Femur

Anterior horn medial meniscus

Tibial spine fracture

Prolene suture

FIGURE 5

PEARLS

- *Remove a small amount of excess sub-chondral cancellous bone from the base of the fracture site to help with over-reduction of the fragment, which better tensions the ACL.*

PITFALLS

- *Avoid removing any bone from the tibial spine fragment itself—it is usually thin and fragile.*

Instrumentation/Implantation

- Mastoid curettes
- A 2.9-mm shaver

PEARLS

- *The tibial spine fragment is often hinged laterally; use the hinge as a key to reduction.*
- *A knee flexion angle of 30–45° and slight posterior pressure on the tibia should take tension off the ACL and allow for the best reduction.*

PITFALLS

- *If arthroscopic visualization is difficult and fragment reduction cannot be confirmed, do not hesitate to proceed with an arthrotomy, which can still be done through a minimally invasive incision and approach.*

STEP 2: PREPARATION OF THE FRAGMENT AND FRACTURE SITE

- Fibrinous clot material is removed from the fracture site using tiny mastoid curettes and a shaver.
- If the fragment is hinged, the surgeon should try to leave the hinge intact.
- A smaller (2.9-mm) shaver can be useful for débriding the tissue in the fracture bed (Fig. 6A).
- The arthroscope can be moved into the fracture site to ensure débridement is complete (Fig. 6B).

STEP 3: REDUCTION OF THE FRAGMENT

- With the arthroscope remaining in the anterolateral portal, a probe or blunt obturator is placed through the anteromedial portal.
- Knee flexion is adjusted to whatever best reduces the displaced fragment (Fig. 7) and places it under the least amount of tension.
- The fragment is reduced and held in place with the probe or blunt obturator (Fig. 8).
  - An attempt should be made to over-reduce the fragment by 1–2 mm.
- Fragment reduction is confirmed by visualizing the medial and lateral walls of the fragment in relation to the medial and lateral tibial plateau surface (Fig. 9).
- If visualization is difficult, the surgeon should proceed with arthrotomy.
  - For arthrotomy, the anteromedial portal is extended 2–3 cm proximally.
  - An Army-Navy retractor is used to retract the patellar tendon and fat pad laterally and the medial retinacular tissue medially.
- Following arthrotomy, the surgeon can visually confirm fragment reduction and use the index finger to hold the fracture reduced.

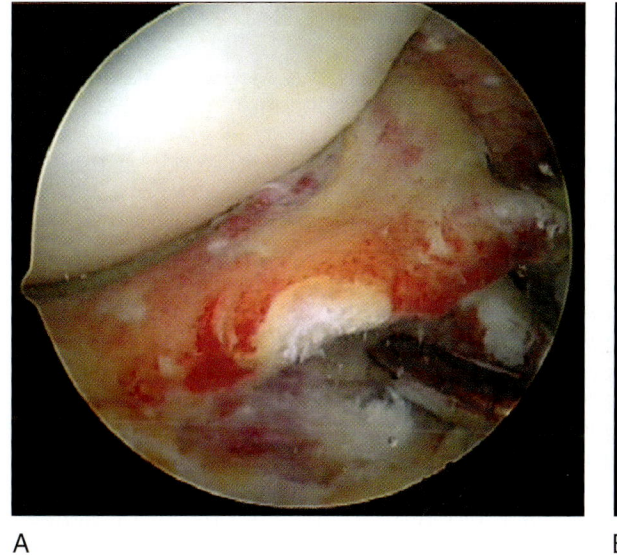

A

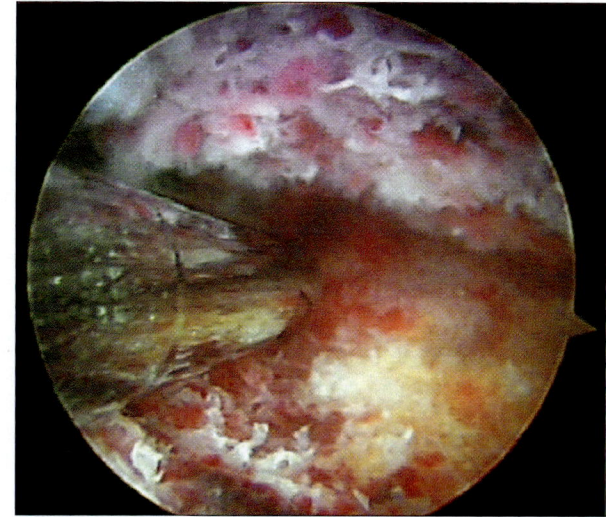

B

FIGURE 6

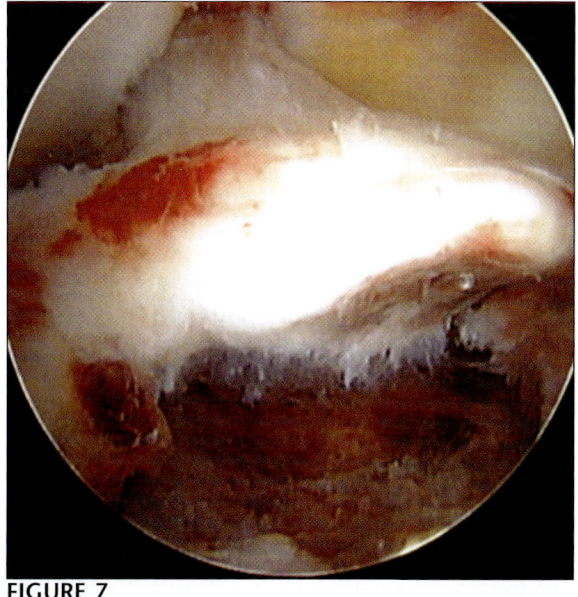

FIGURE 7

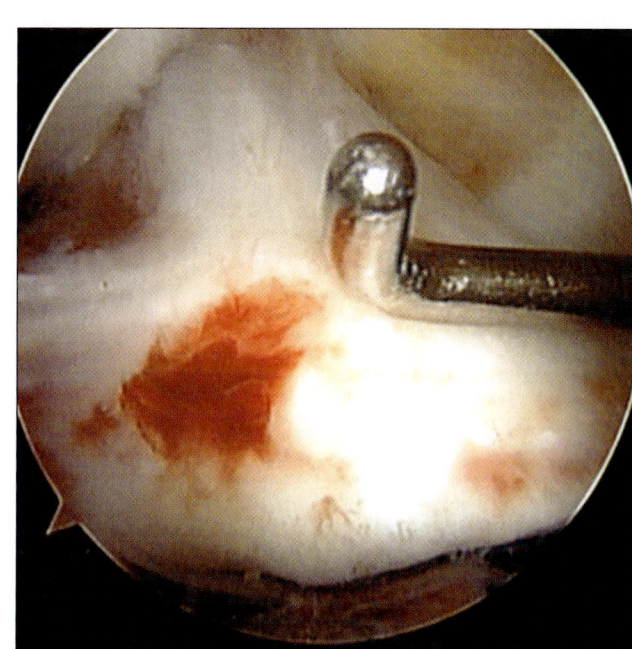

FIGURE 8

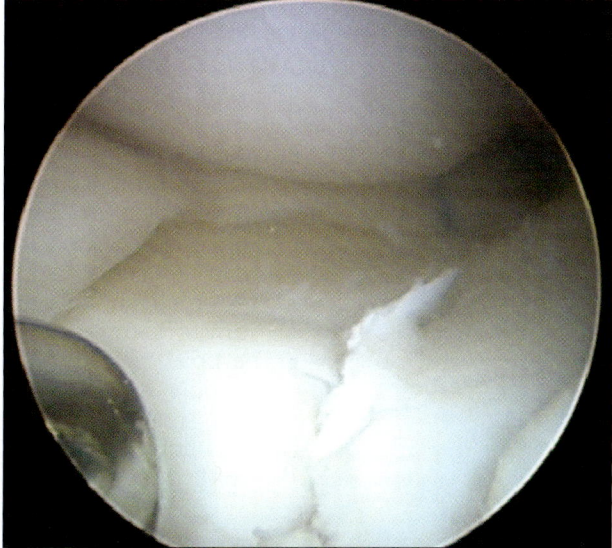

FIGURE 9

STEP 4A: EPIPHYSEAL CANNULATED SCREW FIXATION OF THE FRAGMENT

- One or two 3.5-mm partially threaded cannulated screws are used for fixation of a large, noncomminuted tibial spine fragment (>1 cm^2).
- The first guide pin is placed through the skin at the superomedial border of the patella.
  - An accessory portal is made here to facilitate guide pin passage. The surgeon must stay proximal enough to get the proper angle into the tibia.
- The guide pin is advanced to the fracture fragment by hand.
- The guide pin is drilled across the tibial spine fragment wherever the bone of the fragment is the thickest. This is often at the anterior base of the ACL insertion.
- The guide pin is advanced into the tibia to just past the level of the proximal tibial physis.
  - On a lateral fluoroscopic view, an approximately 30–45° angle for the guide pin into the tibia with the guide pin heading distally and posteriorly is optimal.
- The surgeon should attempt to get a second guide pin across the fracture site, if possible.
  - The ideal starting position for both guide pins is proximal medial.
  - If there is no room at the superomedial border of the patella for a second guide pin, then place the second guide pin percutaneously near the superolateral border of the patella.
  - This would be used for temporary fixation only as it is very difficult to place a screw in the tibial spine fragment from a proximal lateral starting point.
- When two guide pins are in place, reduction and pin position are confirmed with a lateral fluoroscopic image.
  - Our preference is to place the leg in the figure-of-4 position with the foot on the end of the bed and use the mini C-arm to hover over the bed to obtain a lateral image of the knee.
- Screw length (typical = 16 mm) is estimated or checked with a depth gauge.
- The surgeon next drills and taps over the guide pin(s).
- A 3.5-mm cannulated screw is placed up to but not across the proximal tibial physis. A probe is used to hold the tibial spine reduced while the cannulated screw is placed into the tibial spine fragment at the base of the ACL (Fig. 10A), as seen in the lateral radiographic image of screw placement in Figure 10B.
  - Single screw fixation is acceptable if good purchase is obtained.
  - If the fragment is large enough, a second screw is placed.

STEP 4B: SUTURE LASSO TECHNIQUE FOR FRAGMENT FIXATION

- Suture fixation is used for smaller fragments and/or comminution.
- Two sutures are passed around the base of the ACL at its insertion on the tibial spine (Fig. 11A).
  - A special suture punch instrument from a shoulder arthroscopy set, such as the suture lasso (Arthrex, Naples, FL), can be used to help pass the sutures arthroscopically.
  - Alternatively, sutures can be passed with a standard needle driver following an arthrotomy.
- The tibial spine fragment is held reduced with the tip of the ACL tibial tunnel guide (Fig. 11B).
  - The surgeon may consider obtaining temporary fixation at this point by placing a 1-mm K-wire across the fragment as well.

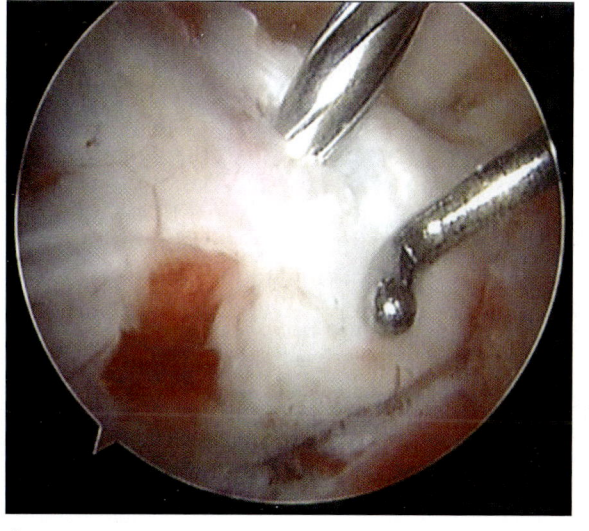

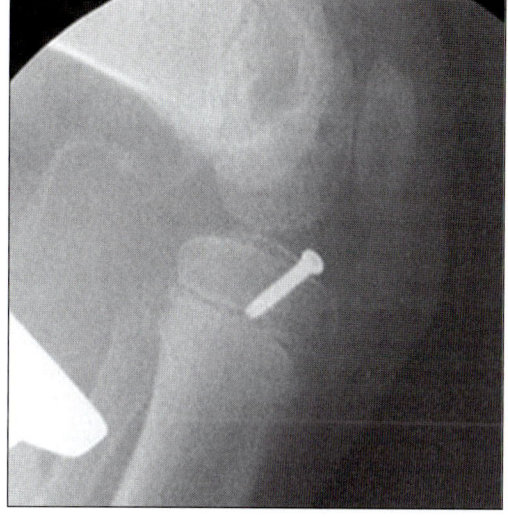

A

B

FIGURE 10

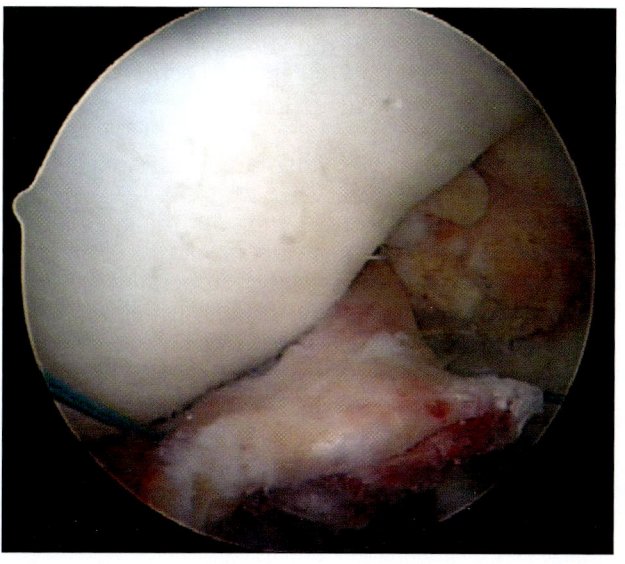

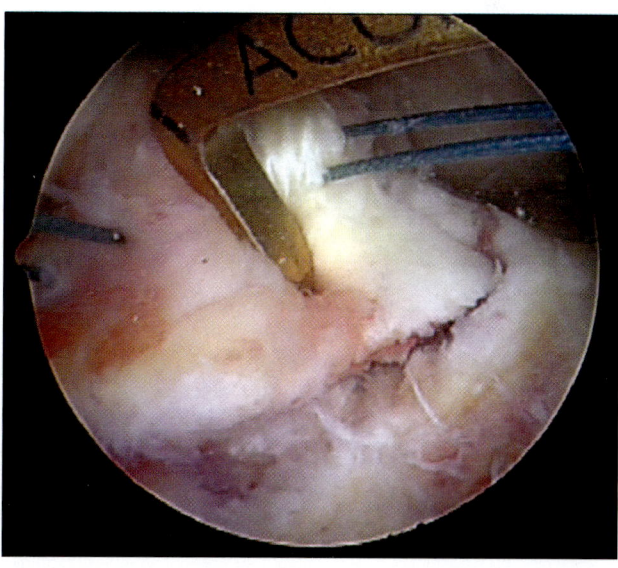

A

B

FIGURE 11

Instrumentation/ Implantation

- Either absorbable or nonabsorbable suture may be used. Our current preference is to use nonabsorbable suture (#5 Ethibond or FiberWire).

Controversies

- The proximal tibial physis is at risk during drilling of the tibial tunnels. While drilling two small tunnels across the physis with a smooth guide pin may be safe, nonabsorbable suture crossing the physis poses a theoretic risk of physeal injury due to tethering.

PEARLS

- *Encourage hamstring strengthening in physical therapy to protect the ACL, which may have some plastic deformation.*

PITFALLS

- *Early diagnosis of extensor lag should be treated with physical therapy for quadriceps strengthening.*
- *Delayed instability can occur following anatomic reduction and fixation if plastic deformation of the ACL occurred at the time of injury.*

Controversies

- Cannulated screws may be removed at 3–6 months postoperatively; alternatively, they can be left in place.

- Reduction is confirmed under fluoroscopy as for the screw fixation technique.
- A 2-cm vertical incision is made over the proximal medial tibia 2 cm distal to the joint line and 1 cm medial to the tibial tubercle.
- Two smooth K-wires and the tibial guide from the ACL reconstruction kit are used to drill two parallel bone tunnels retrograde through the proximal tibia and into the medial and lateral aspects of the ACL insertion point (Fig. 12).
  - There should be a minimum 1-cm horizontal tibial bone bridge between each tunnel at the proximal medial tibia.
  - The medial tibial tunnel enters the knee joint just medial to the base of the ACL while the lateral tibial tunnel enters just lateral to the ACL base.
- K-wires are then sequentially removed and each end of the suture is pulled antegrade through the corresponding bone tunnel using a suture passer.
- Each suture is pulled taut and then tied to itself over the bone bridge of the proximal medial tibia (Fig. 13).
- Figure 14 shows a completed diagram of the repair.

POSTOPERATIVE CARE AND EXPECTED OUTCOMES

- Protocols vary; my preference is presented here.
- A cast or hinged knee brace with the knee in a position of maximal stability (usually 30° of knee flexion) is used for 4 weeks. Partial weight bearing with crutches is permitted during this time.
- Knee range of motion in a hinged knee brace is gradually increased over weeks 5–8.
- The patient may bear weight as tolerated with the knee locked in extension starting at 4 weeks postoperatively.
- Physical therapy is started at 4–6 weeks postoperatively.
- Serial radiographs are obtained to document healing.
- The patient may plan for return to sports in a custom ACL brace at 4 months postoperatively.

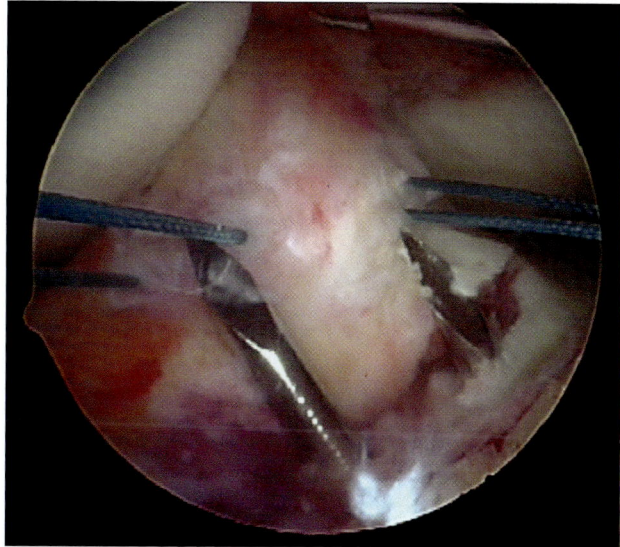

FIGURE 12

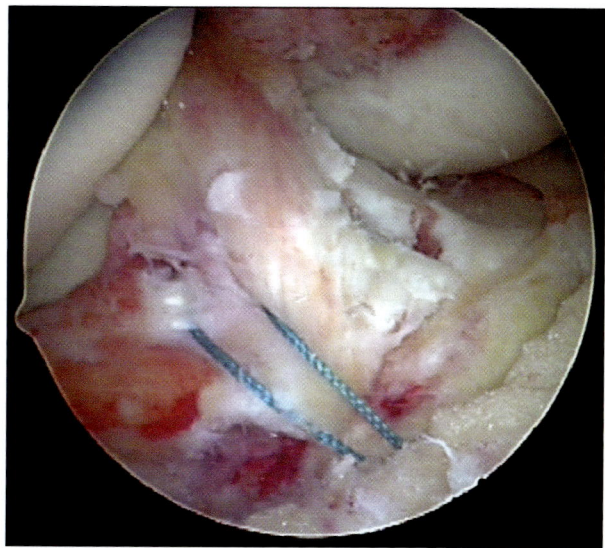

FIGURE 13

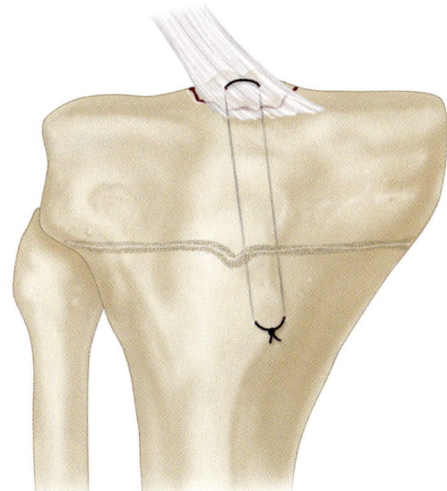

FIGURE 14

EVIDENCE

Ahmad CS, Stein BE, Jeshuran W, Nercessian OA, Henry JH. Anterior cruciate ligament function after tibial eminence fracture in skeletally mature patients. Am J Sports Med. 2001;29:339-45.

The authors use a knee questionnaire and clinical exam to evaluate ACL function, laxity and proprioception following tibial eminence fractures by comparison to patients with ACL deficiency and to patients who have undergone ACL reconstruction. No significant differences were found between the tibial eminence fracture group and the ACL reconstruction group. The ACL deficiency group fared worse in laxity and proprioception. (Level III evidence)

Bong MR, Romero A, Kubiak E, Iesaka K, Heywood CS, Kummer F, Rosen J, Jazrawi L. Suture versus screw fixation of displaced tibial eminence fractures: a biomechanical comparison. Arthroscopy. 2005;21:1172-6.

The authors perform a cadaveric biomechanical study of suture vs. screw fixation for tibial eminence fractures. Suture fixation utilized 3 No. 2 fiberwire sutures and was compared to screw fixation with a 4.0 mm cannulated screw and washer. Suture fixation had higher initial ultimate strength with no difference in stiffness noted.

Eggers AK, Becker C, Weimann A, Herbort M, Zantop T, Raschke MJ, Petersen W. Biomechanical evaluation of different fixation methods for tibial eminence fractures. Am J Sports Med. 2007;35:404-10.

The authors perform a cadaveric biomechanical study assessing the stability of 2 screws, I screw, suture fixation with Ethibond and suture fixation with Fiberwire for tibial eminence fractures. Results showed that under cyclic loading tests suture fixation was better than screw fixation, Fiberwire was better than Ethibond and one screw fixation was better than 2 screw fixation.

Hunter RE, Willis JA. Arthroscopic fixation of avulsion fractures of the tibial eminence: technique and outcome. Arthroscopy. 2004;20:113-21.

The authors describe a technique for treatment and perform a retrospective review of 17 patients with tibial eminence fractures treated with screw or suture fixation. Excellent knee scores were noted at a mean follow-up of 32 months regardless of fixation type. Better knee scores were seen in younger patients. The authors emphasized the need to retract interposed intermenisical tissue to allow anatomic reduction is some cases. (Level IV evidence)

Kocher MS, Foreman ES, Micheli LJ. Laxity and functional outcome after arthroscopic reduction and internal fixation of displaced tibial spine fractures in children. Arthroscopy. 2003;19:1085-90.

The authors perform a retrospective case series in 6 patients to evaluate laxity and functional outcome following arthroscopic reduction and internal fixation of displaced tibial spine fractures. While knee scores improved, persistent laxity by physical exam and KT-1000 measurements in 5 of 6 patients. (Level IV evidence)

Kocher MS, Micheli LJ, Gerbino P, Hresko MT. Tibial eminence fractures in children: prevalence of meniscal entrapment. Am J Sports Med. 2003;31:404-7.

The authors report a consecutive case series of 80 patients who underwent surgery for tibial eminence fractures. Entrapment of the anterior horn of the medial (most common) or lateral meniscus or intermeniscal ligament was seen in 26% (6 of 23) of type 2 fractures and 65% (37 of 57) of type 3 fractures. The authors conclude that surgical intervention should be considered for fractures that do not reduce in knee extension to evaluate for an entrapped meniscus. (Level III evidence)

Mahar AT, Duncan D, Oka R, Lowry A, Gillingham B, Chambers H. Biomechanical comparison of four different fixation techniques for pediatric tibial eminence avulsion fractures. J Pediatr Orthop. 2008;28:159-62.

The authors perform a biomechanical comparison of tibial spine fixation techniques using bovine knees. No significant difference was noted between #2 Ethibond sutures, 3 bioabsorbable nails, a single resorbable screw or a single metal screw. Variability in performance was greatest for resorbable screw and suture constructs. (Level III evidence)

Osteochondritis Dissecans: Arthroscopic Evaluation and Extra-articular Drilling with or without Fixation

Jay C. Albright

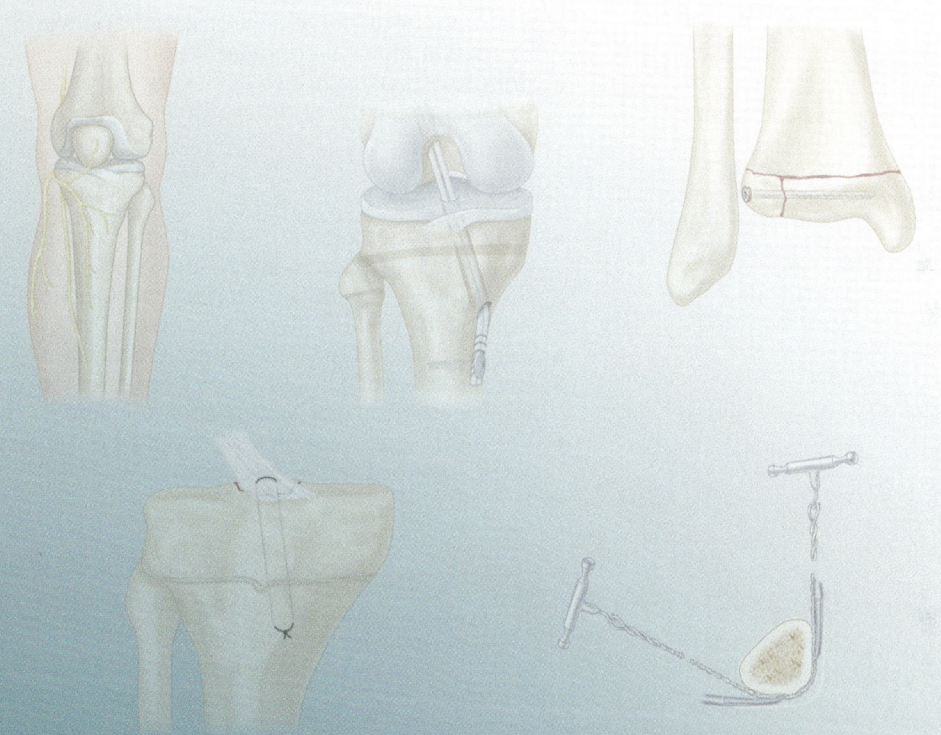

Controversies

• Occasionally, when a patient does not improve symptomatically even with cast or brace immobilization, earlier surgical intervention, prior to 3 months, may be warranted even in stable lesions.

Treatment Options

• Arthroscopic: transarticular drilling

• Open drilling with or without fixation

• Osteochondral autograft transplantation

INDICATIONS

■ Failed nonoperative treatment (3–6 months)
■ Unstable lesion by radiographs or magnetic resonance imaging (MRI)

EXAMINATION/IMAGING

■ Adequate anteroposterior (AP) (Fig. 1A) and lateral (Fig. 1B) radiographs are needed to establish the ability to see stable lesions intraoperatively.
■ MRI imaging (Fig. 2) is essential for evaluation of stability and cartilage integrity.

SURGICAL ANATOMY

■ The saphenous nerve and/or its infrapatellar branches are at risk for medial femoral condylar lesions.
■ The growth plate is also at risk for damage, particularly without radiographic control during drilling.

POSITIONING

■ Supine positioning with a leg holder and 90° flexion off the end of the bed and a well-leg holder is adequate (Fig. 3).
■ Alternatively, supine positioning with a lateral post and a radiolucent table is also reasonable.
■ Standard padding of all extremities is used.
■ The fluoroscope should enter from the nonoperative side at an angle perpendicular to the operative knee.
■ The arthroscopy equipment should be sufficiently positioned out of the way of the fluoroscope.

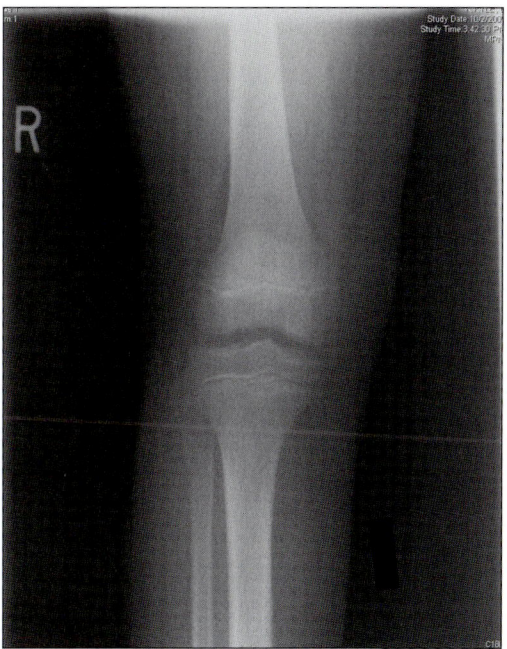 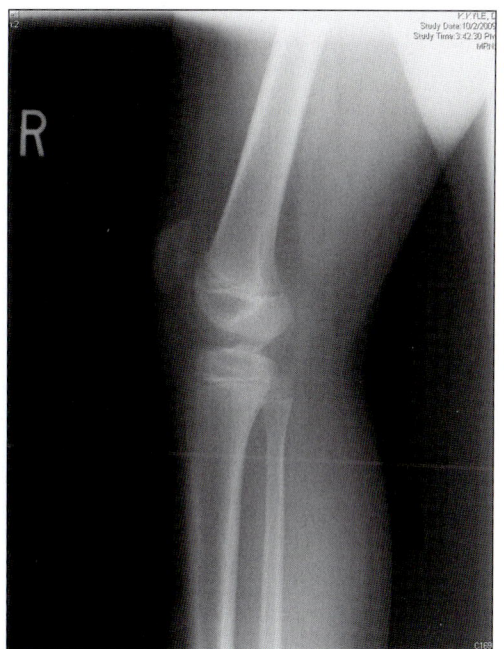

A

B

FIGURE 1

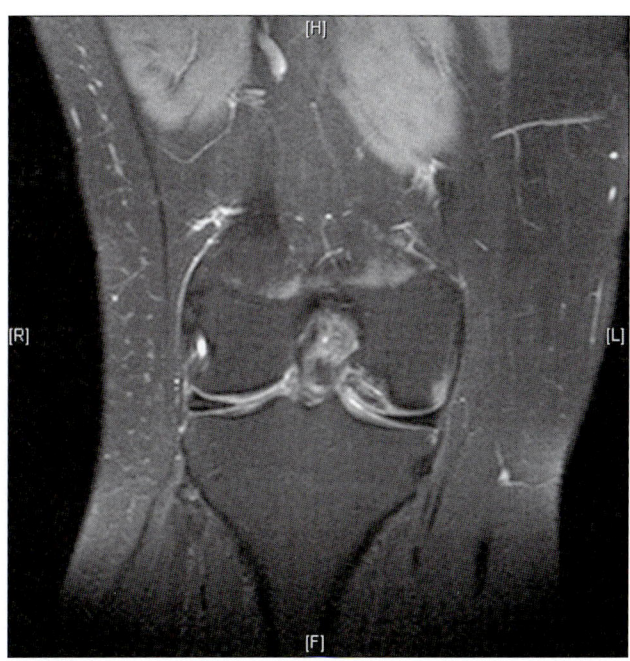

FIGURE 2

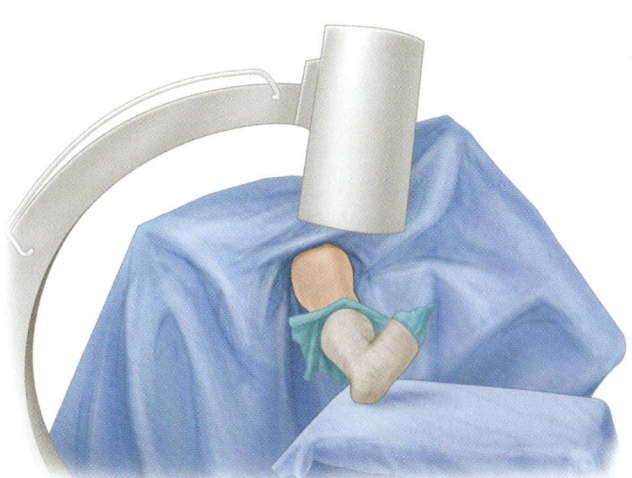

FIGURE 3

Controversies

- Accessory portals may be necessary for placement of fixation for unstable lesions.
- Vertical or horizontal portal incisions may be used.

Controversies

- Bone grafting may or may not be needed for good healing of lesions.

Instrumentation/ Implantation

- Guide wire
- Bioabsorbable headless screw

PORTALS/EXPOSURES

- Standard arthroscopy portals are utilized.
  - Three standard portals
  - Suprapatellar portal (medial or lateral, opposite side of lesion)
  - Inframedial or infralateral peripatellar portal

PROCEDURE

STEP 1

- Systematic evaluation of the joint should be performed to avoid missing other pathology.
- The surgeon should evaluate the integrity of lesion cartilage, and the size and position of the lesion.
- If the lesion is partially detached or flapped, débridement of the poor-quality soft tissue healing at the base of the lesion is performed prior to fixation and drilling.
- Bone grafting of large amounts of bone loss may be performed as well.

STEP 2

- If the lesion is unstable or there is significant cartilage detachment/fissuring, stabilization with internal fixation should be considered (Fig. 4).
- A bioabsorbable headless screw, with variable pitch angles for compression, is the author's preferred device.
- The fragment is reduced and fixed in place with a guide wire.
- The correct size hole to accommodate the implant is drilled and pretapped.
- A screw is placed. Multiple screws may be used in large lesions where use of more than one will not cause weakness or fracture of the lesion.

Controversies

- Prior thinking suggests removal of unstable lesions or lesions with little or no bone on the fragment without attempted fixation.

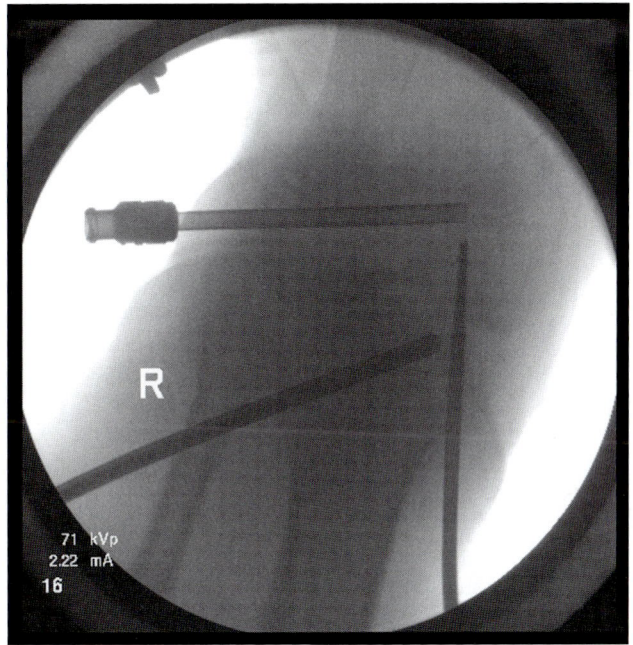

FIGURE 4

STEP 3

■ Extra-articular drilling of the stable or stabilized fragment is performed.

■ A 0.062-inch or a ⁵⁄₆₄ smooth pin or Kirschner wire is placed in the central position on both AP (Fig. 5A) and lateral (Fig. 5B) projections in the epiphysis only.

■ Using a parallel pin drill guide (Fig. 6) as well as image intensification, the skin as well as the hard rind/rim of the lesion into the fragment is penetrated in a 360° pattern.

■ If the lesion is large (more than 2 cm^2), two rows of drillings should be used, creating a double-ringed "bull's-eye" pattern.

POSTOPERATIVE CARE AND EXPECTED OUTCOMES

■ Closure is accomplished with an absorbable suture.

■ A straight leg brace/immobilizer is used for 6 weeks.

■ Crutches or a wheelchair is used for touch-down weight bearing for 6 weeks.

■ Physical therapy is begun immediately for full range of motion and quadriceps activation/strength.

■ The patient may expect to progress to full weight bearing at 6 weeks with radiographic evidence of healing. Return to sport may be expected at 3 months.

■ Figure 7 shows AP (Fig. 7A) and lateral (Fig. 7B) views at 3 months postoperative.

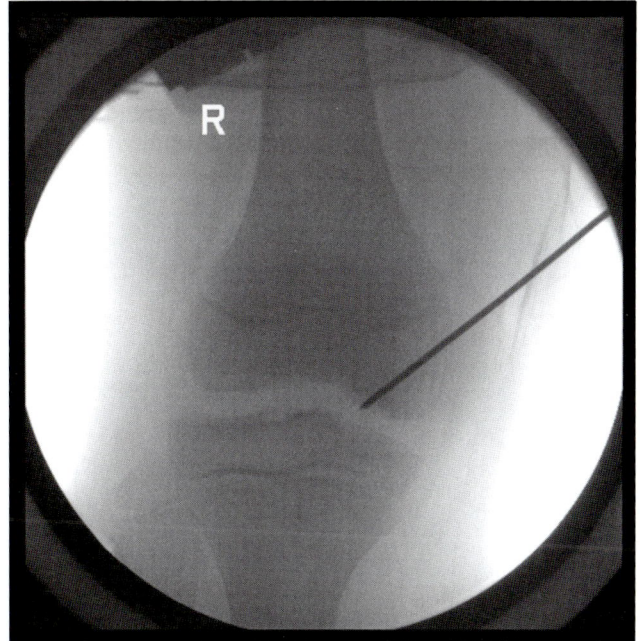

A

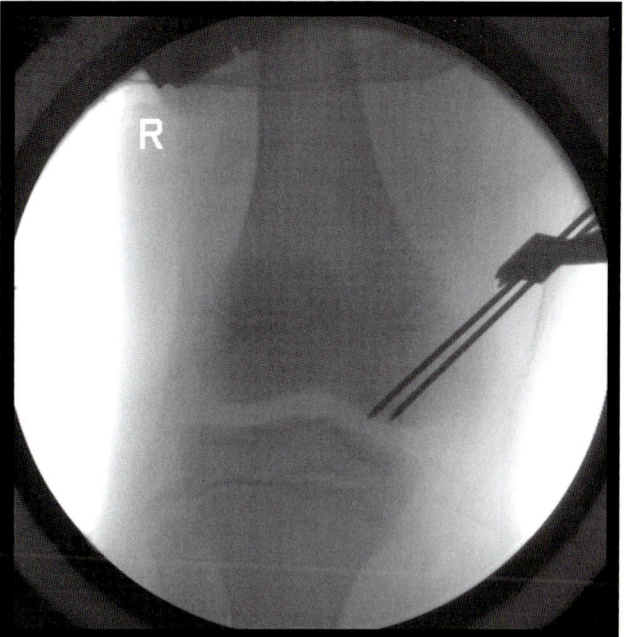

FIGURE 6

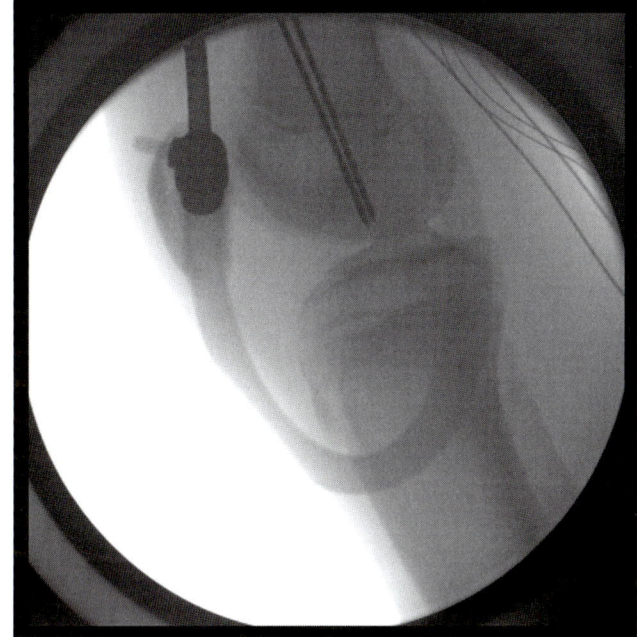

B

FIGURE 5

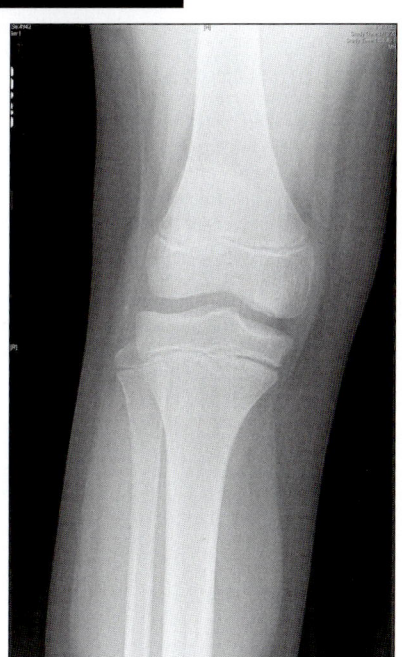

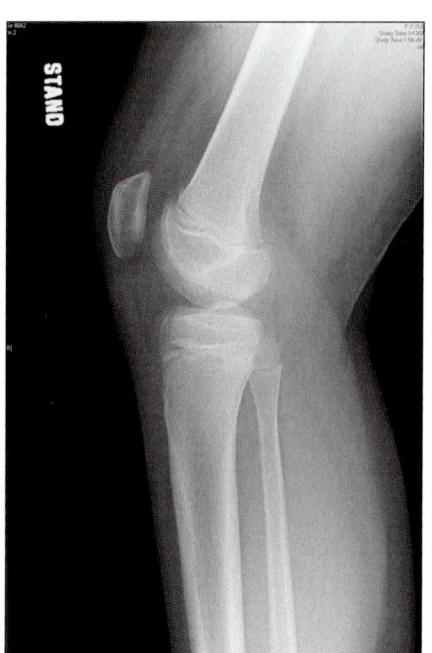

FIGURE 7 A   B

EVIDENCE

Anderson AF, Richards DB, et al. Antegrade drilling for osteochondritis dissecans of the knee. Arthroscopy. 1997;13:319–24.

Twenty-four knees with osteochondritis dissecans of the femoral condyles failed a conservative program and were treated with antegrade drilling. To our knowledge, this represents the largest reported series using this technique. The average age at the time of surgery was 13 years 6 months. The average follow-up was 5 years. Postoperative evaluation included rating by the International Knee Documentation Committee (IKDC) form and the Hughston Rating Scale for osteochondritis dissecans. This operation is not as likely to result in a successful outcome in patients with closed physes; consequently, other methods should be considered in skeletally mature patients.

Dines JS, Fealy S, et al. Outcomes of osteochondral lesions of the knee repaired with a bioabsorbable device. Arthroscopy. 2008;24:62–8.

This article sought to evaluate the functional and radiographic outcome of osteochondral lesions involving the femoral condyle that were arthroscopically repaired via a bioabsorbable fixation device made of self-reinforced poly-L-lactic acid. A retrospective clinical and radiographic evaluation of 9 patients (8 male and 1 female) with a mean age of 18 years at the time of surgery was carried out. This report documents the efficacy of a bioabsorbable nail to internally fix osteochondral lesions. It supports the use of MRI for both preoperative planning and postoperative assessment of fragment healing. (Level IV evidence)

Kawasaki K, Uchio Y, et al. Drilling from the intercondylar area for treatment of osteochondritis dissecans of the knee joint. Knee. 2003;10:257–63.

This paper demonstrates a new method in which a drilling is made from the intercondylar space, and its efficacy in treating osteochondritis dissecans (OCD) of the knee in skeletally immature patients with relatively stable lesions with an intact articular surface, in cases where there was failure of initial non-operative management. The lesions of 16 knees of 12 patients with OCD of the femoral condyles failed to heal by conservative treatment for more than 3 months (average 5–6 months) and thereafter were arthroscopically treated with drilling from not the transarticular but the intercondylar bare area without damaging the articular surface. The authors advocate the new and less invasive procedure of drilling from the bare area of the intercondylar space for OCD in the knee joint of skeletally immature patients who have had failure of initial non-operative management.

Kocher MS, Czarnecki JJ, et al. Internal fixation of juvenile osteochondritis dissecans lesions of the knee. Am J Sports Med. 2007;35:712–8.

This paper presents operative techniques for the management of juvenile osteochondritis dissecans lesions of the knee include drilling, internal fixation, fragment removal, and chondral resurfacing. The study design was a retrospective case series. Twenty-six knees in 24 skeletally immature patients underwent internal fixation of osteochondritis dissecans lesions. Mean follow-up was 4.25 years (range, 2–14.75 years). Mean patient age was 14.7 years (range, 11–16 years). There were 13 boys and 11 girls. Lesions were graded per the Ewing and Voto classification, with 9 stage II lesions (fissured), 11 stage III lesions (partially attached), and 6 stage IV lesions (detached). Given the relatively high healing rate, good functional outcome, and low complication rate, the authors advocate internal fixation of unstable juvenile osteochondritis dissecans lesions of the knee, even for detached lesions and in patients with a history of surgery for the osteochondritis dissecans lesion. (Level IV evidence)

Kocher MS, Micheli LJ, et al. Functional and radiographic outcome of juvenile osteochondritis dissecans of the knee treated with transarticular arthroscopic drilling. Am J Sports Med. 2001;29:562–6.

Management of juvenile osteochondritis dissecans is controversial. The purpose of this study was to evaluate the functional and radiographic outcomes of transarticular arthroscopic drilling for isolated stable, juvenile osteochondritis dissecans lesions of the medial femoral condyle with an intact articular surface after 6 months of nonoperative management had failed. The authors reviewed 30 affected knees in 23 skeletally immature patients (mean age, 12.3 years; range, 8.5 to 16.1) at an average follow-up of 3.9 years (range, 2.0 to 7.2). Functional outcome was determined using the Lysholm score and radiographic outcome was determined using lesion size, and the radiographic score of Rodegerdts and Gleissner. Linear regression analysis revealed that younger age was an independent, multivariate predictor of Lysholm score improvement. There were no apparent surgical complications.

Osteochondritis Dissecans Fixation

Matthew Diltz and Mininder S. Kocher

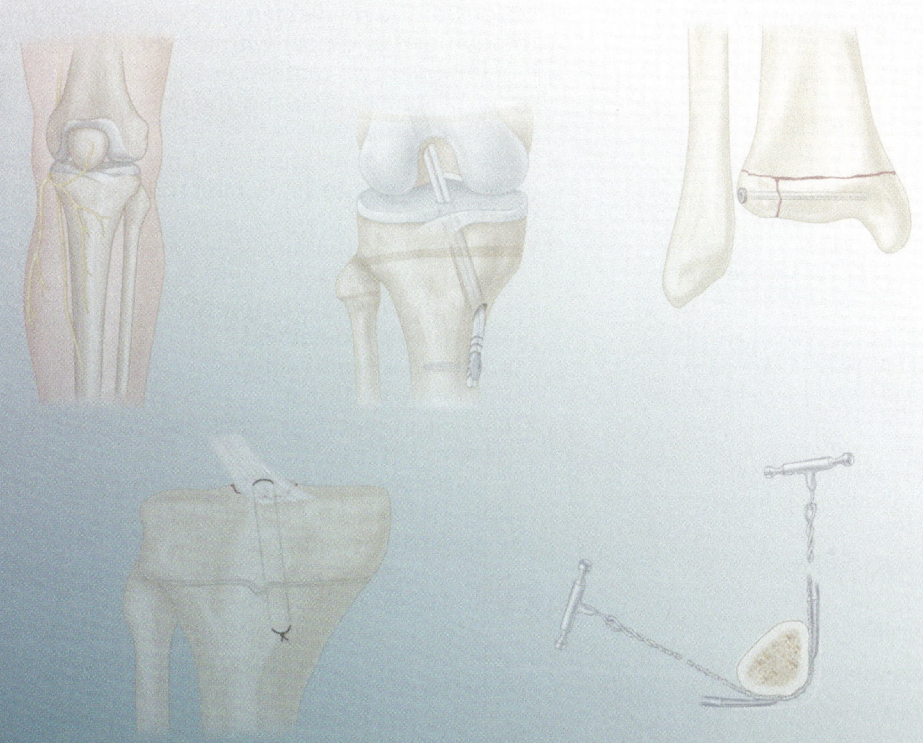

Treatment Options

Three-Phase Nonoperative Management Protocol (Flynn and Kocher, 2004)
- Phase 1 (first 6 weeks)
  - Baseline MRI
  - Crutch-protected partial weight bearing
  - Child should be pain free at the end
  - Repeat radiographs at the end
- Phase 2 (weeks 6–12)
  - Weight bearing as tolerated without immobilization
  - No impact activities
  - Physical therapy for knee range of motion, quad strengthening
- Phase 3 (begins at 3 months)
  - Supervised increase in activities
  - Restrict high-impact and shear activities until several months' pain free
  - Consider repeat MRI
  - Repeat immobilization for lesion progression

Other Treatment Options
- Drilling
- Internal fixation
- Fragment removal
- Chondral resurfacing

INDICATIONS

- Stable osteochondritis dissecans (OCD) lesions that have failed nonoperative management
- Initial treatment of unstable lesions
- OCD in patient with closed physis

EXAMINATION/IMAGING

- The patient often reports aching, activity-related anterior knee pain. The presentation can be quite similar to patellofemoral syndrome. The presence of OCD should be considered when making the diagnosis of patellofemoral stress syndrome.
- Other findings on physical examination include an antalgic gait.
  - With unstable lesions, effusion and mechanical symptoms may be present as well.
- Lesions of the medial femoral condyle can present with external rotation gait and pain with internal rotation (Wilson's sign)
- It is important to remember that 25% of these chondral lesions occur bilaterally, stressing the importance of checking both knees for symptoms.
- Radiographs, bone scans, and magnetic resonance imaging (MRI) are useful to determine the presence and stage of the OCD lesion.
  - Radiographic grading (Berndt and Harty)—anteroposterior, lateral, sunrise, and notch views
    - I—subchondral compression
    - II—partially detached
    - III—detached in situ
    - IV—free fragment
  - Bone scan grading (Cahill and Berg) useful for determining healing potential
    - I—visible on radiograph, normal bone scan
    - II—increased uptake in lesion only
    - III—increased uptake in lesion + femoral condyle
    - IV—increased uptake in lesion + tibial plateau
  - MRI staging (Hefti et al.) (Figs. 1–3)
    - Stage I—small signal change, no clear margins
    - Stage II—fragment with clear margins without fluid between fragment and bone
    - Stage III—fluid partially visible between fragment and bone
    - Stage IV—fluid completely surrounds fragment
    - Stage V—fragment displaced
  - Arthroscopic grading (Ewing and Voto/International Cartilage Repair Society)
    - Grade 1—intact
    - Grade 2—early cartilage separation
    - Grade 3—partially attached
    - Grade 4—loose body + crater

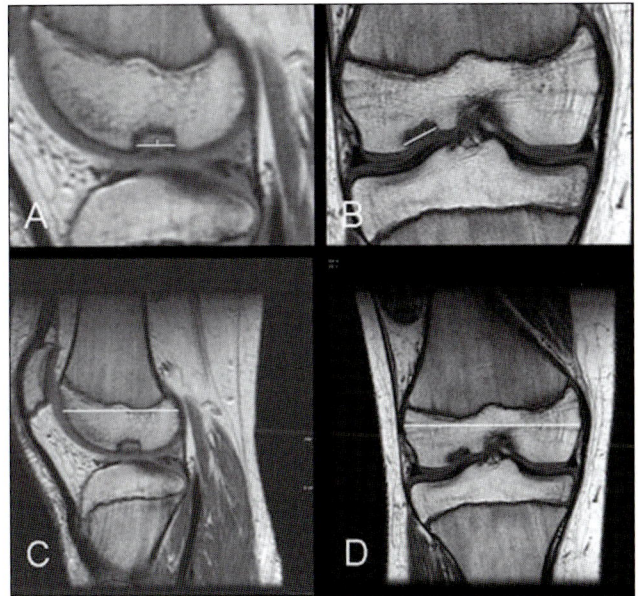

FIGURE 1

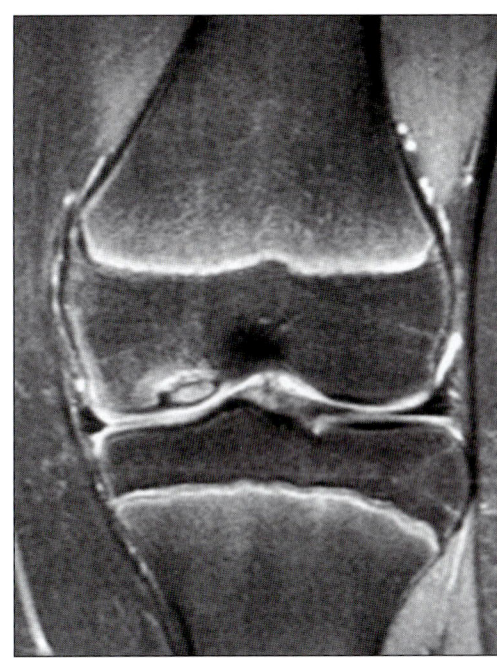

FIGURE 2

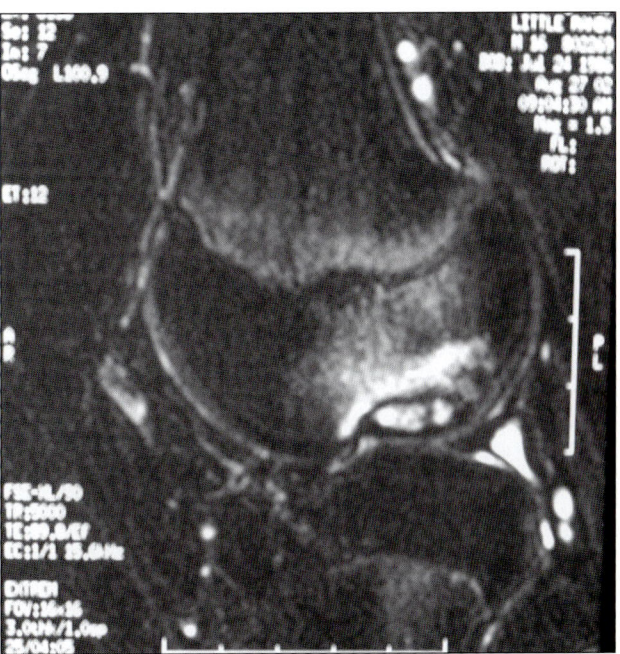

FIGURE 3

SURGICAL ANATOMY

- Most common locations:
  - Posterolateral medial femoral condyle—70% (often only seen on notch view) (Figs. 4 and 5)
  - Inferocentral lateral femoral condyle—20%
  - Patellar—10%
  - Trochlear—1%
  - 25% bilateral
- It is important to perform a complete arthroscopic survey of the knee when evaluating OCD. Fissuring of the chondral surface can lead to loose bodies. These loose bodies should be removed at the time of the operation (Fig. 6)
- Also, we have found that derangement of the chondral surface often predisposes the knee to the development of abundant inflammatory and scar tissue. This can develop into a symptomatic plica or synovial impingement.

POSITIONING

- The patient is placed supine on the operating room table.
- A tourniquet is placed at the proximal thigh.
- It is useful to place a lateral post at the level of the tourniquet. This post can be used to place a valgus force to the knee and evaluate the medial compartment.

PORTALS/EXPOSURES

- Standard knee arthroscopy portals are utilized.
- We establish the anteriolateral portal first.
  - With the knee flexed to 90°, the inferior pole of the patella and lateral border of the patellar tendon are palpated.
  - The surgeon should feel for the soft spot. Skin is marked just lateral to the tendon and 1 cm below the pole of the patella. A 5- to 10-mm vertical incision is made with a #11 blade through the skin, subcutaneous tissue, and capsule.
- The medial portal is established with direct visualization.
- A complete examination of the knee is performed. Any derangements are noted and addressed.
- Additional exposure depends on the location of the lesion.
  - For lesions located at the patellar facet or trochlear groove, a lateral retinacular release assists in mobilization of the patella and exposure of the lesion (Figs. 7 and 8).

PEARLS

- *We place a lateral post at the level of the tourniquet. The post facilitates valgus force to evaluate the medial compartment.*

Equipment

- Standard arthroscopy equipment.
- There is always the possibility of an arthrotomy, so a basic orthopaedic tray should be available.
- Small Kirschner wire (K-wire) or C wire (0.45 inch) to drill the lesion.
- Screw (Herbert) or tack (SmartNail; Conmed) for fixation.
  - We prefer bioasorbable fixation. It allows repeat MRI and avoids the need to remove fixation later.

PEARLS

- *When the OCD lesion is in the lateral compartment of the knee, a slightly more proximal anteriolateral portal aids in visualization.*

PITFALLS

- *Placement of the lateral portal is essential to inspect the entire knee.*
  - *With lateral placement, it is difficult to see the notch.*
  - *Superior placement leads to difficulty with posterior evaluation.*
  - *Inferior placement can lead to damage to the anterior horn of the meniscus and fat pad impingement.*
  - *Medial placement can damage the patellar tendon and lead to fat pad impingement.*

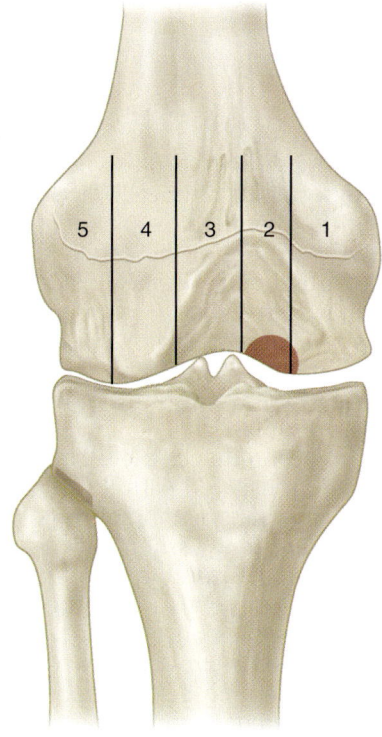

FIGURE 4

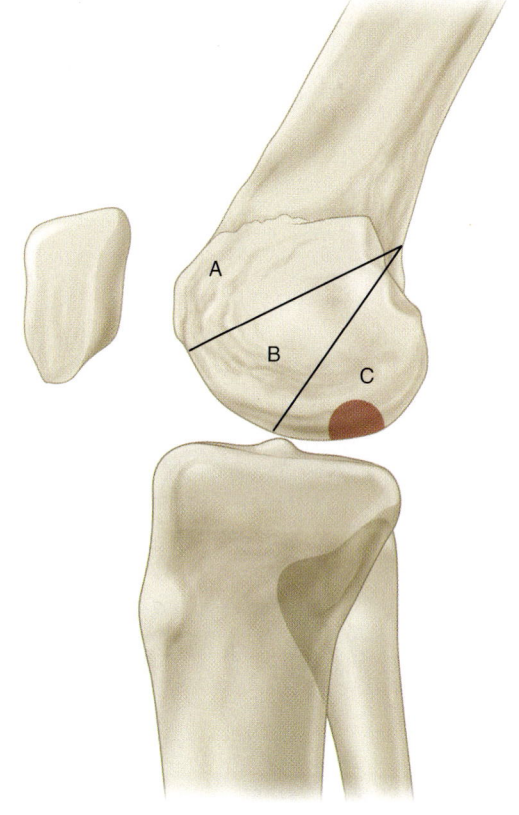

FIGURE 5

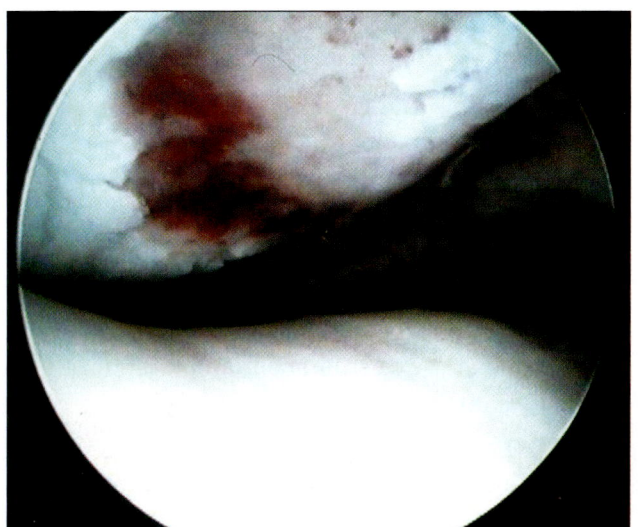

FIGURE 6

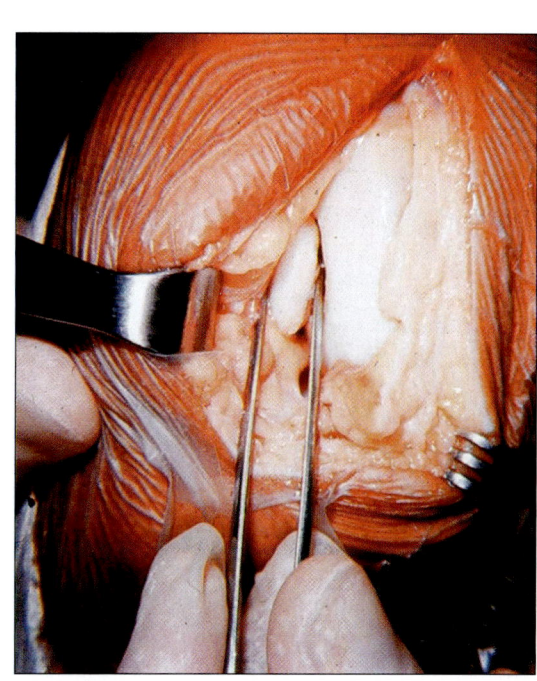

FIGURE 8

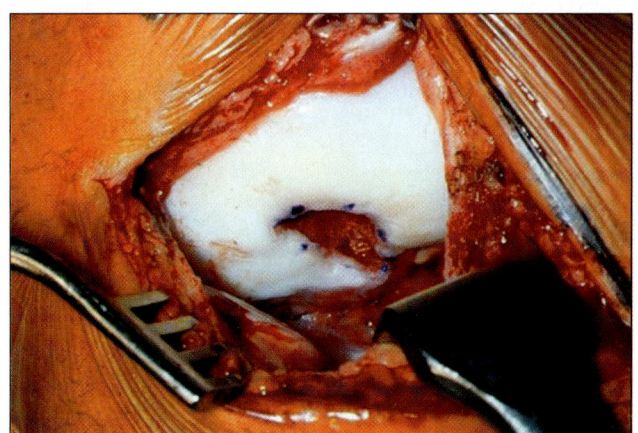

FIGURE 7

PROCEDURE

STEP 1

- For grade 4 lesions, it is often necessary to enlarge the medial or lateral portal for removal of the loose body.
  - Part of the preoperative planning involves determining the optimal exposure of the cartilage defect.
  - The arthroscope is typically placed on the contralateral side of the lesion for viewing (Fig. 9) and the portal on the ipsilateral side is enlarged for removal of the loose body (Fig. 10).
  - There is a low threshold to perform an arthrotomy. The location of the arthrotomy is dependent on the location of the defect.
- The free cartilage defect is evaluated.
  - The size is measured with a ruler and documented.
  - The amount of subchondral bone at the base of the lesion is an important prognostic factor.
  - The presence of fissuring of the cartilage surface is noted.
- The base of the lesion is also inspected. It is important that the defect matches the contours of the base.
  - Typically there is hypertrophy of the free cartilage fragment requiring trimming before fixation.
- Once the fragment is contoured to a precise fit, it is held in place and fixed to the subchondral bone
  - The type of fixation is dependent on the size of the OCD lesion.
  - For large lesions, fixation with two to three screws allows for firm compression and rotation control (Figs. 11 and 12).
  - For smaller lesions, the defect can be held in place with a 0.45-inch K-wire as fixation is placed.
- Large partially detached lesions are fixed in situ to provide compression for healing.
- Supplement drilling with a 0.45-inch K-wire to a depth of 3 cm provides additional blood supply for healing.

STEP 2

- For patients with open growth plates, every attempt should be made to obtain fixation of the OCD lesion.
- In patients with chronic lesions without the presence of subchondral bone at the free fragment and failed fixation, chondral resurfacing is necessary.
- If there is a defect at the time of primary surgery, abrasion chondroplasty is performed.
  - The edges of the cartilage lesion are débrided to stable margins.
  - Picks are then used to micropenetrate the subchondral bone.
  - Four-millimeter-wide subchondral bone bridges preserve the subchondral bone plate integrity and function.
  - When arthroscopic fluid pressure is reduced, bleeding and fat droplets should be present.
- Other salvage procedures include osteoarticular transplant, autologous cultured cartilage transplant, and osteochondral allograft.

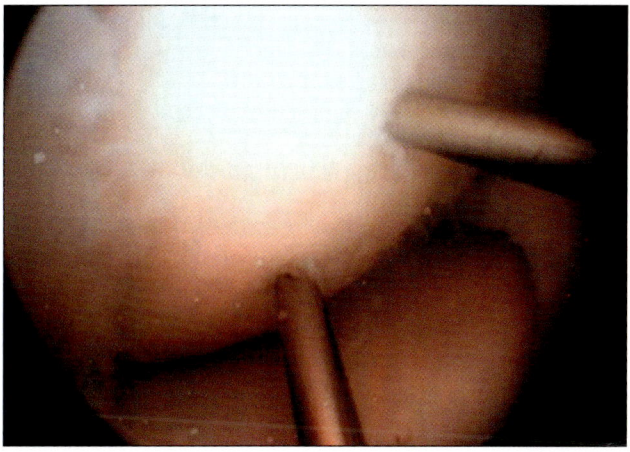

FIGURE 9

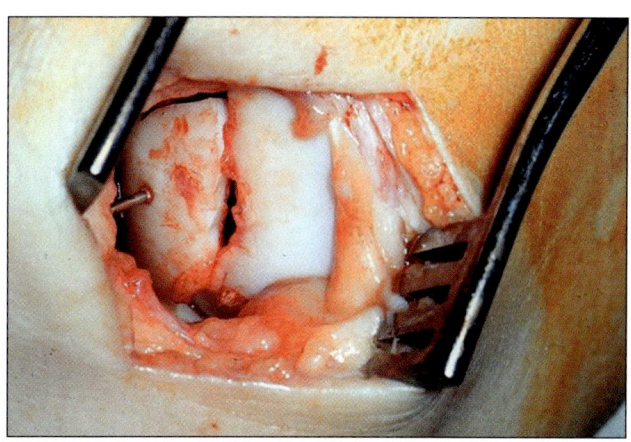

FIGURE 10

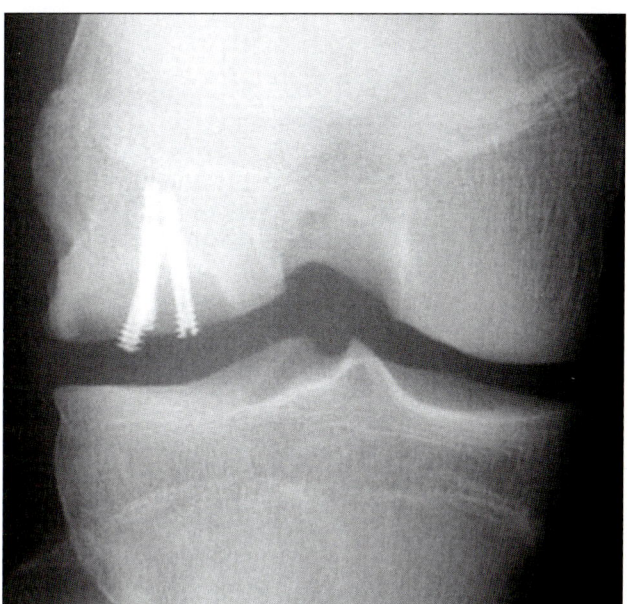

FIGURE 11

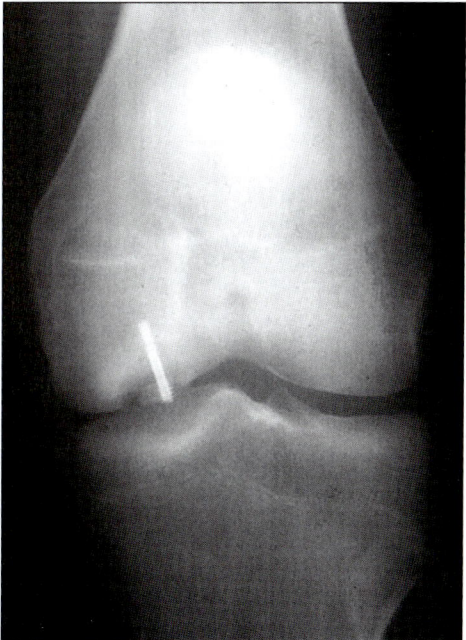

FIGURE 12

Controversies

- We have found that the majority of lesions can be reached arthroscopically through a transarticular approach.
- Another option is transepiphyseal drilling.
  - *Fluoroscopic guidance is employed to open channels from the epiphysis to the cartilage defect.*

STEP 3

- For stable lesions with intact articular surfaces, transarticular drilling provides channels for revascularization.
  - The lesion is first assessed arthroscopically. A "soft spot" in the cartilage is delineated with a probe.
  - With the arthroscope in the contralateral portal, the lesion is visualized.
  - The placement of the 0.45-inch K-wire is determined by the location of the lesion and anatomy of the patient.
- Multiple holes are drilled into the OCD lesion to a depth of 3 cm.
  - The number of holes is dependent on the size of the lesion.

POSTOPERATIVE CARE AND EXPECTED OUTCOMES

- Postoperative protocol
  - First 2 weeks:
    - Partial weight bearing is permitted.
    - A hinged knee brace is applied with range of motion limited to 0–90° for 6 weeks (0–30° for lesions of the patellar facet or trochlea for 2 weeks).
    - Continuous passive motion is used at home.
  - Two weeks:
    - Formal physical therapy is initiated.
    - The Bledsoe is continued at the above range of motion and partial weight bearing is continued.
  - Six weeks:
    - Weight bearing as tolerated is permitted.
    - The brace is discontinued.
    - Radiographs are reviewed.
  - No impact is permitted for 3 months.
  - At 3 months, MRI scans are reviewed. Impact is started based on MRI findings.
- An 85% healing rate for unstable lesions treated with internal fixation was obtained in juvenile patients (Kocher et al., 2007).
- Transarticular drilling of isolated stable juvenile OCD lesions (open physis) of the medial femoral condyle with intact articular cartilage surface has been done after 6 months of failed nonoperative treatment (Kocher, 2001).
  - Radiographic evidence of healing was found in all patients at 4.4 months.
  - A younger age predicted better outcomes.
  - All lesions were stage 1–2.
- Factors associated with failure of treatment:
  - Nonclassic lesion location
  - Multiple lesions
  - Underlying medical problems

EVIDENCE

Berndt AL, Harty M. Transchondral fractures (osteochondritis dissecans) of the talus. J Bone Joint Surg [Am] 1959;41-A:988–1020.

The authors describe a grading system using radiographs for osteochondritis dissecans lesions of the talus.

Cahill BR, Berg BC. 99m-Technetium phosphate compound joint scintigraphy in the management of juvenile osteochondritis dissecans of the femoral condyles. Am J Sports Med. 1983;11:329–35.

The authors followed 18 patients with osteochondritis dissecans of the femoral condyle for 18 months with bone scans every 6 weeks in order to develop a grading system for healing potential.

Ewing JW, Voto SJ. Arthroscopic surgical management of osteochondritis dissecans of the knee. Arhroscopy.1988;4:37–40.

This paper presents a series of 29 patients who were treated surgically for symptomatic osteochondritis dissecans using arthroscopic techniques. The authors describe an arthroscopic grading system for the lesions.

Flynn JM, Kocher MS, Ganley TJ. Osteochondritis dissecans of the knee. J Pediatr Orthop. 2004;24:434–43.

Hefti F, Beguiristain J, Krauspe R, Möller-Madsen B, Riccio V, Tschauner C, Wetzel R, Zeller R. Osteochondritis dissecans: a multicenter study of the European Pediatric Orthopedic Society. J Pediatr Orthop [Br]. 1999;8:231–45.

The authors collected information from 798 cases of osteochondritis dissecans of the knee from 44 hospitals. Based on the findings they developed an MRI grading system that correlates with prognosis.

Kocher MS, Czarnecki JJ, Andersen JS, Micheli LJ. Internal fixation of juvenile osteochondritis dissecans lesions of the knee. Am J Sports Med. 2007;35:712–8.

This is a retrospective case series of 26 knees with juvenile osteochondritis dissecans lesions treated with internal fixation. There was an 84% healing rate, including all 6 detached lesions. The mean time to healing was 6 months. There was no difference between location, implant used, or grade of lesion.

Kocher MS, Micheli LJ, Yaniv M, Zurakowski D, Ames A, Adrignolo AA. Functional and radiographic outcome of juvenile osteochondritis dissecans of the knee treated with transarticular arthroscopic drilling. Am J Sports Med. 2001;29:562–6.

Kocher et al. reviewed 30 cases of OCD of the medial femoral condyle in 23 skeletally immature patients that had failed 6 months of nonoperative management. All lesions were stage 1 or 2. There was significant improvement in the mean Lysholm score (from 58 to 93). There was significant improvement in the mean lesion size on anteroposterior (4.5 ± 5.8 mm decrease) and lateral (8.4 ± 8.1 mm decrease) radiographs. There was also significant improvement in the mean radiographic score (from 3.0 to 1.9). Radiographic healing was achieved in all patients at an average of 4.4 months after drilling (range, 1 to 11 months). Linear regression analysis revealed that younger age was an independent, multivariate predictor of Lysholm score improvement. There were no apparent surgical complications.

Kocher MS, Tucker R, Ganley TJ, Flynn JM. Management of osteochondritis dissecans of the knee: current concepts review. Am J Sports Med. 2006;34:1181–91.

Two review articles that describe findings and classification of osteochondritis dissecans of the knee as well as management options.

Transphyseal ACL Reconstruction in Skeletally Immature Patients Using Autogenous Hamstring Tendon

Mininder S. Kocher, Craig J. Finlayson, and Adam Nasreddine

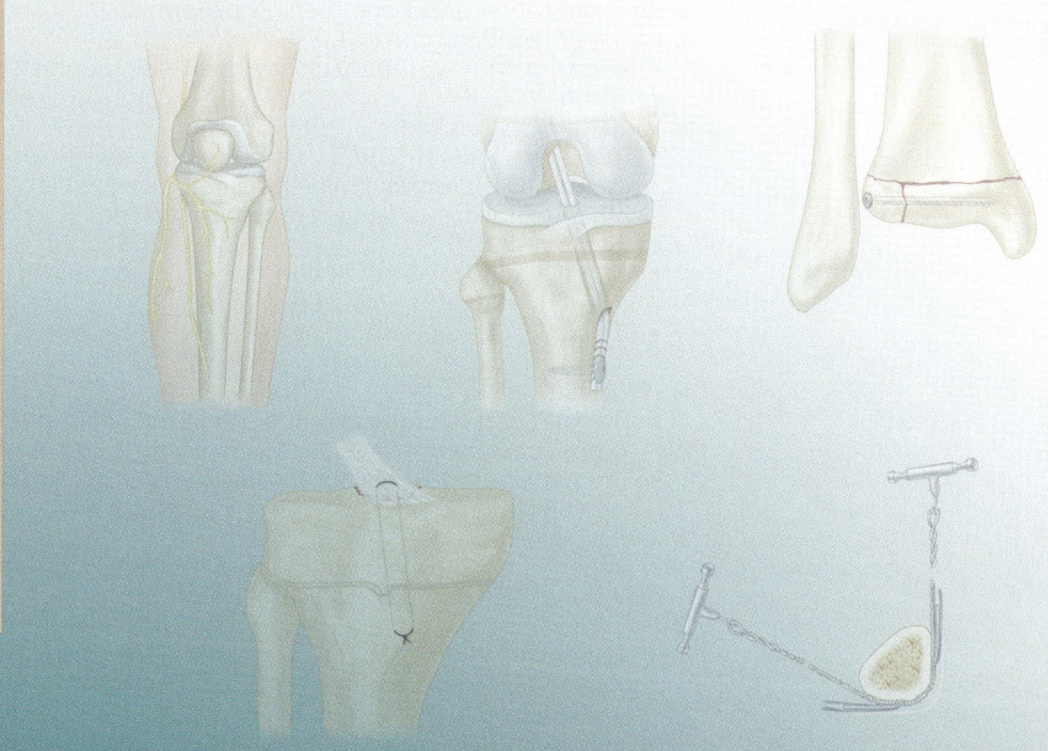

PITFALLS

- *Delaying ACL reconstruction by 3 months is recommended in the case of a meniscal tear that requires extensive repair in order to protect the meniscal repair from early mobilization prescribed by ACL reconstruction.*
- *Patients must be emotionally mature enough to actively participate in the extensive rehabilitation required after ACL reconstruction.*

Treatment Options

- Conservative treatment with activity modification and protective bracing

INDICATIONS

- Adolescent patient with significant growth remaining (Tanner stage 3 or greater) with a complete anterior cruciate ligament (ACL) tear and functional instability (Fig. 1)
- Adolescent patient with significant growth remaining with a partial ACL tear that has failed nonoperative treatment
- Adolescent patient with significant growth remaining with an ACL tear and other injuries such as meniscal tears or chondral injury
- Adolescent patient with significant growth remaining with congenital ACL insufficiency and symptomatic instability despite bracing

EXAMINATION/IMAGING

- An examination under anesthesia is performed.
- Range of motion is checked.
  - Normal range can have slight hyperextension up to 130° of flexion.
- Varus/valgus stress test
  - This test is done at both 0° and 30° of flexion.
  - The surgeon must determine if there is increased laxity of either the medial or lateral collateral ligament.
- Lachman test
  - With the knee at 30° of flexion, the tibia is translated anteriorly without a solid endpoint.
  - The patient is re-evaluated at the end of the case for comparison.
- Pivot shift test
  - The knee is taken from extension to flexion while placing valgus stress on the knee and internally rotating the tibia.
  - The surgeon should feel for a gliding or shifting sensation of the tibiofemoral joint.
- Tanner stage
  - Staging is done by assessing for the presence and distribution of pubic hair and for breast/testicular development.
- Plain radiographs
  - Posteroanterior (PA), lateral, Merchant's, and tunnel views are obtained before surgery to evaluate for any bony abnormalities.
  - Radiographs allow for initial evaluation of the physis before surgery has been completed.
  - A anteroposterior (AP) radiograph of the left hand and wrist is obtained to determine bone age.
- Magnetic resonance imaging (MRI) (Fig. 2)
  - MRI scans are evaluated for edema patterns consistent with recent ACL tear: lateral femoral condyle, posterolateral tibial plateau.
  - Scans are also evaluated for other injuries, such as chondral or meniscal injuries.
  - MRI allows for preoperative planning.

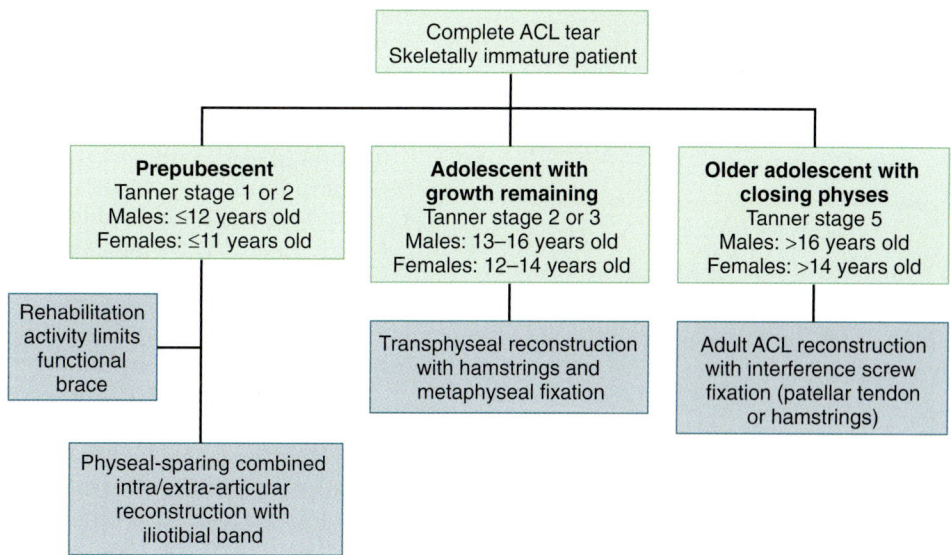

FIGURE 1

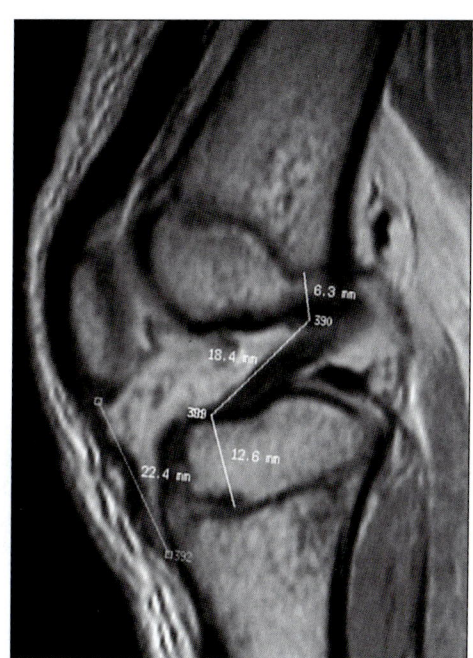

FIGURE 2

Equipment

- A lateral post or leg holder may be used.

SURGICAL ANATOMY

- Anterior cruciate ligament
  - The ACL orginates on the lateral wall of the intercondylar notch of the femur.
  - It inserts on the anterior tibial spine.
- Proximal tibial and distal femoral physes
  - The origin of the ACL is approximately 3–5 mm distal to the femoral physis in adolescents.
- Hamstring tendons (gracilis and semitendinosus)
  - These tendons are palpable at their insertion at the pes anserinus on the medial surface of the proximal tibia.
  - They lie deep to the sartorius fascia.
- Saphenous nerve
  - This nerve runs along the posterior border of the sartorius posterior to the pes anserinus.

POSITIONING

- The patient is positioned supine.
- A tourniquet is placed on the thigh of the operative leg.
- The leg, including the foot, is prepped sterilely.

PORTALS/EXPOSURES

- Two standard arthroscopic portals are used (Fig. 3).
  - The anterolateral portal is the primary viewing portal.
  - The anteromedial portal is the primary working portal.
- Hamstring harvest/tibial tunnel
  - A 4-cm incision is made over the palpable pes anserinus on the proximal medial tibia (see Fig. 3).
  - Dissection is carried down to the level of the sartorius fascia.
  - The sartorius fascia is opened, and the semitendinosus and gracilis tendons are identified.

PROCEDURE

STEP 1: GRAFT HARVEST AND PREPARATION

- A 4-cm incision is made over the palpable pes anserinus tendons.
- Once the gracilis and semitendinosis tendons are isolated, they are released from their distal insertion on the tibia (Fig. 4).
- The free ends of the tendons are whipstitched with #2 or #5 Ethibond suture (Fig. 5).
- The tendons are dissected proximally using sharp and blunt dissection, paying attention to fibrous bands to the medial head of the gastrocnemius (Fig. 6).
- A closed tendon stripper is used to amputate the tendons proximally.
  - Alternatively, the tendons can be left attached distally, amputated proximally with an open tendon stripper, and then released distally.
- On the back table, excess muscle is removed from the tendons, and the remaining ends are whipstitched with #2 or #5 Ethibond suture (Fig. 7).

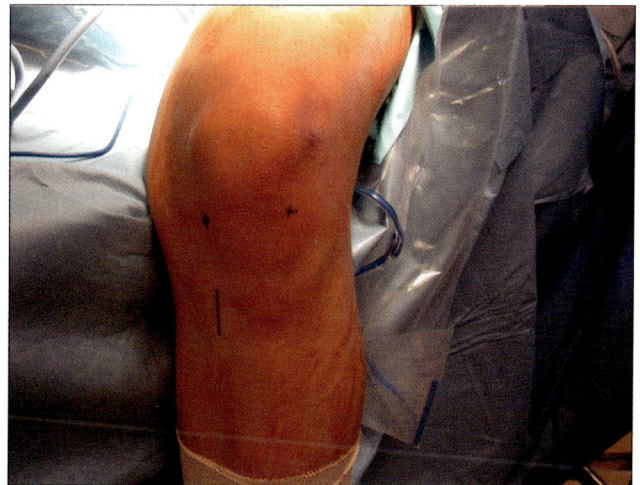

FIGURE 3

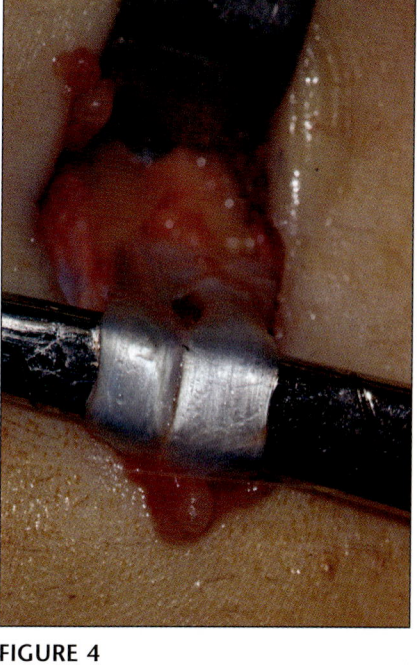

FIGURE 4

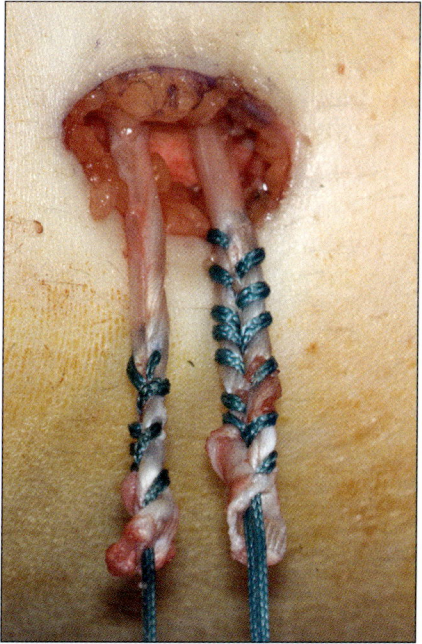

FIGURE 5

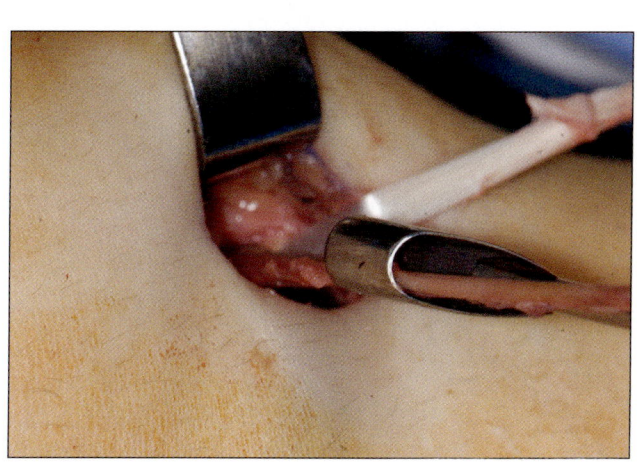

FIGURE 6

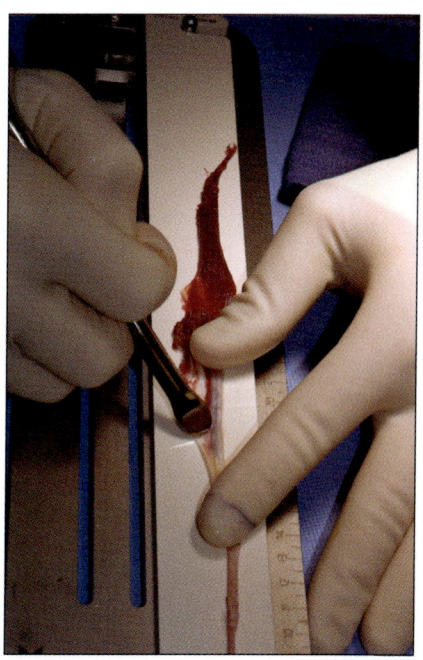

FIGURE 7

PEARLS

- *Typically, the graft is 8–9 mm in adolescent patients.*

- *A closed-loop system with tension applied to the hamstring tendons and pressure applied to the tendon stripper simultaneously with the same hand can provide valuable feedback and decrease harvesting complications.*

PITFALLS

- *Fibrous connections to the medial gastrocnemius must be sought and released in order to prevent premature amputation of the hamstring tendons, especially the semitendinosus.*

PEARLS

- *Minimal notchplasty is performed to avoid iatrogenic injury to the perichondrial ring of the distal femoral physis, which is in very close proximity to the over-the-top position.*

Controversies

- The femoral tunnel can be drilled via a trans-tibial approach or the anteromedial portal.

- The tendons are folded over a closed-loop EndoButton to form a four-stranded graft (Fig. 8).
- The graft diameter is sized to allow for a tight fit in the bone tunnels yet easy passage of the graft.
- The graft is then placed under tension and covered with a moist sponge.

STEP 2: ARTHROSCOPIC EXAMINATION

- An anterolateral viewing portal is established.
- The patellofemoral joint as well as the medial and lateral gutters are evaluated.
- The anteromedial portal is then established under arthroscopic visualization.
- Diagnostic arthroscopy of the medial and lateral compartments is performed.
- Meniscal and chondral pathology is addressed.
- The remaining ACL stump is débrided.
- The over-the-top position on the femur is identified (Fig. 9).

STEP 3: TUNNEL PREPARATION

- A tibial tunnel guide, set at 55°, is used through the anteromedial portal (Fig. 10).
- A guidewire is drilled through the hamstrings harvest incision into the posterior aspect of the ACL tibial footprint.
- The knee is brought into extension to confirm that the graft will not impinge anteriorly on the femur.
- The guidewire is reamed with the appropriate-diameter reamer.
- Excess soft tissue at the tibial tunnel is excised to help prevent arthrofibrosis.
- The trans-tibial over-the-top guide of the appropriate offset to ensure a 1- or 2-mm back wall is used to pass the femoral guide pin at the 10:00–10:30 position of the femoral notch (Fig. 11).
- The femoral guide pin is driven through the anterolateral femoral cortex and overdrilled with the EndoButton reamer.
- The femoral tunnel length is then measured with a depth gauge.
- The guide pin is replaced and brought through the skin of the lateral thigh.
- The femoral socket is reamed to the appropriate depth (Fig. 12).

PEARLS

- *The tibial tunnel should be kept medial to avoid injury to the tibial tubercle apophysis.*

- *The tibial tunnel should be relatively more vertical to provide adequate tunnel length distal to the physis for interference screw fixation.*

- *Femoral socket length = femoral tunnel length − EndoButton length + 7 mm to flip the EndoButton*

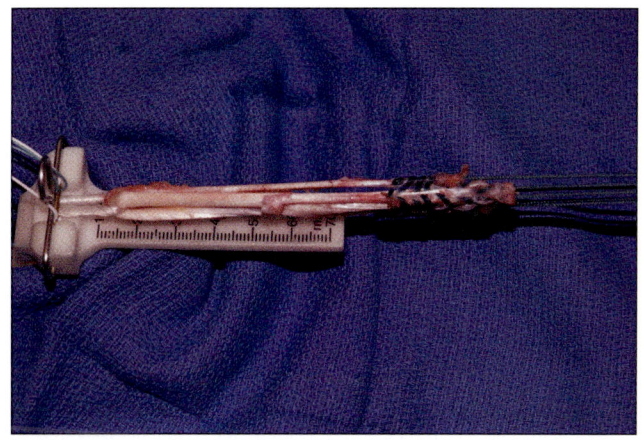

FIGURE 8

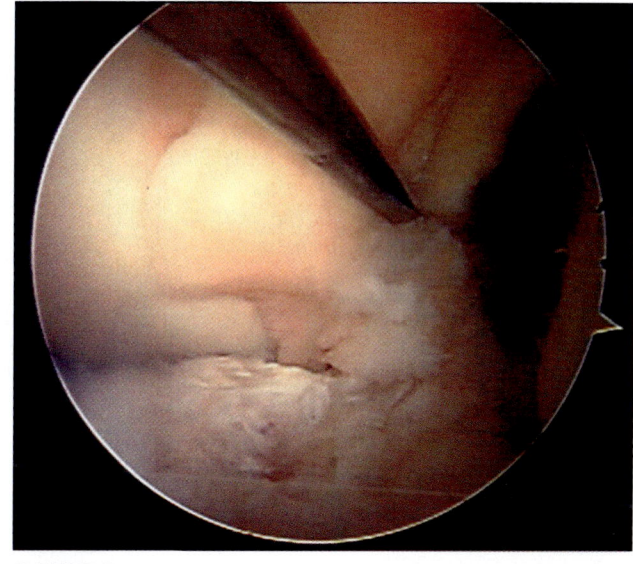

FIGURE 9

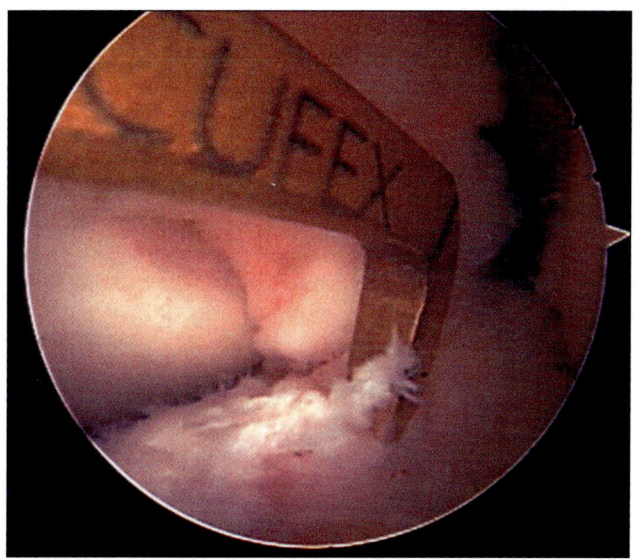

FIGURE 10

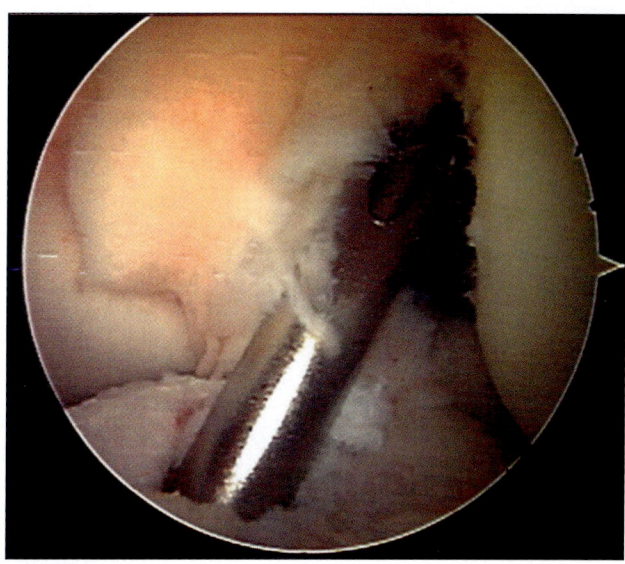

FIGURE 11

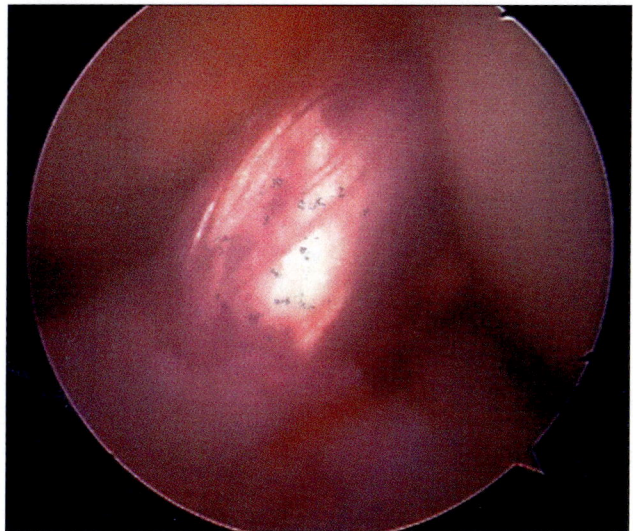

FIGURE 12

STEP 4: GRAFT PASSAGE AND FIXATION

- The #5 Ethibond sutures on the EndoButton are placed in the slot of the guidewire and pulled through the tibial tunnel, through the femoral tunnel, and out of the lateral thigh.
- The sutures are then pulled to bring the EndoButton and graft through the tibial tunnel and into the femoral tunnel.
  - One set of sutures is used to "lead" the EndoButton, while the other set of sutures is used to "follow."
- Once the graft is fully seated in the femoral tunnel, the "follow" sutures are pulled to flip the EndoButton on the femoral cortex.
- The flipping of the EndoButton can be palpated in the thigh, and tension is applied distally to ensure solid proximal fixation on the femoral cortex.
- The knee is extended to evaluate for graft impingement anteriorly. Additional notchplasty may be performed if necessary.
- The knee is cycled approximately 10 times with tension applied to the graft.
- The graft is then fixed on the tibial side with the knee in 20–30° of flexion.
- Firm tension is applied to the graft, and a posterior force is placed on the tibia.
- The graft is fixed with a soft tissue interference screw if there is adequate tunnel distance (at least 25 mm) below the physis to ensure metaphyseal placement of the screw (Fig. 13) or with a post and spiked washer if tunnel distance is insufficient (Fig. 14).
- Fluoroscopy can be used to ensure that the fixation is away from the physes.
- The tibial incision is closed in layers with subcutaneous Vicryl followed by a running subcuticular Monocryl suture.
- Arthroscopic portals are closed with inverted Monocryl suture.
- Figure 15 shows a 1-month postoperative radiograph.
- Figure 16 shows a 4-year postoperative radiograph.

POSTOPERATIVE CARE AND EXPECTED OUTCOMES

POSTOPERATIVE CARE

- Incisions are covered with sterile dressings and an elastic bandage.
- A cryotherapy unit is applied to the knee.
- A hinged knee brace is applied with range of motion limited to 0–90°.
- Continuous passive motion (CPM) from 0° to 90° for 6 hr/day along with cryotherapy are used for 2 weeks postoperatively.
- Touch-down weight bearing is permitted for 2 weeks postoperatively, followed by weight bearing as tolerated.
- Formal physical therapy is initiated at 2 weeks postoperatively.
- A hinged knee brace is used for 6 weeks with range of motion 0–90°. A simple hinge brace is then used from 6 weeks until 6 months postoperatively with unlimited motion.
- The patient may begin straight-ahead running at 3 months.
- Return to full activity, including cutting sports, is usually allowed at 6 months.
- An ACL brace is worn for high-risk activities for 1–2 years after return to sport.
- Radiographs of the knee are obtained to assess for growth disturbance at 6 months postoperatively and annually thereafter until skeletal maturity.

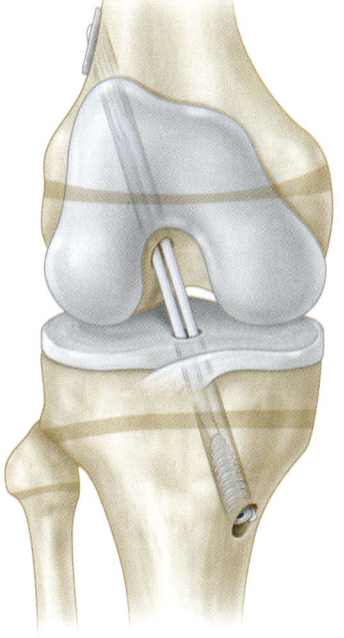

FIGURE 13

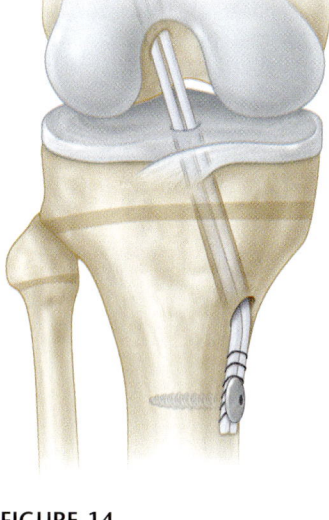

FIGURE 14

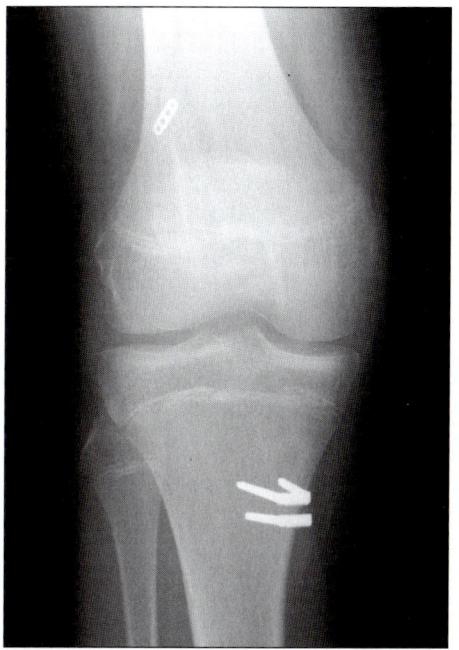

FIGURE 15

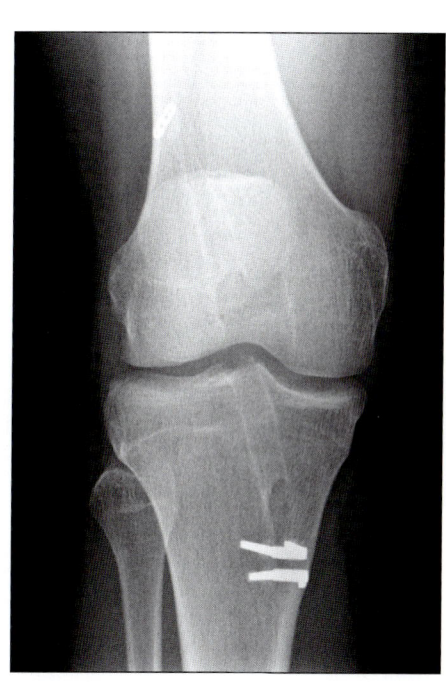

FIGURE 16

RESULTS AND COMPLICATIONS

- This procedure has an excellent functional outcome with a low revision rate and minimal risk of growth disturbance.
- Poor tunnel placement can lead to graft impingement, stiffness, graft failure, and physeal damage.
- Care should be taken to avoid injury to the vulnerable tibial tubercle apophysis and perichondrial ring of the distal femur.
- Large tunnels should be avoided as the likelihood of arrest is associated with greater violation of the epiphyseal plate cross-sectional area.

EVIDENCE

Most clinical studies on ACL injury in the adolescent population are retrospective case series. Anatomic studies of the ACL in the skeletally immature knee have also been performed.

Aichroth PM, Patel DV, Zorrilla P. The natural history and treatment of rupture of the anterior cruciate ligament in children and adolescents: a prospective review. J Bone Joint Surg [Br]. 2002;84:618–9.

The authors presented a prospective review of skeletally immature patients with ACL injuries. Nonoperative treatment resulted in poor functional outcomes with instability and a high rate of new meniscal tears and degenerative changes in the knee. (Level IV evidence)

Behr CT, Potter HG, Paletta GA Jr. The relationship of the femoral origin of the anterior cruciate ligament and the distal femoral physeal plate in the skeletally immature knee: an anatomic study. Am J Sports Med. 2001;29:781–7.

This anatomic study of immature knees demonstrated that the origin of the ACL is approximately 3 mm from the femoral physis.

Kocher MS, Saxon HS, Hovis WD, Hawkins RJ. Management and complications of anterior cruciate ligament injuries in skeletally immature patients: survey of the Herodicus Society and The ACL Study Group. J Pediatr Orthop. 2002;22:452–7.

The authors presented case reports of complications following ACL reconstruction in skeletally immature patients. Growth disturbances were reported in association with fixation hardware across the lateral femoral physis, bone plugs of a patellar tendon graft across the distal femoral physis, large (12-mm) tunnels, fixation hardware across the tibial tubercle apophysis, lateral extra-articular tenodesis, and dissection about the over-the-top femoral position. (Level V evidence)

Kocher MS, Smith JT, Zoric BJ, et al. Transphyseal anterior cruciate ligament reconstruction in skeletally immature pubescent adolescents. J Bone Joint Surg [Am]. 2007;89:2632–9.

In this case series of 61 knees in 59 patients treated with transphyseal ACL reconstruction with hamstrings autograft, excellent functional outcome was obtained, with a failure rate of 3% at 3.6-year follow-up. No growth disturbances were reported. (Level IV evidence)

Physeal-Sparing ACL Reconstruction in Skeletally Immature Patients Using Iliotibial Band Technique

James A. Krcik and Mininder S. Kocher

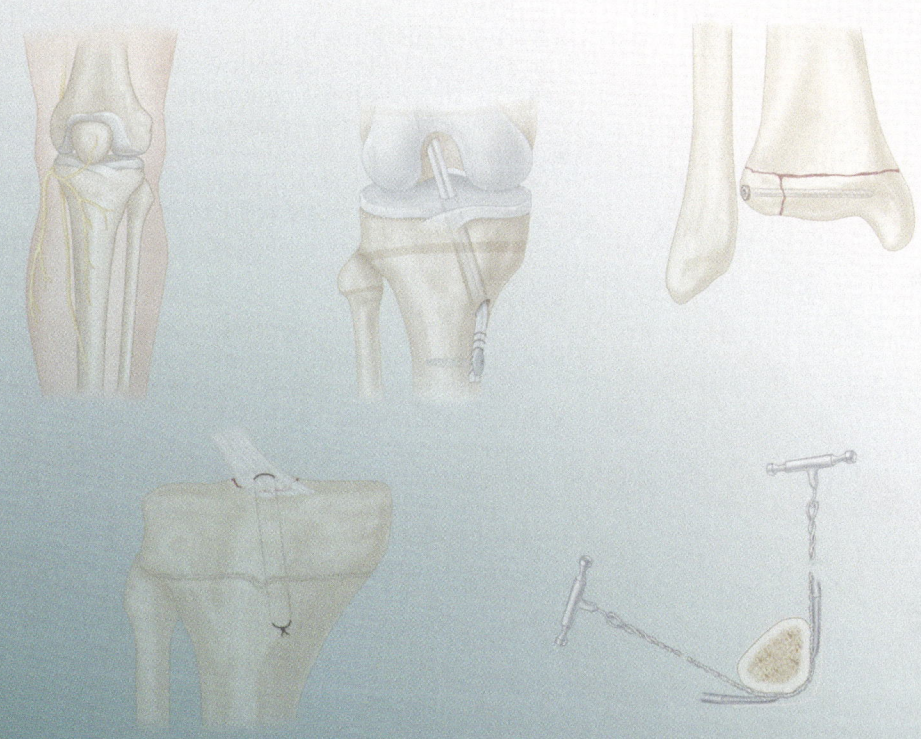

Controversies

- Other surgical options in the skeletally immature prepubescent patient include all-epiphyseal reconstruction and transphyseal reconstruction.

INDICATIONS

- Prepubescent skeletally immature patient with anterior cruciate ligament (ACL) tear who is Tanner stage 1 or 2 who has failed nonoperative treatment (Fig. 1)
- Prepubescent skeletally immature patient with ACL tear and other injuries, such as meniscal tears or chondral injury and functional instability
- Prepubescent skeletally immature patient with congenital ACL insufficiency with symptomatic instability recalcitrant to bracing

EXAMINATION/IMAGING

- An examination under anesthesia is performed.
- Range of motion is checked.
  - Normal range can have slight hyperextension up to 130° of flexion.
- Varus/valgus stress test
  - This test is done at both 0° and 30° of flexion.
  - The surgeon must determine if there is increased laxity of either the medial or lateral collateral ligament.
- Lachman's test
  - With the knee at 30° of flexion, the tibia is translated anteriorly without a solid endpoint.
  - The patient is re-evaluated at the end of the case for comparison.
- Pivot shift test
  - Pivot shift is very difficult to assess in the clinic.
  - The knee is taken from extension to flexion while placing valgus stress on the knee and observing for subluxation.
- Tanner stage (Fig. 2)
- Plain radiographs
  - Posteroanterior, lateral, Merchant's, and tunnel views are obtained before surgery to evaluate for any bony abnormalities.
  - Radiographs allow for initial evaluation of the physis before surgery has been completed .
  - An anteroposterior radiograph of the left hand and wrist is obtained to determine bone age.

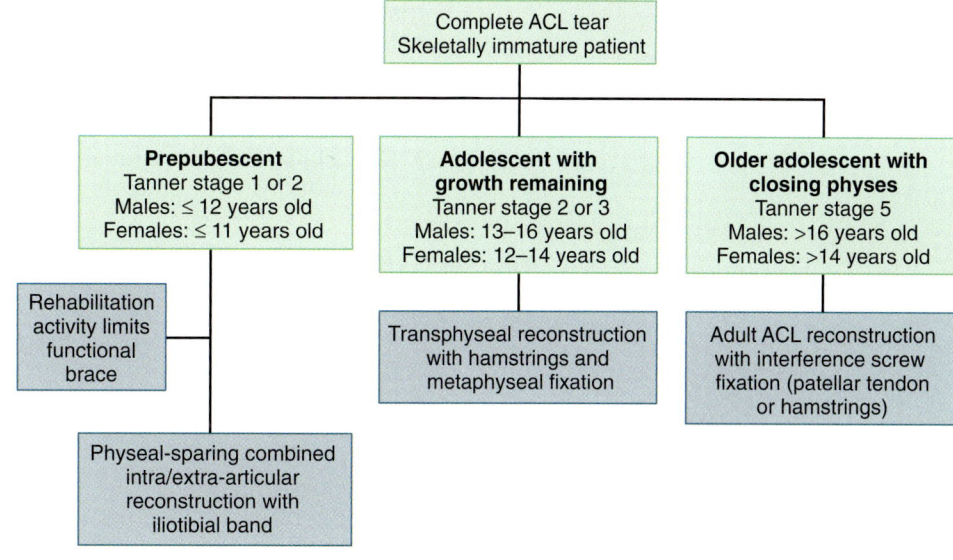

FIGURE 1

Tanner Stage		Males	Females
Stage 1 (Prepubertal)	Growth	5–6 cm/yr	5–6 cm/yr
	Development	Testes <4mL or <2.5cm No pubic hair	No breast development No pubic hair
Stage 2	Growth	5–6 cm/yr	7–8 cm/yr
	Development	Testes 4mL or 2.5–3.2cm Minimal pubic hair at base of penis	Breast buds Minimal pubic hair on labia
Stage 3	Growth	7–8 cm/yr	8 cm/yr
	Development	Testes 12mL or 3.5cm Pubic hair over pubis Voice changes Muscle mass increases	Elevation of breast; areolae enlarge Pubic hair on mons pubis Axillary hair Acne
Stage 4	Growth	10 cm/yr	7 cm/yr
	Development	Testes 4.1–4.5cm Pubic hair as adult Axillary hair Acne	Areolae enlarge Pubic hair as adult
Stage 5	Growth	No growth	No growth
	Development	Testes as adult Pubic hair as adult Facial hair as adult Mature physique	Adult breast contour Pubic hair as adult
Other		Peak height velocity: 13.5 years	Adrenarche: 6–8 years Menarche: 12.7 years Peak height velocity: 11.5 years

FIGURE 2

- Magnetic resonance imaging (MRI)
  - MRI scans are evaluated for edema patterns consistent with recent ACL tear.
  - Scans are also evaluated for other injuries, such as chondral or meniscal injuries.
  - MRI allows for preoperative planning and discussion of expectations with patients and their families.

SURGICAL ANATOMY

- Iliotibial band (ITB)
  - The ITB is located laterally along the leg and inserts into Gerdy's tubercle.
  - The ITB is a tendinous structure, which is the important reason why meniscotomes or a modified closed tendon stripper is used.
- Intermeniscal ligament
  - The intermensical ligament is located anterior to the medial aspect of the tibia.
  - It is the structure that helps maintain the ligament reconstruction in an anatomic manner.
- Figure 5 shows pediatric ACL anatomy. Note the proximity of the over-the-top position to the perichondrial ring of the distal femoral physis.

POSITIONING

- The patient is placed in the supine position.
- The extremities are padded.
- The tourniquet is placed on the operative leg as proximal as possible and the leg is prepped circumferentially from foot to tourniquet.
- A leg holder not used, but a retractable post can be placed on the side of the operative leg to aid with valgus stressing when having difficulty evaluating the medial compartment.

PORTALS/EXPOSURES

- Two standard arthroscopic portals are used.
  - The anterolateral portal is the primary viewing portal.
  - The anteromedial portal is the primary working portal.
- ITB harvest
  - A 6-cm incision is made laterally ending just short of the ITB insertion at Gerdy's tubercle.
- Proximal tibia incision
  - Approximately 3 cm medial and 2 cm inferior to the tubercle, a 2- to 3-cm incision is made to the bone and later through the periosteum.

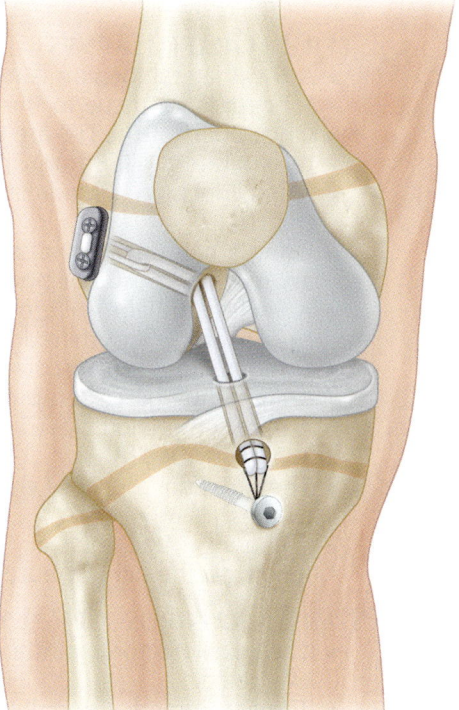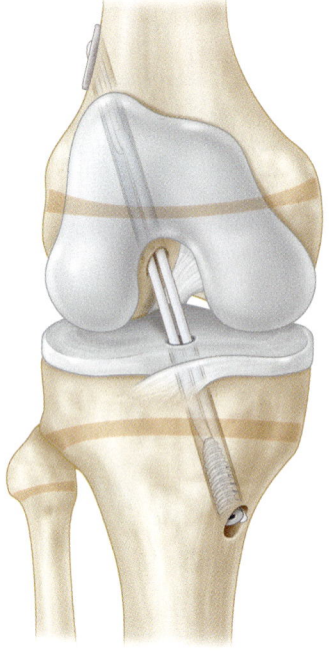

FIGURE 4

FIGURE 3

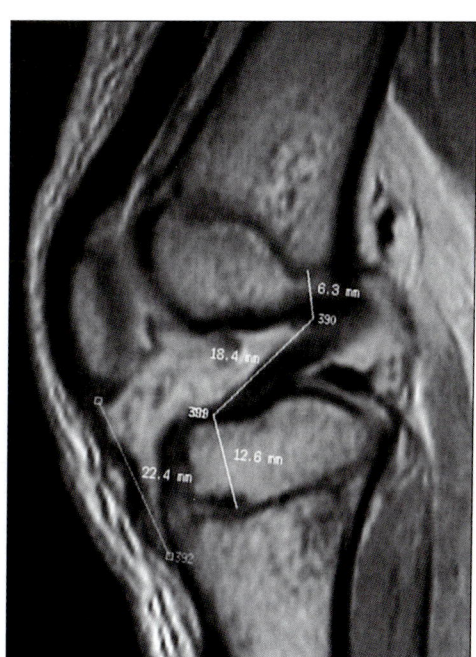

FIGURE 5

PEARLS

- *Harvest an adequate graft.*
- *A second incision can be made proximally if needed in order to harvest enough length of the ITB.*

PITFALLS

- *Avoid opening the capsule when obtaining length of the ITB; this helps to maintain the joint when arthroscopy is performed.*

PEARLS

- *Remember to make the anteromedial portal slightly larger to allow for the clamp later.*

PITFALLS

- *Avoid aggressive notchplasty.*
- *Avoid injuring the physis when placing the clamp in the over-the-top position.*

PROCEDURE

STEP 1: GRAFT HARVEST

- A 6-cm lateral incision is made through the skin and subcutaneous tissue to the ITB (Fig. 6).
- Once fibers of the ITB are visualized, a periosteal elevator is used to separate the ITB from the subcutaneous tissue.
- A small incision is made in the anterior and posterior border of the ITB.
- Using a pair of Mayo scissors, the ITB is elevated between the anterior and posterior border.
- A Smiley cartilage knife/meniscotome is run up the anterior border of ITB and then again up the posterior border.
- Using a curved meniscotome up the anterior border, the ITB graft can be harvested proximally (Fig. 7).
  - A new modified closed tendon stripper can also be used to harvest the ITB.
- The proximal aspect of the graft is whipstitched using Ethibond sutures.
- The graft is traced distally toward Gerdy's tubercle to add length to the harvest but must be left attached.

STEP 2: ARTHROSCOPIC EXAMINATION

- The patellofemoral joint and the medial and lateral gutters are evaluated.
- The anteromedial portal is then established, and the shaver is placed into the joint to increase visualization by shaving the ligamentum mucosum.
- The medial and lateral compartments are evaluated, and if there are meniscal tears, they are repaired if necessary.
- The notch is evaluated and the remaining ACL stump is then débrided.
- The intermeniscal ligament is located anterior to the medial meniscus.
- The full-length clamp is taken through the anteromedial portal and pushed through the joint to the over-the-top position, spreading to help make room for the graft to fit through the knee joint.

STEP 3: GRAFT PASSAGE AND FIXATION

- The full-length clamp is passed out the joint capsule at the over-the-top position (Fig. 8).
- The suture is passed from the graft into the clamp.
- The graft is retrieved from the over-the-top position to inside the knee joint.
- A 3-cm incision is now made at the proximal medial tibia metaphysis down to the periosteum; this is approximately 2 fingerbreadths medial to the tibial tubercle and approximately 2–3 cm below the joint.
- A snit-type clamp is then placed in the proximal tibial incision and passed along the anterior tibia up through the intermeniscal ligament. Spreading of the clamp may be helpful to create some space to allow the graft to be passed.
- A rat tail rasp is then used through the proximal tibia incision and used to rasp the proximal medial epiphysis area to allow the graft to seat somewhat posterior in a more anatomic position (Fig. 9).
- The clamp is then placed through the proximal tibia incision and used to grasp the sutures at the end of the graft through the intermeniscal ligament and out the proximal tibia incision (Fig. 10).
- Tension is now placed on the graft with the knee flexed at 90° and externally rotated at 30°.

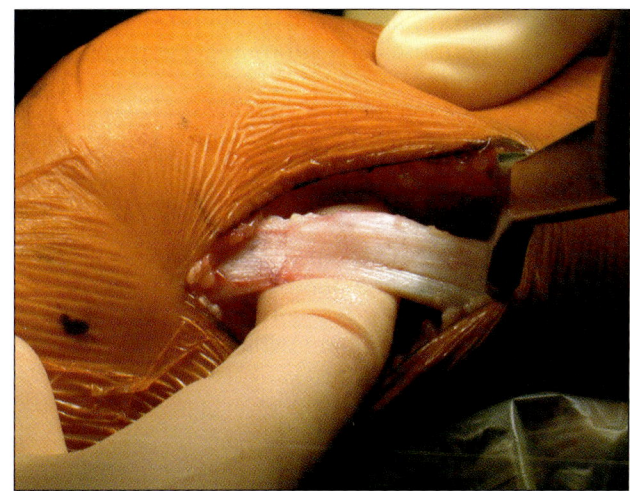

FIGURE 6

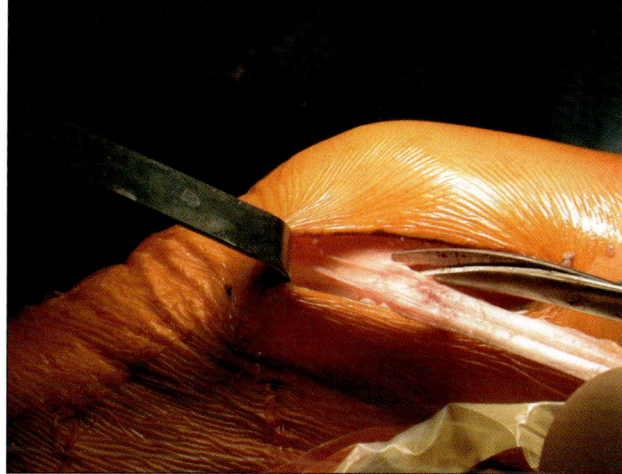

FIGURE 7

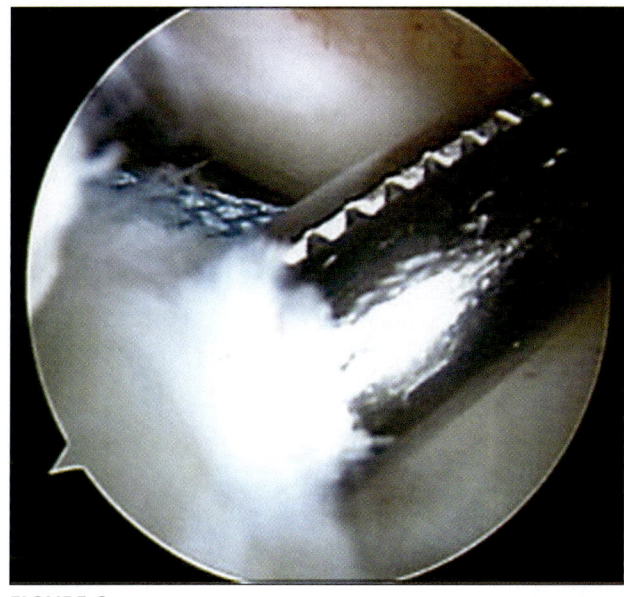

FIGURE 8

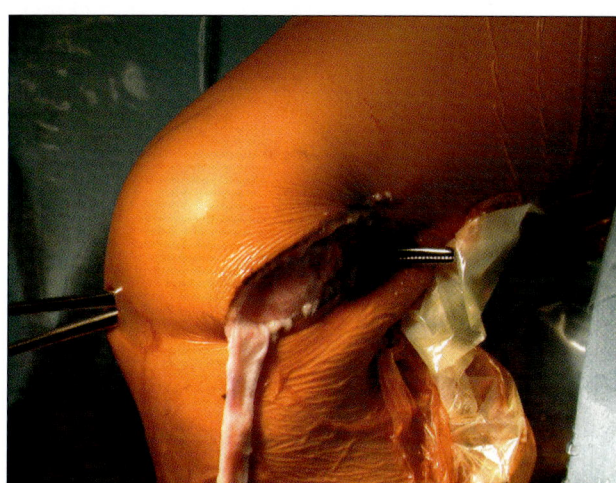

FIGURE 9

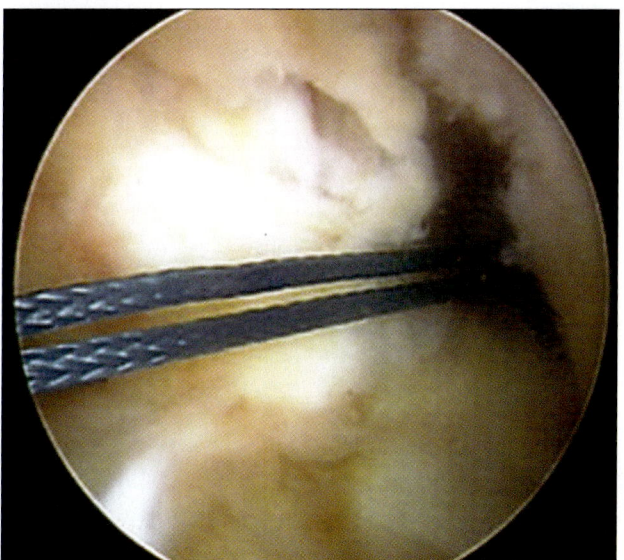

FIGURE 10

- Multiple mattress-type sutures are placed at the proximal end of the graft through the intermuscular septum and the periosteum of the femur (Fig. 11).
- The periosteum of the proximal tibia is then incised.
- The edge of the periosteum is then elevated with a Cobb elevator.
- The bone is decorticated with a small burr.
- The graft is tensioned down as much as possible.
- The knee is placed in 20–30° of flexion.
- Using Ethibond suture through the periosteum and then the graft, the distal aspect of the graft is secured (Fig. 12).
- The incisions are closed in layer fashion with Vicryl and then Monocryl.
- Figure 13 shows a schematic of the reconstruction.
- Figure 14 shows the postoperative MRI appearance; Figure 15 shows the postoperative arthroscopic appearance.

POSTOPERATIVE CARE AND EXPECTED OUTCOMES

- Incisions are covered with a dressing and an Ace bandage, then a Cryo-cuff is placed.
- The patient is then placed in a hinged knee brace set at 0–30° range of motion.
- Continuous passive motion, also set at 0–30°, is used 6–8 hours daily for 2 weeks postoperatively.
- Touch-down weight bearing is permitted for 6 weeks postoperatively.
- A hinged knee brace is used for 6 weeks.
- A follow-up clinic visit is scheduled at 2 weeks.

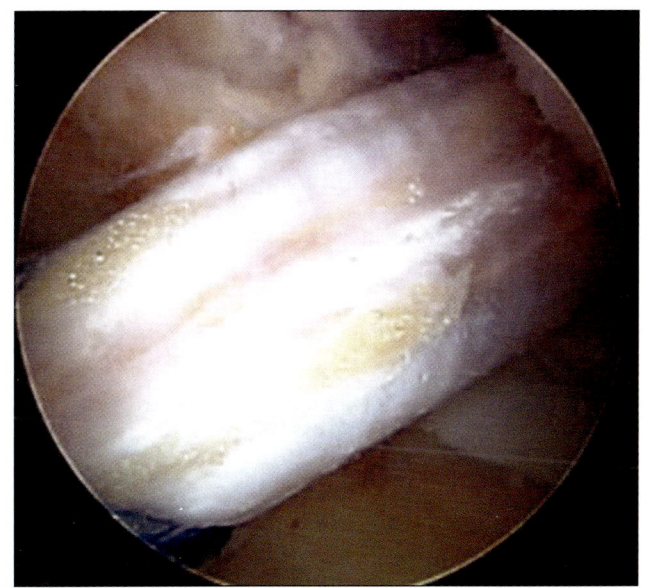

FIGURE 11

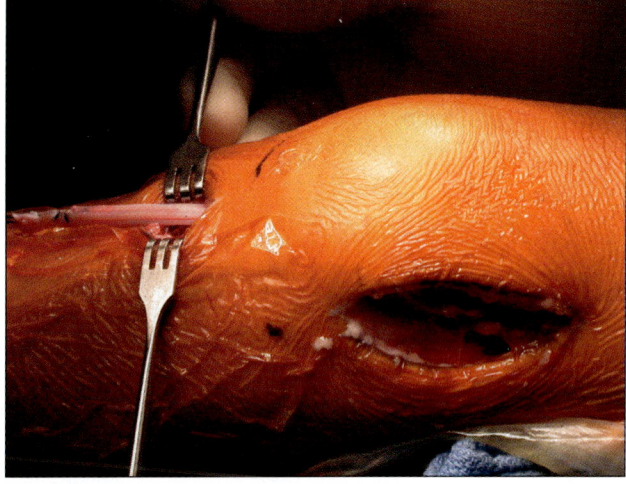

FIGURE 12

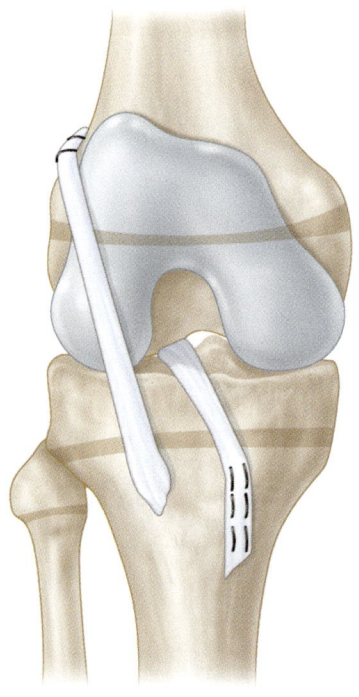

FIGURE 13

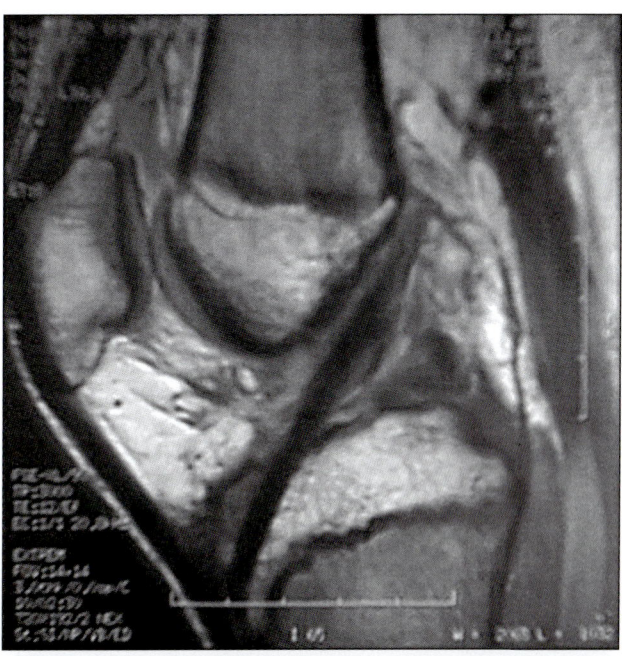

FIGURE 14

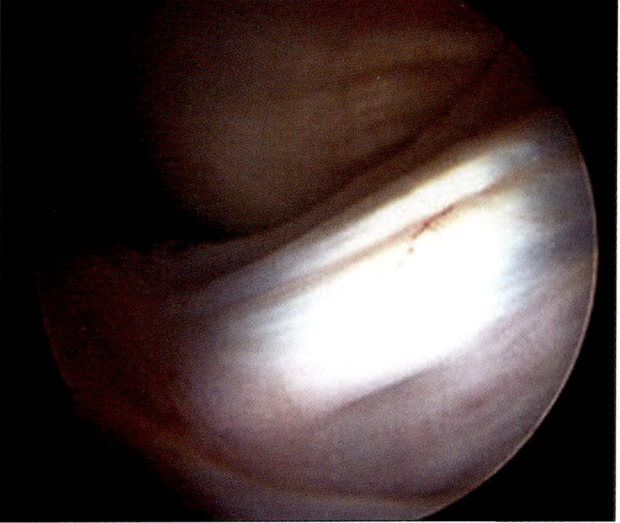

FIGURE 15

EVIDENCE

Angel KR, Hall DJ. Anterior cruciate ligament injury in children and adolescents. Arthroscopy. 1989;5:197–200.

Review of 27 cases showed there was associated pathology in 41% patients with ACL tears in patients 8–18 years of age.

Graf BK, et al. Anterior cruciate ligament tears in skeletally immature patients: meniscal pathology at presentation and after attempted conservative treatment. Arthroscopy. 1992;8:229–33.

Twelve skeletally immature patients with ACL tears were all treated with brace. Seven of 12 developed meniscal tears from the time of their initial nonoperative treatment. Brace did not prevent further injuries.

Guzzanti V, et al. The effect of intra-articular ACL reconstruction on the growth plates of rabbits. J Bone Joint Surg [Br]. 1994;76:960–3.

Study of ACL in rabbits. Using 2 mm tunnels for ACL reconstruction, 3 of 21 of the rabbits noted to have disturbances at the physes.

Janarv PM, et al. Anterior cruciate ligament injuries in skeletally immature patients. J Pediatr Orthop. 1996;16:673–7.

Twenty-eight skeletally immature patients with ACL tears were followed after being treated nonoperatively. Twenty of 28 eventually underwent surgery to allow for return to previous activity level.

Kocher MS, Garg S, Micheli LJ. Physeal sparing reconstruction of the anterior cruciate ligament in skeletally immature prepubescent children and adolescents. J Bone Joint Surg [Am]. 2005;87:2371–9.

Description of ITB physeal sparing ACL reconstruction done at Children's Hospital of Boston. Forty-four patients were studied. Only 2 required revision of ACL reconstruction. No significant growth disturbances were noted in this study.

Kocher MS, Saxon H, Hovis WD, Hawkins RJ. Management and complications of anterior cruciate ligament injuries in skeletally immature patients: survey of the Herodicus Society and The ACL Study Group. J Pediatr Orthop. 2002;22:452–7.

Survey conducted of members of Herodicus society regarding complications in skeletally immature patients treated with surgery for their ACL injuries. Fifteen complications were noted by the members in the survey. Valgus deformities with and without bar as well as leg length and recurvatum were the complications reported.

Lipscomb AB, Anderson AF. Tears of the anterior cruciate ligament in adolescents. J Bone Joint Surg [Am]. 1986;68:19–28.

Twenty-four patients aged 12–15 years of age underwent transphyseal ACL reconstruction with hamstring autograft. Fifteen of 24 patients returned to sport.

McCarroll JR, Rettig AC, Shelbourne KD. Anterior cruciate ligament injuries in the young athlete with open physes. Am J Sports Med. 1988;16:44–7.

Forty patients under 14 with open physes and ACL tears were studied. Twenty-four underwent surgery and 22 returned to sports. Sixteen patients treated non-operatively only 7 returned to sports while having pain, effusions, and knee giving away not reported in the surgically treated group.

Millett PJ, Willis AA, Warren RF. Associated injuries in pediatric and adolescent anterior cruciate ligament tears: does a delay in treatment increase the risk of meniscal tear? Arthroscopy. 2002;18:955–9.

Retrospective study on 39 patients under 14 years of age who had ACL injuries. Results showed that associated injuries were common in the ACL injured patient. Delay in surgery was associated with increased incidence of medial meniscal tears.

Mizuta H, et al. The conservative treatment of complete tears of the anterior cruciate ligament in skeletally immature patients. J Bone Joint Surg [Br]. 1995;77:890–4.

The authors followed 18 skeletally immature patients for 36 months initially treated nonoperatively. Six patients underwent ACL reconstruction during study period. Only one of the 18 patients treated nonoperatively returned to sport. Degenerative changes were noted in x-rays of 11 of 18 patients.

Open Reduction and Internal Fixation of Tibial Tubercle Fractures

Brian K. Brighton and Yi-Meng Yen

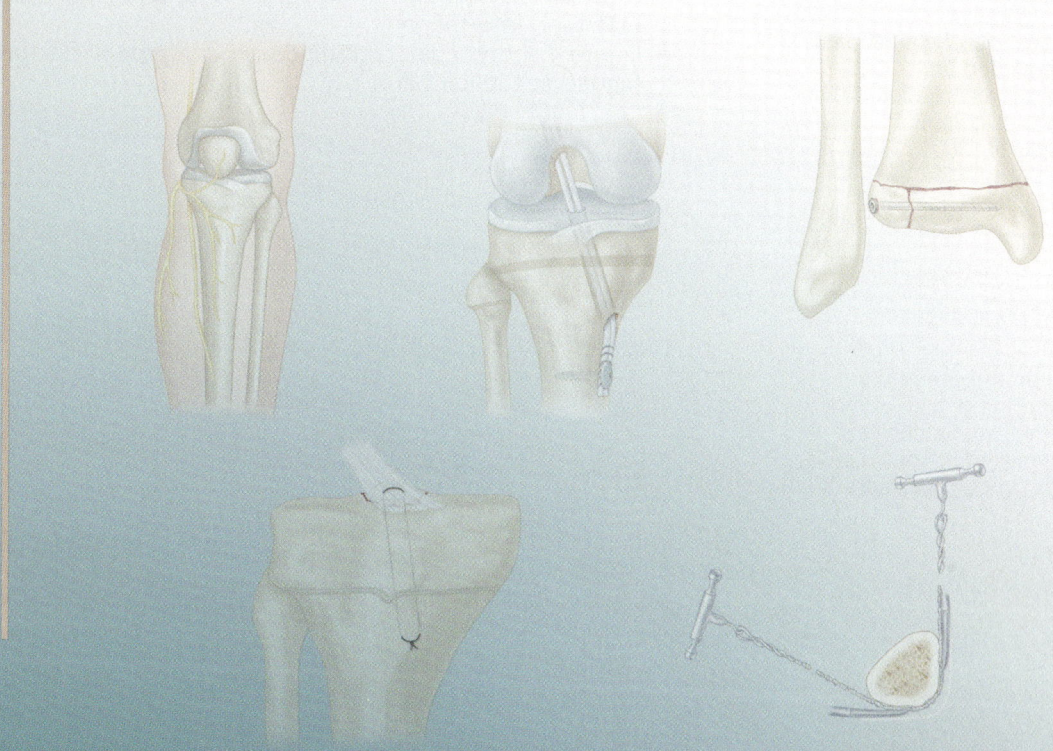

Controversies

- Some fractures may be amendable to closed reduction and percutaneous screw fixation if there is not significant comminution or fracture displacement.

Treatment Options

- Open reduction and internal fixation of the fracture fragment.
- Depending on the size of the fragment and the degree of comminution, fixation choices include cannulated or solid screws, staples, pins, wires, and suture.

INDICATIONS

- Displaced type I and types II, III, and IV fractures are best treated with open reduction and internal fixation.

EXAMINATION/IMAGING

- Fractures can be described by the Ogden modification of the Watson-Jones classification to emphasize both degree of proximal fracture extension and amount of comminution. Figure 1A–E illustrates types I through V, respectively.
- Lateral radiographs of the knee in slight internal rotation provide an adequate view of the tibial tubercle to assess fracture displacement.
  - Figure 2 shows a lateral radiograph of a type I fracture.
  - Figure 3 shows a lateral radiograph of a type II/III with extension into the joint.
  - Figure 4 shows a lateral radiograph of a type III fracture hinged at the joint line.

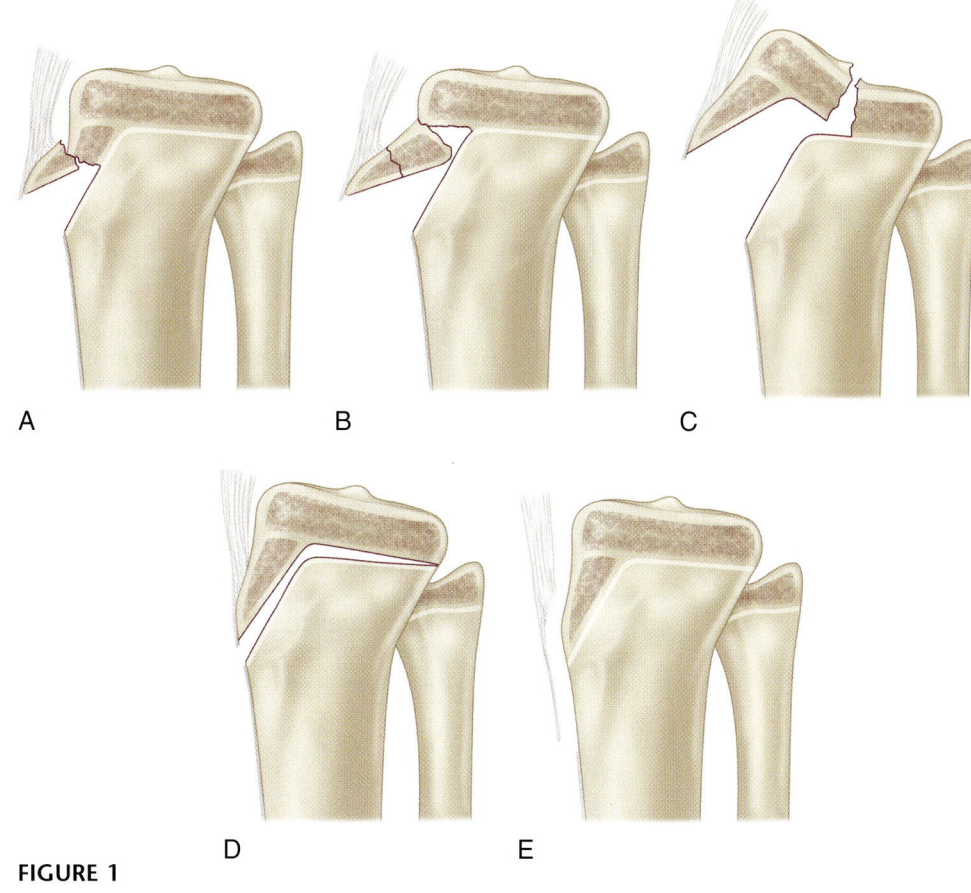

A   B   C

D   E

FIGURE 1

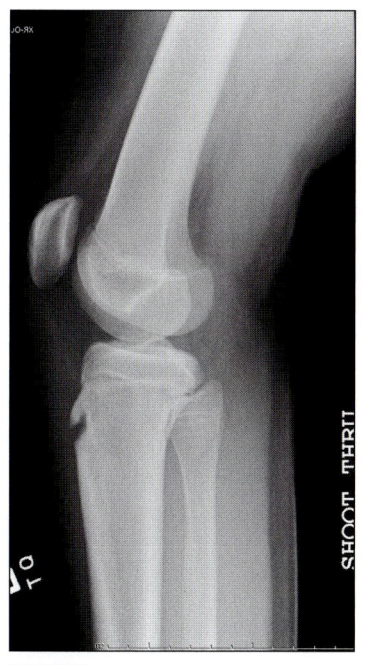

FIGURE 2

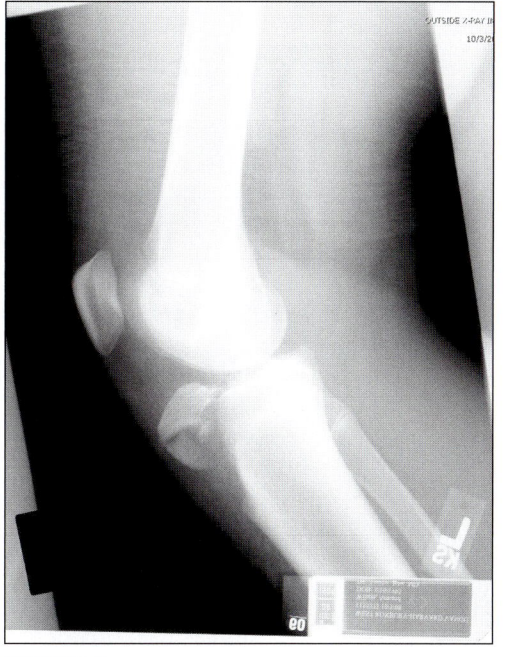

FIGURE 3

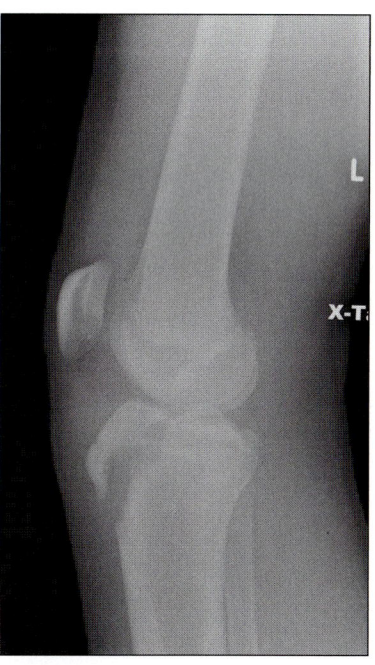

FIGURE 4

- Figure 5 shows a lateral radiograph of a type IV fracture.
■ Magnetic resonance imaging of the knee can show the presence of a nondisplaced fracture line extending into the proximal tibial epiphysis (Fig. 6).

SURGICAL ANATOMY

■ The patellar ligament inserts on the tibial tubercle and has attachments into the deep fascia of the proximal tibia.
  • When injured, this results in varying degrees of soft tissue disruption to the periosteum, extensor retinaculum, and deep fascia adjacent to the tibial tubercle, which often necessitates repair.
■ Along the lateral aspect of the tibial tubercle, there are branches of the anterior tibial recurrent artery that may retract laterally and distally into the musculature of the anterior compartment at the time of injury, resulting in hematoma formation and increasing the risk of developing compartment syndrome (Fig. 7).
■ Medial branches of the infrapatellar branch of the saphenous nerve may be observed, and care should be taken to preserve this nerve to avoid a large area of anesthesia.

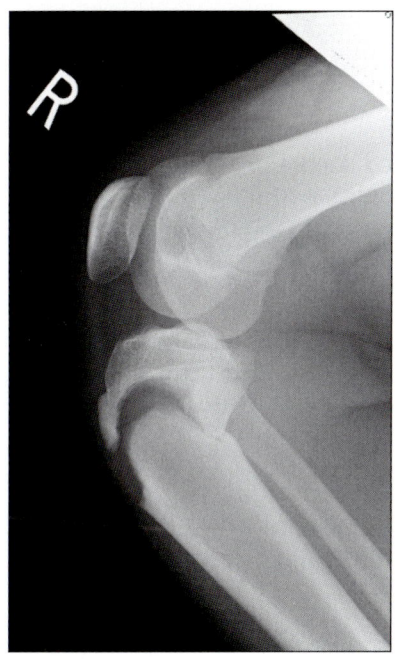

FIGURE 5

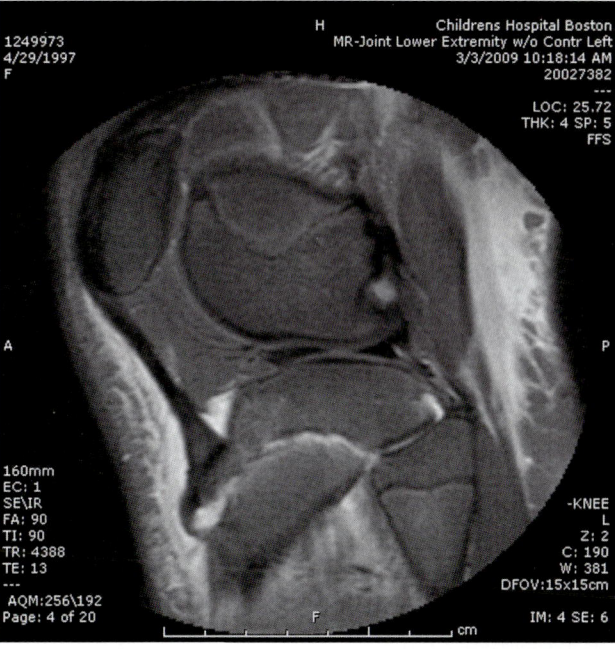

FIGURE 6

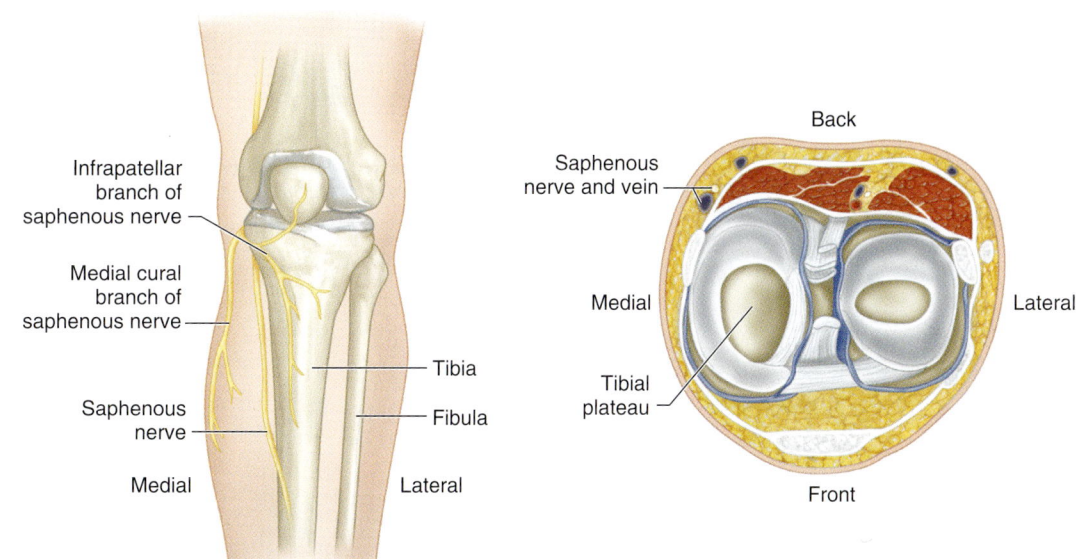

Infrapatellar branch of saphenous nerve

Medial cural branch of saphenous nerve

Saphenous nerve

Medial

Tibia

Fibula

Lateral

Back

Saphenous nerve and vein

Medial

Tibial plateau

Lateral

Front

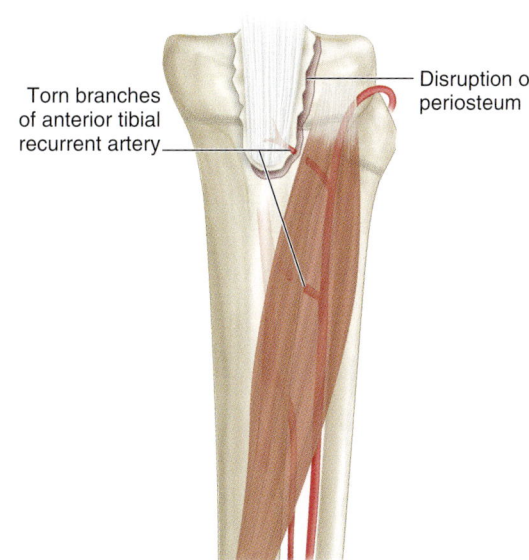

Torn branches of anterior tibial recurrent artery

Disruption of periosteum

FIGURE 7

Equipment

• Radiolucent table

Controversies

• Some authors advocate a lateral parapatellar approach to avoid the infrapatellar branch of the saphenous nerve (Fig. 10).

POSITIONING

■ The patient is positioned supine on a radiolucent table with a padded sterile tourniquet placed around the proximal thigh (Fig. 8).

PORTALS/EXPOSURES

■ Exposure is achieved through a longitudinal midline incision extending distally over the displaced tibial tubercle fragment.
■ Flaps medial and lateral to the fracture fragment are developed.

PROCEDURE

STEP 1: EXPOSURE OF FRACTURE SITE

■ Often there is tearing of the periosteum and deep fascia that can be repaired later but needs to first be cleared from the fracture site (Fig. 11).
■ Any fracture hematoma is irrigated and débrided to clear the fracture bed.

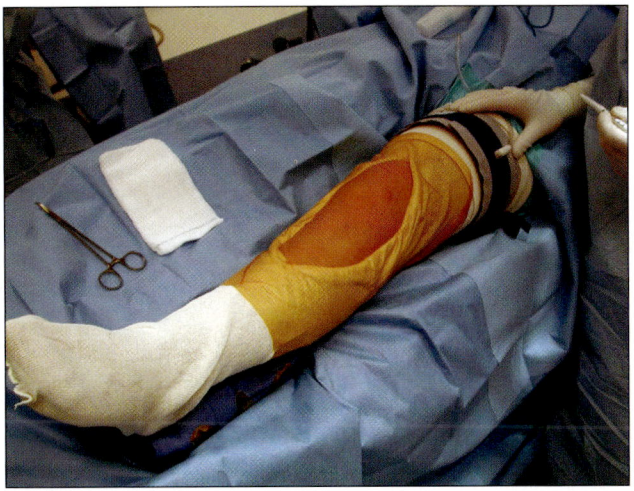

FIGURE 8

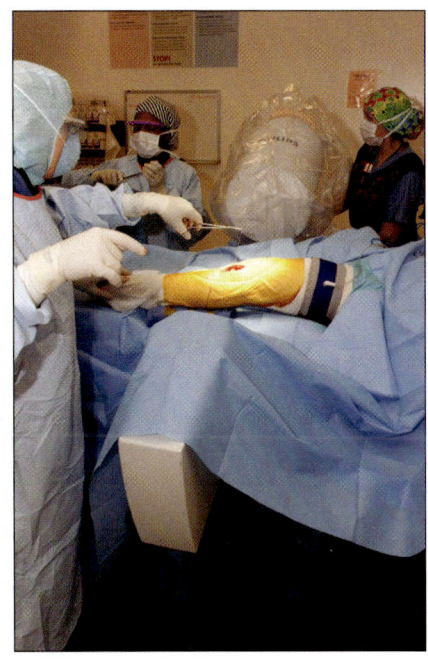

FIGURE 9

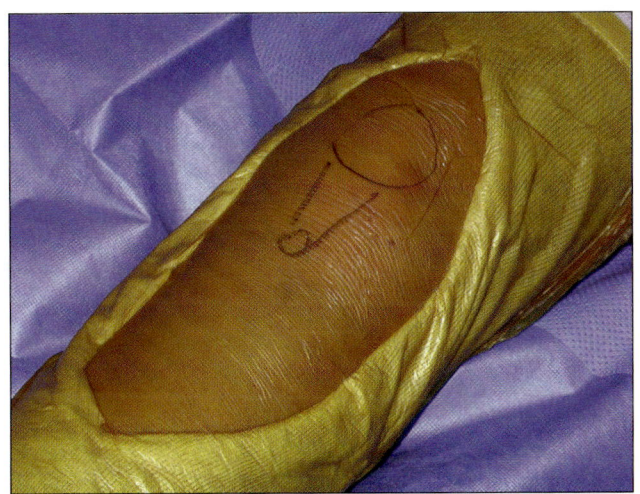

FIGURE 10

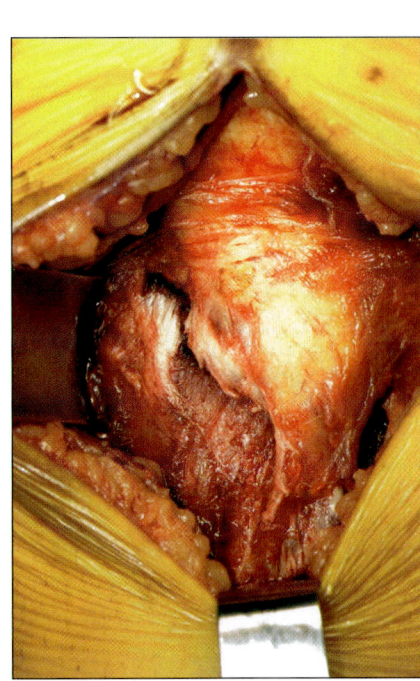

FIGURE 11

Instrumentation/Implantation

- Screw sizes vary from 4.0- to 4.5-mm cannulated cancellous screws for smaller fragments and individuals to 6.5- to 7.3-mm screws for larger fragments.

Controversies

- Using smooth pins in children with more than 3 years of growth remaining may be preferable to prevent premature closure of the tibial tubercle.

STEP 2: REDUCTION AND FIXATION OF FRACTURE

- The fracture is reduced with the knee in extension.
- Depending on the size and number of fracture fragments, several guidewires can be placed parallel through the fracture fragments in either the metaphysis or epiphysis (Figs. 12 and 13).
- The direction, location, and length of the guidewires is confirmed with fluoroscopy (Fig. 14).
- The guidewires are measured for the appropriate-length screws (Fig. 15).
- The guidewires are then overdrilled for the selected screw size.
- Washers may be added to the screws for additional fixation (Fig. 16).
- The screws can approach the posterior cortex but do not have to be bicortical (Fig. 17).

PEARLS

- *A ball-tipped pushing spike can be used to help hold the fracture reduced while placing guidewires across the fracture (see Fig. 13).*

- *Additional fixation may be added with wires, pins, or nonabsorbable suture.*

PITFALLS

- *Failure to obtain an adequate reduction at the joint line in type III fractures requires an arthrotomy.*

- *Patients may complain of pain over prominent screw heads with the use of larger screws.*

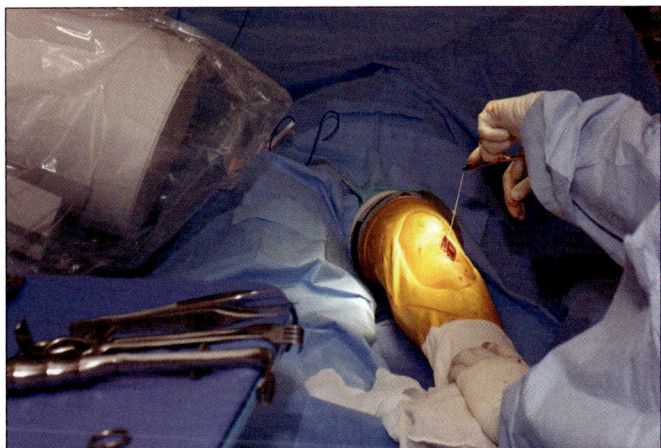

FIGURE 12

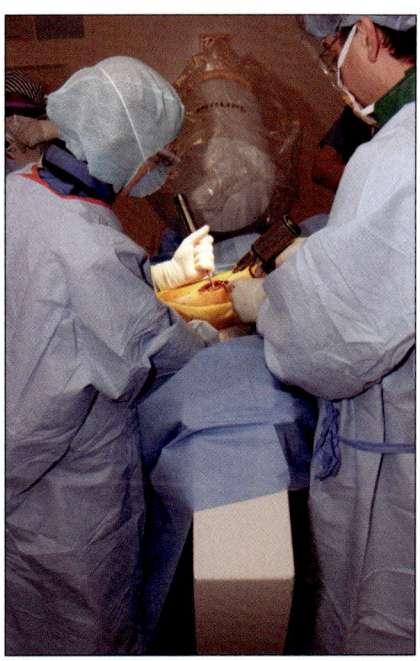

FIGURE 13

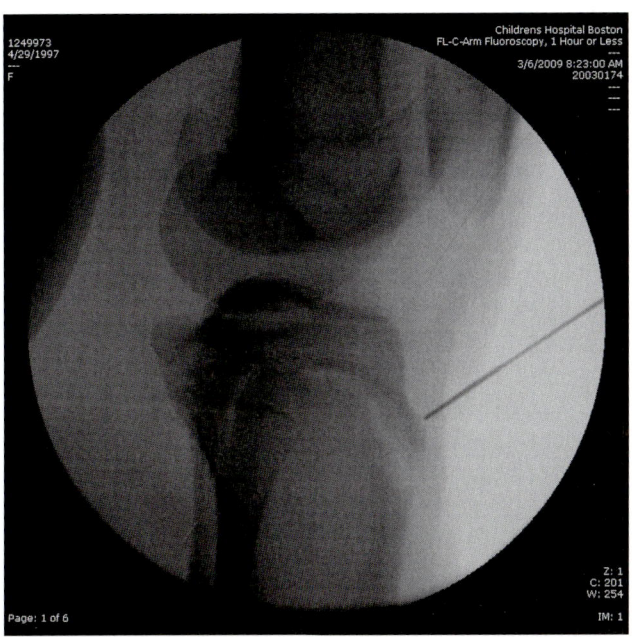

FIGURE 14

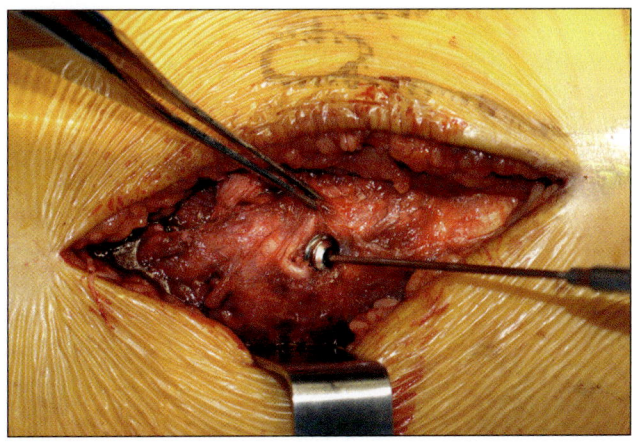

FIGURE 16

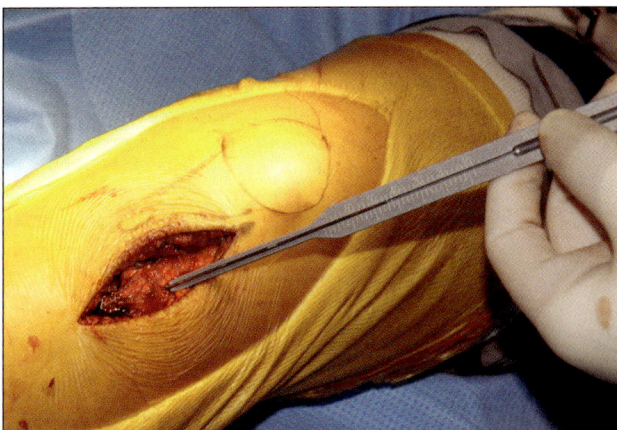

FIGURE 15

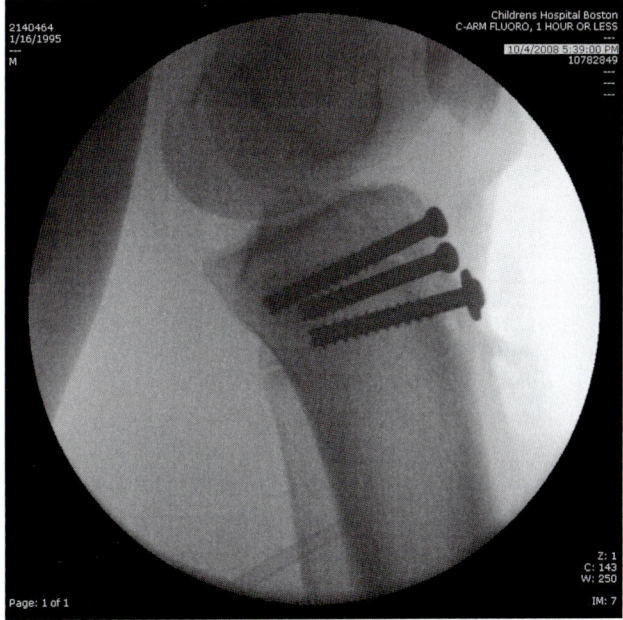

FIGURE 17

STEP 3: SOFT TISSUE REPAIR AND CLOSURE

- The torn periosteum and retinacular extensions need to be repaired with heavy nonabsorbable suture (Figs. 18–20).
- Repairing the soft tissue supplements the fracture repair.
- Figure 21 shows a preoperative lateral radiograph; Figure 22 shows an intraoperative fluoroscopic image, and Figure 23 shows anteroposterior (Fig. 23A) and lateral (Fig. 23B) postoperative radiographs.

POSTOPERATIVE CARE AND EXPECTED OUTCOMES

- Patients are placed into an above-the-knee long-leg or cylinder cast in full extension.
- Patients are kept either toe-touch or non–weight bearing for 6 weeks in the cast with crutches.
- Once the cast is removed, physical therapy and weight bearing are initiated with the use of a hinged knee brace.
- During the first 2 weeks out of the cast, patients are allowed active flexion and passive knee extension with weight bearing in the brace locked in full extension.
- After 2 weeks of physical therapy have been completed, patients are allowed to begin active extension and weight bearing with the brace unlocked.
- Range-of-motion and strengthening exercises are then progressed.
- Once sports-specific rehabilitation goals have been met, the patient can return to sports activity, typically by 3–4 months.

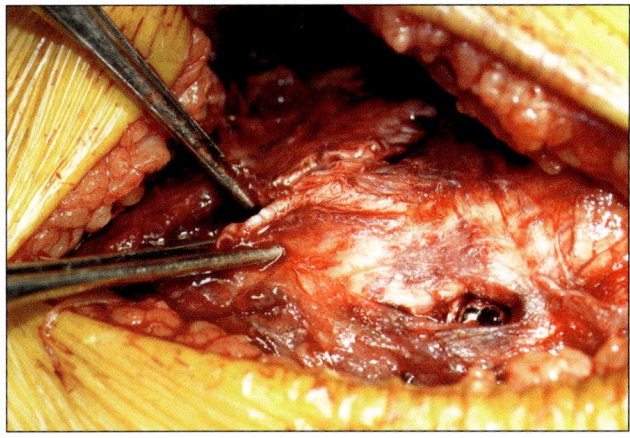

FIGURE 18

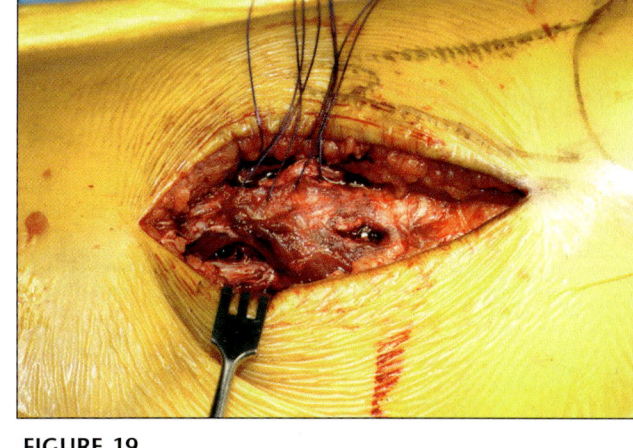

FIGURE 19

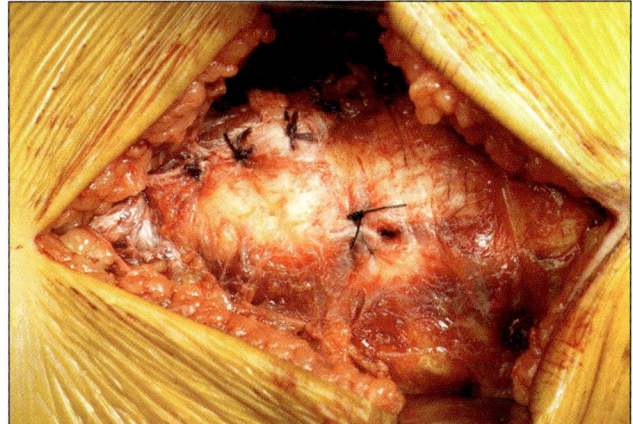

FIGURE 20

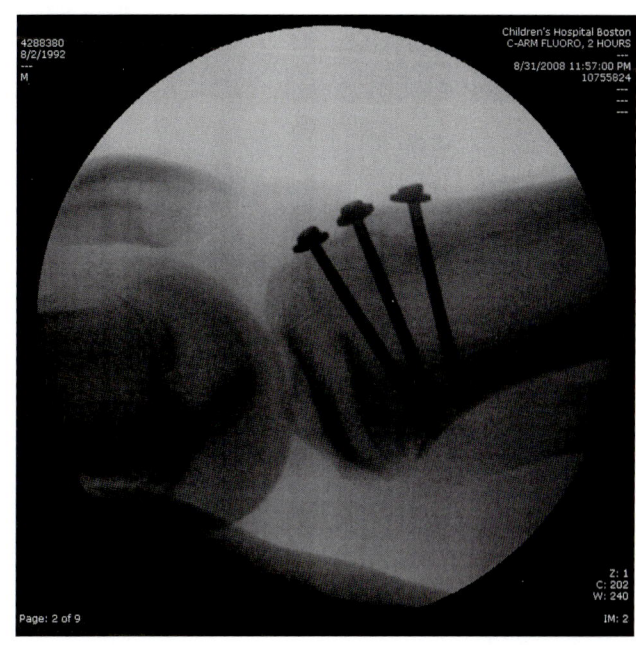

FIGURE 22

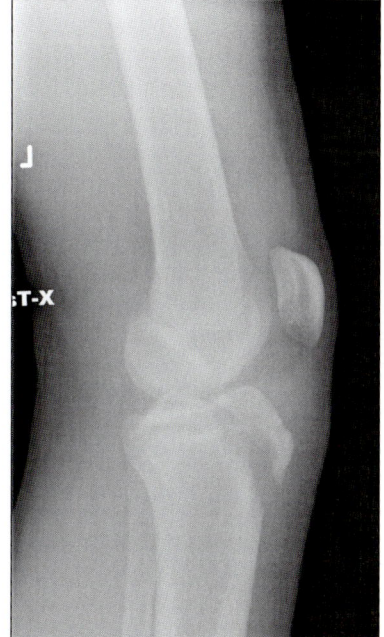

FIGURE 21

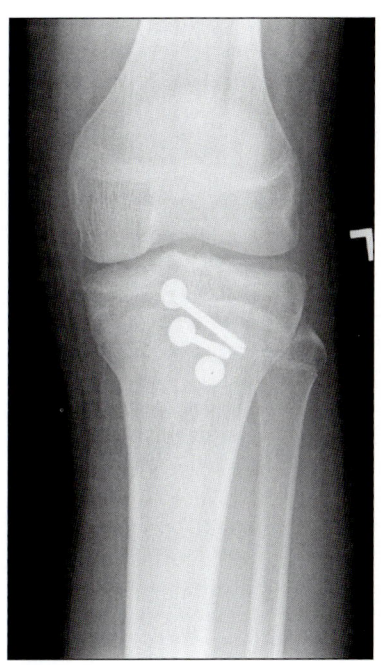

A

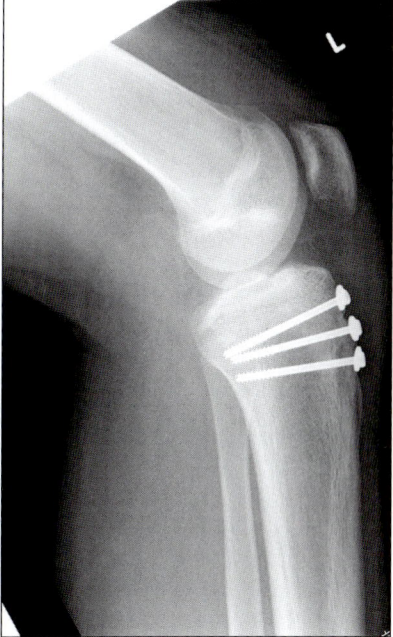

B

FIGURE 23

EVIDENCE

Mosier SM, Stanitski CL. Acute tibial tubercle avulsion fractures. J Pediatr Orthop. 2004;24:181–4.

The authors presented a retrospective review of 19 tibial tubercle fractures with operative fixation on 15 fractures. (Level IV evidence)

Ogden JA, Tross RB, Murphy MJ. Fractures of the tibial tuberosity in adolescents. J Bone Joint Surg [Am]. 1980;62:205–15.

This paper presented a classification system of tibial tubercle fractures. (Level IV evidence)

Pape JM, Goulet JA, Hensinger RN. Compartment syndrome complicating tibial tubercle avulsion. Clin Orthop Relat Res. 1993;(295):201–4.

The authors presented a retrospective review of tibial tubercle fractures with the complication of compartment syndrome. (Level IV evidence)

Zrag M, Annabi H, Ammari T, Trabelsi M, Mbarek M, Ben Hassine H. Acute tibial tubercle avulsion fractures in the sporting adolescent. Arch Orthop Trauma Surg. 2008;128:1437–42.

The authors described recent operative intervention of acute tibial tubercle fracture, with satisfactory results at 4.5 years. (Level IV evidence)

Proximal Tibial Osteotomy for Blount's Disease

Deborah F. Stanitski

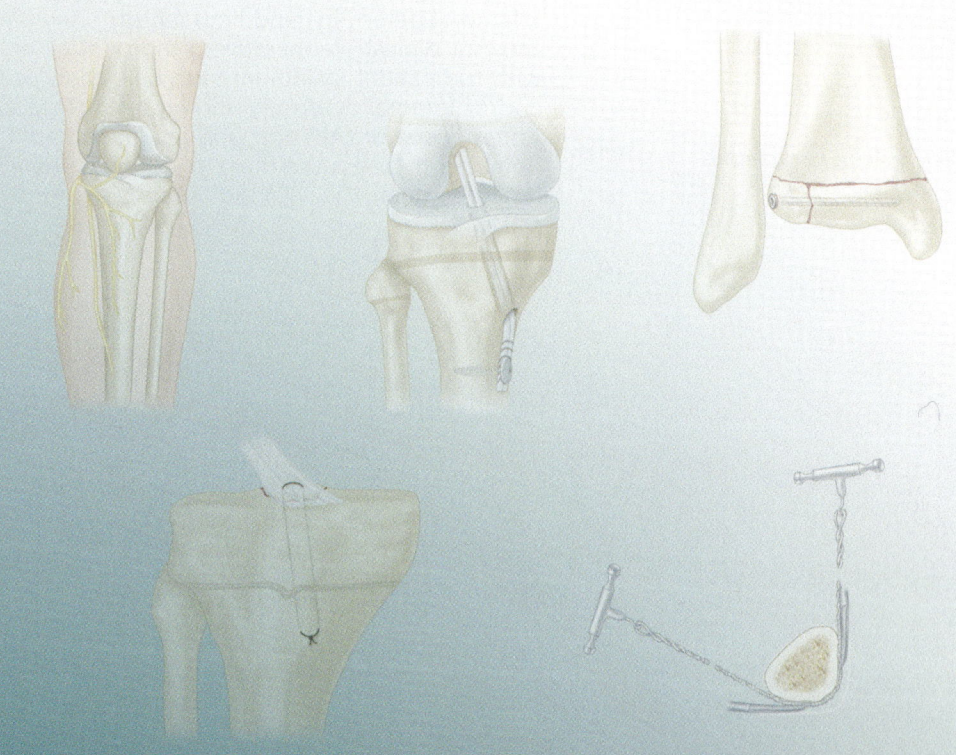

PITFALLS

- *Recurrence in young patients with significant growth remaining*
- *Abnormal bone density (e.g., history of renal disease)*
- *Possible concomitant SCFE*

Controversies

- Depression of tibial plateau
- Treatment of varus alone by stapling

Treatment Options

- Dependent on patient size, degree of deformity, ± joint depression

INDICATIONS

- Progressive tibial varus deformity
- Infantile, juvenile, or adolescent disease
- Associated limb-length inequality

EXAMINATION/IMAGING

- Complete physical examination with emphasis on:
  - Limb-length symmetry
  - Knee range of motion
  - Presence/absence of rotational abnormality
  - Hip examination for possible slipped capital femoral epiphysis (SCFE)
- Imaging studies
  - An orthoroentgenogram is obtained to assess alignment, ± femoral deformity, and limb length discrepancy. Figure 1 shows a typical preoperative orthoroentgenogram, obtained with the patient facing anterior, delineating coronal tibial and/or femoral deformity and limb length discrepancy.
  - Anteroposterior (AP) and frog-leg lateral radiographs are obtained to assess the hips. In Figure 2, the AP (Fig. 2A) and frog-leg lateral (Fig. 2B) radiographs demonstrate a right SCFE.

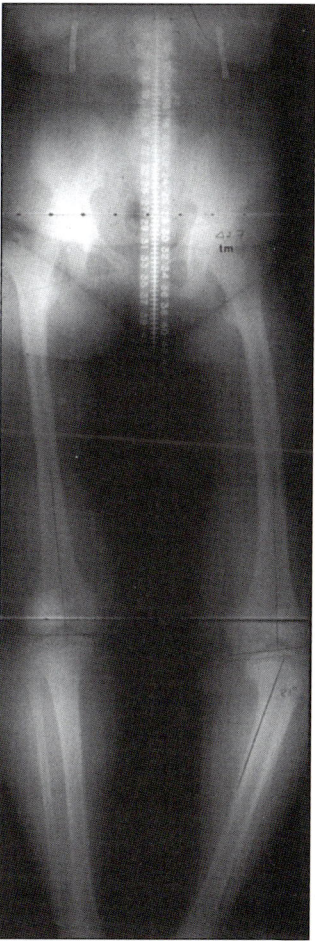

FIGURE 1

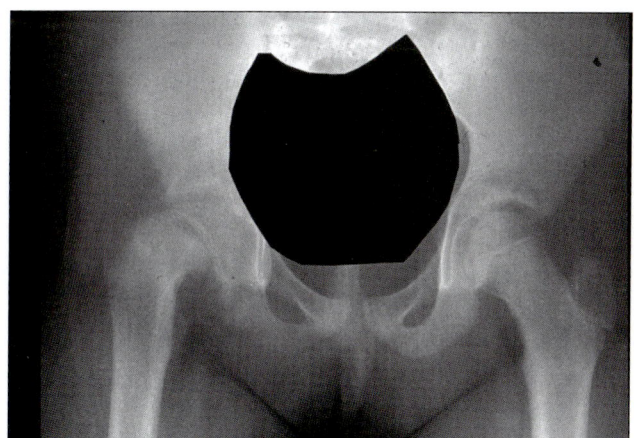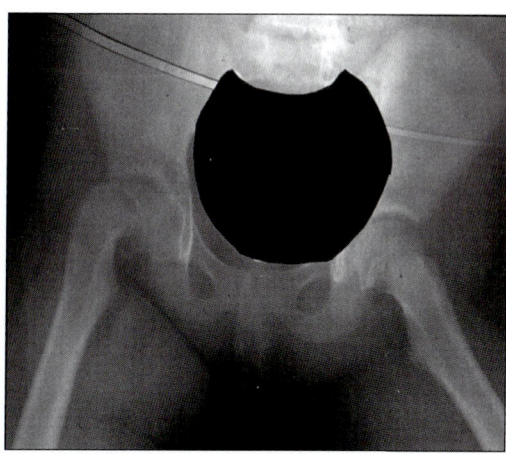

A
FIGURE 2
B

- An AP/lateral radiograph is obtained of the entire tibia, including the ankle joint. Figure 3 shows an orthoroentgenogram and lateral radiograph of the tibia in a 6-year-old.
- Computed tomography (CT) or magnetic resonance imaging (MRI) can be done if the patient is young or in a patient with long-standing problems to assess the joint surface. Figure 4 shows an MRI of the right proximal tibia delineating both the joint contour and the proximal physis.
- CT or MRI is also used for possible growth plate assessment.

SURGICAL ANATOMY

- The sural nerve is at risk when lengthening the gastrocnemius-soleus and on approach to the calcaneus and cuboid laterally.

POSITIONING

- The patient is placed supine with the patellae anterior and a tourniquet on the thigh. Draping is just distal to the tourniquet, leaving both legs visible for comparison, especially in acute correction (Fig. 5).
- General anesthesia is used.
- The involved leg is prepped distal to the tourniquet.
- The C-arm is placed perpendicular to the end of the bed, allowing both the surgeon and the assistant access from either side, as shown in Figure 5.

PORTALS/EXPOSURES

- The limb is exsanguinated.
- The tourniquet is elevated to 350 mm Hg.
- A distal fibular osteotomy (> 5 cm proximal to mortise) is performed. Bone is subcutaneous in this location, and osteotomy ≥ 5 cm from the joint will not interfere with the ankle.
- Two small Hohmann retractors facilitate the exposure.
- Bone is transected with a narrow oscillating saw with irrigation.
- The tourniquet is not released until after wound closure.

PITFALLS

- *Spinal anesthesia is not recommended in young patients due to anxiety.*
- *The patient should not be paralyzed; spinal anesthesia would not allow a neural response alerting the surgeon to any wire proximity to a motor nerve (e.g., the peroneal nerve).*

Controversies

- There is a controversy concerning the possible contribution of spinal anesthesia to compartment syndrome.

PEARLS

- *A distal, not proximal, fibular osteotomy is performed unless tibiofibular synostosis is present, to avoid peroneal nerve injury.*
- *Removal of a piece of fibula is unnecessary.*

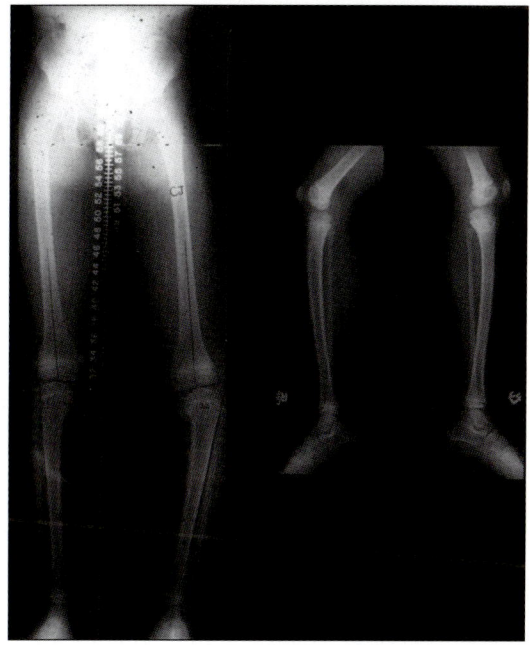

FIGURE 3

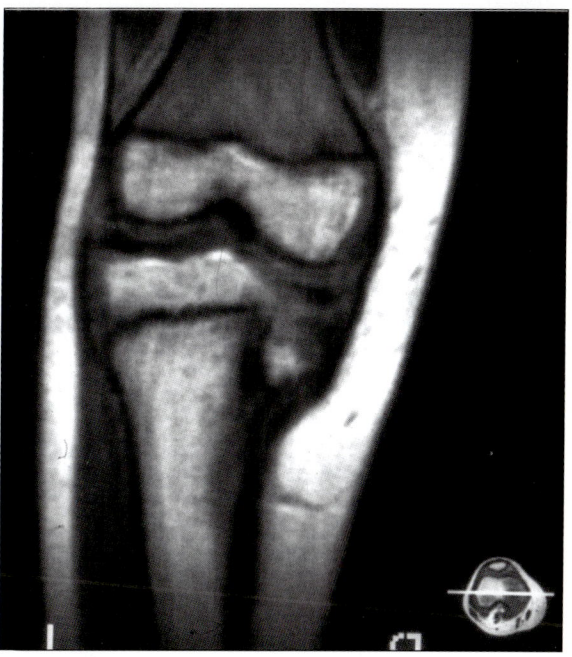

FIGURE 4

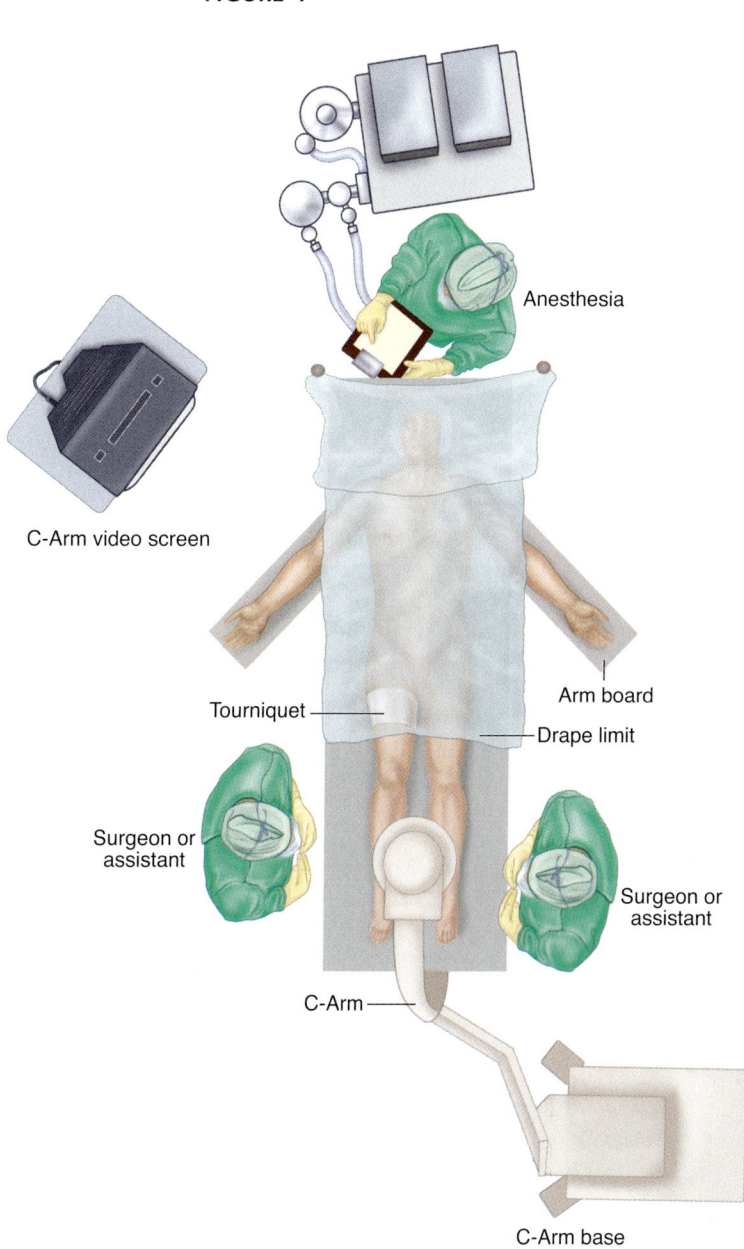

FIGURE 5

PROCEDURE: SMALL WIRE CIRCULAR FIXATORS

STEP 1

- Preoperative construction is based on patient size (ring size choice) and radiographs.
- The initial wire (when using wire fixators) should be smooth (Fig. 6) and is placed parallel to the proximal tibia just distal to the capsular insertion so as not to be intra-articular. The wire is tightened and tensioned appropriately.
- The second wire is again smooth and is placed distally parallel to the ankle joint and tightened and tensioned as was the first wire.
- The ring fixator is thus "hung" on the leg. It should be confirmed at this point, prior to additional wire insertion, that the fixator "fits" appropriately and that there is adequate soft tissue clearance, especially posterolaterally.
- Two additional smooth wires (one proximal and one distal) should be introduced at at such an angle as to transfix both the fibula and tibia (posterolateral to anteromedial).
- Two additional wires (stoppered or "olive" wires; see Fig. 6) are applied from anteromedial to posterolateral. These two wires should be closer together than the final two wires and are placed distal to the second ring and proximal to the third ring from the knee joint.
- Finally, the last two stoppered wires are placed posterolateral to anteromedial proximal to the second ring and distal to the third ring from the knee.

STEP 2

- The tibial osteotomy itself can be done in a number of ways.
- Predrilling the cortices with irrigation through a 1-cm longitudinal incision and then completing the osteotomy with a narrow osteotome is one option.
  - The benefit of this technique is one small incision.
  - The disadvantage is the necessity of disconnecting the proximal and distal ring complexes and the potential of a nonlinear osteotomy.
- The other option is an osteotomy using a Gigli saw requiring two incisions (Fig. 7A) but producing a linear osteotomy without disconnecting the rings (Fig. 7B). One must be careful when coming through the anterior cortex not to damage the anterior skin (Fig. 7C).

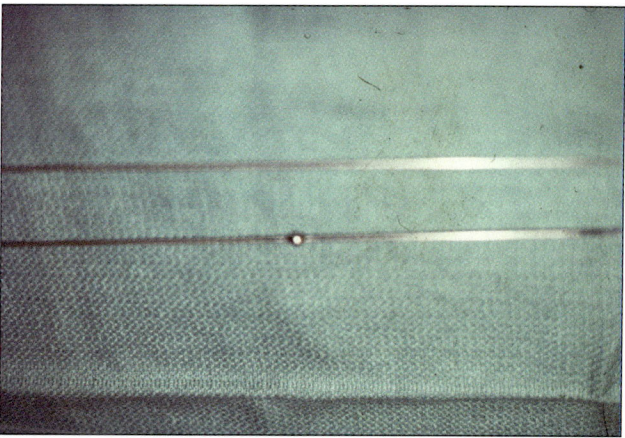

FIGURE 6

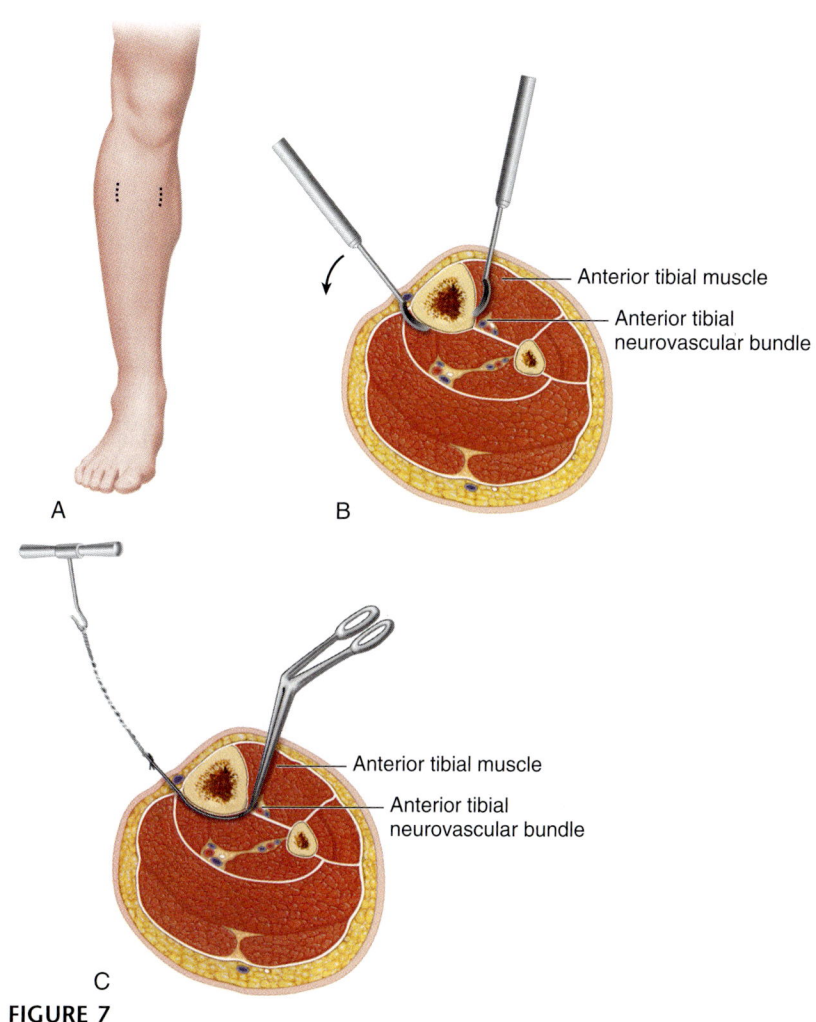

A

B

Anterior tibial muscle

Anterior tibial
neurovascular bundle

C

Anterior tibial muscle

Anterior tibial
neurovascular bundle

FIGURE 7

STEP 3

- A template of plexiglass is used to ensure anatomic correction if done acutely in the operating room.
  - The template can be purchased and modified with 2-mm Kirschner wires glued or taped to produce the appropriate distal femoral and proximal tibial anatomic axes.
  - A template can be created for the right or the left leg by flipping it over.
- Acute correction to the 87° proximal tibial angle can be performed, checking the final position using the C-arm with the plexiglass template.
- Acute correction of > 20° is probably unwise due to the delayed healing potential, even in a child, with an opening wedge type osteotomy.
- Hinge location (at or lateral to the lateral cortex) is critical if lengthening is either desired or not. Figure 8A shows pure angular correction (triangular regenerate of new bone). Figure 8B shows angular correction plus lengthening (trapezoidal regenerate bone).

PROCEDURE: HALF-PIN MONOLATERAL FIXATORS

STEP 1

- Two half-pins are inserted proximally (size is dependent on patient size; type is dependent on fixator type).
  - The pins are placed parallel to the knee joint line anteromedial to posterolateral and anterolateral to posteromedial (Fig. 9).
  - Ideally these should not be at exactly the same level in order to facilitate bony purchase.
- Two half-pins are placed distally, parallel to each other and parallel to the ankle joint (location is fixator-dependent). They are directed from anterior to posterior (see Fig. 9).

STEP 2

- Bleeding from the tibial osteotomy is decreased by tourniquet use temporarily.
- Tibial oteotomy can be achieved by various methods (see Small Wire Circular Fixators, Step 2).

STEP 3

- Acute correction of angulation can be performed again using the plexiglass template to check the position.
- The pin-skin junction is stabilized by wrapping the entire pin group (one group proximal and one distal) with a 2-inch Kling bandage.

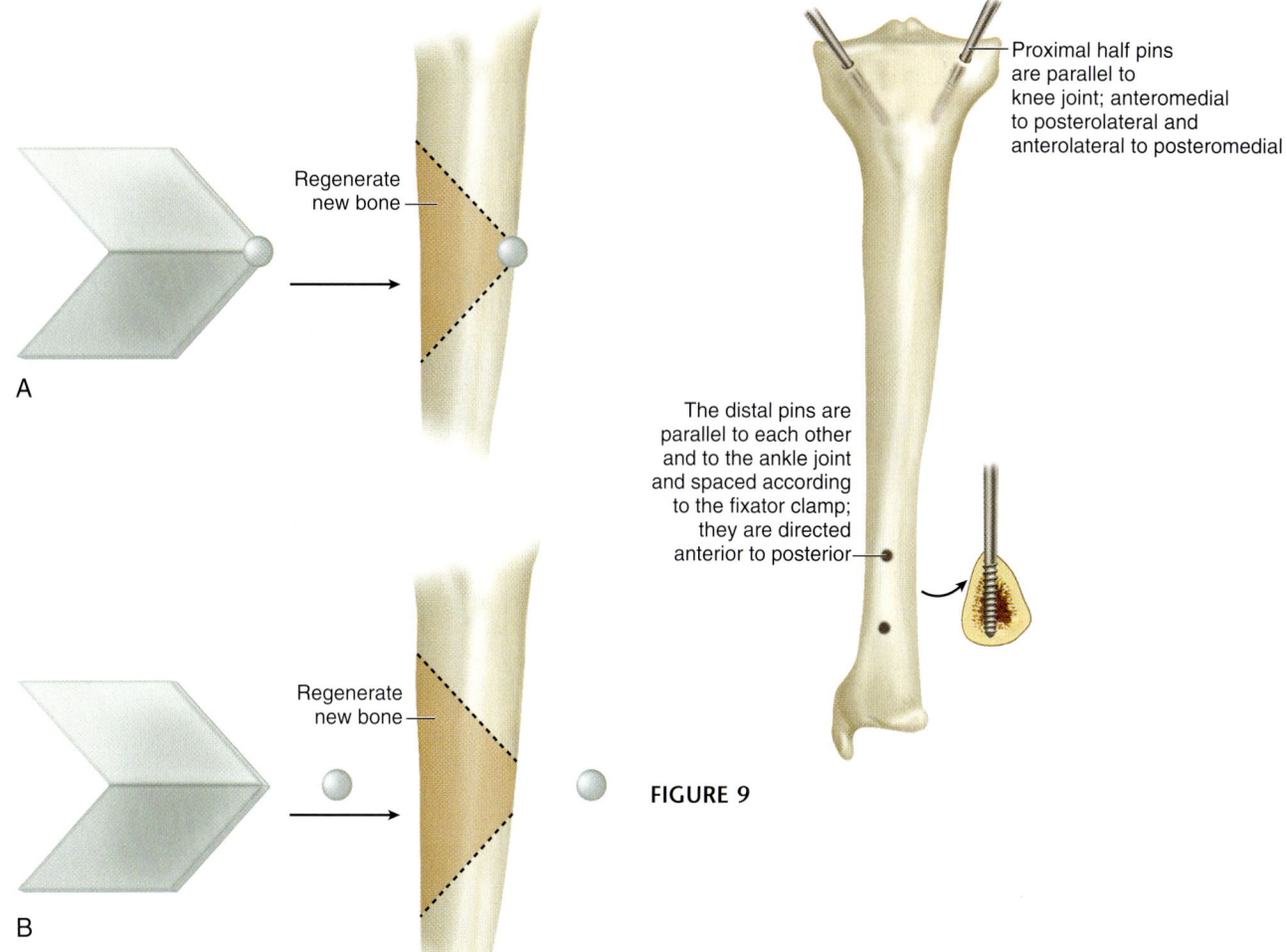

Regenerate
new bone

A

Regenerate
new bone

B

FIGURE 8

Proximal half pins
are parallel to
knee joint; anteromedial
to posterolateral and
anterolateral to posteromedial

The distal pins are
parallel to each other
and to the ankle joint
and spaced according
to the fixator clamp;
they are directed
anterior to posterior

FIGURE 9

PITFALLS

- *Pin site inflammation or infection occurs in 100% of patients and usually responds to 7 days of broad-spectrum oral antibiotics.*

- *Noncompliance with ROM and/or weight bearing is common.*

POSTOPERATIVE CARE AND EXPECTED OUTCOMES

- All patients receive 24 hours of intravenous antibiotic prophylaxis.
- Pin care is performed once daily.
  - Solution used is not important.
  - Removing crusts is important.
- Showers are encouraged. Bathing is discouraged, as are hot tubs.
- Use of chemically treated cold swimming pools is encouraged for pin hygiene and limb use (Fig. 10).
- Weight bearing as tolerated is encouraged *throughout* treatment with both small wire and large pin fixators (Fig. 11). Initially this is often in the parallel bars at physical therapy (Fig. 12A) but progresses to a walker, crutches, or cane (Fig. 12B).
- All patients are seen by a physical therapist postoperatively to encourage knee and ankle range of motion (ROM), weight bearing, and crutch or walker use.
- Lengthening or gradual angular correction commences 5–7 days postoperatively.

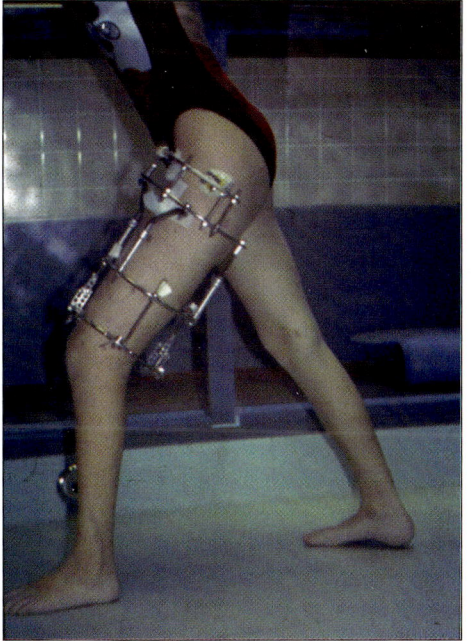

FIGURE 10

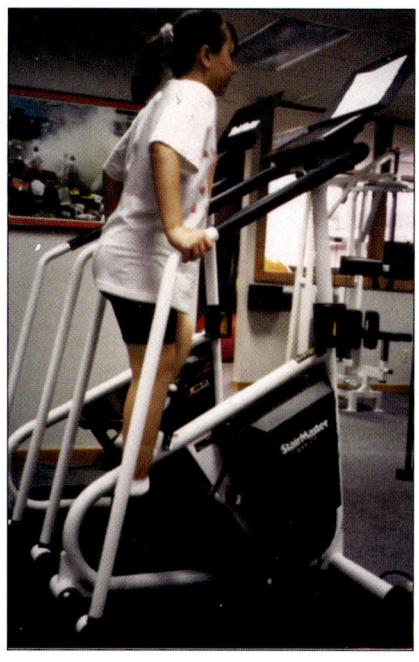

FIGURE 11

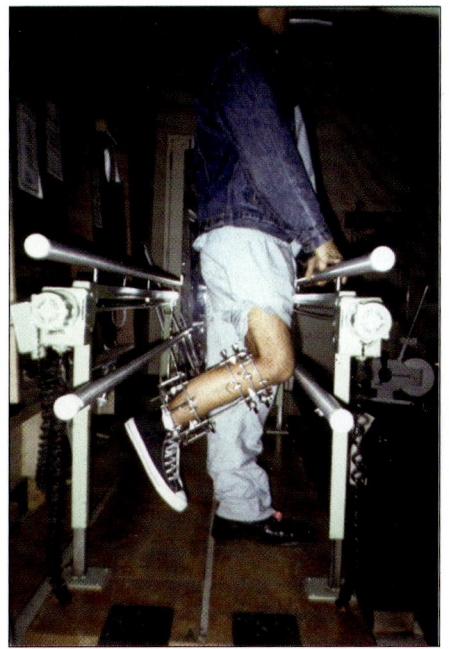

A

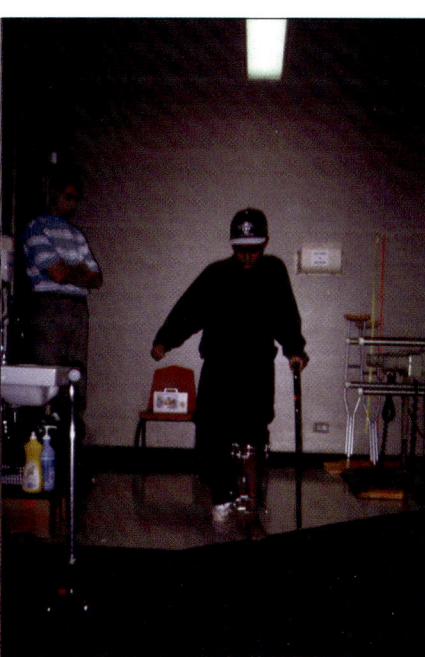

B

FIGURE 12

■ Outpatient follow-up is dependent on patient compliance and specific treatment plans, but usually is scheduled no more often than every 2 weeks during angular or rotational correction or lengthening, and monthly during consolidation.

• Figure 13 shows a preoperative photograph (Fig. 13A) and radiographs (Fig. 13B) of a 12-year-old boy demonstrating tibial deformity and minimal limb-length inequality. The patient is shown postoperatively with crutches in Figure 13C. A final radiograph is shown in Figure 13D.

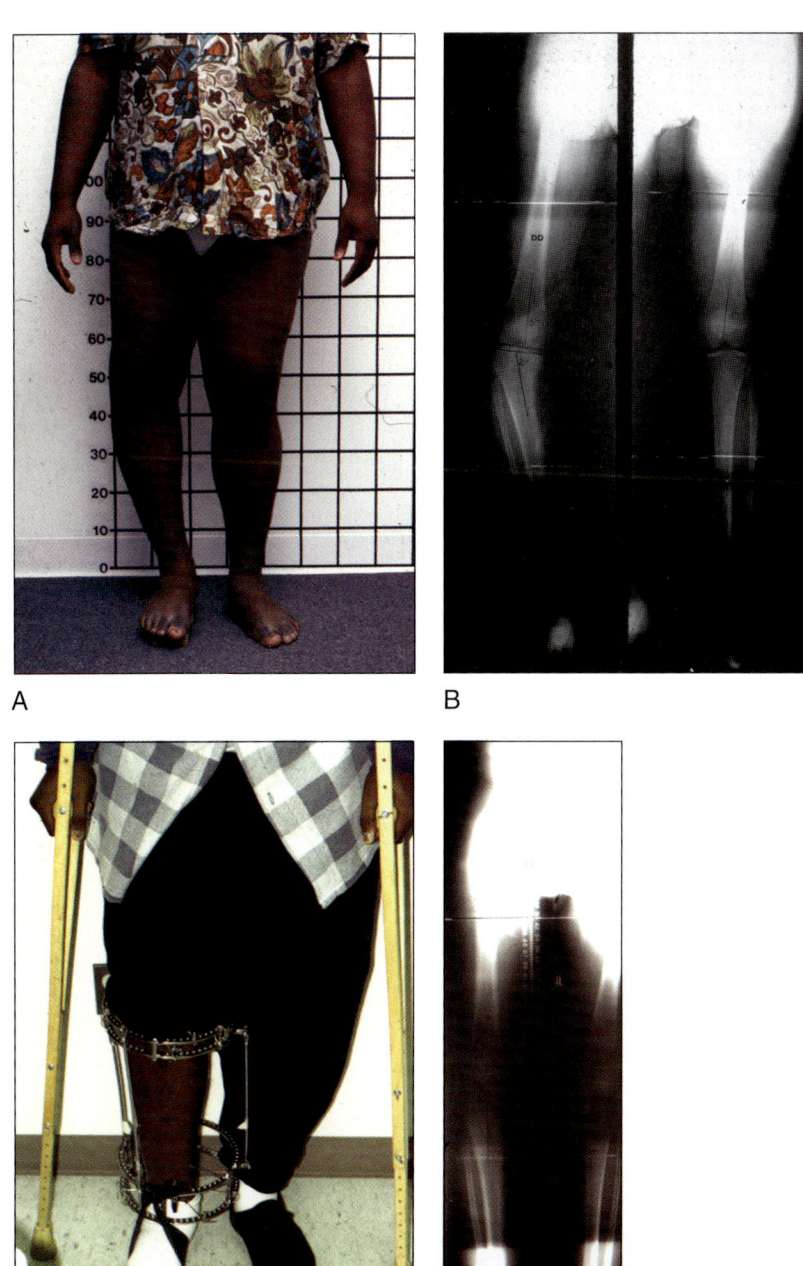

A

B

C

D

FIGURE 13

- Figure 14 shows a preoperative photograph (Fig. 14A) and radiograph (Fig. 14B) of a 14-year-old boy demonstrating mild tibial deformity. An intraoperative radiograph demonstrates converging proximal pins and tibial osteotomy (Fig. 14C). A photograph (Fig. 14D) and radiograph (Fig. 14E) show results following fixator removal.

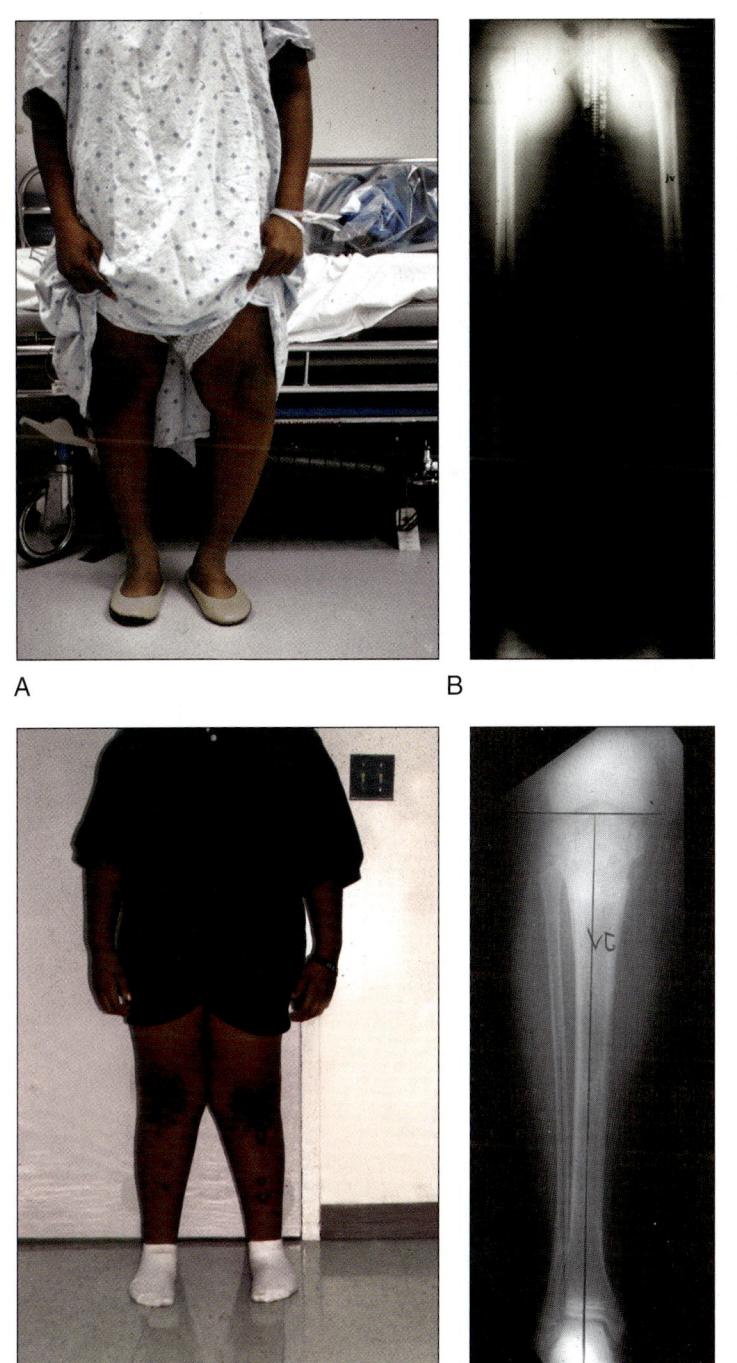

A

B

C

D

E

FIGURE 14

EVIDENCE

Kim YH, Kang TS, Koo KK, Liong BTL, Hua KG, Inoue N, Chao ED. Simulation of tibial osteotomy execution under unilateral external fixation. Presented at the 2003 Summer Bioengineering Conference, Key Biscayne, FL.

A model of varus tibial deformity was created and mathematical modeling performed. The purpose of the study was to determine whether the deformity could be defined preoperatively and whether an adjustable unilateral external fixator, when applied according to these parameters, could completely resolve the deformity. The study was predicated on the premise, confirmed by prior clinical studies, that unadjustable fixation ran a real risk of inadequate deformity correction as intraoperative radiographic assessment is not as precise as that which can be obtained postoperatively or in a standing position. The study did not define the number of deformities created; however, it confirmed the ability of an adjustable unilateral fixator to correct deformity and that deformity can be accurately assessed preoperatively. (Level I evidence)

Price CT, Scott DS, Greenberg DA. Dynamic axial external fixation in the surgical treatment of tibia vara. J Pediatr Orthop. 1995;15:236–43.

Twenty-three patients were treated for tibia vara with a large pin external fixator and an opening wedge corrective osteotomy. Seventeen (78%) had what would be considered either juvenile or adolescent tibia vara. Seven (30.4%) were bilateral and the remainder unilateral, thus consisting of 30 tibiae. Twelve of the 23 patients (52%) were considered obese, having weights exceeding the 95th percentile for their height. Pre- and postoperative radiographs assessing limb mechanical axes were assessed. All corrections were acutely performed. Three of the patients had had prior operative intervention with either recurrent deformity or inadequate initial correction. Preoperative mechanical axes ranged from 4° to 46° of varus (average, 20°). Postoperative mechanical axes varied from 17° of varus to 13° of valgus. There were no infections, nonunions, or compartment syndromes. Two patients had transient neurapraxia and nine had pin site infections treated with oral antibiotics. This was the first report of opening wedge osteotomy with external fixations and no adjunctive fixation. (Level IV evidence)

Felman DS, Madav SS, Ruchelsman DE, Sala DA, Lehman WB. Accuracy of correction of tibia vara: acute versus gradual correction. J Pediatr Orthop. 2006;26:794–8.

Fourteen tibiae in 14 patients underwent acute intraoperative deformity correction (AC), and 18 tibiae in 18 patients underwent gradual postoperative deformity correction (GC). The mean age was 11.4 (range, 3–17) in the AC group and 10.2 (range, 3–16) in the GC group. The mean preoperative proximal tibial, posterior tibial, and lateral distal femoral angles and mechanical axis deviations were also similar and nearly identical in the two groups. The Fisher exact test was used to compare the two groups with respect to the accuracy of both translational and angular correction based on assessment of long-leg standing radiographs. In both groups, rotational correction, when needed, was accurate. The frequency of accurate translational correction was only 50% (7/14 tibiae) in the AC group but 100% (18/18) in the GC group. The frequency of accurate angular correction was significantly grater (17/18) in the GC group than in the AC group (7/14). The authors' conclusion was that gradual deformity correction is more accurate than acute correction. (Level III evidence)

Operative Treatment of Tillaux Fractures of the Ankle

Brian G. Smith

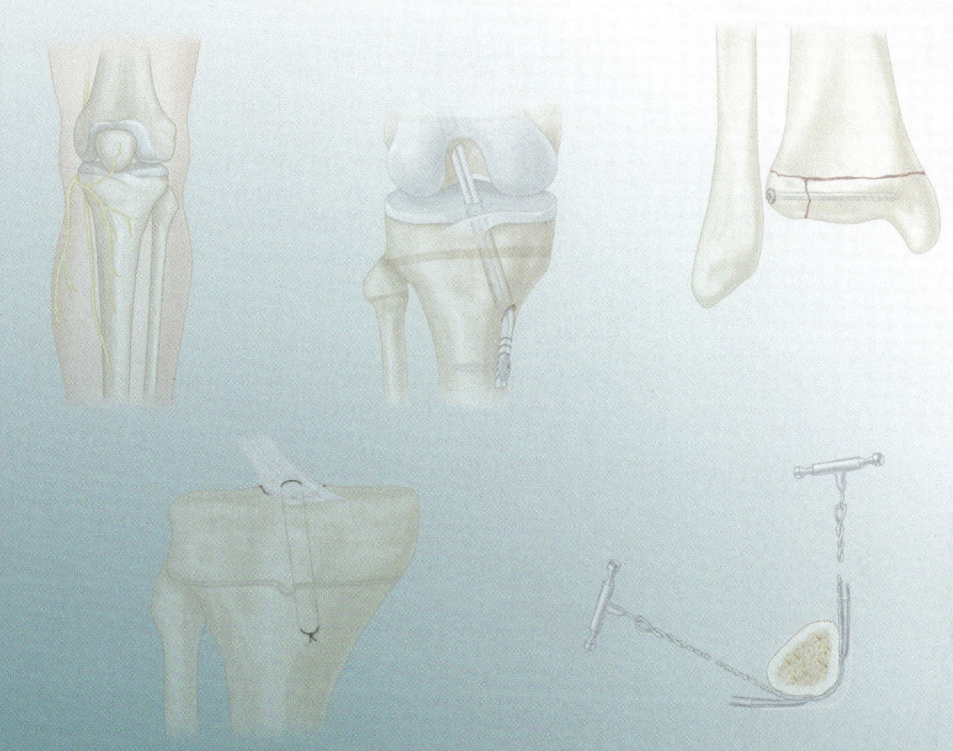

Controversies

• Borderline displaced fractures not evaluated with computed tomography scanning

Treatment Options

• Closed reduction and casting for nondisplaced fractures

• Open reduction and internal fixation for displaced fractures

• Arthroscopically aided percutaneous reduction and internal fixation

Equipment

• Bolster to elevate affected-side buttock

INDICATIONS

■ Displaced fractures of the distal tibial plafond
■ Tibial intra-articular fractures displaced more than 2 mm

EXAMINATION/IMAGING

■ Three radiographic views of the affected ankle should be obtained demonstrating a displaced intra-articular fracture.
  • The mortise view is best to visualize the fracture.
■ Computed tomography (CT) scan should be done to assess displacement if there is any question
  • Figure 1 shows a Tillaux fracture assessed by CT scan, including anteroposterior (Fig. 1A), lateral (Fig. 1B), and axial (Fig. 1C) images demonstrating displacement of the fracture on the anterolateral aspect of the distal tibia.

SURGICAL ANATOMY

■ An intra-articular tibial plafond fracture requires anatomic realignment.
■ Attachment of the anterior inferior tibiofibular ligament should be preserved on the fracture fragment (Fig. 2).
■ The superficial peroneal nerve should be preserved on exposure.
■ The physis of the distal tibia may need to be spared if still open.

POSITIONING

■ The patient is placed in supine position with a bolster beneath the ipsilateral buttock (Fig. 3).
■ The patient's foot should be near the end of the bed to facilitate access and imaging.
■ A radiolucent table enables fluoroscopic imaging and confirmation of internal fixation and reduction.

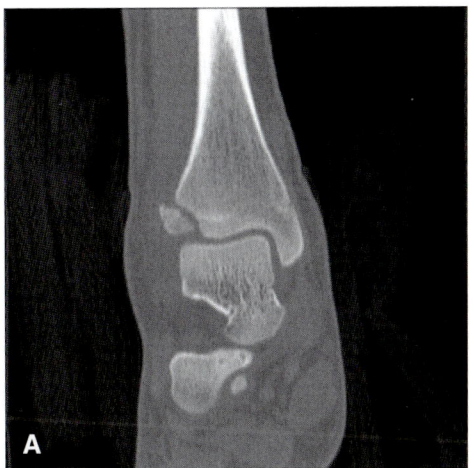
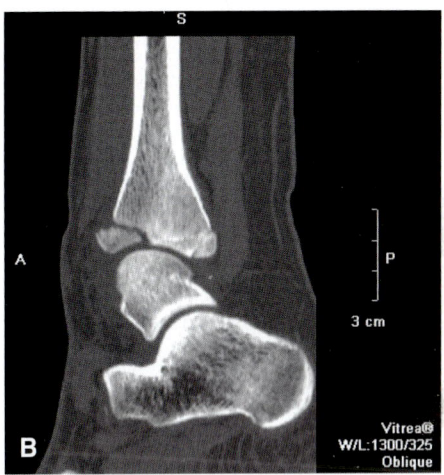
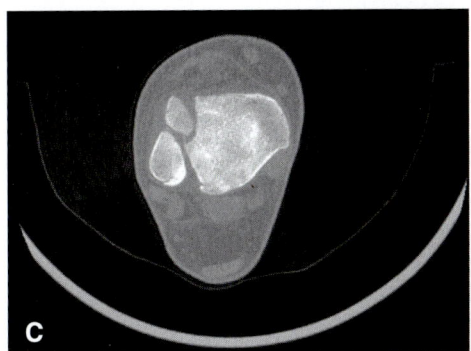

FIGURE 1

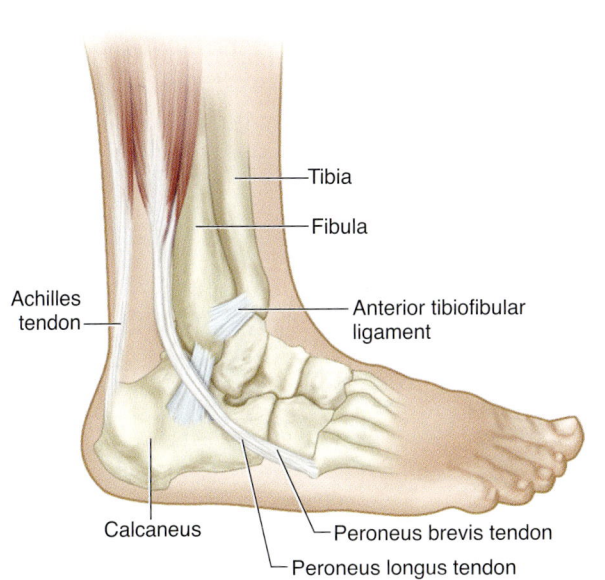
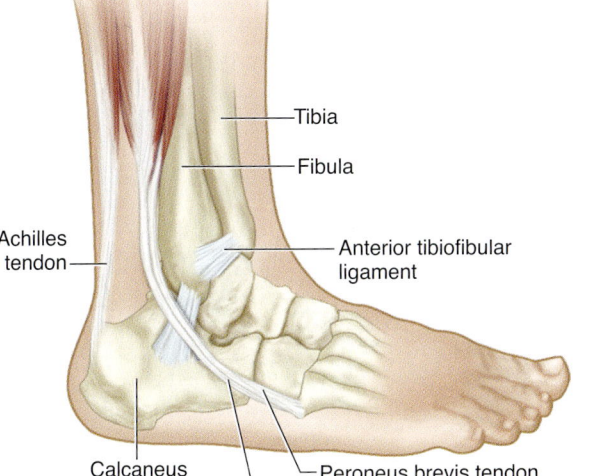

Tibia

Fibula

Achilles
tendon

Anterior tibiofibular
ligament

Calcaneus

Peroneus brevis tendon

Peroneus longus tendon

FIGURE 2

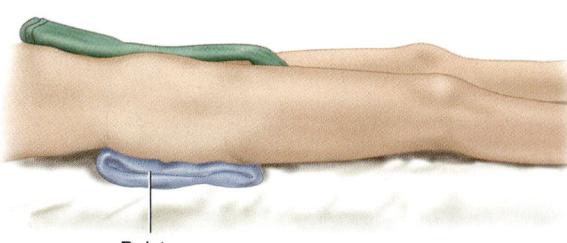

Bolster

FIGURE 3

Instrumentation/ Implantation

- Dental pick
- Guide pins for cannulated screws
- Reduction forceps

Controversies

- Inability to reduce fracture

PORTALS/EXPOSURES

- Closed reduction may be attempted in the operating room and percutaneous screw fixation performed through a small anterolateral incision over a guide pin.
- A small anterolateral incision may be needed to reduce and hold the fragment internally prior to screw fixation (Fig. 4).

PROCEDURE

STEP 1

- Fracture reduction is done after evacuating any hematoma.
- A percutaneous pin or dental pick is used to reduce the fracture, and if necessary a fracture reduction clamp (Fig. 5) is applied to hold the fracture reduced.

STEP 2

- Place a guide pin from a cannulated screw set across the reduced fracture.
- Place a second pin if the fragment is large enough to accommodate it (Fig. 6).

Instrumentation/Implantation

- Guide pin from cannulated screw set

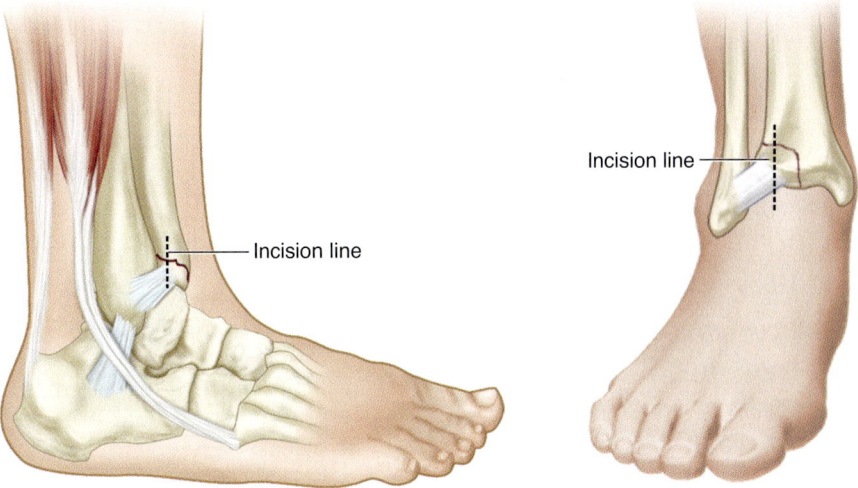

Incision line

Incision line

FIGURE 4

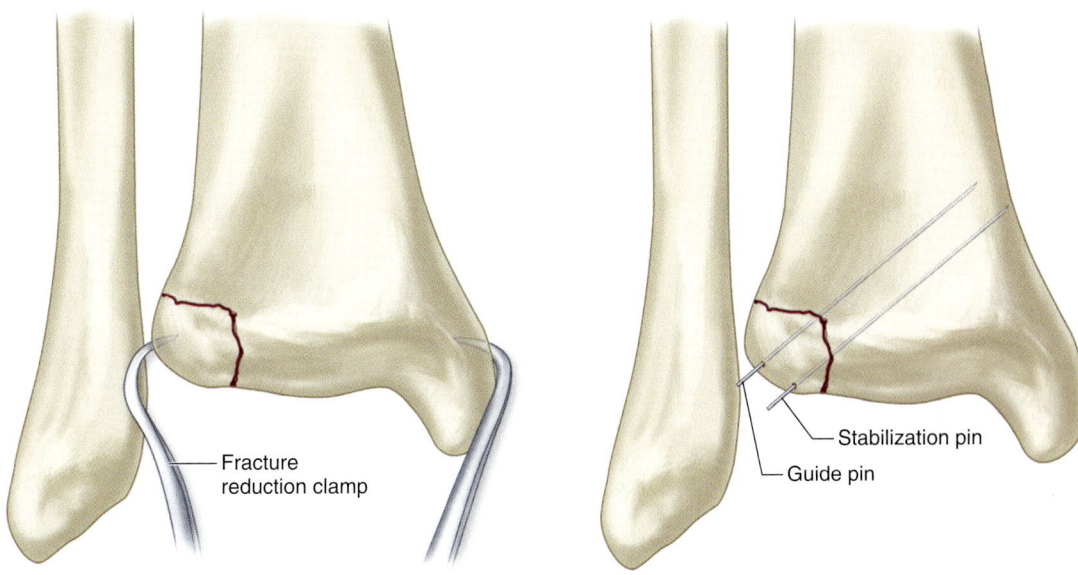

Fracture
reduction clamp

FIGURE 5

Stabilization pin

Guide pin

FIGURE 6

Instrumentation/ Implantation

- Cannulated drill bit for 4.0 cannulated screw system

Controversies

- Is a washer necessary?
- Does the screw need to engage a far cortex or is cancellous purchase enough?

STEP 3

- Drill over the guide pin to prepare the tract for the screw (Fig. 7).

STEP 4

- Place a screw over the guide pin (first pin) and tighten it securely (Fig. 8).
- Remove the rotational control pin (second pin).

POSTOPERATIVE CARE AND EXPECTED OUTCOMES

- A cast is applied for 2–3 weeks.
- A walker boot may then be used to permit range of motion while protecting the ankle.
- The patient is kept non–weight bearing with crutches for 4–6 weeks.
- Range of motion is started when the patient is out of the cast.

Controversies

- When to start range of motion
- When to start weight bearing

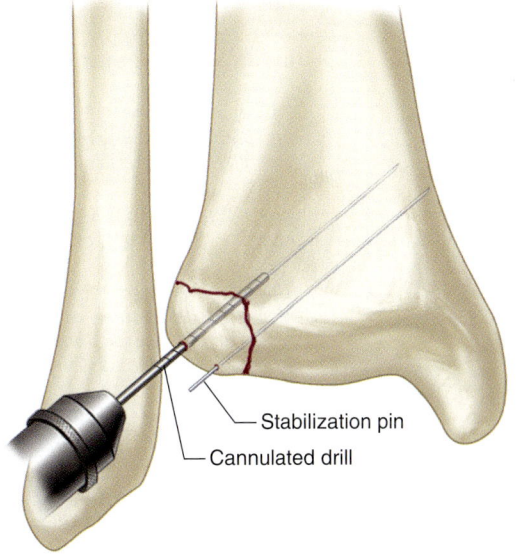

Stabilization pin
Cannulated drill

FIGURE 7

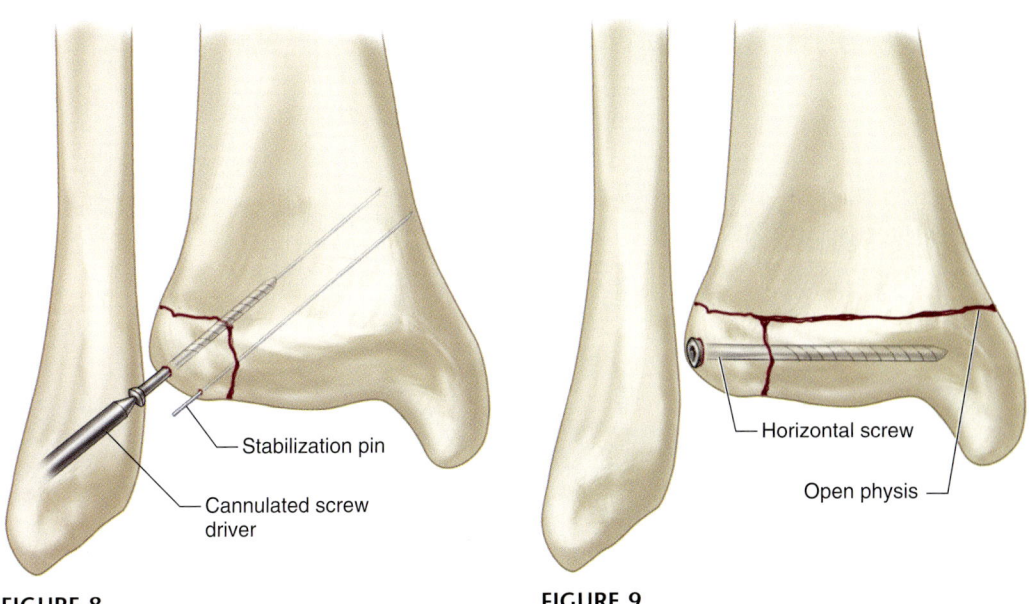

Stabilization pin

Cannulated screw driver

FIGURE 8

Horizontal screw

Open physis

FIGURE 9

EVIDENCE

Horn B, Crisci K, Krug M, et al. Radiographic evaluation of juvenile Tillaux fractures of the distal tibia. J Pediatr Orthop. 2001;21:162–4.

This study compared CT scans and plain radiography for the evaluation of displaced Tillaux fractures in cadaver specimens. While CT was superior in detecting displacement, neither modality was completely accurate in assessing these fractures. (Level II evidence)

Kaya A, Altay T, Ozturk H, Karapinar L. Open reduction and internal fixation in displaced juvenile Tillaux fractures. Injury. 2007;38:201–5.

This paper reviewed 10 patients treated with open reduction and internal fixation of displaced Tillaux fractures, with an average follow-up of 54 months and assessment with the American Orthopaedic Foot and Ankle Society scoring scale. This is one of the few studies to provide long-term follow-up using an outcome scoring measure. (Level III evidence)

Leetun D, Ireland M. Arthroscopically assisted reduction and fixation of juvenile Tillaux fracture. Arthroscopy. 2002;18:427–9.

This paper described an alternative arthroscopic technique for evaluation, reduction, and fixation of the Tillaux fracture. (Level V evidence)

Tibial Lengthening with Circular External Fixation

John E. Herzenberg and Shawn C. Standard

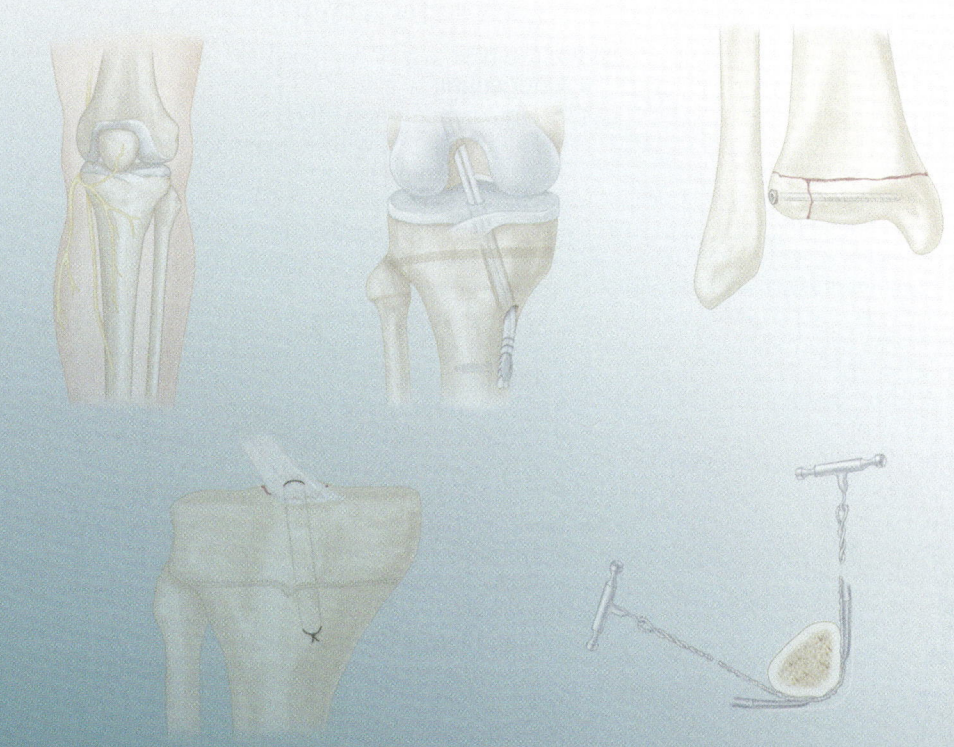

INDICATIONS

- Tibial shortening with or without limb deformity
  - Deformity correction can be performed simultaneously with gradual distraction for lengthening at the same osteotomy site, provided the osteotomy is at or near the apex of the deformity.
  - Double-level tibial osteotomies can be performed in older children, especially if there are multiple apices of deformity.
- Tibial shortening greater than 7 cm may be more easily accomplished with staged lengthenings or a combination of lengthening and epiphysiodesis.
- Tibial shortening greater than 3 cm that cannot be treated with more conservative methods (shoe lifts or epiphysiodesis)
  - Contraindications to epiphysiodesis:
    - Short predicted overall height
    - Inadequate growth remaining

ETIOLOGIES

- Congenital
  - Fibular hemimelia (FH)
  - FH associated with congenital short femur
  - Tibial hemimelia
  - Hemihypertrophy
    - Neurofibromatosis
    - Beckwith-Wiedemann syndrome
    - Idiopathic
    - Proteus syndrome
    - Klippel-Trénaunay-Weber syndrome
  - Hemiatrophy
  - Congenital banding syndrome (Streeter's dysplasia)
  - Clubfoot-related leg length discrepancy
  - Posteromedial bowing
  - Congenital pseudarthrosis of the tibia
- Neuromuscular
  - Hemiplegic cerebral palsy
  - Polio
- Traumatic
  - Malunion with shortening
  - Growth arrest
  - Bone loss
  - Overgrowth after fracture
- Infection
  - Septic arthritis
    - Growth arrest or bone loss
    - Neonatal
  - Osteomyelitis
    - Growth arrest or bone loss
  - Meningococcal septicemia
- Developmental
  - Blount disease
  - Ollier's enchondromatosis
  - Multiple hereditary exostosis
  - Rickets
  - Renal osteodystrophy
  - Skeletal dysplasia/achondroplasia
  - Osteogenesis imperfecta
  - Juvenile rheumatoid arthritis (JRA)

SURGICAL PITFALLS

- Fibular hemimelia
  - Possible valgus procurvatum of the diaphysis—Requires simultaneous angular correction with slight overcorrection of valgus

Controversies

- LLD less than 1.5–2 cm
  - Considered within normal variation
  - Easily treated with internal shoe lift
  - No evidence of long-term sequelae
- Severe deformities requiring extensive lengthening
  - Reconstruction with lengthening should be performed at specialized centers.
  - Limb ablation with prosthetic reconstruction can be considered if total tibial predicted LLD is greater than 20 cm. Associated joints are not amenable to reconstruction.
- LLD less than 5 cm in the skeletally immature patient
  - Long-leg epiphysiodesis if there is adequate growth remaining and height prediction is within normal range
- LLD less than 5 cm in the skeletally mature patient
  - Femoral shortening of long leg
  - Acceptable to have knees at different levels, but not more than 5 cm difference

- Instability of the knee—May need crossing of the knee with the fixator for stabilization (fixation to femur with external fixation or cast brace linked to tibial fixator)
- Fixed equinovalgus of the ankle—Peroneal/Achilles tendon lengthening plus supramalleolar osteotomy or subtalar osteotomy to realign the hindfoot/ankle (can be staged or simultaneous)
- Intrinsic soft tissue contractures—Vulpian lengthening of the gastrocnemius-soleus at the time of tibial lengthening
- Concurrent instability of the ankle joint
  - The ankle joint should always be bridged from the tibia to the foot with external fixation components during tibial lengthening in the face of instability or contracture.
- Tibial hemimelia
  - The knee is often unstable, requiring the external fixator frame to be extended to the femur with hinges.
  - Foot equinovarus needs simultaneous correction (supramalleolar osteotomy for ankle diastasis type).
- Posteromedial bowed tibia
  - Typically has proximal varus and distal valgus/recurvatum; check for compensatory subtalar varus contracture
- Russell-Silver syndrome
  - It is difficult to predict the final limb length inequality during growth.
  - The surgeon should wait until skeletal maturity to equalize limb lengths.
    - One may proceed with initial lengthening if leg length discrepancy (LLD) is greater than 5 cm.
    - Parents must be warned to expect possible recurrence and need for further treatment.
- Juvenile rheumatoid arthritis (JRA)
  - Type V growth pattern with upward slope–plateau–downward slope with improvement without intervention.
  - Final LLD should be assessed at skeletal maturity and then corrected.
- Achondroplasia
  - Limb lengthening at ages less than 8 years can result in growth inhibition.
  - Staged lengthenings should be planned to gain functional height.
- Polio
  - Delayed regenerate bone formation and healing—Plan decreased rate of distraction.
  - Slight ankle equinus and residual LLD may be desireable to aid knee extension in the face of weak quadriceps.
- Blount's disease
  - May need medial hemiplateau elevation as preliminary staged procedure, followed by metaphyseal osteotomy for lengthening and residual varus correction
- Ollier's enchondromatosis
  - Ollier's disease always has angular deformities.
  - Angular deformities recur with subsequent growth until skeletal maturity.
  - The leg may be lengthened through the edge of the Ollier lesion.
  - Bone healing may be premature, requiring faster rate of lengthening.
- Rickets, renal osteodystrophy, JRA
  - Delayed regenerate bone formation and healing—Plan decreased rate of distraction.

EXAMINATION/IMAGING

PHYSICAL EXAMINATION

- Range of motion of the hip, knee, and ankle and subtalar joints
  - Contractures or joint/bony abnormalities must be documented.
    - ◆ Special consideration must be given to knee and ankle fixed flexion deformity. The cause (soft tissue contracture vs. bony deformity) must be determined
  - Concurrent joint instabilities and ligamentous deficiencies must be documented.
    - ◆ FH is often associated with congenital short femur, with absence of anterior and posterior cruciate ligaments.
- Clinical alignment
  - Coronal plane: varus deformity vs. valgus deformity
  - Sagittal plane: recurvatum vs. procurvatum
- Rotational profile
  - The presence of internal or external tibial torsion and femoral version must be determined.
- Clinical limb-length assessment
  - One-centimeter blocks are placed under the short leg until the pelvis is level.
- Neurologic examination
  - The patient's strength and sensation should be noted.

RADIOGRAPHIC EXAMINATION

- Anteroposterior (AP) standing long-leg radiographs are obtained (taken at a distance of 10 feet using a 51-inch cassette).
  - Malalignment and malorientation tests are performed to determine concurrent deformity and location of deformity.
  - Limb lengths are assessed (the pelvis should be leveled with blocks and the number of blocks noted on the radiograph).
- Standing long-leg lateral radiographs (with maximum knee extension) are obtained.
  - The radiographs are checked for fixed flexion deformity of the knee.
  - A malorientation test is performed to determine the presence and location of sagittal plane deformity.
  - The radiographs are checked for joint subluxation (significant anterior-posterior instability).
- AP and lateral standing ankle radiographs to include the tibia are obtained to help measure ankle malalignment.
  - Figure 1 shows a preoperative radiograph of an 11-year-old girl with FH and valgus knee, with 5-cm LLD.
  - Figure 2 shows a preoperative radiograph of a 14-year-old girl with Ollier's disease, demonstrating shortening of the femur and tibia, with angular deformity in both.
- Additional views of the foot and heels (Saltzman view) are obtained as needed to assess deformity.

Treatment Options

- LLD less than 2 cm
  - No treatment
  - Shoe lift

- LLD less than 5 cm (see Fig. 2): shoe lift or epiphysiodesis
  - A shoe lift should be avoided during sports (risk of ankle sprain).
  - For lifts of greater than 5 cm, the patient may need an ankle-foot orthosis to stabilize the ankle.
  - For lifts of greater than 8 cm, a platform prosthesis should be used.
  - Epiphysiodesis is done percutaneously by drills and curettes without need for implants. Figure 3 shows a contralateral distal femoral epiphysiodesis in a patient undergoing an ipsilateral tibial lengthening.

- Extreme LLD
  - Amputation with prosthetic reconstruction if predicted tibial LLD greater than 20 cm, with severe dysplasia or absence of associated joints (ankle and knee), or in patient not a candidate for lengthening

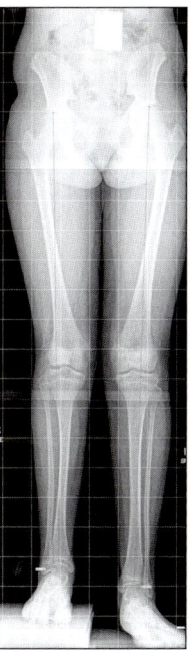

FIGURE 1

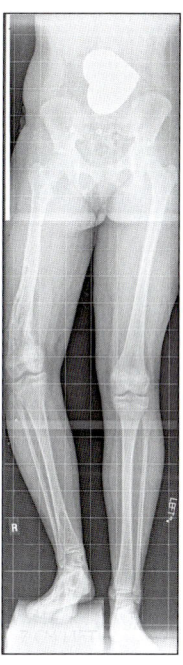

FIGURE 2

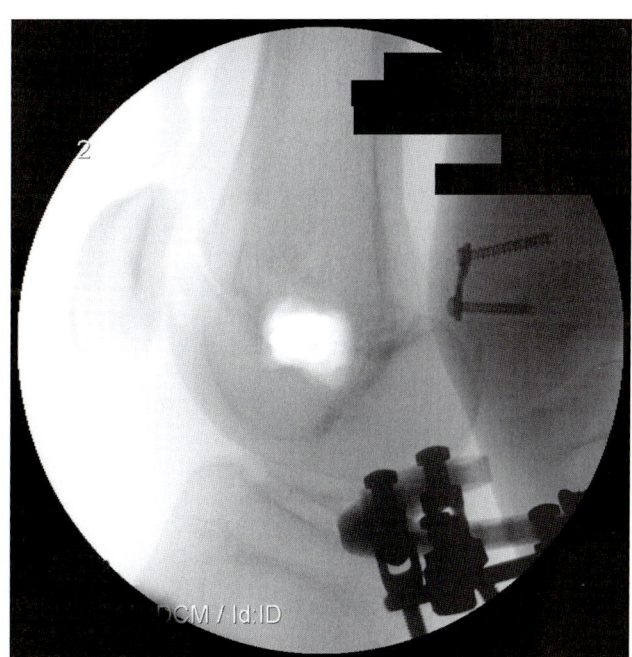

FIGURE 3

SURGICAL ANATOMY

- **Fibula**
  - The surgical approach for osteotomy is through the internervous interval (peroneals/soleus).
  - It is safer to perform the fibular osteotomy in the distal half to avoid traction injury to the nerve to the extensor hallucis longus.
- **Crural fascia**
  - A prophylactic anterior compartment fasciotomy is safe, and can give a larger diameter appearance to an atrophic leg.
    - A small incision, with combined longitudinal and transverse fasciotomy, will result in better decompression.
- **Achilles tendon**
  - Prophylactic Vulpian gastrocnemius-soleus recession helps the Achilles tendon to stretch to accommodate the tibial lengthening.
    - The sural nerve, which is lateral to the tendon, should be protected.
    - The midline raphe usually needs to be cut.
- **Peroneal nerve**
  - This nerve is at risk during the external fixation application if wires are placed near the fibular neck or slightly below, or if the fibular osteotomy is high.
  - Rapid lengthening or concurrent deformity correction can place tension on the peroneal nerve.
    - Peroneal nerve tension or irritation initially will result in pain on the anterior aspect of the lower leg and dorsum of the foot.
    - Further tension causes decreased sensation.
    - Late findings include weakness of the dorsiflexors or a drop foot.
    - Young patients will often hold the toes up with their hands or continuously rub their foot.
    - Treatment involves slowing the rate of distraction, allowing the hip to extend and the knee to flex, and decompression of the peroneal nerve.
  - The superficial peroneal nerve may be entrapped by distal tibial wires.
- **Posterior tibial nerve**
  - This nerve is at risk during the external fixation application if wires are passed posteromedially in the distal tibia.
  - Tarsal tunnel syndrome may occur from swelling, or traction during distal tibial deformity correction, requiring release of fascia over the tarsal tunnel.
- **Knee joint**
  - Intrinsic instability will result in increased risk of joint subluxation or dislocation.
    - Contracted posterior fascia in FH can result in knee flexion contracture.
    - A contracted gastrocnemius can create a flexion contracture with posterior translational subluxation of the femur on the tibia.
  - Severe knee instability should be addressed with ligamentous reconstruction prior to tibial lengthening.
- **Ankle joint**
  - Pre-existing ankle equinus will be worsened with lengthening.
    - Achilles tendon lengthening or Vulpian recession is needed.

Equipment

• Sterile bumps under the distal thigh and lower leg allow lateral fluoroscopic visualization of the operative leg, and elevate the leg off the table to allow for positioning of a circular fixator.

• A sterile tourniquet is needed.

POSITIONING

■ The patient is placed supine on a radiolucent table that allows visualization from the hips to the ankles.
■ A small bump is placed under the ipsilateral sacrum to allow the lower extremity to rest in a patella-forward position.
■ The entire lower extremity is prepped and draped to include the groin area, gluteal region, and iliac crest to the subcostal margin.
  • This allows the extremity to be manipulated during the procedure.
  • All aspects of the hip, femur, and knee are accessible.
  • Seeing from hip to ankle allows better assessment of alignment.

PROCEDURE: EXTERNAL FIXATOR PLACEMENT

STEP 1

■ The limb is held with patella forward for a true AP image intensifer view.
■ The level of the knee, ankle, and each growth plate is marked.
■ The level of the intended osteotomy sites (tibia and fibula) is marked.
  • Metaphyseal tibial osteotomy about 6–7 cm distal to the knee joint typically produces the best bone.
  • Fibular osteotomy is best at the junction of middle and distal third.
  • If an abnormal mechanical axis is present, then preoperative planning is required to determine the level of the deformity.
    ◆ The osteotomy level will be influenced by the level of the center of rotation of angulation (CORA) of the deformity
    ◆ Deformity correction with concurrent lengthening can be performed through either a single or double osteotomy

STEP 2: TIBIOFIBULAR FIXATION

- Using image intensifier guidance, a 1.5-mm wire is passed from the distal lateral fibula into the tibia, aiming proximally about 15° (not perpendicular).
  - The lateral view is checked to confirm centrality of the wire in the fibula and tibia.
  - Figure 4 shows tibiofibular proximal and distal stabilization with internal screws, demonstrated in an adolescent with achondroplasia undergoing tibial lengthening. The distal tibiofibular wire is shown inclined proximally.
- A 1-cm incision is made on the medial side, where the wire exits the tibia, and then a 3.2-mm cannulated drill is used to drill retrograde through all four cortices (tibia and fibula).
  - The length of the screw is measured with a second wire or depth gauge.
- A 4.5-mm solid (not cannulated) screw is inserted from the medial side of the tibia to the lateral side of the fibula. Position is confirmed on a lateral image intensifier view (Fig. 5).
- These steps are repeated for the proximal tibiofibular fixation.
  - In proximal tibiofibular syndesmosis, the screw should be perpedicular to the long axis of the tibia on the AP view, not inclined like the distal screw.
  - Care is taken not to start the initial wire too posterior in the fibular head, as this is close to the peroneal nerve.
  - It is sufficient to capture three cortices (tibia medial, tibia lateral, and fibular head medial) (Fig. 6).
  - The position of the proximal screw is checked on a lateral view (Fig. 7) to ensure it is in both the tibia and the fibula.

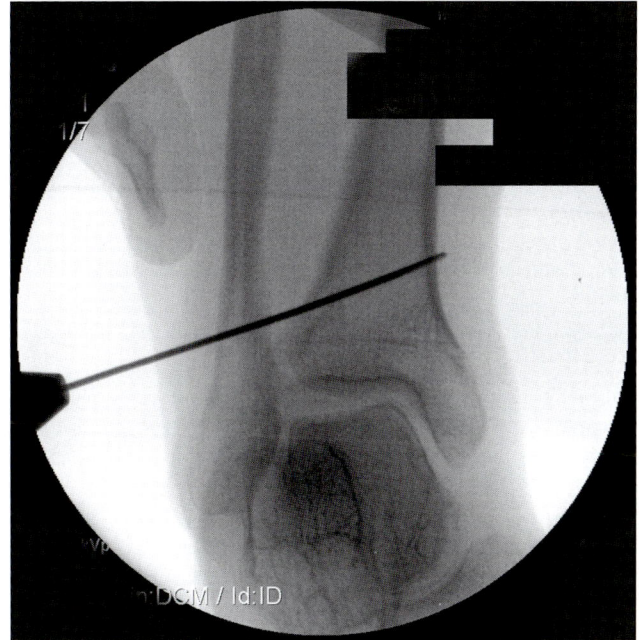

FIGURE 4

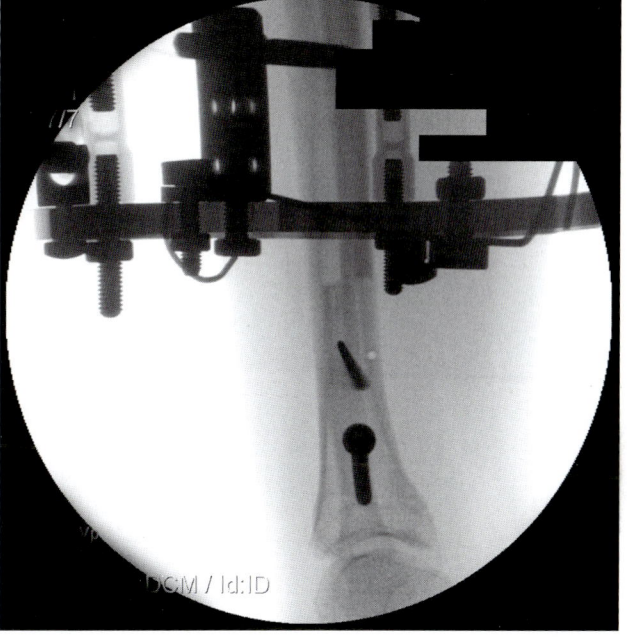

FIGURE 5

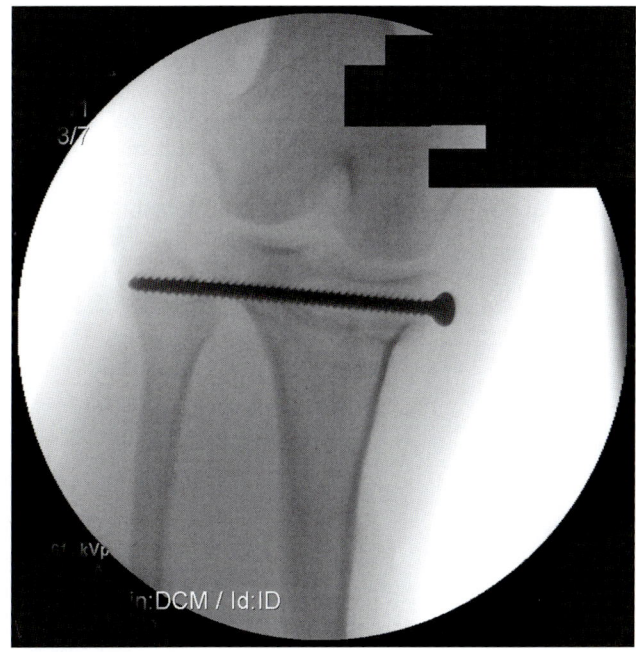

FIGURE 6

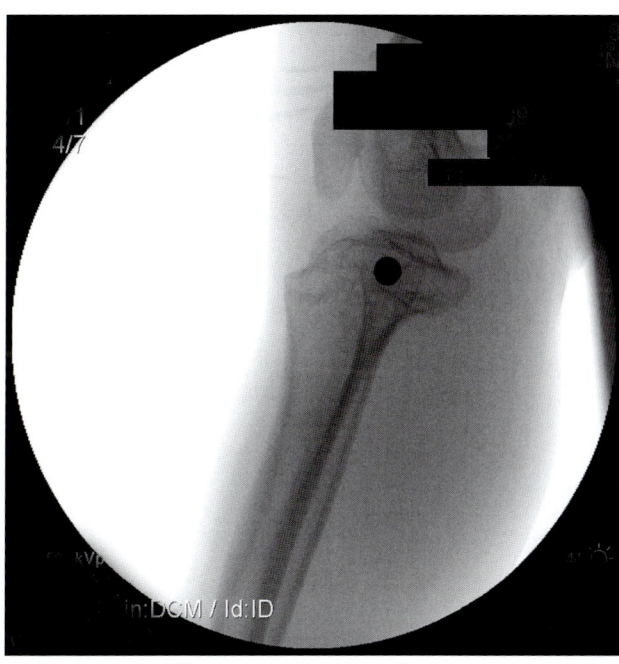

FIGURE 7

STEP 3: FIBULAR OSTEOTOMY

- The limb is exsanguinated and the sterile tourniquet elevated. A 3- to 4-cm incision is made over the palpable interval between the soleus and the peroneal muscles in the mid-tibia.
  - This interval is dissected longitudinally and deeper retractors are used to pull the peroneals anteriorly, to expose the fibula. A narrow subperiosteal dissection is made around the fibula and small Hohmann retractors are applied.
  - Multiple (~5) passes are made with a 1.8-mm wire to initiate the fibular osteotomy. It is completed with a 10-mm osteotome. The surgeon should confirm under image intensification that the osteotomy can be translated.

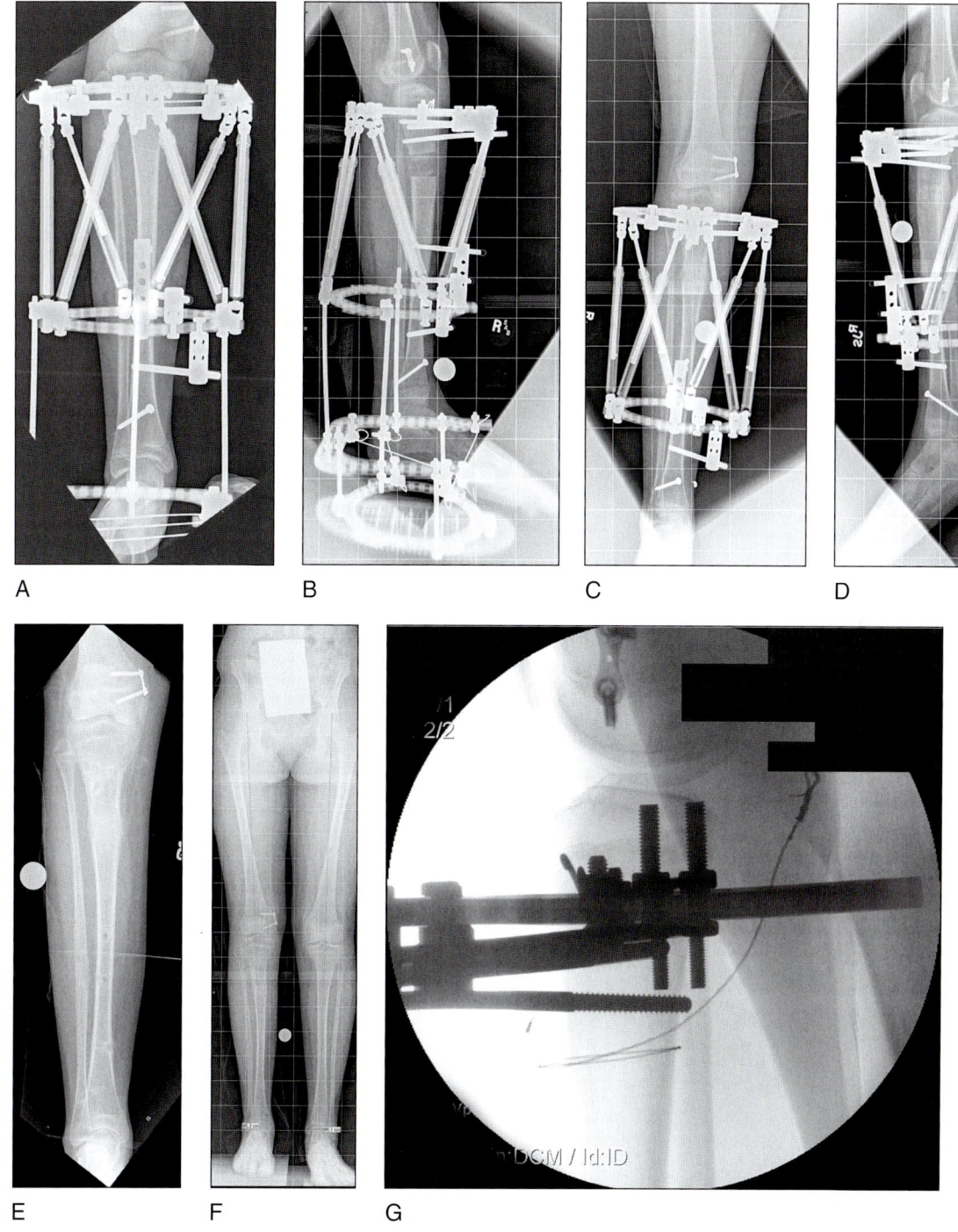

A

B

C

D

E

F

G

FIGURE 8

- Figure 9 depicts the proper incision, muscle retraction, and drilling of the fibula for a complete osteotomy.

STEP 4: PASSING THE GIGLI SAW

- The ideal level for Gigli saw osteotomy is about 6 cm below the knee, just distal to the tibial tubercle, in metaphyseal bone. A Gigli saw osteotomy should never be done for lengthening in diaphyseal bone. If a Gigli saw is chosen over a more classical osteotome technique, the Gigli saw should be passed in the beginning of the surgery, before the external fixator is applied.

- The skin is marked under image intensification. Two incisions are made: one anterior and one posteromedial, each transverse in direction and 1 cm in length.

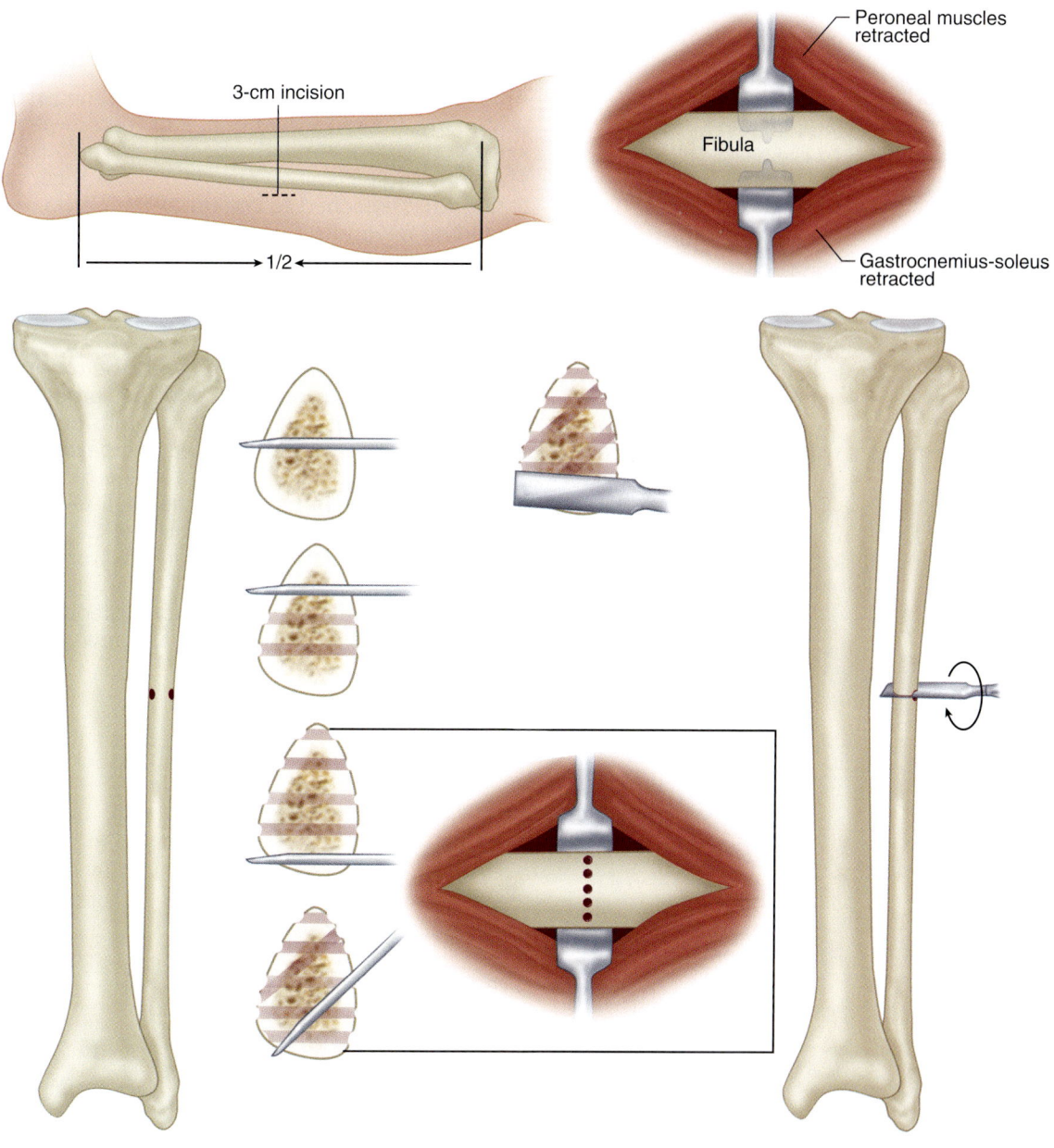

FIGURE 9

Instrumentation/Implantation

- The ideal Gigli saw should be flexible and long. Some are short and stiff. We prefer the Gigli saw marketed by DePuy. These Gigli saws are also strong enough to cut an aluminum carbon fiber ring if needed.
- Commercially available Gigli saw passers from Pega Medical may be useful as an alternative to using solely the right-angle clamp and tonsil clamp.

Controversies

- Gigli saw osteotomy allows a very proximal osteotomy without risk of making butterfly fragments that would break into the proximal pin sites posteriorly.
- Healing of a Gigli saw osteotomy is satisfactory in the metaphysis but not the diaphysis. For diaphyseal osteotomies, it is preferable to use multiple drill holes and an osteotome to break the bone.

- A subperiosteal dissection is made with a small sharp periosteal elevator 360° around the tibia (anteromedial and anterolateral from the anterior wound, and posterior from the posteromedial wound) (Fig. 10).
  - A right-angle clamp is passed from the medial incision posteriorly, hugging the bone, and then turned 90° on its axis to "hook" the lateral aspect of the tibia (see Fig. 10).
  - The right-angle clamp is removed and a thick suture (#2 Ethibond) is attached to the tip of the clamp, with a piece extending beyond the tip. This right-angle clamp is reinserted as before (see Fig. 10).
  - A slightly curved tonsil clamp is inserted from the anterior wound subperiosteally, feeling for the tip of the right-angle clamp (see Fig. 10).
  - By "feel," the suture is grasped with the tonsil clamp, the right-angle clamp is released, and the surgeon should try to pull the suture out anteriorly. If it comes out, the two clamps may be removed. If not, this step is repeated (see Fig. 10).
- Once the suture is passed, the end is tied to the Gigli saw, a slight bend is made in the tip of the Gigli saw, and it is passed from posteromedial to anterolateral. The Gigli saw should not be activated until after the entire ring fixator has been applied (Fig. 11).
- The tourniquet is released. The fibular osteotomy wound, and the small wound over the tibiofibular screws, are irrigated and closed.

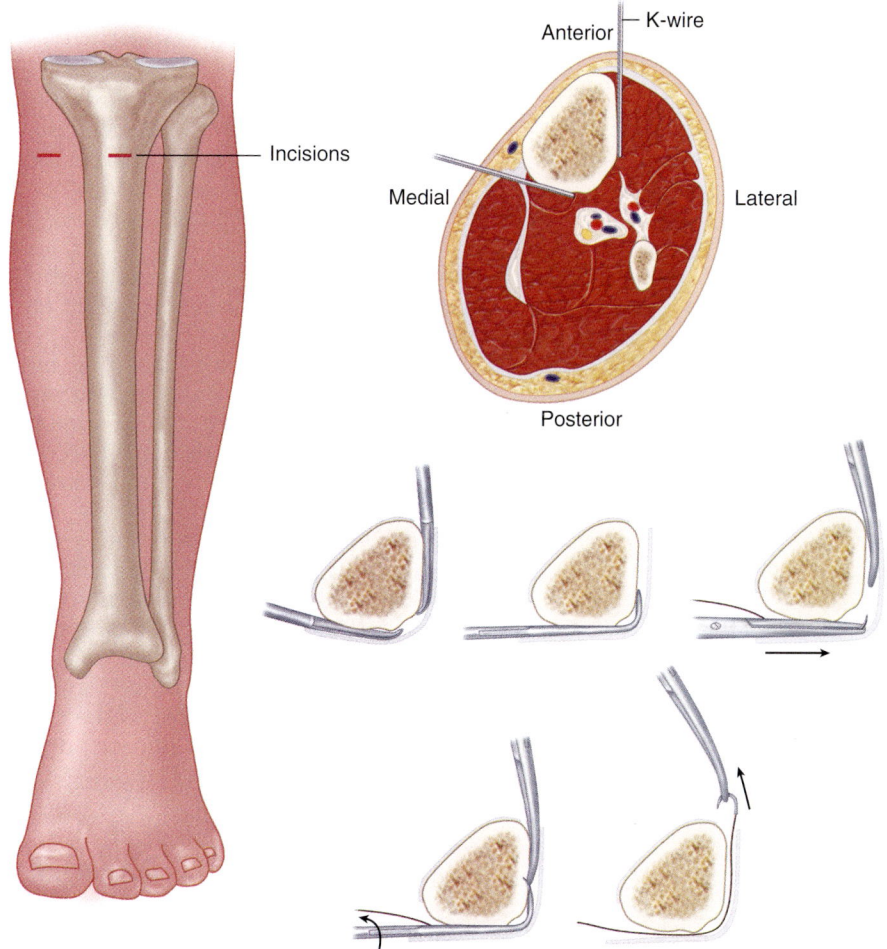

Anterior — K-wire

Medial

Lateral

Posterior

FIGURE 10

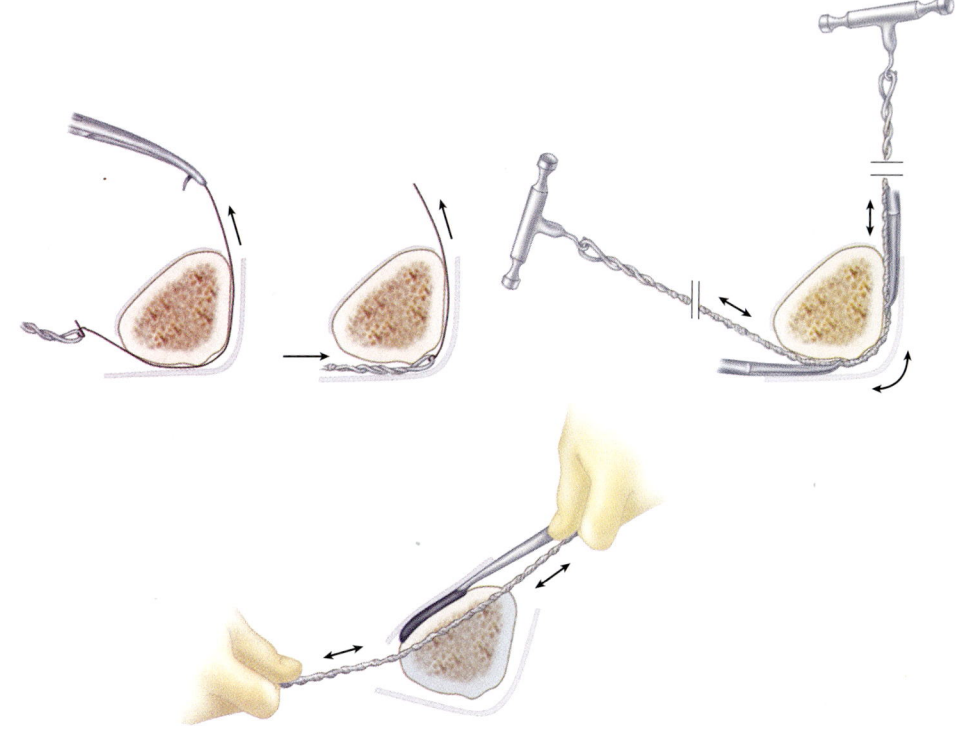

FIGURE 11

■ Later, when the osteotomy is complete, the Gigli saw is cut to extract it (Fig. 12).

STEP 5: PROXIMAL REFERENCE RING APPLICATION

■ For this procedure, we are illustrating the mounting of a six-axis deformity correction circular external fixator.
■ A 1.8-mm wire is inserted perpendicular to the mechanical axis of the upper tibia, just below the proximal tibial physis.
  • The limb is held patella forward, checked with the image intensifier.
  • The wire should be parallel to the horizontal plane/floor.
■ A proximal TSF ring is suspended above this wire, with the front tab directly anterior. The wire is tensioned and tightened.
  • Adequate soft tissue clearance, at least 1.5 cm circumferentially, must be ensured. A ⅔ TSF ring opened posteriorly allows for more knee flexion.
■ A pin fixation cube, typically two or three holes in height, is added to the anterior central hole of the TSF ring.
■ The image intensifier is brought to the lateral position, and the ring swiveled on the wire until it is perpendicular to the long lateral axis of the tibial diaphysis.
  • For proximal metaphyseal deformities, this ring should be positioned at an ~ 9° tilt to the knee joint line to simulate a normal posterior proximal tibial angle (81°).
■ With the ring in this position, an anterior-to-posterior half-pin is inserted in the distal hole of the cube.
■ This fixes the proximal ring orthogonal to the upper tibia.

Instrumentation/Implantation

• Ilizarov wires (1.8 and 1.5 mm) (Smith and Nephew)
• Drill bits
  ■ 4.8-mm and 3.2-mm cannulated (Orthofix)
  ■ 3.8-mm cannulated (Smith and Nephew)
• Half-pins
  ■ 6.0-mm HA-coated pins (Orthofix; Smith and Nephew)
  ■ 4.5-mm HA-coated pins (Smith and Nephew)
  ■ 3.5- to 4.5-mm tapered HA-coated pins (Orthofix)

PEARLS

• *Half-pin size is determined by the diameter and location of pin placement.*
  ■ *Half-pin diameter should be approximately ⅓ the diameter of the bone.*
  ■ *In pediatric tibias, the metaphyseal ends of the bone can accommodate larger half-pins (6 mm).*
• *Preferences for wire/drill/pin size combinations are as follows:*
  ■ *1.8-mm wire/4.8-mm cannulated drill/6.0-mm half-pin*
  ■ *1.5-mm wire/3.8-mm cannulated drill/4.5-mm half-pin*
  ■ *1.5-mm wire/3.2-mm cannulated drill/3.5- to 4.5-mm tapered half-pin*
• *All half-pins are hydroxyapatite (HA) coated.*
• *Using the wire/cannulated drill method results in more accurate pin placement in small, pediatric tibias.*

PITFALLS

• *Failure to use cannulated drill technique can result in:*
  ■ *Unicortical pin placement with poor fixation or pin cutout*
  ■ *Unused preliminary drill holes that can be stress risers for potential fractures*
• *Non–HA-coated half-pins have higher rates of pin loosening and pin site infections*

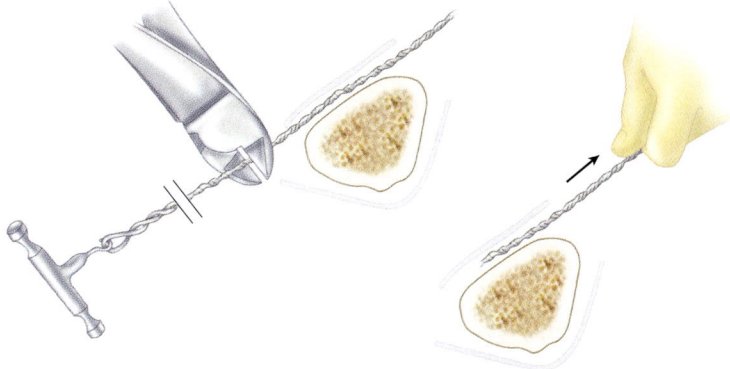

FIGURE 12

STEP 6: APPLYING THE DISTAL RING AND STRUTS

- A pin is inserted in the diaphysis of the tibia, perpendicular to the bone in the lateral view.
  - A full TSF ring is suspended from this pin off the central tab with a four- or five-hole pin fixation cube.
  - Circumferential skin clearance must be ensured.
  - The image intensifier is placed in the AP view and the ring rotated around the pin side to side until the ring is perpendicular to the long axis of the diaphysis. All connections are tightened. Now the distal ring is orthogonal to the distal segment.
- Six oblique TSF struts are added, starting at the anterior tab, so that they exactly fit between the two rings that have been placed.
- The struts are labeled, with the #1 and #2 strut meeting at the proximal anterior "master tab" in the front of the tibia and proceeding clockwise, as viewed from the bottom of the foot.
- Once the TSF struts are in place, the available free corridors for placement of additional half-pins can now be seen (Fig. 13).
  - A total of three half-pins are inserted in the proximal fixation block and three in the distal fixation block. If the foot is to be included in the fixator, then two half-pins are sufficient in the distal block. For very young children (<5 years old), two half-pins in each block may be adequate.
  - The proximal pin pattern is one anterolateral, one anteromedial, and one directly anterior.
  - The distal pin pattern is anteromedial and anterior. The surgeon should strive for a spread to ensure a "delta" configuration for more stability. The distal pins should be suspended above and below the distal ring with four- or five-hole cubes in each direction (less in small children) to ensure maximum spread, but not too close to the osteotomy site for longer lengthenings.
  - The surgeon must ensure that all the struts spin freely (not too long or too short).
- The ring sizes, strut sizes, and strut lengths are recorded for later planning purposes.

Instrumentation/Implantation

- Our preference for circular external fixation devices is the Smith and Nephew TSF ring fixator. Wire guides, drill guides, and drill bits are contained in the standard instrument trays.

- An alternate approach is to use TSF rings connected by straight perpendicular Ilizarov rods. This can provide better radiographic visualization (compared to TSF struts that can block x-rays). At the end of lengthening, the Ilizarov rods may be swapped out for TSF struts if needed (to correct deformity).

- Monolateral fixations such as the Orthofix LRS can also be used for straight tibial lengthening.

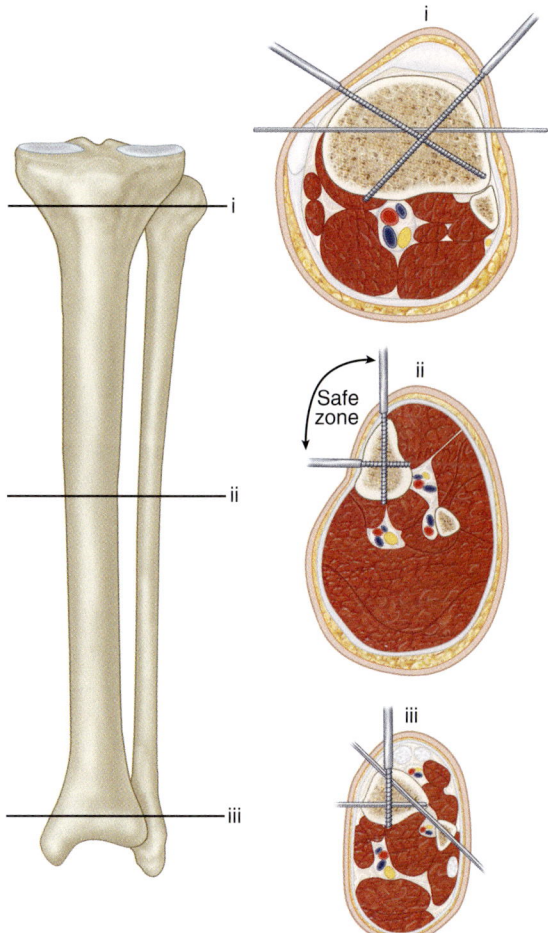

Safe
zone

FIGURE 13

STEP 7: OSTEOTOMY

- If the Gigli saw has been passed, it may now be activated.
  - The anterior three struts are disconnected and the table is lowered.
  - The Gigli handles are attached. Ideally, there are two assistants with small retractors to protect the skin at each opening for the Gigli saw, and one assistant holding the leg down.
  - The Gigli saw is activated, first at 90°, and gradually lowering the angle as one cuts, reaching the anteromedial face of the tibia last. The surgeon must be careful not to cut the skin bridge.
  - The surgeon must demonstrate that the bone ends can translate, indicating a complete osteotomy. The struts are reattached orthotopically, and reduction is confirmed with the image intensifier.
  - Figure 8A shows a postoperative view of patient following nondisplaced Gigli saw corticotomy.
- If using a drill/osteotome technique, all six of the struts are removed. A 1-cm vertical incision is made over the crest of the tibia.
  - A hole is drilled front to back with a 4.8-mm solid drill bit.
  - The drill back is pulled, the flutes are cleaned, and the drill is reinserted at a slight angle medially, and then laterally to make a total of three posterior perforations.
  - A 10-mm osteotome is inserted to cut first the lateral and then the medial cortex. Finally, the central area of the bone is cut, and the osteotome blade rotated 90° with a wrench, to complete the osteotomy.
  - The surgeon must confirm with the image intensifier that the osteotomy is complete.
  - The osteotomy is reduced, the struts are reapplied orthotopically, and then reduction is confirmed with the image intensifier.
  - The leg and frame are cleansed of blood. Sponge pressure dressings are applied to the pins and wires. Final permanent radiographs are obtained (AP, lateral of the tibia centered on the reference ring).
- Figure 14 provides an illustration of the osteotomy.

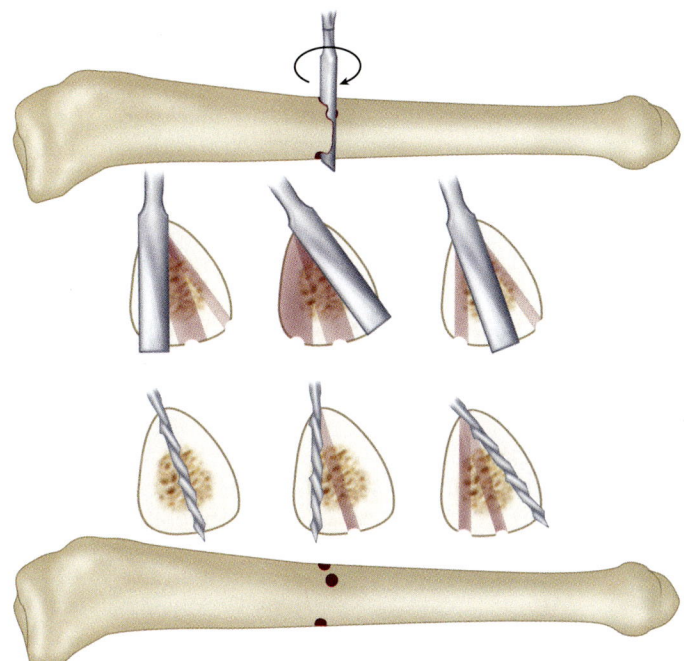

FIGURE 14

POSTOPERATIVE CARE AND EXPECTED OUTCOMES

- Elevate the leg on pillows for the first night after surgery. After the first night, the pillows should be placed under the distal ring and foot in order to keep the knee straight. Keeping the knee bent encourages a flexion contracture.
- After surgery, the TSF program (Internet based) is filled out with the deformity parameters, mounting parameters, frame parameters, and the structures at risk in order to generate the computerized printout and turn schedule for the patient. It is beyond the scope of this procedure to describe the intricacies of the Internet-based software for the TSF total residual program.
- Figure 8F presents a lateral view showing mounting parameters of the Gigli saw. For magnification calculation, the known length of the AP screw threads is used.

PAIN MANAGEMENT AND ANTIBIOTICS

- Postoperative epidural analgesia is used for the first 48 hours, with gradual conversion to oral pain medications.
- Perioperative antibiotics
  - Prophylactic antibiotics are given for 24 hours.
  - IV antibiotics continue after the initial 24 hours for as long as the epidural catheter is present.
- Muscle spasms are controlled with oral Diazepam (0.4–0.8 mg/kg/day)

DISTRACTION STRATEGY

- Distraction rate
  - 0.75 mm/day for children less than 6 years of age
  - 1.0 mm/day for children greater than 6 years of age
- Distraction begins 5–7 days after the osteotomy, which is termed the latency period.
  - The latency period allows the bone to recover from the trauma of the osteotomy, enabling early bone healing.
  - Increased latency periods of 10 days may be used for overtly traumatic osteotomies.
- The distraction rate is adjusted during the lengthening period depending on regenerate bone formation and joint range of motion.
  - Distraction rates are decreased:
    - If the regenerate bone becomes narrow or hypotrophic
    - If the fibrous interzone is greater than 5–6 mm in width
    - If there is a significant decrease in the ankle or knee joint range of motion
    - If there is a nerve stretch injury during lengthening
  - Distraction rates are increased:
    - If the regenerate bone becomes hypertrophic with a width greater than the normal bone diameter
    - If early preconsolidation of the osteotomy is becoming apparent on radiographs
  - Figure 8B shows a lateral view of 11-year-old girl with FH and procurvatum after 3-cm distraction.
  - The follow-up EL (see Fig. 8D) shows correction of procurvatum following 4-cm lengthening.

POSTOPERATIVE PHYSICAL THERAPY

- Physical therapy is essential for a successful tibial lengthening.
- Physical therapy is required:
  - 5 days per week (1–2 hr/day) during the distraction period of the lengthening treatment
  - 2–3 days per week (1 hr/day) during the consolidation period of the lengthening treatment
- Physical therapy can include both land and hydrotherapy.
- Weight bearing:
  - Patients less than 6 years of age are allowed weight bearing as tolerated.
  - Patients greater than 6 years of age are allowed 50% weight bearing.
- Range-of-motion requirements:
  - Patients must maintain a full or nearly full knee extension and ankle dorsiflextion to be able to continue the distraction process.
    - ◆ No more than 10° equinus contracture
    - ◆ Maintenance of full knee extension
  - **Continued distraction despite inadequate range of motion will result in joint contractures requiring extensive surgical and physiotherapeutic intervention.**

FRAME MAINTENANCE AND PIN CARE

- Preoperative and perioperative education is essential for the family.
- An external fixation education manual is provided for each family.
- A patient education nurse performs an education session with the family about the specific external fixator and its adjustment schedule.
  - Daily reinforcement of external fixator specifics and care is performed during the hospital stay.
- Pin care
  - The initial pin dressing change is performed 24 hours after surgery by nursing staff with instructions to the parents.
  - Pin care is performed daily by the family.
    - ◆ For the first week, the pin sites are cleaned with sterile normal saline daily and wrapped with rolled gauze or "marshmallow" sponges.
    - ◆ After the first week, the pins are cleaned using antibacterial soap when the patient performs the daily shower.
    - ◆ Patients should keep the proximal pin sites wrapped with rolled gauze or "marshmallow" sponges to reduce skin motion and protect the sites from the environment. Distal pin sites should be wrapped if the ankle is free.

PIN SITE INFECTIONS

- Pin site infections are very common.
- The vast majority of pin site infections are superficial skin infections easily treated with oral antibiotics.
- The earliest sign of pin site infection is increasing pain at the pin site.
  - This pain rapidly increases over the ensuing 6–12 hours.
  - Other pin site qualities such as drainage, mild erythema, and crusting can be misleading for parents and are not diagnostic of infection unless pain is also present.
- Oral antibiotic treatment is initiated at the earliest sign of pin infection.

PEARLS

- *Ensure that there is no significant skin tension or adherence around the pin site.*

- *Skin tension equals skin necrosis, which will lead to an environment that promotes pin infections. Skin releases should be performed if there is significant skin tension or obvious necrosis*

- *Chronically irritated or problematic pin sites should be stabilized with gauze wraps and treated with water-based polymicrobial ointment (Bactroban).*

- *Granulomatous reactions can occur around pin sites that cause tremendous concern for the patient and family.*

  - *Reassure the family that this does not signify infection.*

  - *The pin site should be wrapped to provide slight pressure to the skin.*

  - *Silver nitrate sticks can be applied to the granulomatous tissue to desiccate and cauterize.*

- Primary antibiotic tier
  - Keflex (50–100 mg/kg/day) qid for 10 days
  - Bactrim DS (penicillin-allergic patients) bid for 10 days
- Secondary antibiotic tier (patients who fail with the primary antibiotic tier)
  - Bactrim DS bid for 10 days
  - Clindamycin (10–25 mg/kg/day) tid for 10 days
- Tertiary antibiotic tier
  - Ciprofloxacin (10–20 mg/kg/dose) bid, not to exceed 750 mg/dose no matter the child's size.
  - Tailor antibiotics according to sensitivities from pin swab culture taken for difficult pin sites.
- Organism identification
  - The vast majority of pin site infections are treated empirically.
  - Difficult pin sites that are resistant to routine oral antibiotic treatment may undergo swab culture.
    - Culture results must be analyzed with the correct perspective of the routine skin flora.
    - Swab results are helpful to identify unusual organisms such as *Pseudomonas* or resistant organisms such as methicillin-resistant *Staphylococcus aureus.*
    - Swab results are used to tailor antibiotic treatment.
- Severe pin site infections are rare and usually deeper.
  - Severe infections begin as a typical pin site infection with pain and eventual progressive erythema.
  - They cause constitutional symptoms such as fever, lethargy/malaise, and nausea.
  - Symptoms must not be ignored, and the patient must be treated immediately.
  - The patient is admitted to the hospital for IV antibiotics.
  - If the infected pin site does not respond within 24 hours to the IV antibiotics, the pin is removed and the site is débrided and curetted in the OR.
  - Rarely, toxic shock syndrome or necrotizing fasciitis may occur. The surgeon should look for systemic signs of illness! Treat aggressively!

CLINICAL FOLLOW-UP STRATEGY

- The patient is seen within 2 weeks from hospital discharge.
- Clinical follow-up visits occur every 2 weeks during the distraction or lengthening phase of the treatment for clinical and radiographic examination.
- Clinical examination and review of physical therapy notes:
  - Normal neurovascular status of the limb is ensured.
  - Overall clinical alignment in the coronal and sagittal plane is checked.
  - Joint motion measurements recorded during physical therapy are reviewed.
  - The frame and distraction device are checked for stability and position (i.e., overall mechanical check of frame and connections).
  - Pin sites and pin stability are checked.
- Radiographic examination
  - Anteroposterior and lateral radiographs of the tibia are obtained; these must include the knee and the ankle.
    - Radiographs are checked to ensure that the knee and ankle are in normal position with no contracture or subluxation.
    - The length of distraction and quality of the regenerate bone are evaluated.
    - The joint orientation measurements for both the knee and the ankle are evaluated to ensure that malalignment is not occurring.

- A bilateral standing AP radiograph of the legs, to include hips to ankles, is obtained.
  - An overall measurement of LLD and extremity alignment is performed.
  - This is done at the end of the lengthening to evaluate the global position and alignment.
- Clinical follow-up is done every month during the consolidation/healing phase of the treatment.
- When the follow-up radiographs demonstrate complete consolidation, the surgical removal of the external fixator is scheduled.

PROCEDURE: EXTERNAL FIXATOR REMOVAL

- The timing of external fixation removal must be determined.
  - The consolidation phase is completed when three of four cortices have healed on radiographs (see Fig. 8C and 8D).
  - Estimated total frame time equals one month for every centimeter gained in bone length.
- Dynamization is recommended in the last month of treatment. Tension is reduced on the struts until they all spin freely.
  - Another dynamization technique is to "decommission" one or more of the half-pins. If three half-pins were used on the proximal or distal ring segments, one may be detached from the ring by removing the pin cube.

Step 1

- The patient is placed under general anesthesia.
- The pin sites are cleaned and external fixator pin clamps loosened.
- The half-pins are removed through the pin clamp to reduce torque on the tibia.
- The frame is removed from the last half-pin and the tibia is supported while this pin is removed.

STEP 2

- Anteroposterior and lateral radiographs are obtained.
  - The quality of regenerate bone and the half-pin sites are checked radiographically.
  - If the regenerate bone is narrowed or the half-pin sites are at risk for a post-lengthening fracture, then intramedullary support (Rush rod) may be considered, or at least a long-leg cast is applied.
  - Figure 8E shows an AP view 1 week after removal; note that there is no evidence of fracture.
- Figure 15 shows a 12-year-old girl with Ollier's disease and complex multilevel deformity involving the femur and tibia, and LLD of 7 cm. EL image (A) during correction with TSF on tibia and TSF on femur. An EL image (B) is shown after frame removal. The malalignment and LLD have been corrected.
- If radiographs demonstrate adequate healing, then bulky sterile dressings are applied with mild compression.

POSTOPERATIVE CARE AND EXPECTED OUTCOMES

- Dressings are removed 48 hours after surgery.
- The patient is allowed partial weight bearing and continues with gentle range of motion for 4 weeks after external fixator removal.
- Residual LLD is to be made up by contralateral distal femoral epiphysiodesis (see Fig. 3).

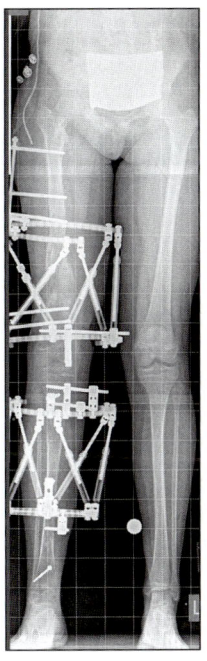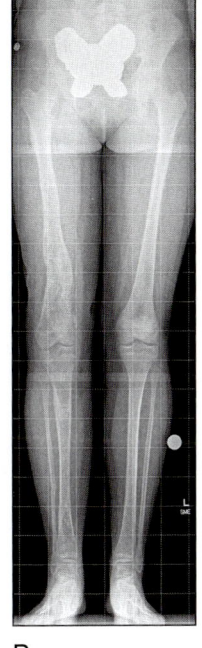

A B

FIGURE 15

EVIDENCE

Bhave A, Paley D, Herzenberg JE. Improvement in gait parameters after lengthening for the treatment of limb-length discrepancy. J Bone Joint Surg [Am]. 1999;81:529–34.

This prospective study compared objective gait parameters before and after lengthening, including the stance time, the second peak of the vertical ground-reaction-force vector, and the rate of loading with use of two force-plates arranged in a series. Lengthening of the shorter limb of patients who have limb-length discrepancy can normalize symmetry of quantifiable stance parameters and eliminate a limp.

Eralp L, Kocaoğlu M, Ozkan K, Türker M. A comparison of two osteotomy techniques for tibial lengthening. Arch Orthop Trauma Surg. 2004;124:298–300.

Forty-four tibias of 41 patients were lengthened with the Ilizarov device using either a percutaneous Gigli saw osteotomy or one with multiple drill holes and an osteotome. The mean length discrepancy was 5.7 cm (range, 2–12 cm). The mean healing index (HI) of the whole group was 1.65 month/cm (range, 1.1–2.4 month/cm). The multiple-drill-hole group had a mean HI of 1.98 month/cm (range, 1.4–2.4 month/cm), while the Gigli saw group had a mean HI of 1.37 month/cm (range, 1.1–1.8 month/cm) (p = .022).

Hahn SB, Park HW, Park HJ, Seo YJ, Kim HW. Lower limb lengthening in Turner dwarfism. Yonsei Med J. 2003;44:502–7.

Twelve tibiae and two femora were lengthened in six patients using the Ilizarov method for the tibia and a gradual elongation nail for the femur. The mean age at the time of surgery was 19 years, and the patients were followed up for a minimum of 2 years. The average gain in the tibial length was 6.2 cm. The average HI of the tibia was 1.9 months. The overall rate of complications was 100%. Turner's dwarfism lengthening requires management in a specialist unit in order to prevent complications during the lengthening procedure.

Hatzokos I, Drakou A, Christodoulou A, Terzidis I, Pournaras J. Inferior subluxation of the fibular head following tibial lengthening with a unilateral external fixator. J Bone Joint Surg [Am]. 2004;86:1491–6.

Inferior subluxation of the head of the fibula may occur with distraction osteogenesis of the tibia. Thirty tibiae in 17 patients underwent tibial lengthening of 8.1 cm (range, 3.5–13 cm) without proximal tibial-fibular stabilization. All cases developed an inferior shift of the fibular head, ranging from 0.4 to 3.3 cm, proportional to the amount of tibial lengthening.

Herzenberg JE, Paley D. Leg lengthening in children. Curr Opin Pediatr. 1998;10:95–7.

The authors discussed leg-lengthening techniques derived from Russia and Europe that have revolutionized treatment of LLD and even stature lengthening in dwarfism. Long-term follow-up studies are forthcoming, and there is still extensive room for basic research. Precise indications and limits for lengthening in femoral hypoplasia and fibular hemimelia are unclear. Future research needs to include outcome studies, hardware improvements, implantable lengthening devices, and a better understanding of the basic science behind lengthening of both bone and soft tissues.

Nogueira MP, Paley D, Bhave A, Herbert A, Nocente C, Herzenberg JE. Nerve lesions associated with limb-lengthening. J Bone Joint Surg [Am]. 2003;85:1502–10.

In this retrospective study of 814 limb-lengthening procedures, 76 of the limbs (9.3%) had a nerve lesion. Eighty-four percent occurred during gradual distraction, and 16% occurred immediately following surgery. The pressure-specified sensory device showed 100% sensitivity and 86% specificity in the detection of nerve injuries. Patients undergoing double-level tibial lengthening and those with skeletal dysplasia were at higher risk for nerve lesions (77% and 48%, respectively). Nerve decompression was performed in 53 cases (70%). The time between the diagnosis and surgical decompression was strongly associated with the time to recovery (p = .0005). Complete clinical recovery was achieved in 74 of the 76 cases.

Paley D, Bhave A, Herzenberg JE, Bowen JR. Multiplier method for predicting limb-length discrepancy. J Bone Joint Surg [Am]. 2000;82:1432–46.

In congenital LLD, the short limb grows proportional to the normal limb. These authors described the multiplier method, which is based on existing databases of children's bone lengths, dividing the femoral and tibial lengths at maturity by the femoral and tibial lengths at each age. The multipliers for the femur and tibia were equivalent in all percentile groups, varying only by age and gender. The discrepancy at maturity can be calculated as the current discrepancy times the multiplier for the current age and the gender. This calculation can be performed with use of a single measurement of limb-length discrepancy. Multiplier calculations correlated well with the Moseley straight line graph method.

Paley D, Herzenberg JE, Tetsworth K, McKie J, Bhave A. Deformity planning for frontal and sagittal plane corrective osteotomies. Orthop Clin North Am. 1994;25:425–65.

This article presented a universal system of x-ray deformity planning based on the mechanical or anatomic axes. Intersection of the proximal and distal axes is called the center of rotation angulation (CORA). This type of planning is applicable to both frontal and sagittal plane deformities. Adherence to the rules of planning espoused here prevented secondary translational deformities.

Sabharwal S, Paley D, Bhave A, Herzenberg JE. Growth patterns after lengthening of congenitally short lower limbs in young children. J Pediatr Orthop. 2000; 20:137–45.

This study evaluated growth after lengthening of the congenitally short femur or tibia in children younger than 6 years. Twenty children underwent 28 bone segment lengthenings (13 femora and 15 tibiae) by distraction osteogenesis. Femoral lengthening in children younger than 6 years does not lead to growth inhibition, whereas isolated femoral lengthening may be associated with growth stimulation. Isolated tibial lengthening in children younger than 6 years does not lead to growth inhibition, whereas simultaneous femoral and tibial lengthening or two tibial lengthenings in close succession can lead to tibial growth inhibition.

Saleh M, Bashir HM, Farhan MJ, McAndrew AR, Street R. Tibial lengthening: does the fibula migrate? J Pediatr Orthop B. 2002;11:302–6.

In this study, 32 patients underwent tibial lengthening. In 16 patients the lower tibiofibular syndesmosis was stabilized, and in the other 16 no stabilization was done. All showed some proximal migration of the distal fibula, but those without stabilization demonstrated more severe migration associated with a valgus tendency. The difference between the groups was statistically significant (p < .001), confirming the need for fibular fixation.

Yasui N, Kawabata H, Kojimoto H, Ohno H, Matsuda S, Araki N, Shimomura Y, Ochi T. Lengthening of the lower limbs in patients with achondroplasia and hypochondroplasia. Clin Orthop Relat Res. 1997;(344):298–306.

In this study, 35 lengthening patients with achondroplasia and 7 patients with hypochondroplasia were reviewed. Mean age at the time of first operation was 14.5 years. Mean age at follow-up was 18.8 years. Mean lengthening was 7.2 cm in the femur (range, 4.5–12 cm) and 7.1 cm in the tibia (range, 4.5–13 cm). The function of lengthened limbs, evaluated by physical strength tests, was better at follow-up than before lengthening in the growing children, despite some mechanical axis deviation.

Arthroscopic Management for Juvenile Osteochondritis Dissecans of the Talus

Craig J. Spurdle and Michael Busch

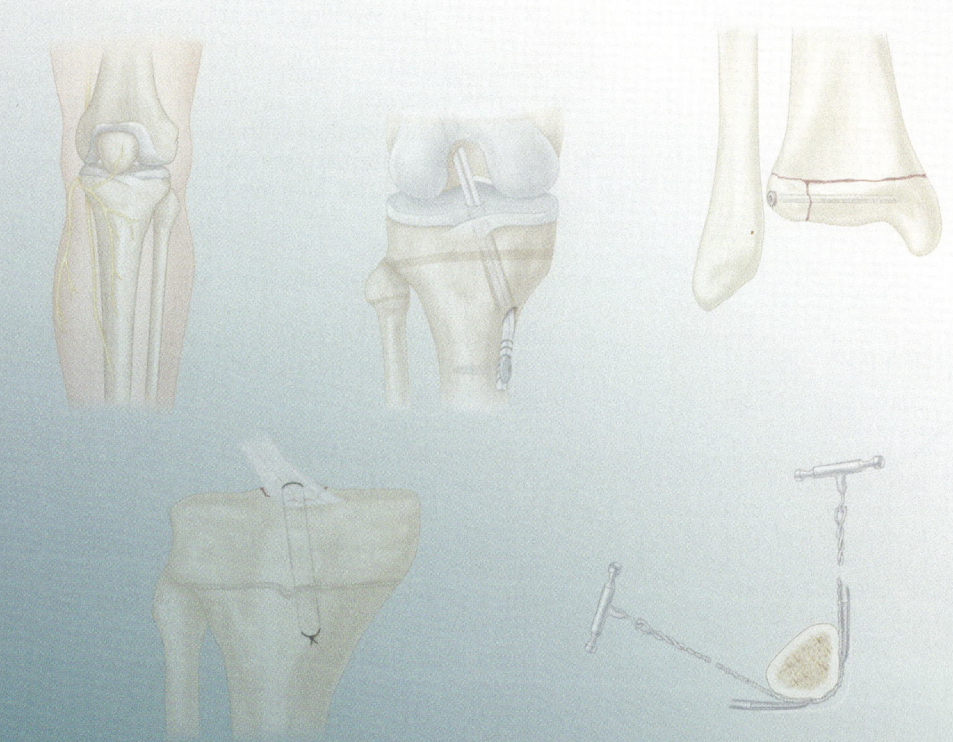

INDICATIONS

- Failed conservative treatment for 6 months, including casting and weight-bearing restriction
- Unstable osteochondritis dissecans (OCD) lesions at presentation
  - All Berndt and Harty stage 4 and anterolateral stage 3 lesions (Canale and Belding, 1980; Pettine and Morrey, 1987)
- Relative indications
  - Early surgery for symptomatic stage 3 (posteromedial and central) and all stage 4 lesions
  - Early surgery for symptomatic stage 2, 3, and 4 in patients nearing skeletal maturity (age > 12) (Letts et al., 2003; Perumal et al., 2007; Pettine and Morrey, 1987)

EXAMINATION/IMAGING

- Ankle pain and swelling are the most common complaints with OCDs.
- A standard ankle examination should be performed, including a thorough neurovascular and motor examination, and a range-of-motion examination with comparison to the opposite side.
- Lateral ankle instability should be assessed with the anterior drawer test and the talar tilt test. These tests examine the anterior talofibular ligament and calcaneofibular ligaments, respectively.
- Medially, the deltoid ligament should also be examined for tenderness and laxity.
- Other sources of ankle pain should be excluded: peroneal tendon pathology, flexor hallucis longus pathology, and os trigonum pain.
- Plain radiographs
  - Anteroposterior (AP), lateral, and mortise views are obtained.
  - OCD lesions are usually diagnosed by radiographs (Fig. 1).
- Magnetic resonance imaging (MRI)
  - MRI provides valuable information regarding the stability of the lesion.
  - The size, location (posteromedial, anterolateral, or central), and stability can be evaluated.
  - The arthroscopic surgical approach (anterior vs. posterior portals) is chosen from the location of the OCD on MRI (Fig. 2).

Treatment Options

- OCDs with arthroscopically determined intact articular cartilage (stable) and less than 1 cm in size are treated with extra-articular drilling.
- OCDs with arthroscopically determined intact articular cartilage (stable) and greater than 1 cm in size are treated by extra-articular drilling and placement of autograft.
- OCDs with disrupted articular cartilage (unstable) are treated by débridement and marrow perforation.
- Alternatives for rare large lesions of the talus (2 cm or greater) include internal fixation, osteoarticular allograft/autograft, and autologous chondrocyte implantation.
  - Note: Medial malleolar osteotomy is contraindicated in the skeletally immature patient.

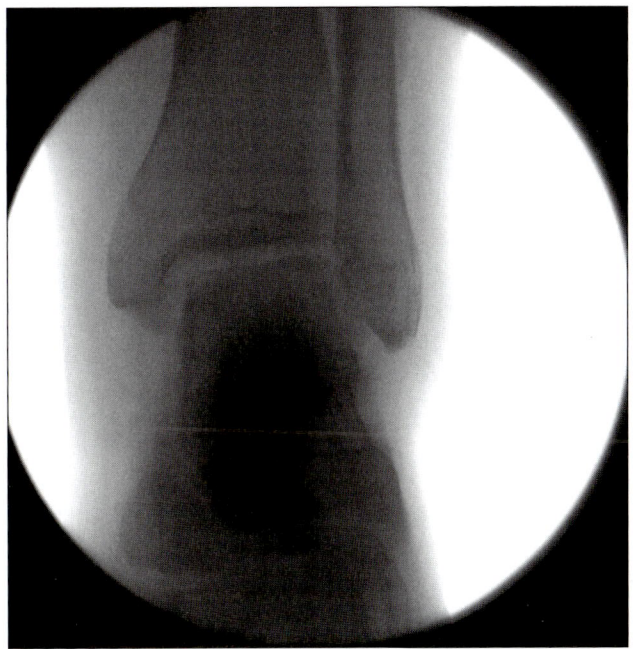

FIGURE 1

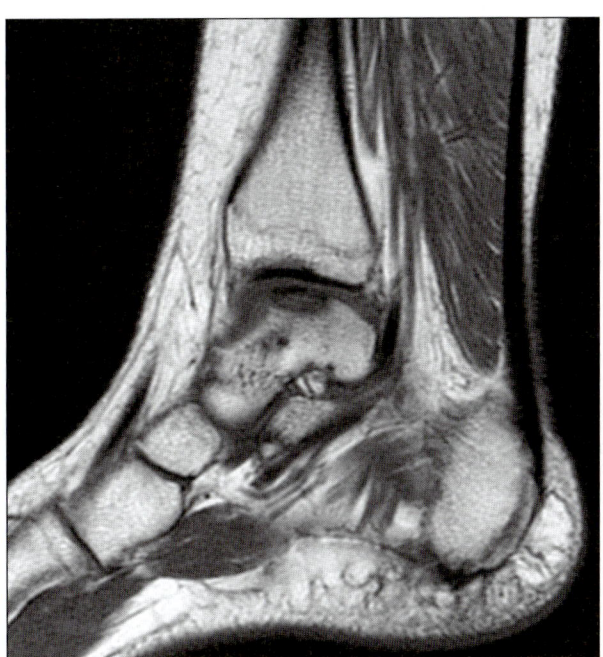

FIGURE 2

Equipment

• A mini C-arm is used for this procedure.

• An arthroscopy leg holder is used on the surgical side and an Allen stirrup is used for the well leg.

Controversies

• Using coaxial posterior portals for the ankle allows us the use of one position for both anterior and posterior ankle arthroscopy. Any intraoperative change using conventional posterior portals requires repositioning of the patient.

SURGICAL ANATOMY

■ Anterior structures at risk (Fig. 3)
  • Lateral portal: The intermediate branch of the superficial peroneal nerve is at risk.
  • Medial portal: This portal is near the saphenous vein and nerve.
■ Posterior structures at risk using the coaxial posterior portals (Fig. 4)
  • Medial portal: The posterior tibial artery and nerve are near this portal.
  • Lateral portal: This portal is located just posterior to the peroneal tendons. The sural nerve is near this portal.

POSITIONING

■ We position all patients supine, and our table setup is the same as for a standard knee arthoscopy (Fig. 5).
■ The foot is placed on the surgeon's thigh during the surgery, and we do not use traction (Fig. 6).

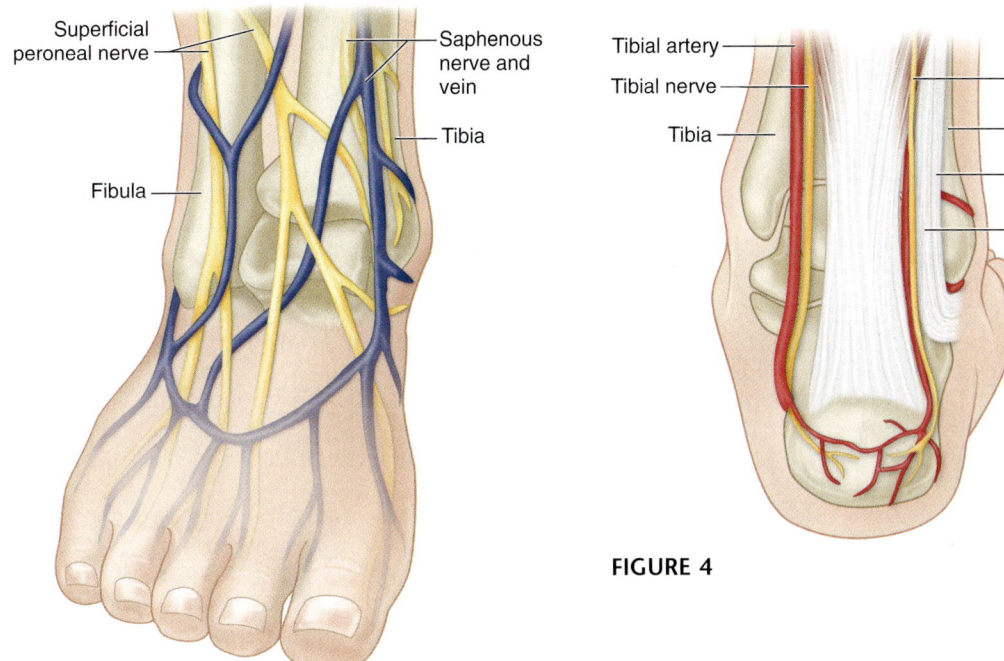

FIGURE 3

FIGURE 4

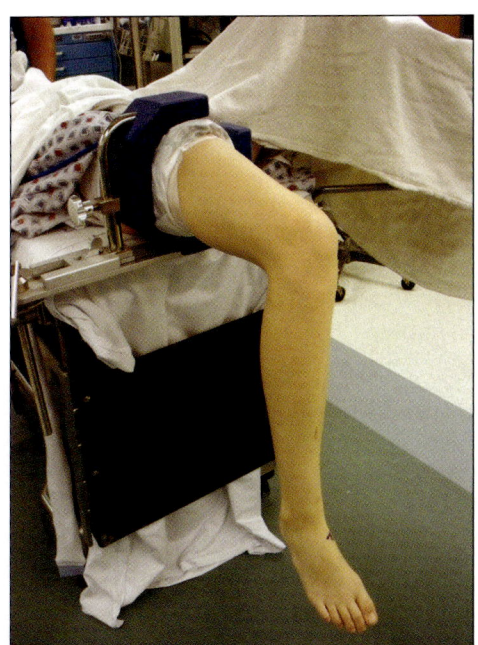

FIGURE 5

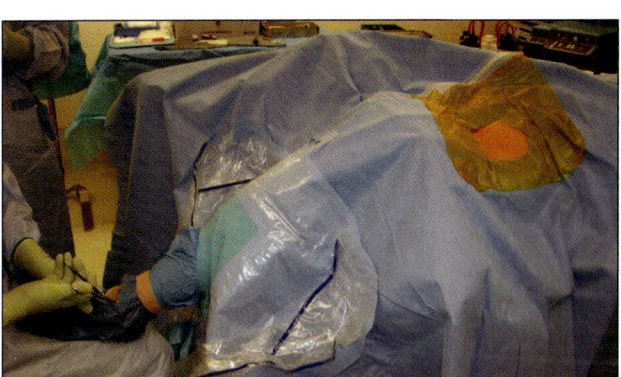

FIGURE 6

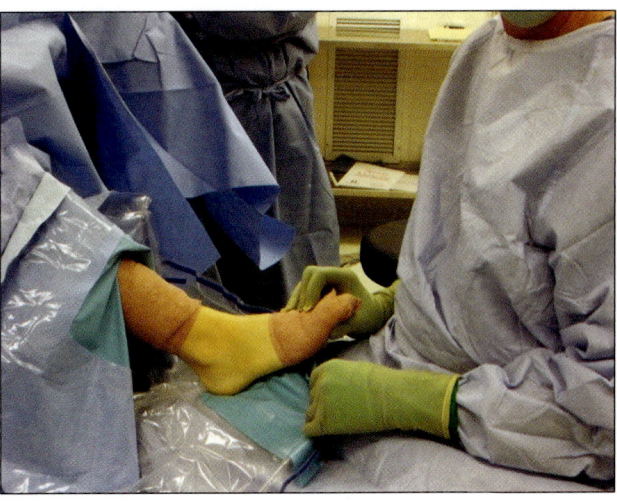

FIGURE 7

Instrumentation

- We use a 2.7-mm arthroscope.

Controversies

- The use of coaxial posterior portals avoids the need for skeletal distraction. To our knowledge, there are no available data that confirm the safety of using distraction during ankle arthroscopy in the skeletally immature patient.

PORTALS/EXPOSURES

- In general, we utilize standard anterior arthroscopic portals for anterolateral lesions and coaxial posterior portals described by Acevedo and colleagues (2000) for posteromedial lesions. We have found that these posterior coaxial portals have several advantages when treating OCD lesions of the talus:
  - First, they provide access for both anterior and posterior ankle arthroscopy with one patient position.
  - They also offer more direct access to débride and perform marrow perforation for the difficult posteromedial lesions.
  - Additionally, they avoid skeletal traction in these skeletally immature patients. Alternatively, conventional posterior portals can used.
- For anterior arthroscopy, the standard medial and lateral portals are established.
  - The joint is insufflated with normal saline using an 18-gauge spinal needle.
  - The medial portal is established first and the lateral portal is established with arthroscopic assistance.
  - The medial portal is placed at the level of the ankle joint between the medial malleolus and the anterior tibial tendon, avoiding the saphenous vein and nerve.
  - The lateral portal is placed at the level of the ankle joint and just lateral to the peroneus tertius tendon, taking care to avoid injuring the dorsal intermediate branch of the superficial peroneal nerve (see Fig. 3).
- For coaxial posterior arthroscopy, we have modified the originally described technique in two important ways. We now establish the medial portal first, and then the lateral portal. In addition, the medial portal is now located between the posterior tibial tendon and the flexor digitorum (Acevedo et al., 2000).
  - After the joint is insufflated, a palpable joint effusion is easily located posterior and proximal to the medial malleolus (Fig. 8).
  - The medial portal lies at the joint line between the posterior tibial tendon and the flexor digitorum. This is approximately 2 cm posterior and 1 cm proximal to the distal tip of the medial malleolus.
  - The skin is incised and blunt dissection with a straight hemostat is directed onto the capsule. The capsule is penetrated, and some saline solution should flow out, indicating access to the joint capsule (Fig. 9A and 9B).
  - The portal is gently spread and the sheath for a 2.9-mm arthroscope (3.5-mm sheath with blunt obturator) is introduced through the same path. The scope is inserted, the joint distended, and the intra-articular location confirmed (Fig. 10).
  - Next, the posterolateral portal is established directly posterior to the peroneal tendons using an inside-out technique.
  - The tip of the scope and scope sheath are directed posteriorly, beneath the posterior capsular fold and positioned adjacent to the posterolateral capsule. This lies between the transverse tibiofibular ligament and the posterior talofibular ligament.
  - The scope is removed while leaving the sheath in place. The obturator is then reinserted through the sheath and both the sheath and obturator are advanced through the capsule just behind the fibula. The skin is tented by the obturator and all other tissues are swept aside (Fig. 11).

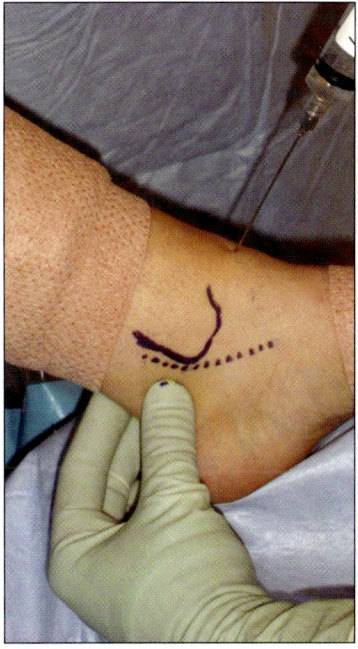

FIGURE 8

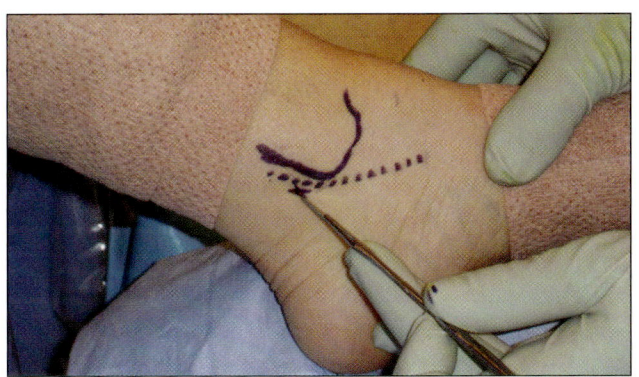

FIGURE 9 A

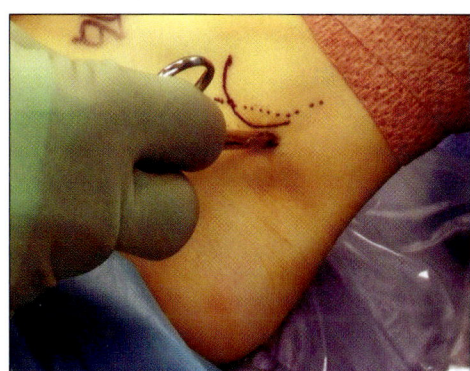

B

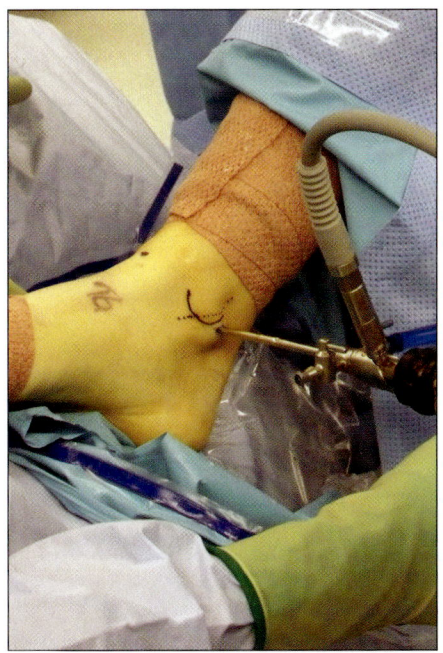

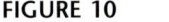

FIGURE 10

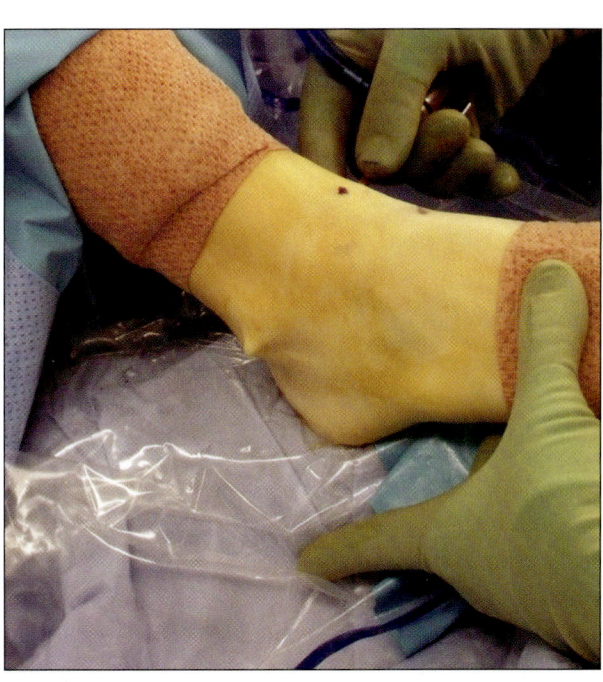

FIGURE 11

- The skin is then incised, taking care not to injure the sural nerve, and the tip of the scope sheath and the obturator are pushed through this portal.
- The obturator is removed while holding the sheath in place. The tip of a 3.5-mm shaver is placed (retrograde) into the tip of the sheath and both are returned to the joint together (Fig. 12).
- Next, the sheath is pulled back about 0.5 cm while leaving the shaver in position and the scope is reinserted. The tip of the shaver should now be directly visualized.
- Hypertrophic synovium is now débrided to improve visualization in the posterior ankle joint.

PROCEDURE

STEP 1

- For arthroscopically confirmed OCD lesions with intact articular cartilage (stable) that are less than 1 cm, our treatment plan uses extra-articular drilling with a 0.62-inch Kirschner wire (K-wire).
- A mini C-arm is used to visualize the lesion in both the AP and lateral planes. We then perforate the lesion in a retrograde fashion (Fig. 13A and 13B).
- The entry point for the K-wire is the distal lateral portion of the talus, just proximal to the sinus tarsi.

Instrumentation/ Implantation

- We use a mini C-arm for localizing these lesions. It is safer with regard to radiation exposure compared to a regular C-arm and easier to manipulate when performing arthroscopy of the ankle.

PEARLS

- *Subchondral bone of OCD lesions has sclerosis and provides a tactile resistance while drilling. This "feel" may be helpful when trying to locate the lesion.*
- *Have the MRI up and available for reference in the operating room to help localize the lesion.*

PITFALLS

- *Avoid penetrating the articular cartilage. The drilling is performed with arthroscopic visualization and/or radiographic visualization to avoid this in both the AP and lateral planes.*

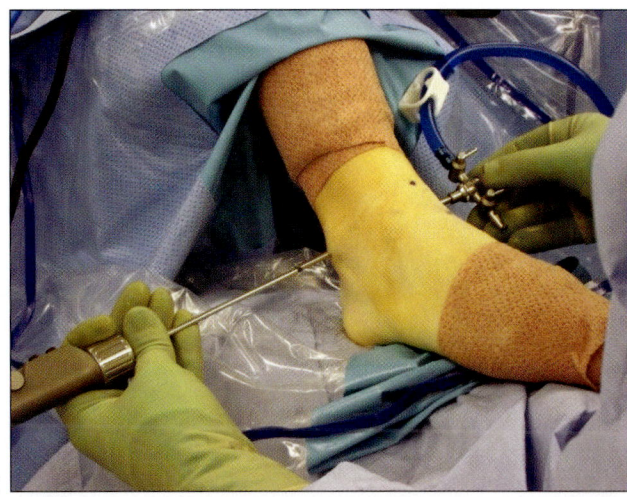

FIGURE 12

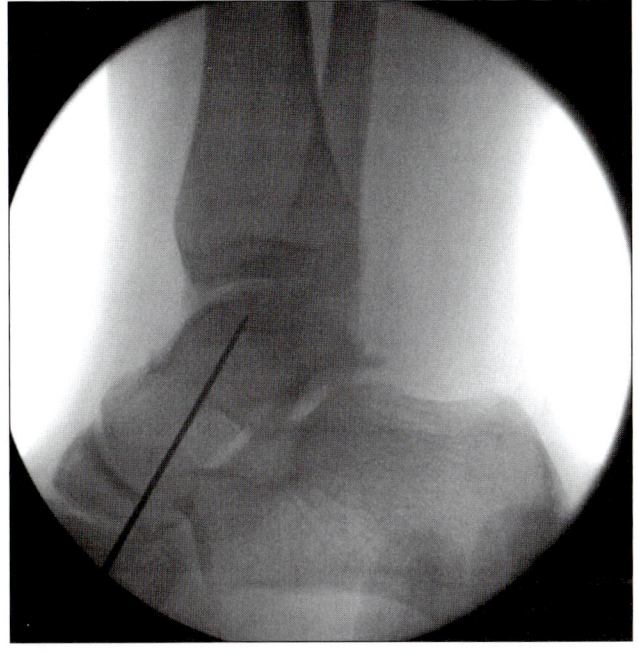

A

FIGURE 13

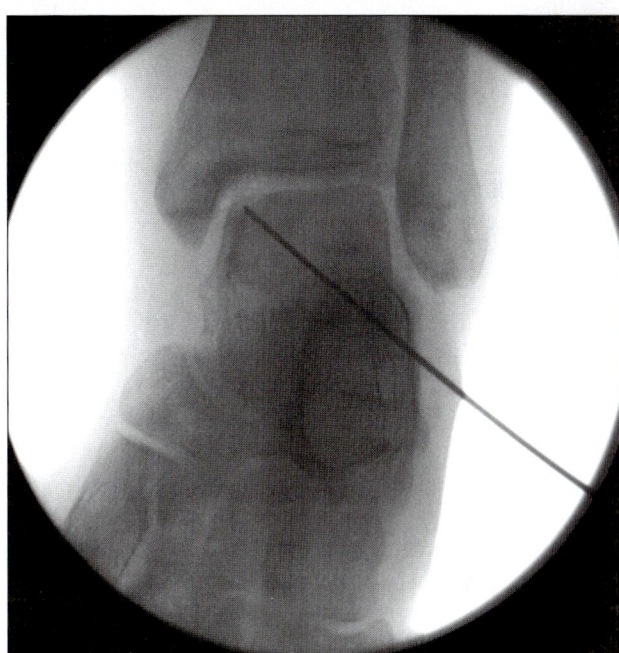

B

PEARLS

- *Radiopaque dye can be injected into the tunnel in the talus prior to the graft insertion. This may allow better visualization of the graft position on fluoroscopy before deploying it.*

PITFALLS

- *Avoid cartilage penetration with drilling.*

Controversies

- There is limited literature support for this specific technique, but the use of autograft for OCDs is well established (Perumal et al., 2007).

- The goal is to perforate the subchondral bone in both planes in at least a 2×2 array with the K-wires without violating the articular cartilage.
  - This can be performed "freehand" or with an intra-articular guide (Fig. 14A and 14B).

STEP 2

- For arthroscopically confirmed OCDs with intact articular cartilage (stable) that are greater than 1 cm, we use extra-articular drilling and autograft.
- A single guidewire (cannulated 4.0-mm set) is introduced into the center of the lesion in a retrograde fashion as described in Step 1.
- A small skin incision is made and blunt dissection is completed down to bone. The surgeon must be careful to avoid any injury to the superficial peroneal sensory nerve branches here.
- Using a 4.0-mm cannulated drill over the guidewire, the lesion is drilled through the subchondral bone. Care is taken to not violate the articular cartilage. The guidewire is then removed (Fig. 15A and 15B).

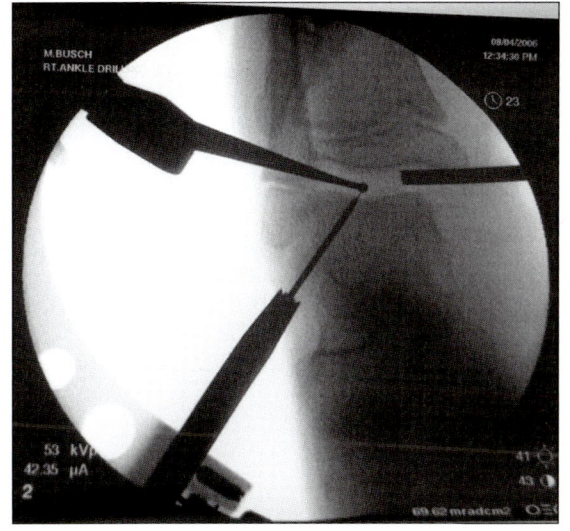

A
FIGURE 14

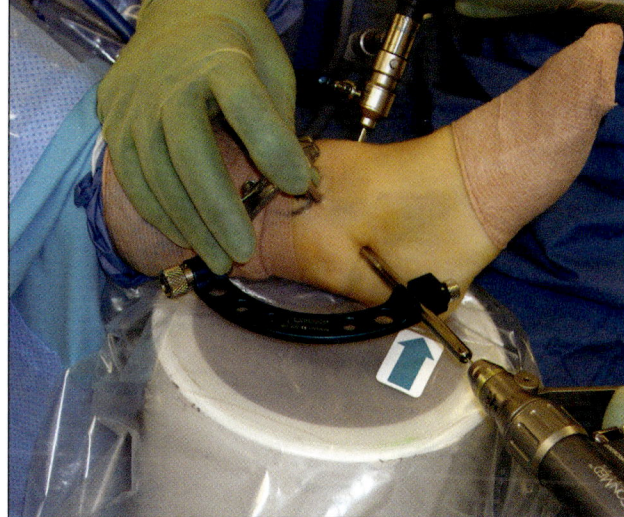

B

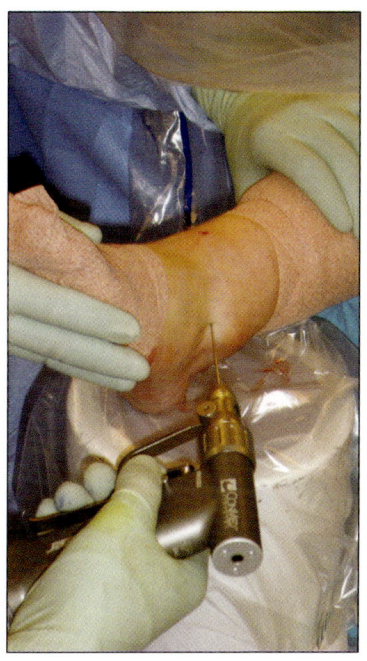

A

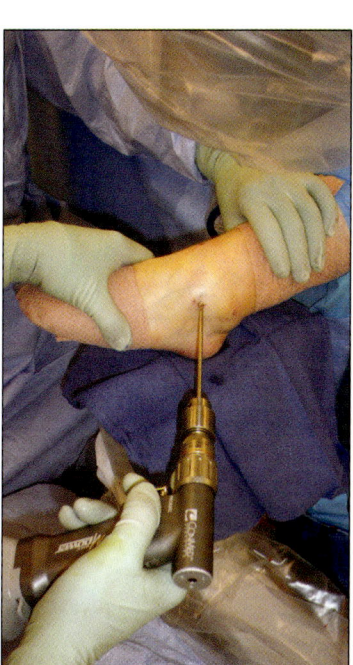

B

FIGURE 15

- Graft material is then harvested from the iliac crest using a Gallini needle (Biomed biopsy needle, 8 gauge × 15 cm).
  - A 1-cm incision is made 3 cm posterior to the anterior superior iliac spine along the iliac crest. Blunt dissection is performed down to the crest to preserve any small branches of the lateral femoral cutaneous nerve (Fig. 16A).
  - Using the Gallini biopsy needle, a core of bone is taken and inspected. It should be at least 1.5 cm in length and composed of bone (cartilage should be removed if present). This is then reinserted into the needle (Fig. 16A–C).
  - This biopsy needle is inserted into the OCD lesion using the drilled pathway in a retrograde fashion (Fig. 17).
- The graft material is deployed in the OCD lesion under fluoroscopic control.

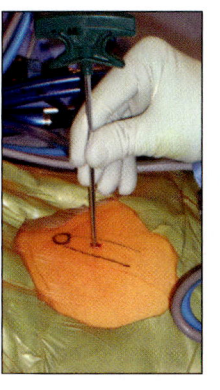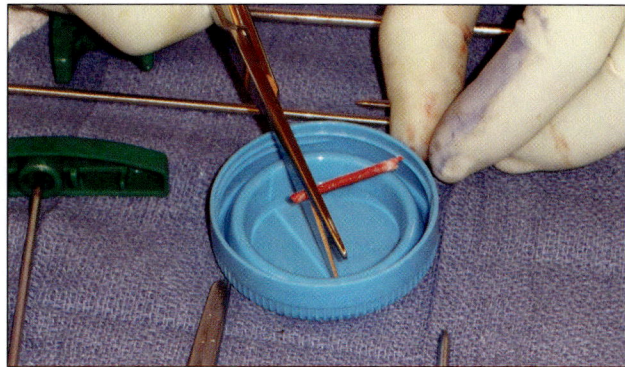

A   B

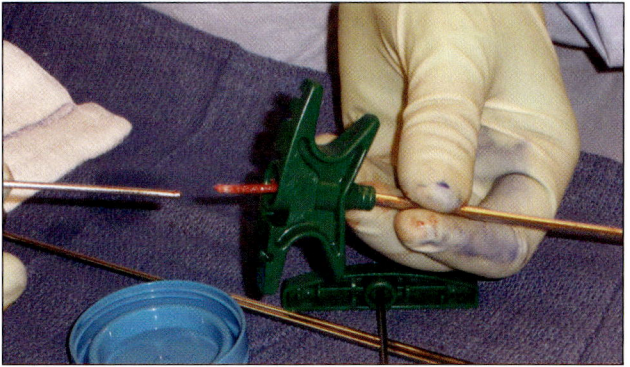

C

FIGURE 16

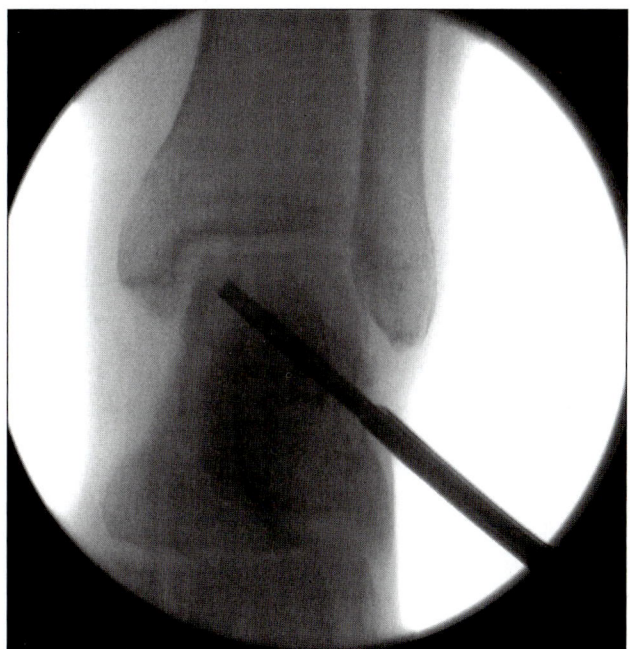

FIGURE 17

PEARLS

- *Some advocate reducing the intra-articular fluid pressure to visualize bleeding from the marrow perforation sites prior to the termination of surgery.*

PITFALLS

- *Additional portals can be helpful to avoid unwanted iatrogenic articular damage.*

Instrumentation/ Implantation

- We use microfracture awls and curettes.

STEP 3

- For arthroscopically confirmed lesions with disrupted articular cartilage (unstable), we use débridement and marrow perforation.
- The lesion is débrided to stable margins and any necrotic bone is débrided from the bed of the lesion with curettes and a shaver.
- Marrow perforation is then performed with microfracture awls spaced about 2–3 mm apart (Fig. 18).
  - Care is taken to remove all loose fragments from the joint.

STEP 4

- Once the surgery is complete, the wounds are irrigated and closed with 3-0 nylon interrupted sutures.
- Sterile dressings are applied.
- An Ace bandage is lightly applied.

POSTOPERATIVE CARE AND EXPECTED OUTCOMES

- A Cryo-cuff or other cooling device is used for the first 24–48 hours.
- We keep the patients non–weight bearing for 4 weeks and begin a general ankle physical therapy program in the first postoperative week.
- At 3 months, a sports-specific training and running program is initiated if symptoms are resolved and there are signs of radiographic healing.
  - If at 3 months there is no sign of healing on radiographs, a computed tomography (CT) scan is obtained.
  - If there is no sign of healing on CT and the symptoms persist, we consider a revision surgery.
- The average time to symptomatic recovery is variable (3–9 months or longer).

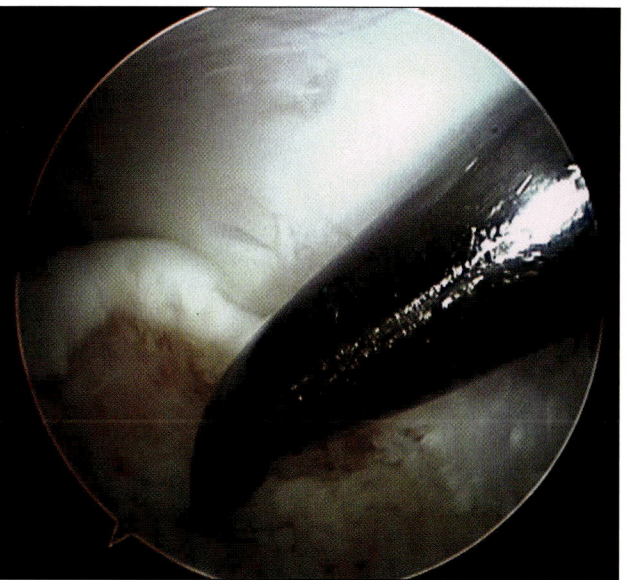

FIGURE 18

EVIDENCE

Acevedo J, Busch M, Ganey T, Hutton W. Coaxial portals for posterior ankle arthroscopy: an anatomic study with clinical correlation on 29 patients. Arthroscopy. 2000;16:836–42.

In this anatomical study, coaxial portals were used in 10 cadaveric ankles for posterior ankle arthroscopy, with an additional clinical cohort of their use in 29 patients.

Canale S, Belding R. Osteochondral lesions of the talus. J Bone Joint Surg [Am]. 1980; 62:92–102.

This retrospective review of 29 patients with OCD lesions of the talus described treatment plans with respect to the Berndt and Hardy classification and location of lesion. This provided the basis of the generally accepted conservative management.

Donaldson L, Wojtys E. Extraarticular drilling for stable osteochondritis dissecans in the skeletally immature knee. J Pediatr Orthop. 2008;28:831–5.

This retrospective review of 15 patients treated with extra-articular drilling for OCD of the knee provided a technical basis for this procedure used in the talus.

Kay R, Tang C. Pediatric foot fractures: evaluation and treatment. J Am Acad Orthop Surg. 2001;9:308–19.

This literature review included OCD of the talus. It described the classification, etiology, and management of OCD lesions.

Kumai T, Takakura Y, Higashiyama I, Tamai S. Arthroscopic drilling for the treatment of osteochondral lesions of the talus. J Bone Joint Surg [Am]. 1999;81:1229–35.

This retrospective study evaluated drilling of OCD lesions. It provided evidence that OCD drilling can be effectively performed without a medial malleolar osteotomy.

Lahm A, Erggelet C, Steinwach M, Reichett A. Arthroscopic management of osteochondral lesions of the talus: results of drilling and usefulness of magnetic resonance imaging before and after treatment. Arthroscopy. 2000;16:299–304.

This retrospective study provided evidence for retrograde drilling for all OCD stages (1–4). It also called into question the accuracy of preoperative MRIs in determining OCD stability. This provided support for diagnostic arthroscopy when finalizing the operative plan.

Letts M, Davidson D, Aboubaker A. Osteochondritis of the talus in children. J Pediatr Orthop. 2003;23:617–25.

This retrospective study, which included only pediatric patients with OCD lesions, provided support for early surgical management of OCD lesions in older children.

Perumal V, Wall E, Babekir N. Juvenile osteochondritis dissecans of the talus. J Pediatr Orthop. 2007;27:821–5.

This was one of the largest retrospective groups of juvenile OCDs published to date. It provided support for the early treatment of older children with OCD lesions and provided outcome results that are lower than previously reported. It also provided anecdotal support for the autograft technique we presented.

Pettine K, Morrey B. Osteochondral fractures of the talus. J Bone Joint Surg [Br]. 1987; 69:82–92.

This retrospective study provided support for the early surgical management of unstable OCD lesions.

Pritsch M, Horoshovski H, Farine I, Tel-Hashomer I. Arthroscopic treatment of osteochondral lesions of the talus. J Bone Joint Surg [Am]. 1986;68:862–5.

This retrospective study provided support for arthroscopic evaluation prior to a final treatment plan. It also advocated drilling of intact lesions and débridement of unstable lesions.

Triplane Fractures

Kathryn A. Keeler and Scott J. Luhmann

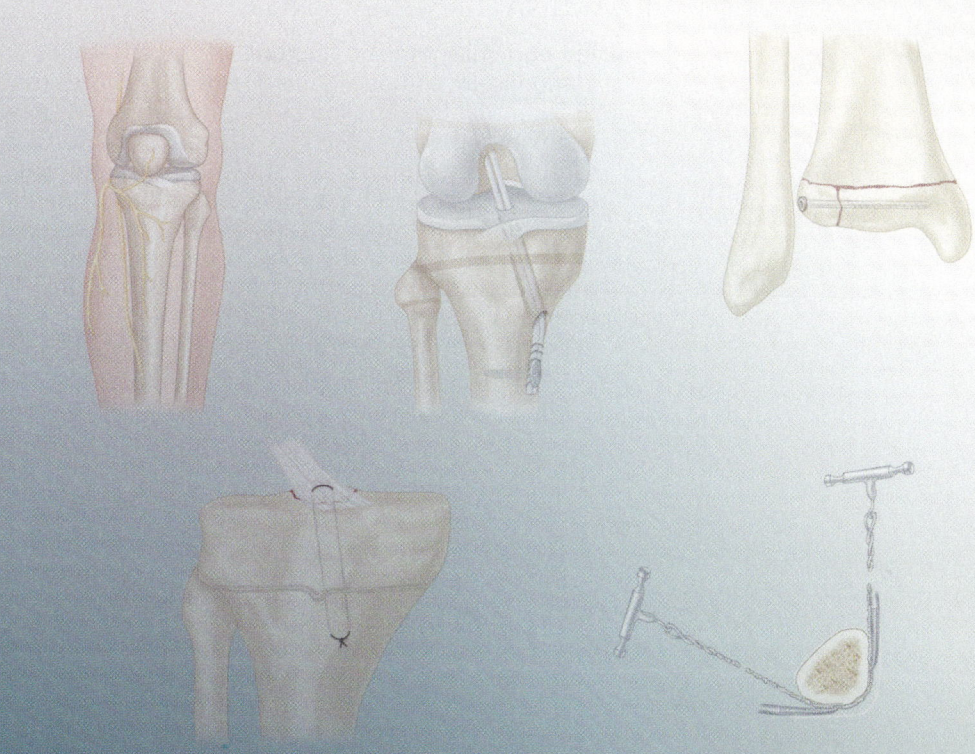

Treatment Options

- Nonmanipulative closed treatment
- Closed reduction and percutaneous fixation
- Open reduction and internal fixation

INDICATIONS

- Nondisplaced fractures are managed nonoperatively with a long-leg cast. Weekly radiographs should be obtained for the first 2 weeks after casting to assess for fracture displacement.
- Fractures with ≥ 2 mm of intra-articular displacement require anatomic reduction to avoid articular incongruity and posttraumatic arthritis.
- Extra-articular triplane fractures extending into the epiphysis of the medial malleolus can occur. Since these fractures do not disrupt the tibial articular surface, nonoperative management can be used in fractures with 2 mm or more of displacement. Treatment guidelines for nonarticular distal tibial fractures can be used.

EXAMINATION/IMAGING

- Intra-articular triplane fractures of the distal tibia are anatomically complex Salter-Harris IV fractures usually consisting of a coronal fracture line in the metaphysis, a transverse fracture line within the physis, and a sagittal, intra-articular fracture through the epiphysis. On the anteroposterior (AP) view, the fracture appears to be a Salter-Harris III fracture; on the lateral view, it appears to be a Salter-Harris II fracture.
- The mortise view of the ankle is the key plain radiographic view used to assess the sagittal, intra-articular fracture line in the epiphysis.
  - Figure 1 shows anteroposterior (AP) (Fig. 1A), mortise (Fig. 1B), and lateral (Fig. 1C) radiographs of a three-part triplane fracture.

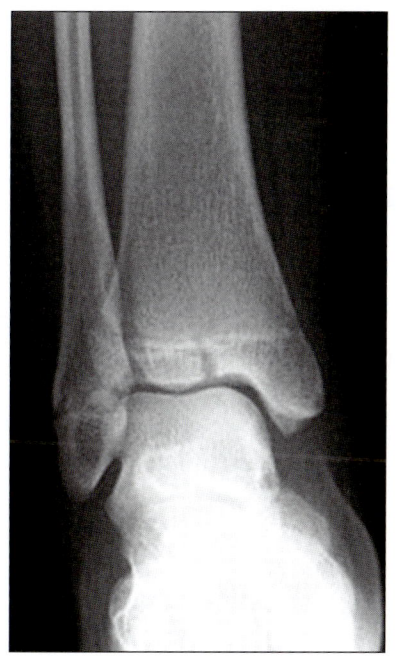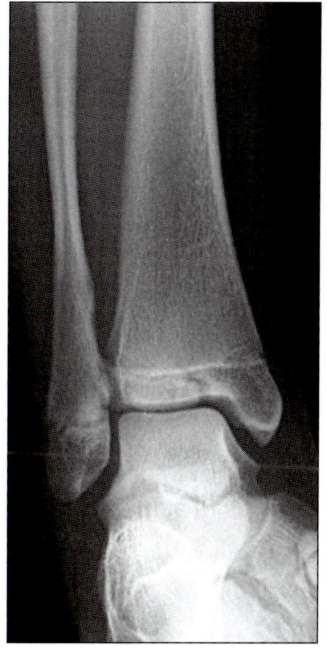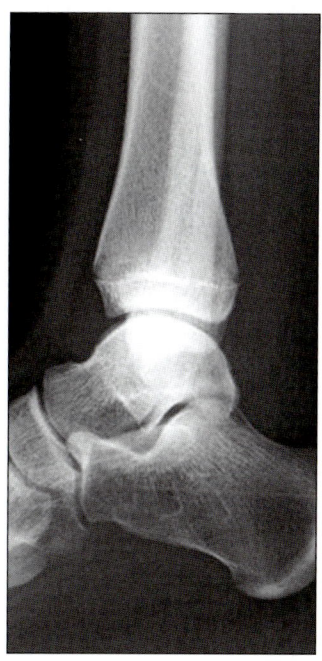

A   B   C

FIGURE 1

- Figure 2 shows AP (Fig. 2A), mortise (Fig. 2B), and lateral (Fig. 2C) radiographs of an extra-articular medial triplane fracture.
- Computed tomography (CT) permits identification of the number and location of fracture fragments.
  - Coronal (Fig. 3) and axial views should be used to accurately measure displacement (stepoff and gap) of the distal tibial articular surface.

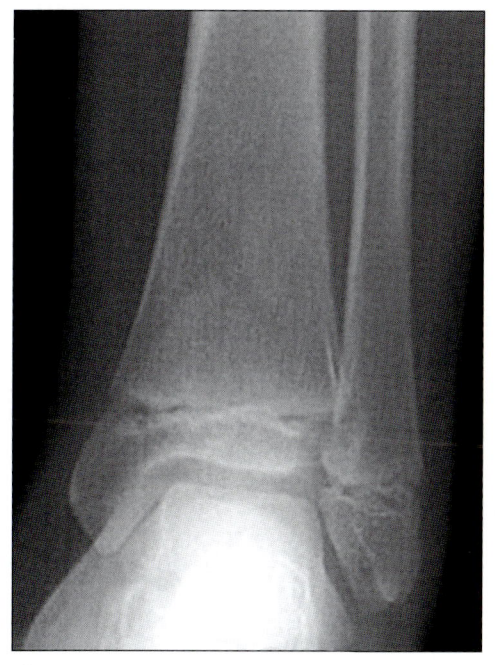

A

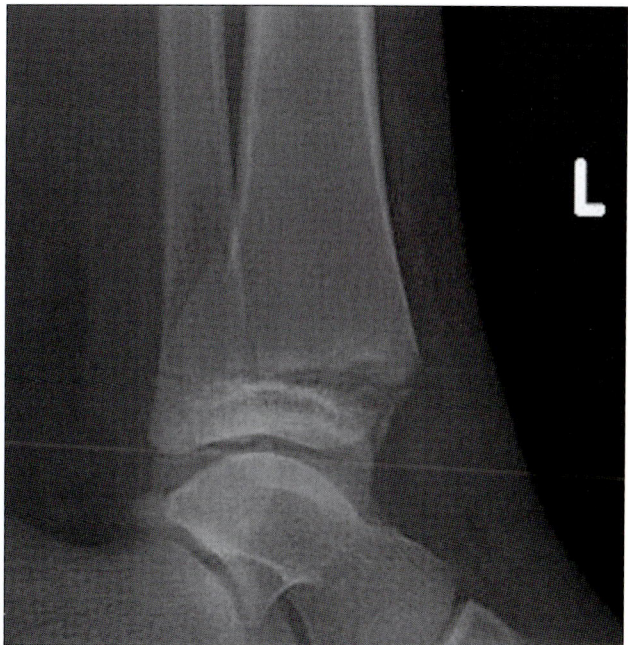

B

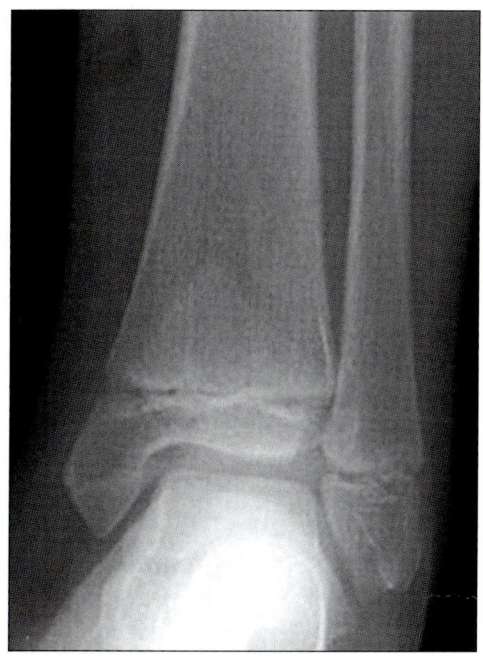

C
FIGURE 2

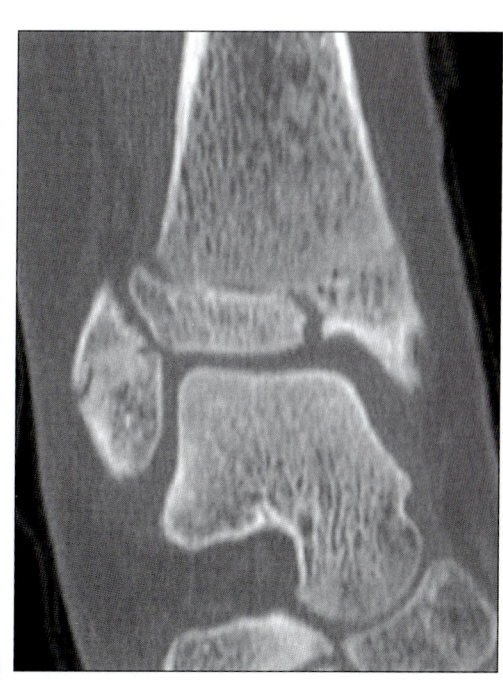

FIGURE 3

- Furthermore, coronal, axial, and sagittal CT views enable the surgeon to preoperatively plan the placement of internal fixation (i.e., screw trajectory) based on the fracture pattern, thus allowing for limited exposure of the fracture fragments. Figure 4 illustrates the use of axial CT images in surgical planning of screw placement at the epiphyseal (Fig. 4A) and metaphyseal (Fig. 4B) levels.

SURGICAL ANATOMY

- The neurovascular bundle, consisting of the anterior tibial artery and the deep peroneal nerve, traverses the ankle joint dorsal to the extensor hallucis longus (EHL) tendon.
- Proximal to the ankle joint, the neurovascular bundle lies between the anterior tibialis and EHL tendons (Fig. 5).

POSITIONING

- The patient is placed in the supine position on a radiolucent operating table with a bump under the ipsilateral hip to internally rotate the limb and permit easy medial and lateral access to the ankle (Fig. 6).
- A nonsterile tourniquet is placed around the ipsilateral thigh.

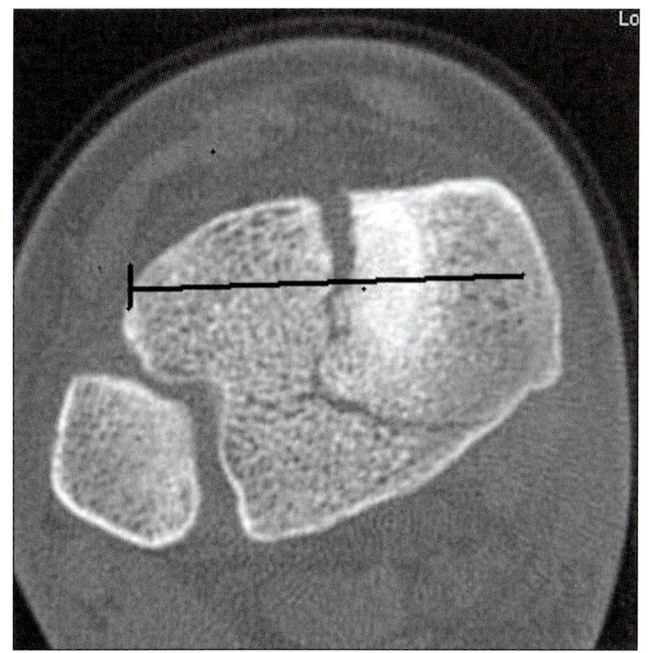

A

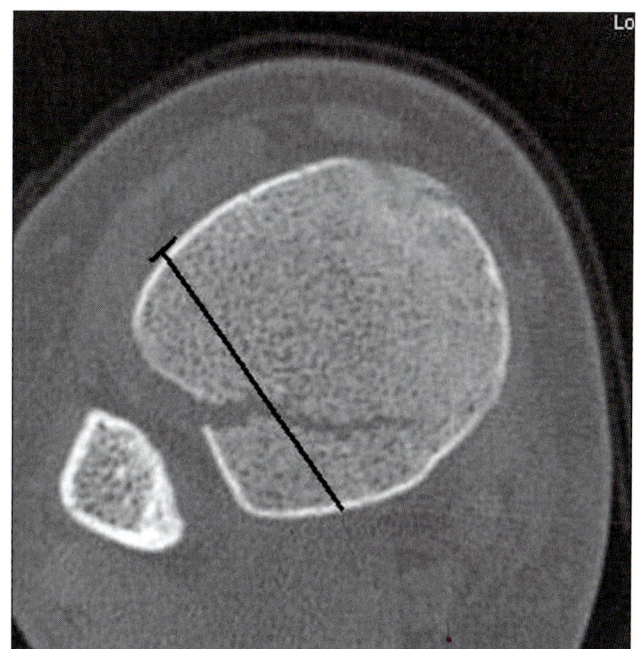

B

FIGURE 4

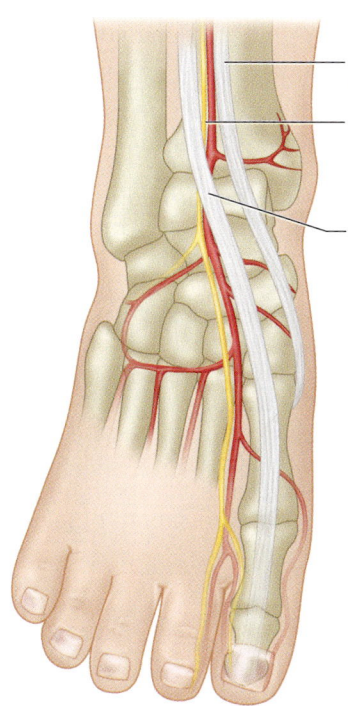

Tibialis anterior
tendon

Anterior tibial
artery and
deep peroneal
nerve

Extensor hallucis
longus tendon

FIGURE 5

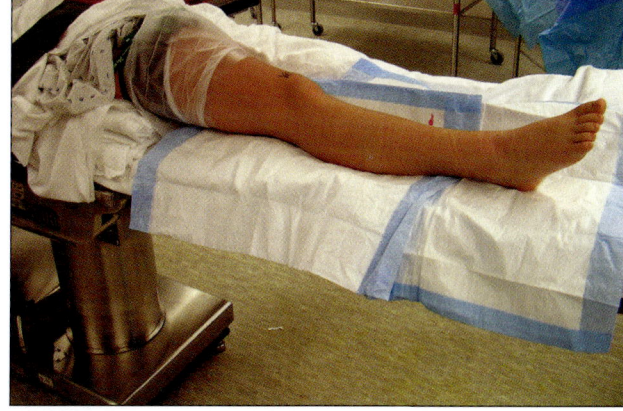

FIGURE 6

Instrumentation/ Implantation

• Large bone reduction forceps

PORTALS/EXPOSURES

■ Anterior exposure is accomplished by dissection lateral to the long toe extensors (Fig. 7).
■ This approach facilitates epiphyseal screw placement from anterolateral to posteromedial and permits visualization of the intra-articular fracture line and the joint surface.

PROCEDURE

STEP 1

■ The intra-articular epiphyseal fracture line is examined.
  • The intraoperative photograph in Figure 8 demonstrates the vertical epiphyseal fracture line (*blue arrow*) and the transverse physeal fracture line (*green arrow*).
■ Interposed periosteum and soft tissues should be removed from the fracture site; however, the surrounding periosteum should not be disturbed.

STEP 2

■ The anterolateral epiphyseal fracture fragment is reduced to the remainder of the epiphysis.
■ Internal rotation of the foot and ankle allows for indirect reduction of the fracture.
■ A large bone reduction forceps is placed directly onto the anteromedial epiphyseal fragment, with the other tine placed percutaneously onto the medial malleolus, to directly reduce the fracture to anatomic position.
  • In Figure 9, the lateral tine of the bone reduction forceps is in the epiphyseal fragment through the incision and the medial tine is percutaneously placed onto the medial malleolus.

STEP 3

■ A small threaded guidewire is placed obliquely through the anterolateral epiphyseal fragment to secure the fragment to the remainder of the epiphysis.
  • Correct orientation of the wire is confirmed using fluoroscopy; the oblique radiograph in Figure 10 shows the bone reduction forceps in place and epiphyseal screw guidewire placement.
  • A partially threaded, cannulated cancellous screw is then placed over the guidewire.
■ Fixation of the anterolateral epiphyseal fragment converts the fracture to a Salter-Harris type II fracture.
■ Since these injuries occur in late adolescence, at the time of physiologic closure of the distal tibial physis, angular deformities rarely develop secondary to physeal arrest. Therefore, screws can be placed across the physis if this is necessary to obtain fixation.

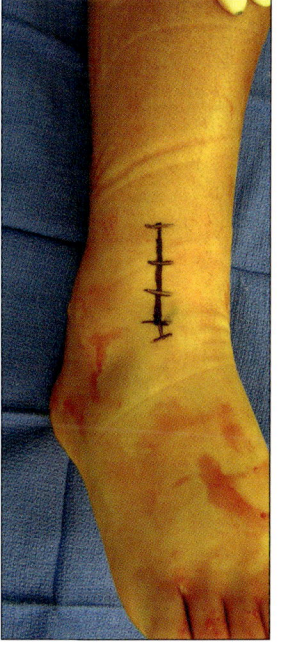

FIGURE 7

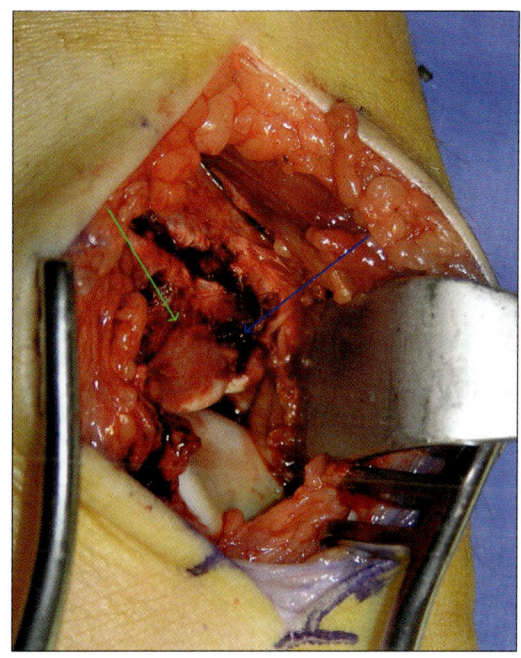

FIGURE 8

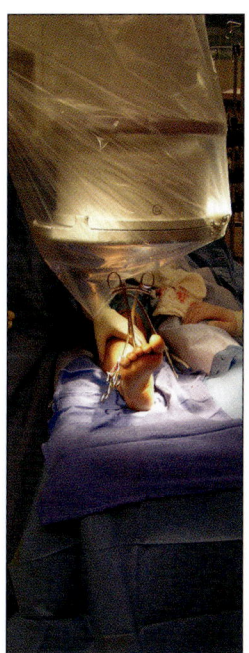

FIGURE 9

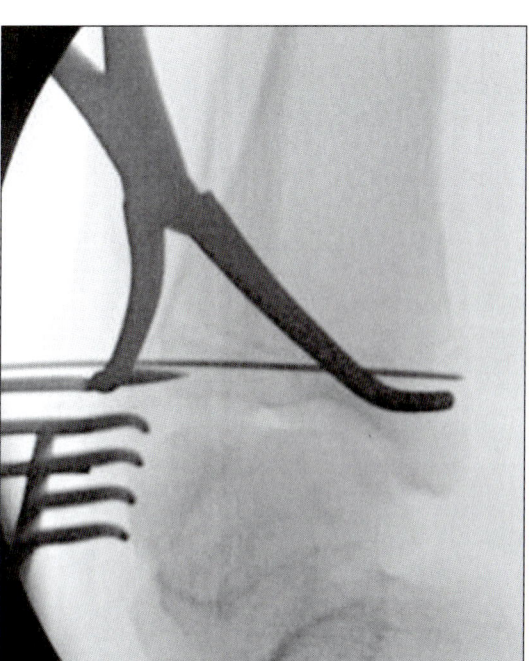

FIGURE 10

Instrumentation/Implantation

- 4.0- or 4.5-mm cancellous screws

Controversies

- Anatomic reduction of the articular surface is paramount. The use of ankle arthroscopy to evaluate articular congruity after reduction and fixation of the fracture has been described. However, limited exposure of the fracture site as described above allows for direct examination of the joint surface without the need for an additional surgical procedure.

PEARLS

- *Fixation of concomitant fibular fractures is infrequently necessary.*

PEARLS

- *Screw trajectory can be optimized by preoperative CT scan analysis of fracture configuration. These images should be available in the operating room.*

- *Alternatively, the screw can be placed from posteromedial to anterolateral.*

PITFALLS

- *Fracture fixation can be negatively impacted if the precise fracture configuration is not appreciated by placing screws into the fracture line or in an area of suboptimal bone quality.*

- *Failure to use partially threaded screws or fully threaded screws in a lag fashion will prevent optimal intra-articular fracture compression and correction.*

STEP 4

- Reduction and fixation of the posterior/posteromedial metaphyseal-epiphyseal fragment to the tibial metaphysis is performed.
  - The intraoperative radiograph in Figure 11 demonstrates epiphyseal screw position and metaphyseal screw guidewire position.
- Dorsiflexion, internal rotation, and distal traction aid in reduction of the fracture.
- A partially threaded, cannulated 4.0- or 4.5-mm cancellous screw placed from anterior to posterior secures the metaphyseal fragment.
  - Figure 12 shows intraoperative AP (Fig. 12A), mortise (Fig. 12B), and lateral (Fig. 12C) radiographs after fixation of a fracture with two screws.

POSTOPERATIVE CARE AND EXPECTED OUTCOMES

- Patients are placed into short-leg non–weight-bearing casts postoperatively for 6 weeks.

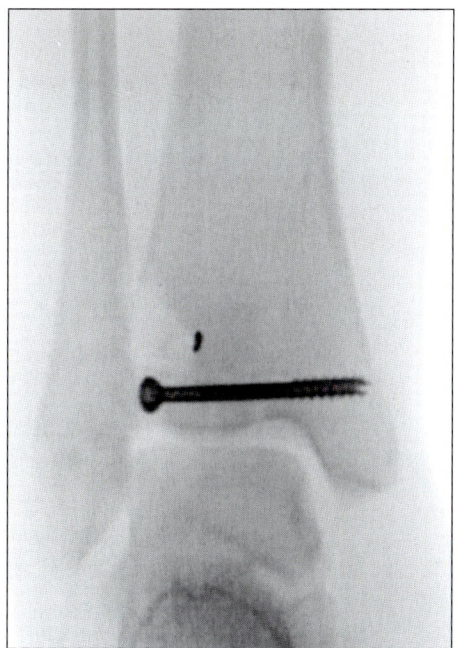

FIGURE 11

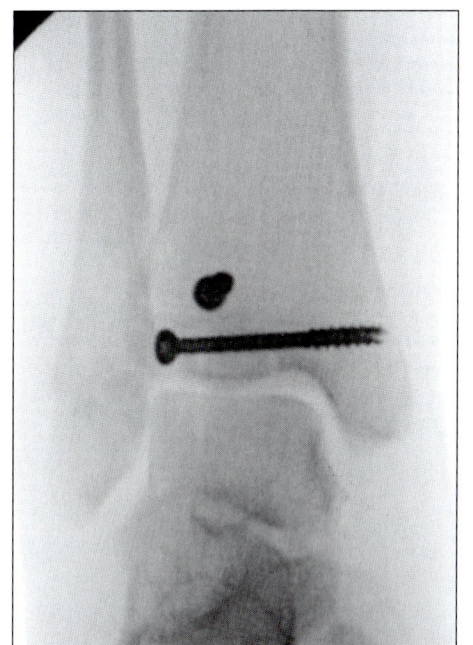

A

FIGURE 12

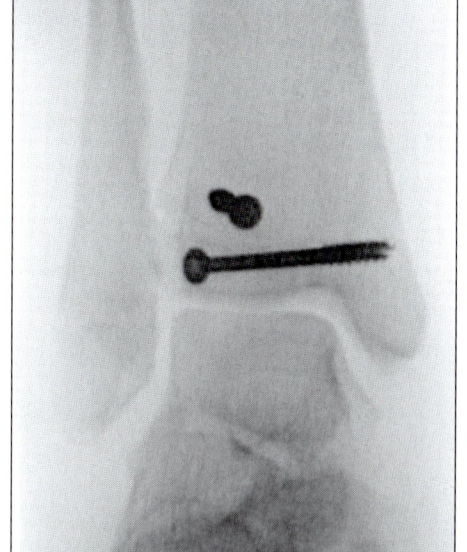

B

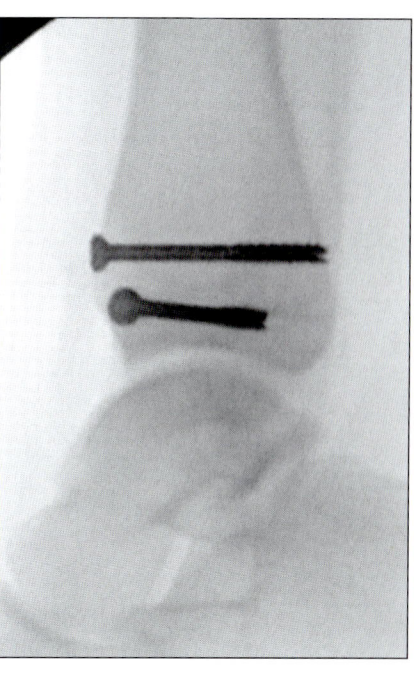

C

EVIDENCE

Ertl JP, Barrack RL, Alexander AH, VanBuecken K. Triplane fractures of the distal tibial epiphysis: long-term follow-up. J Bone Joint Surg [Am]. 1988;70:967–76.

In this retrospective review of 23 patients with triplane fractures, the authors noted that plain radiographs alone did not accurately demonstrate the configuration of the fracture. Twenty patients were asymptomatic when they were evaluated 18–36 months after the injury, but only 8 of 15 patients were asymptomatic when they were evaluated 38 months to 13 years after the fracture. Residual displacement of 2 mm or more after reduction was associated with a less than optimum result unless the epiphyseal fracture was outside the primary weight-bearing area of the ankle.

Feldman DS, Otsuka NY, Hedden DM. Extra-articular triplane fractures of the distal tibial epiphysis. J Pediatr Orthop. 1995;15:479–81.

The authors described the extra-articular intramalleolar fracture pattern. Based on the nature of the fracture, nonoperative management was recommended since anatomic reduction is unnecessary.

Imade S, Takao M, Nishi H, Uchio Y. Arthroscopy-assisted reduction and percutaneous fixation for triplane fracture of the distal tibia. Arthroscopy. 2004;20:e123–8.

In this case report of a 14-year-old male with a displaced (5-mm) triplane fracture, the authors treated the patient with a closed reduction and percutaneously placed cannulated, cancellous screw. Concomitant ankle arthroscopy was performed to view the articular surface. A "second-look" arthroscopy performed 1 year after surgery demonstrated joint congruity.

McGillion S, Jackson M, Lahoti O. Arthroscopically assisted percutaneous fixation of tri-plane fracture of the distal tibia. J Pediatr Orthop B. 2007;16:313–6.

In this case series, four patients with triplane fractures were treated with closed reduction and percutaneous screw placement with concomitant ankle arthroscopy. The authors described the use of ankle arthroscopy to ensure anatomic reduction with minimal soft tissue disruption. All four patients regained full ankle range of motion within 6 weeks of surgery.

Rapariz JM, Ocete G, Gonzalez-Herranz P, Lopez-Mondejar JA, Domenech J, Burgos J, Amaya S. Sistal tibial triplane fractures: long-term follow-up. J Pediatr Orthop. 1996;16:113–8.

In this retrospective review of 35 patients treated for triplane fractures, the authors recommended the use of CT to accurately assess fracture configuration and the amount of displacement. Degenerative changes were seen at long-term follow-up (>5 years) in patients with 2-mm or more displacement at the articular surface.

FOOT

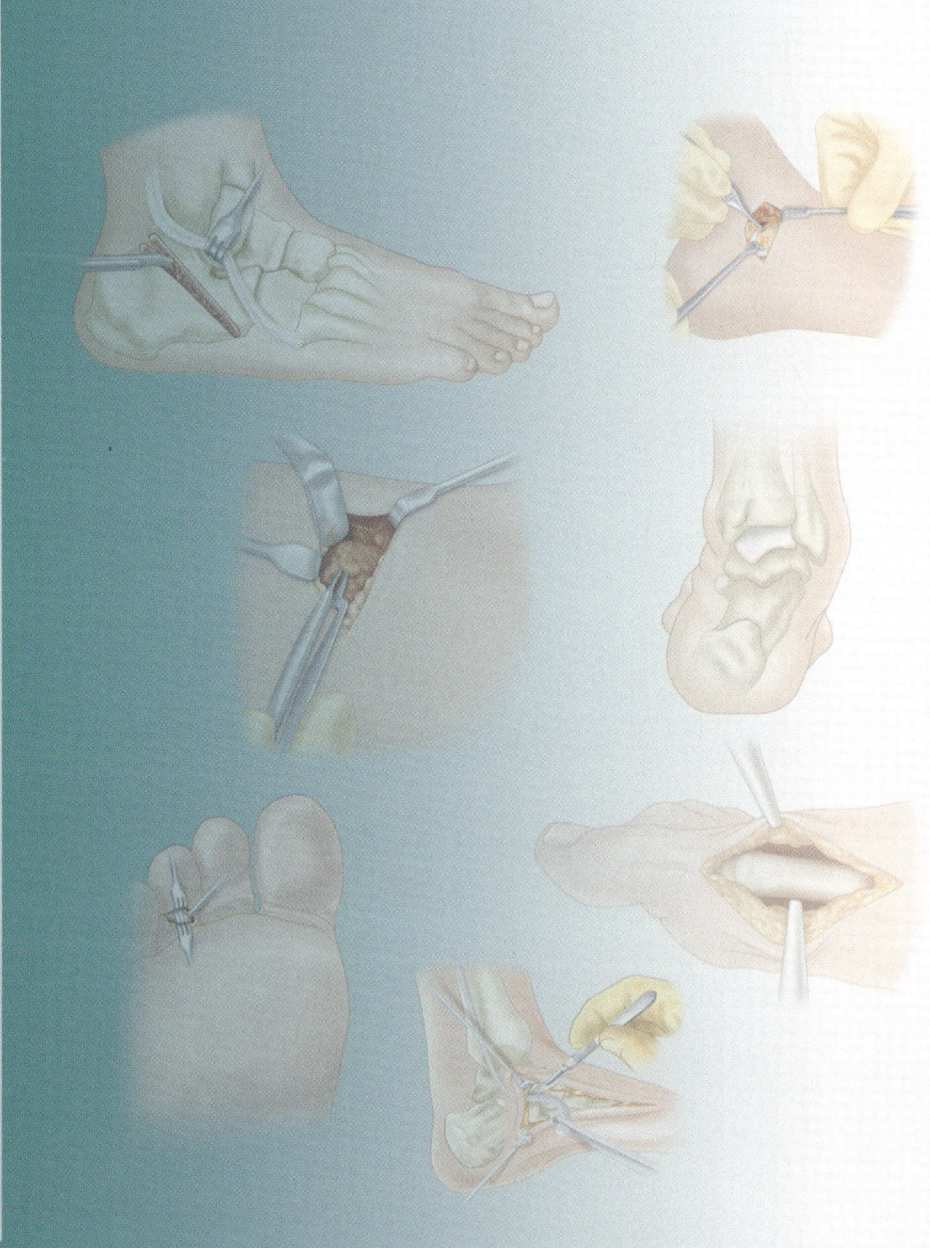

Ponseti Method for Idiopathic Clubfoot Deformity

Constantine A. Demetracopoulos and David M. Scher

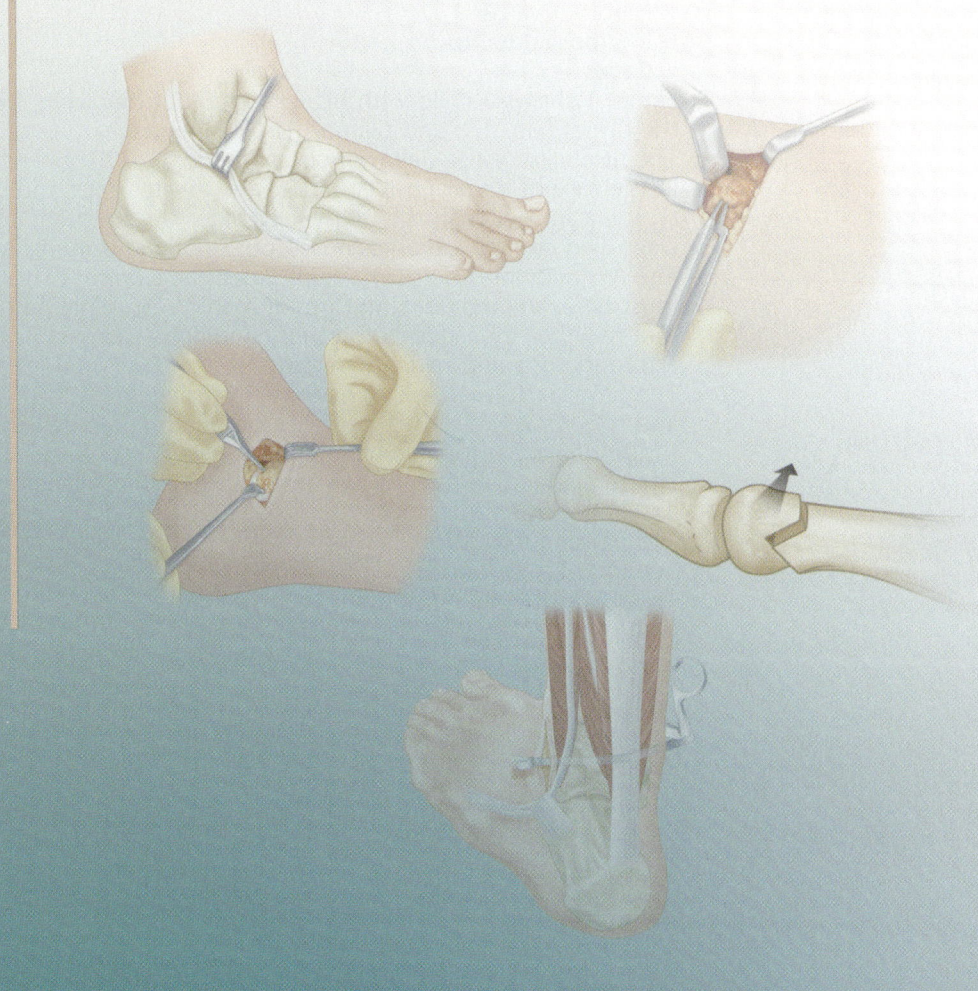

Controversies

• The French physiotherapy method has also been shown to be an effective treatment for idiopathic clubfeet.

Treatment Options

• Initial treatment of a congenital clubfoot deformity is nonoperative regardless of the severity of the deformity.

• Although various forms of serial manipulation and casting have been advocated for clubfoot, the Ponseti method has proven to be the most reproducible and effective method of deformity correction.

• The French physiotherapy method is based on a dynamic method of deformity correction. It relies on daily manipulations and brief periods of immobilization with adhesive taping.

• Early, aggressive surgical intervention consisting of posteromedial releases has resulted in overcorrection, stiffness, increased rates of recurrence, and poor long-term outcomes.

INDICATIONS

■ Nonoperative management is indicated in all patients with an idiopathic clubfoot.

■ Treatment is best initiated shortly after birth; however, the Ponseti technique has been shown to be successful in older infants and children. The upper age limit of this technique has not been defined.

■ The goal of treatment is a functional, plantigrade foot that is flexible, pain free, and without need for modified shoewear.

EXAMINATION/IMAGING

■ Examination of the foot will demonstrate four components to the deformity:
  • Equinus
  • Hindfoot varus
  • Midfoot adductus
  • Cavus

■ Figure 1 shows a child with bilateral clubfoot deformity from the dorsal (Fig. 1A) and plantar (Fig. 1B) views.

■ The flexibility of the deformity is assessed.

■ In the case of a unilateral clubfoot, the affected foot and calf are typically smaller than the uninvolved side.

■ Deep skin creases are often noted posteriorly and medially.

■ The flexibility of other joints (hips, knees and upper extremities) must be examined, looking for neurologic and spinal pathology that may be associated with other conditions such as arthrogryposis and myelomeningocele.

■ The physician should examine for active movement of the foot and toes to assess for the presence of a neurologic deficit, suggesting a neuropathic clubfoot.

■ The remainder of the lower extremity is assessed for deformities and limb-length discrepancies, which may be indicative of a limb reduction disorder, such as fibular hemimelia, tibial hemimelia, or a bowing deformity.

■ There is little role for imaging in the diagnosis of a clubfoot deformity.

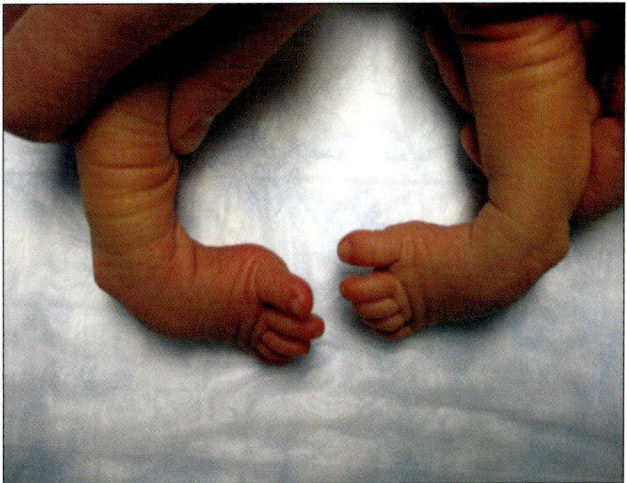

A

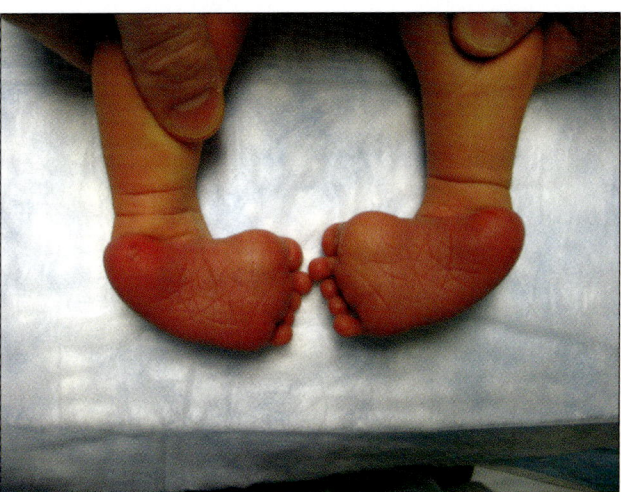

B
FIGURE 1

ANATOMY

- The navicular is subluxed medially and plantar to the head of the talus.
- There is decreased distance between the medial malleolous and the navicular, which can be detected by palpation on physical examination.
- The talar head is palpable laterally just distal and medial to the lateral malleolous.
- The first ray is plantar flexed.
- The forefoot is supinated relative to the floor, but pronated relative to the calcaneus, which is typically in more varus than the forefoot.

POSITIONING

- The patient is placed supine on an examination table.
- Manipulation and casting is best performed when the child is distracted or feeding.

PROCEDURE

STEP 1

- Manipulations must always be gentle and never painful.
- Approximately 1 minute is spent manipulating the foot.
- Five or six manipulations and long-leg casts are typically needed. They are performed at 5- to 7-day intervals.
- Figure 2 demonstrates the first manipulation in an anteroposterior (AP) (Fig. 2A) and lateral (Fig. 2B) view. The forefoot is supinated in line with the hindfoot, and the first ray is dorsiflexed.
- Cast #1
  - The forefoot is placed in supination in line with the hindfoot, and the first ray is dorsiflexed.
  - Cast padding is applied to cover the toes distally (Fig. 3A). A plaster cast is applied using a 2-inch plaster roll (Fig. 3B). Cast should be cut distally so that all five toes are visible (Fig. 3C).
  - This will correct the cavus deformity.

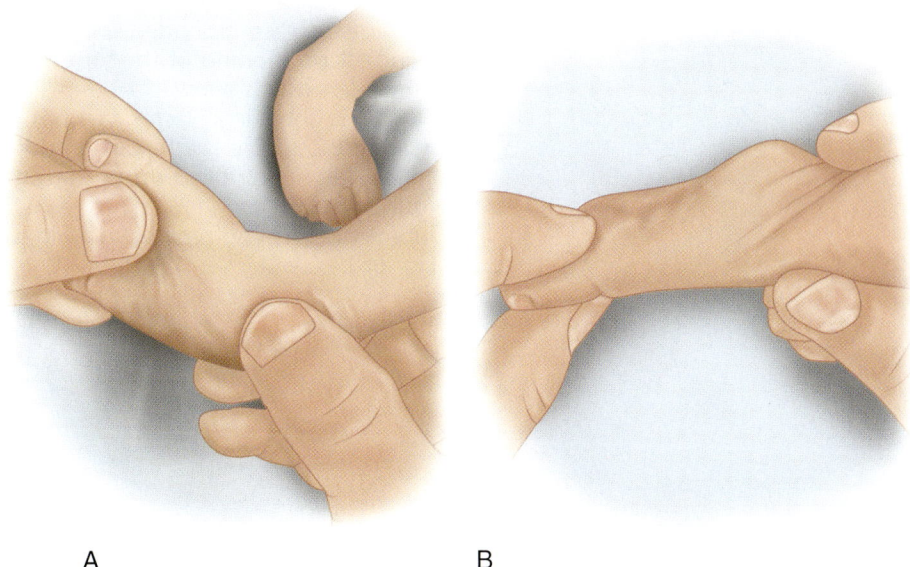

A   B

FIGURE 2

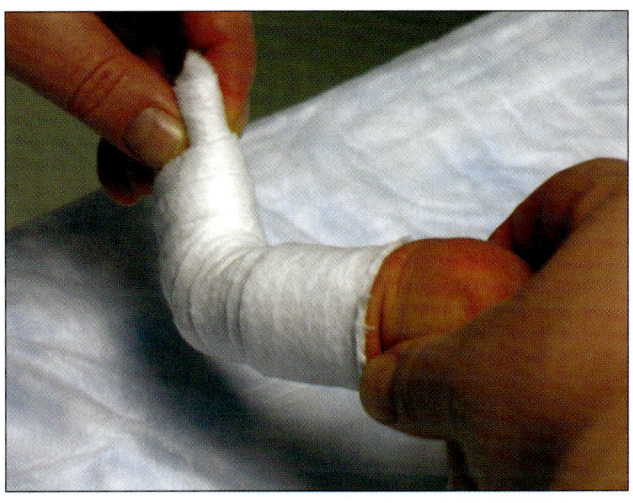

A

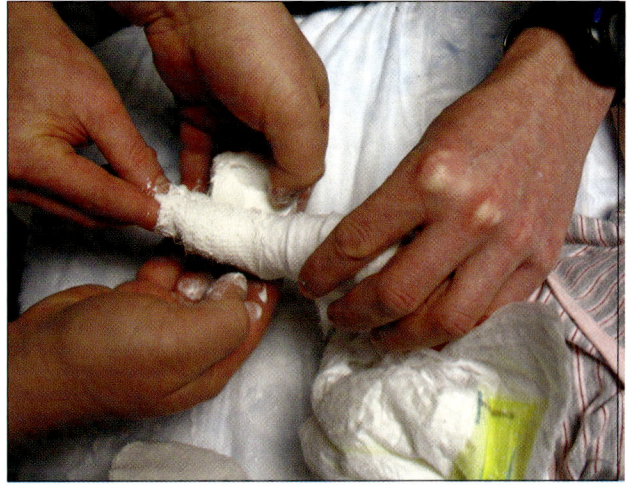

B

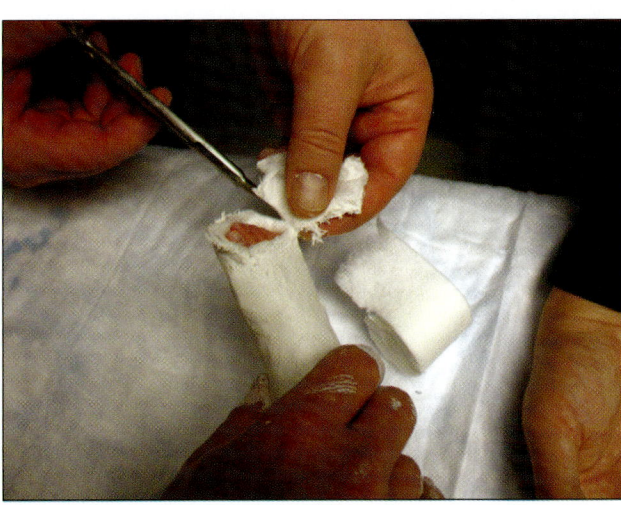

C

FIGURE 3

- A short-leg plaster cast is placed first, allowed to dry, and then extended up the thigh to create a long-leg cast. This technique is recommended for all subsequent casts.
  - Correct positioning of the foot is maintained while the short-leg cast is allowed to dry (Fig. 4).
  - One the short-leg plaster cast has hardened, the cast is extended up the thigh. Cast padding is applied first (Fig. 5A). Plaster is applied up to the proximal thigh (Fig. 5B).
- Figure 6 shows the first cast for a patient with bilateral clubfoot deformity from below (Fig. 6A) and from above (Fig. 6B).

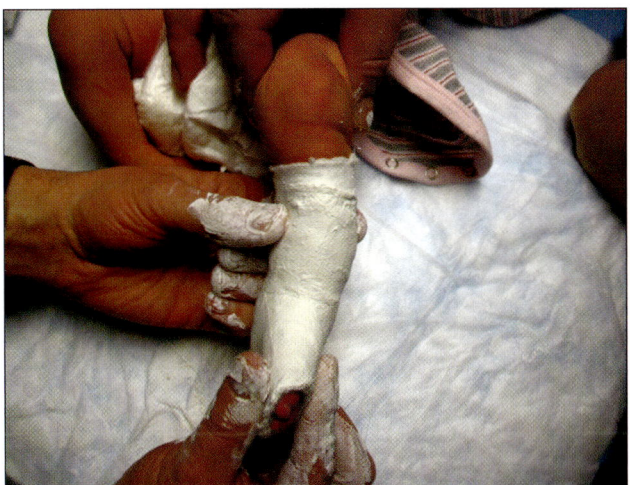

FIGURE 4

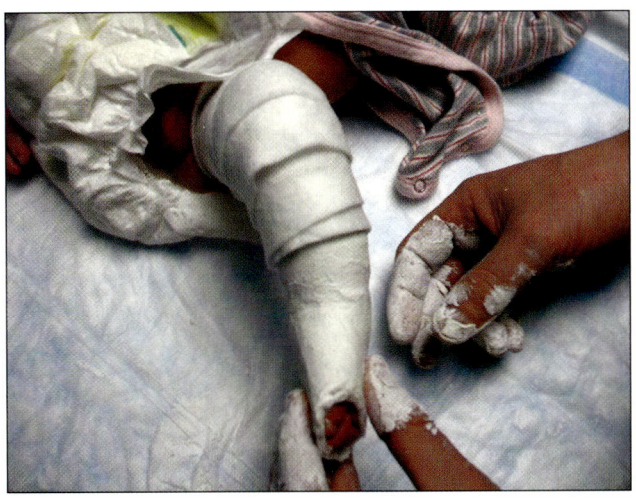

A

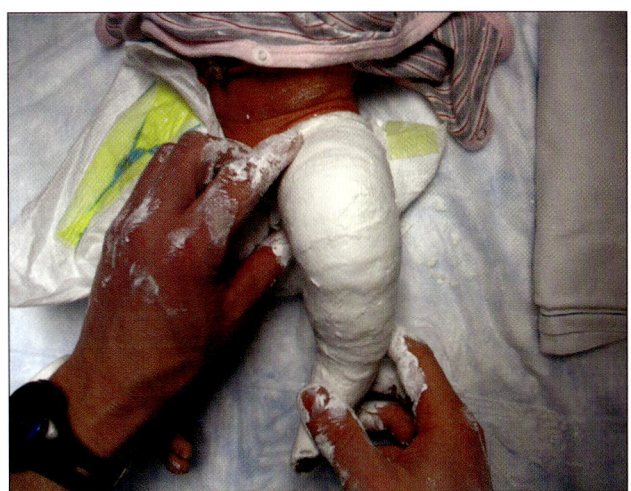

B

FIGURE 5

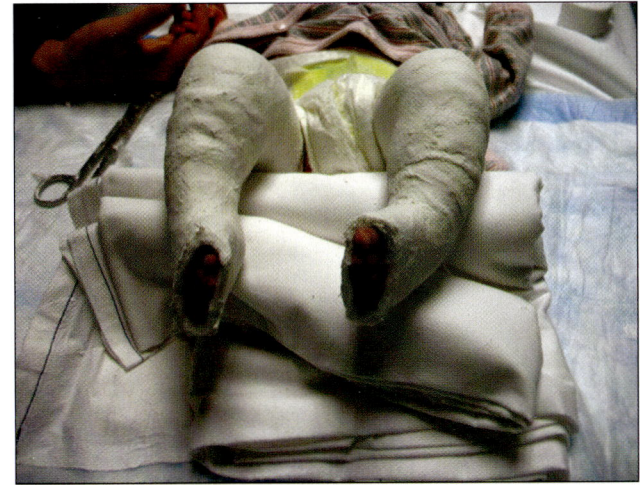

A

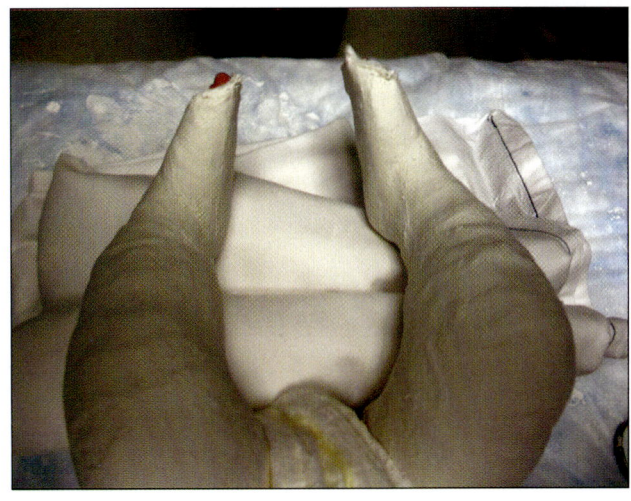

B

FIGURE 6

PEARLS

• *After the first cast is applied, make sure the forefoot is in line with the hindfoot and is neither pronated nor supinated during the manipulations and castings.*

PITFALLS

• *Do not apply counterpressure on the calcaneocuboid joint.*

• *The heel must not be manipulated. The talonavicular, calcaneocuboid, and talocalcaneal joints must be allowed to reduce simultaneously as the forefoot is abducted across the talus. This will bring the heel into valgus.*

STEP 2

■ With the cavus deformity corrected, the next few casts are placed so that the foot is gradually abducted around the head of the talus.

■ The foot is manipulated prior to placement of the second cast.
  • A thumb is placed laterally on the talar head. It will act as the fulcrum (Fig. 7A).
  • Gentle abduction force is transmitted under the head of the first metatarsal (Fig. 7B).
  • The final position is shown in Figure 7C.

■ Cast #2
  • The foot is simultaneously abducted across the Lisfranc line, the naviculocuneiform joints, the Chopart line, and the subtalar joint.
  • Figure 8 shows the maintenance of gentle abduction force while the second short-leg cast is allowed to harden. Thumb remains on the head of the talus.

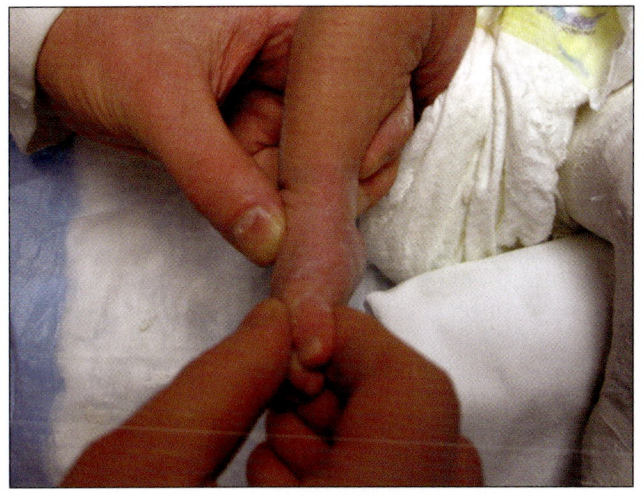

A

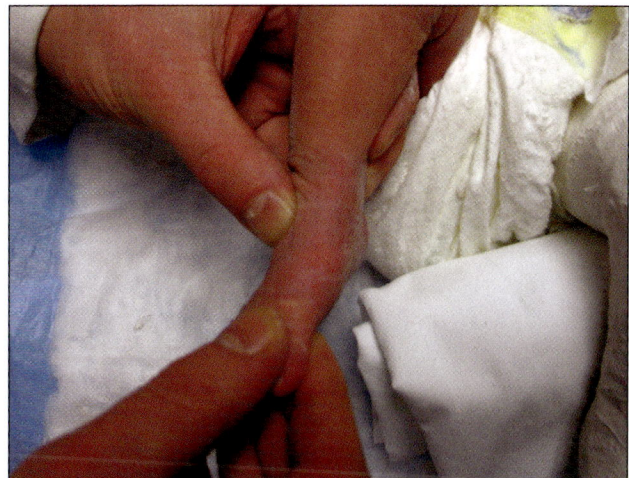

B

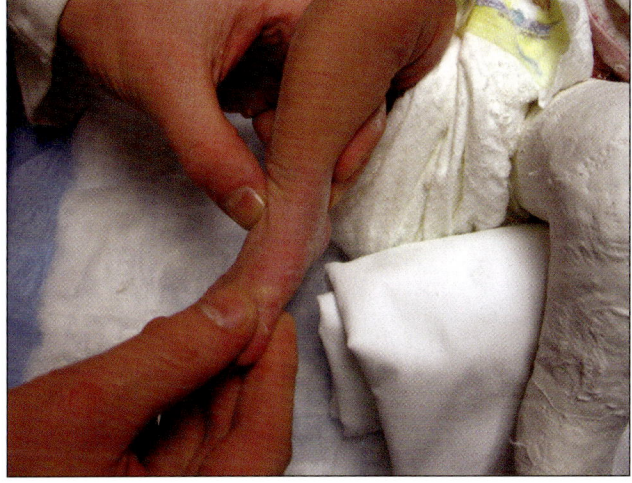

C

FIGURE 7

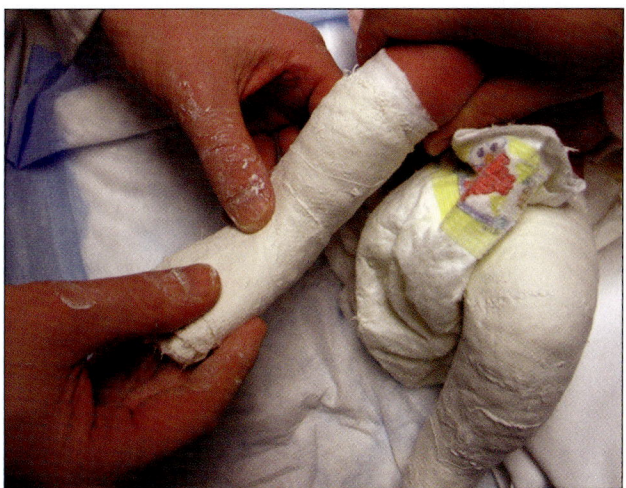

FIGURE 8

- Figure 9 shows final images of the second long-leg cast from AP (Fig. 9A) and lateral (Fig. 9B) views.
- A total of 70° of abduction is achieved at the end of these sets of casts.
- The foot remains in equinus.
- The heel will correct into valgus without being directly manipulated, following abduction of the forefoot.
  - Cast #3
    - The third cast is applied following approximately 1 minute of manipulation.
    - The same hand position is used for manipulation.
      - The thumb is placed on the talus, and the opposite hand grasps the first metatarsal (Fig. 10A).
      - The foot is maintained in equinus (Fig. 10B).
      - A gentle abduction force is applied to the first metatarsal (Fig. 10C).

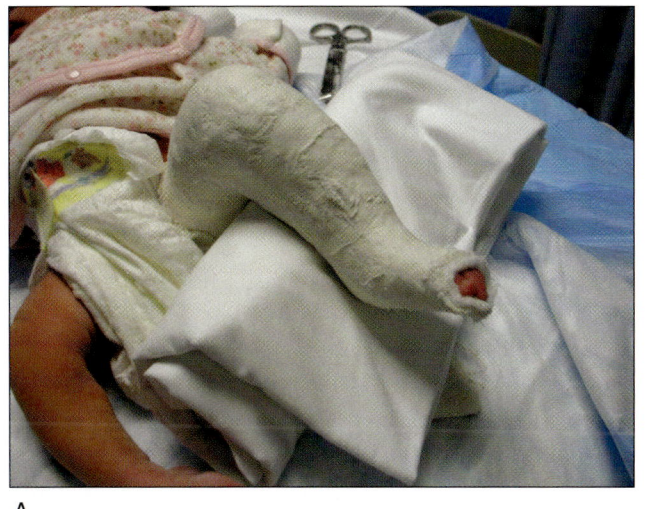

A

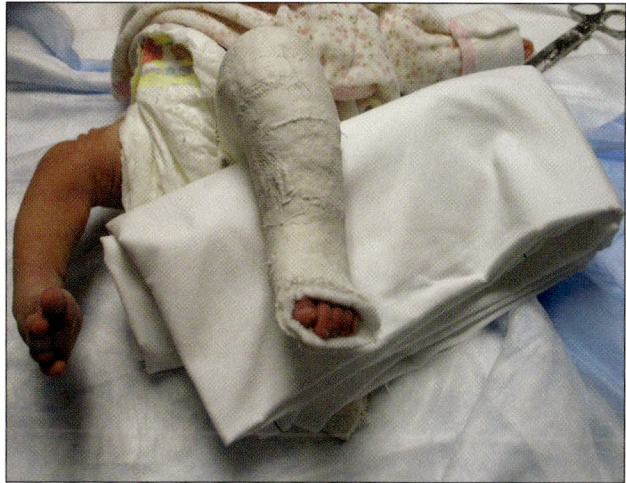

B

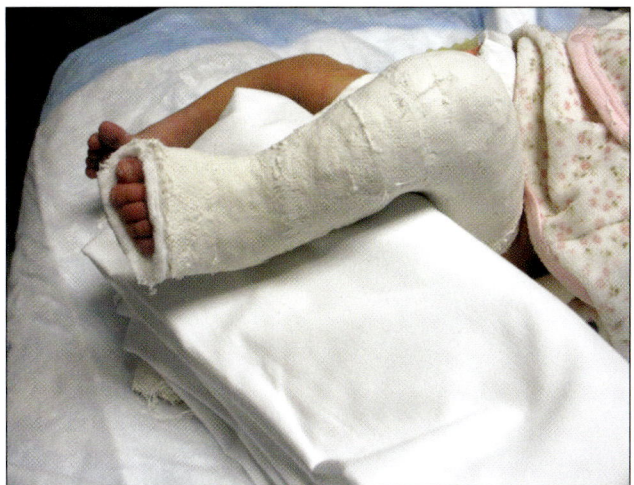

C

FIGURE 9

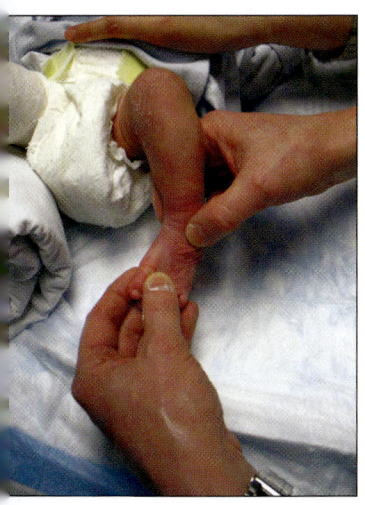

A

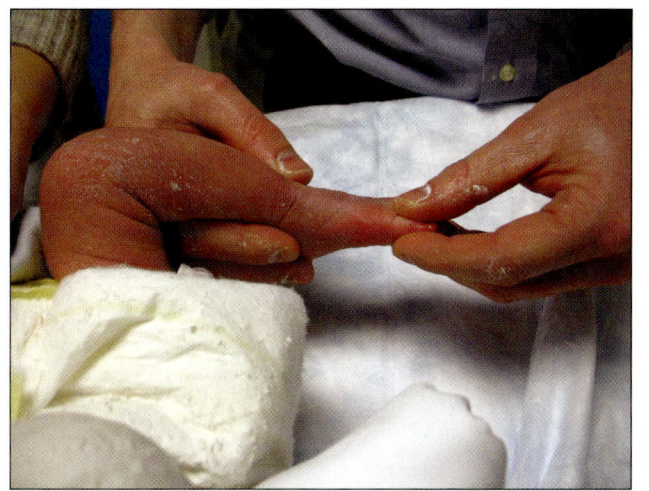

B

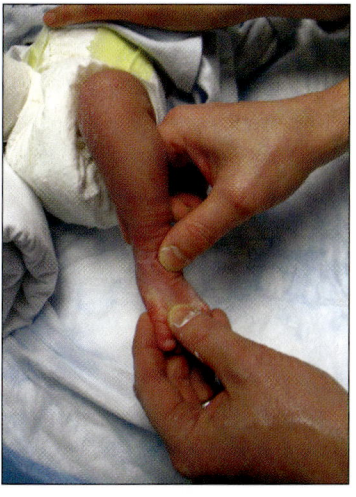

C

FIGURE 10

- Correct foot position is maintained while the cast padding is applied (Fig. 11A) and the short-leg cast is allowed to harden (Fig. 11B).
- Figure 12 shows final images of the third long-leg cast from AP (Fig. 12A), medial (Fig. 12B), and lateral (Fig. 12C) views.

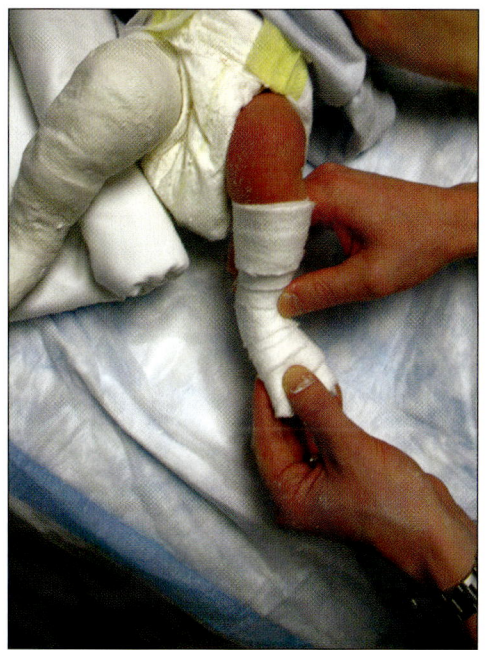

A

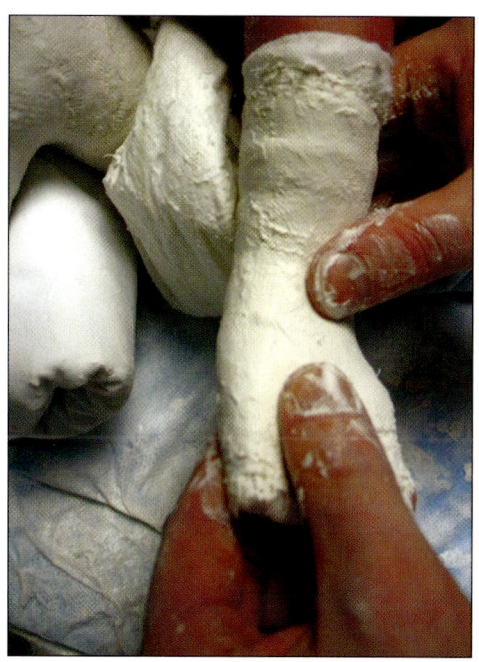

B

FIGURE 11

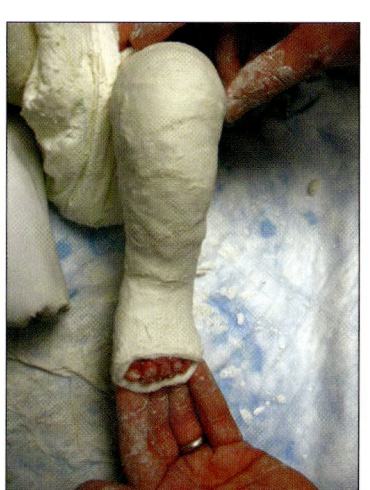

A

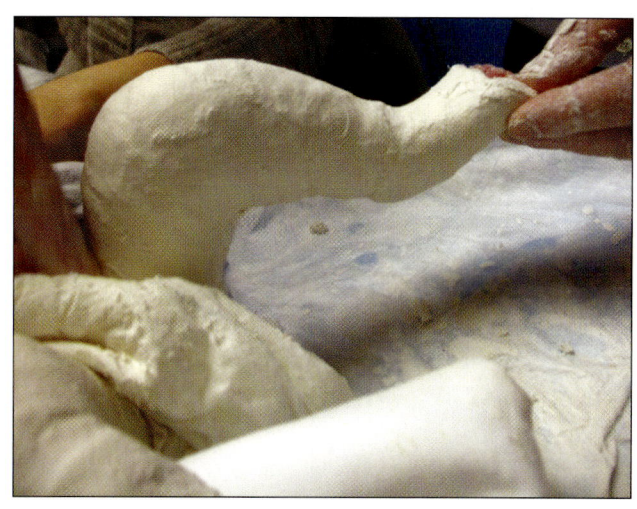

B

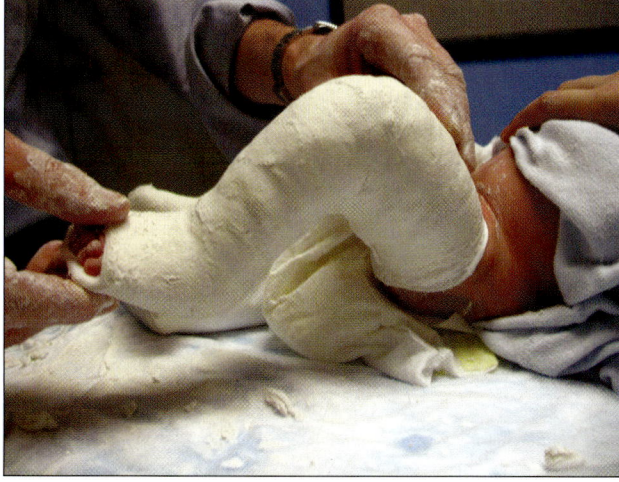

C

FIGURE 12

■ Cast #4
  • The foot is manipulated prior to application of the fourth cast.
    ◆ The thumb is placed on the talus, and the opposite hand grasps the first metatarsal (Fig. 13A).
    ◆ The final position is shown in Figure 13B.
  • Correct foot position for the fourth cast is maintained while the short-leg cast is allowed to harden (Fig. 14).
  • Figure 15 shows final images of the fourth cast for a patient with bilateral clubfoot deformity in the AP view (Fig. 15A) and from below (Fig. 15B).

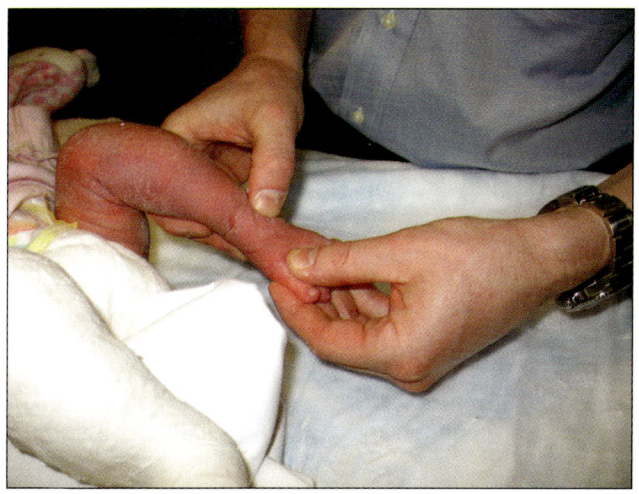

A

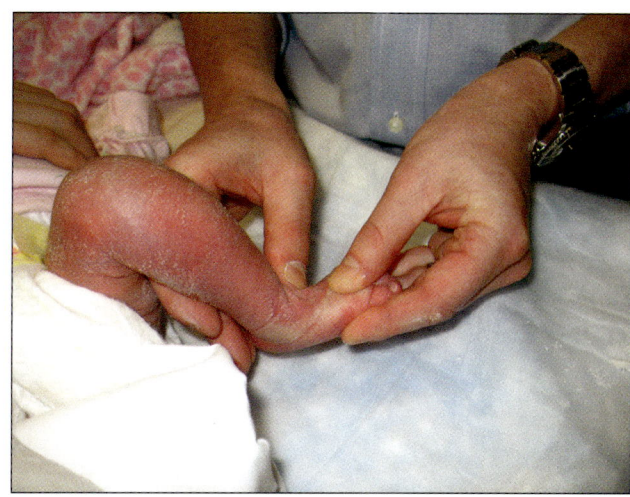

B

FIGURE 13

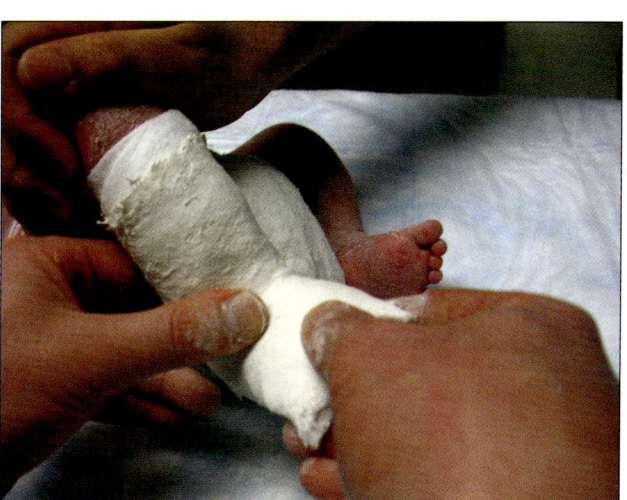

FIGURE 14

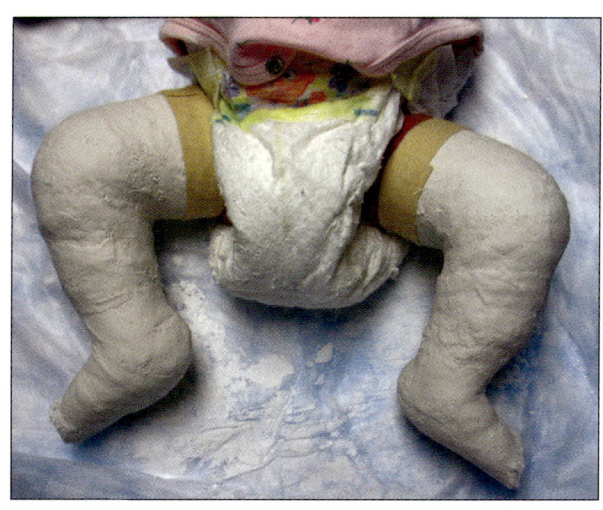

A

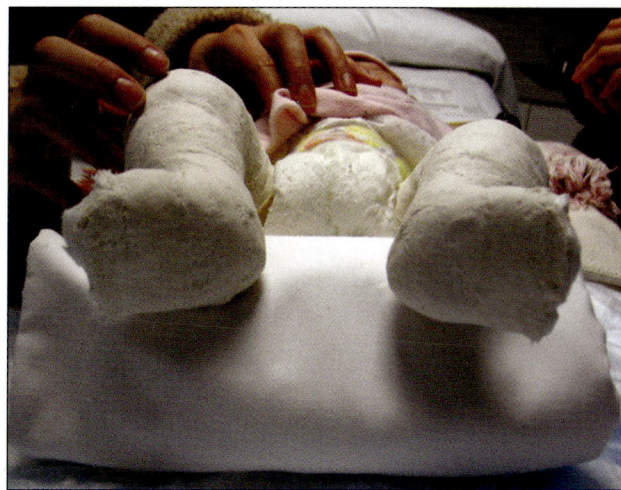

B

FIGURE 15

PEARLS

- *The tenotomy is best performed with the foot in dorsiflexion to place the Achilles tendon under tension.*

STEP 3

- Prior to the final cast, all elements of the clubfoot deformity have been corrected except the equinus. In Figure 16, dorsiflexion is limited to 0°.
- The final cast is intended to correct the equinus deformity. The foot is assessed for passive dorsiflexion. If less than 15–20° of dorsiflexion is achieved, an Achilles tenotomy is necessary.
- Percutaneous Achilles tenotomy
  - This procedure can be performed under local anesthesia in the office setting or under sedation in the operating room or sedation suite, depending on physician preference and institutional policies.
  - A small scalpel blade is recommended. Options include a cataract blade, a round-tipped beaver blade, or a standard #11 blade. Additional necessary equipment includes Betadine prep solution, 1% lidocaine, a tuberculin syringe with a 25-gauge needle, and 2 × 2 gauze pads (Fig. 17).
  - The posterior ankle is prepped with Betadine (Fig. 18).
  - Approximately 0.5 ml of 1% lidocaine is infiltrated into the subcutaneous tissue overlying the tendon (Fig. 19).
  - The tenotomy is performed approximately 1 cm above the insertion of the Achilles tendon.
  - The scalpel blade is inserted from the medial side of the Achilles tendon and positioned anterior (deep) to the tendon. The tendon is then transected by moving the blade in a posterior and lateral direction, away from the neurovascular bundle and through the tendon toward the skin. In this manner, the tendon is completely transected (Fig. 20).
  - Figure 21 shows the tenotomy incision.

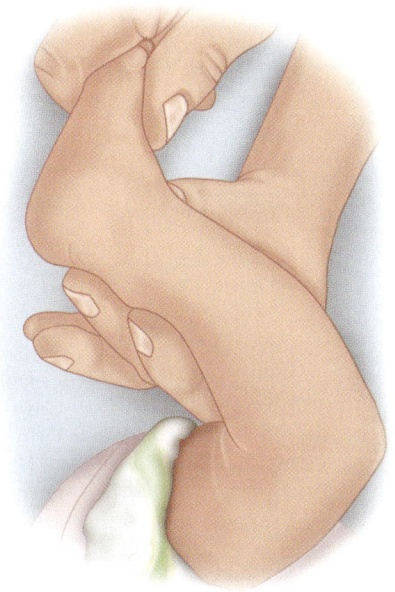

FIGURE 16

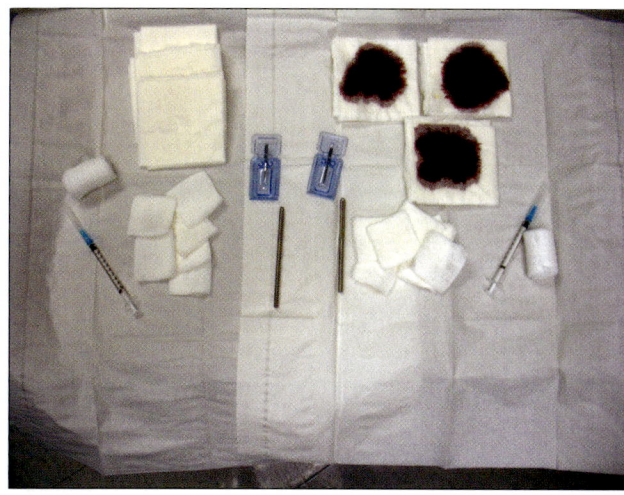

FIGURE 17

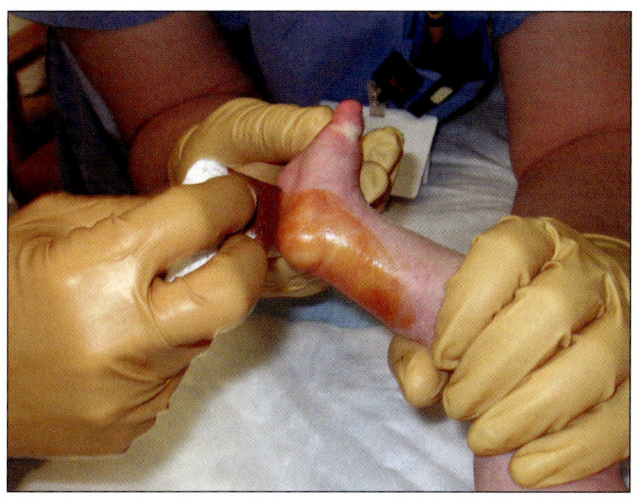

FIGURE 18

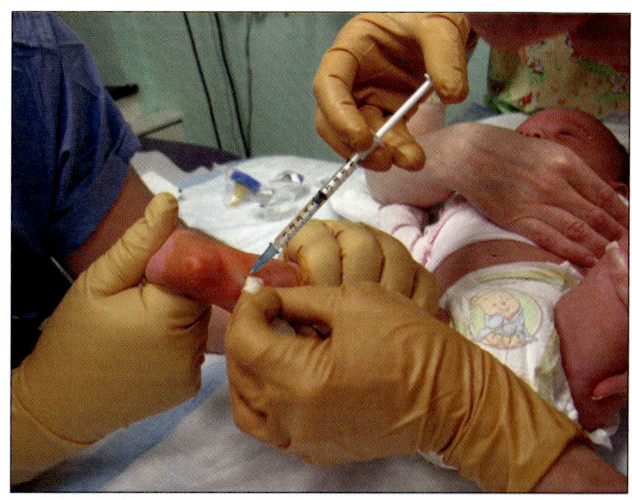

FIGURE 19

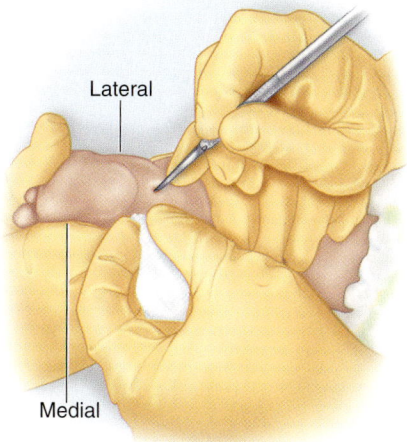

Lateral

Medial

FIGURE 20

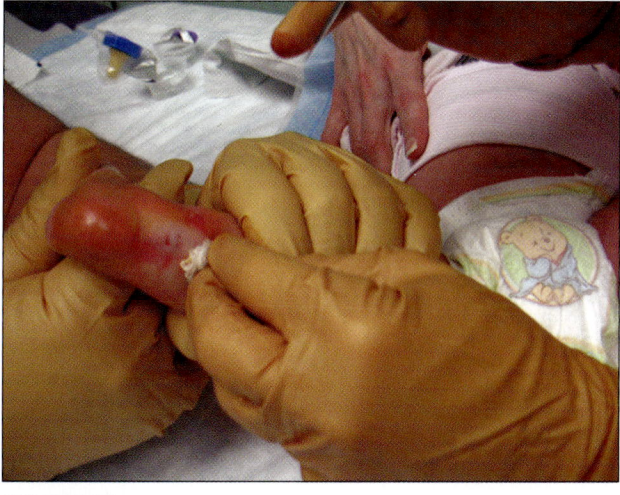

FIGURE 21

- Cast #5
  - The final cast is placed with the foot in 15–20° of dorsiflexion.
  - Figure 22 shows images of the final cast from the lateral side (Fig. 22A), the front (Fig. 22B), and the medial side (Fig. 22C).
  - This cast will remain for 3 weeks.

STEP 4

- Upon removal of the final cast, the patient is placed in a foot abduction orthosis.
  - The shoes are straight-laced and are attached to a bar set at a distance apart that is 1 inch greater than the width of the shoulders.
  - The shoes are dorsiflexed 10° and externally rotated 60–70°.
  - If the deformity is unilateral, the contralateral normal foot is placed in approximately 45° of external rotation.
- The brace is worn for 23 hours each day for the first 3 months. It is then worn at nighttime for several years.
- In a child treated shortly after birth, the deformity is corrected and the child is wearing the brace only while sleeping by approximately 5 months of age.
- Figure 23 demonstrates a patient wearing a foot abduction orthosis. Note that since this child has a right clubfoot only, the brace is set to 60° of external rotation on the right and 40° of external rotation on the left.

Complications

- Recurrence of deformity and need for an anterior tibial tendon transfer and/or repeat Achilles lengthening
- Bleeding complications associated with the percutaneous Achilles tenotomy
- Skin irritation associated with casting

POSTOPERATIVE CARE AND EXPECTED OUTCOMES

- The Ponseti method successfully corrects clubfoot deformity in greater than 90% of cases in all series.
- Eighty percent to 90% of patients will require a percutaneous Achilles tenotomy.
- Recurrence of deformity is most closely associated with intolerance of the foot abduction orthosis.
- In the event of a recurrence, additional manipulation and casting can be curative. The upper age limit for repeat casting has not been defined.
- In patients with appropriate treatment who tolerate the brace, the rate of surgical procedures for correction of the deformity is as low as 1–4%.

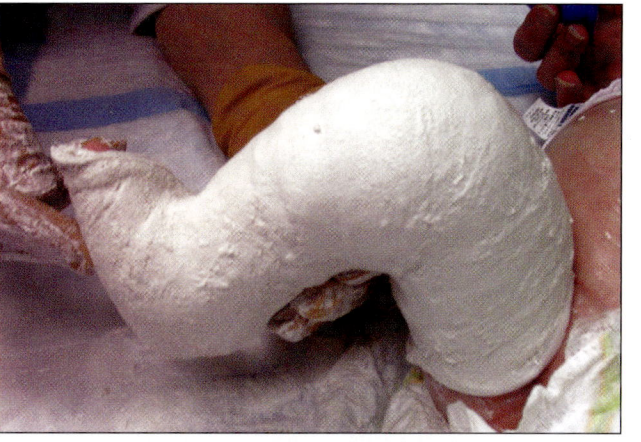

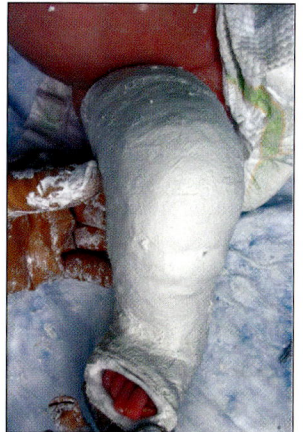

A

B

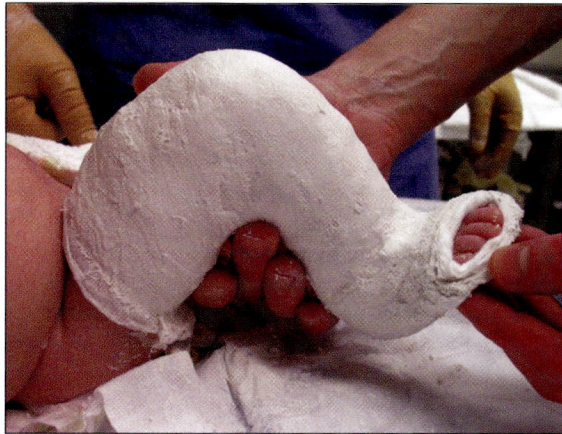

C

FIGURE 22

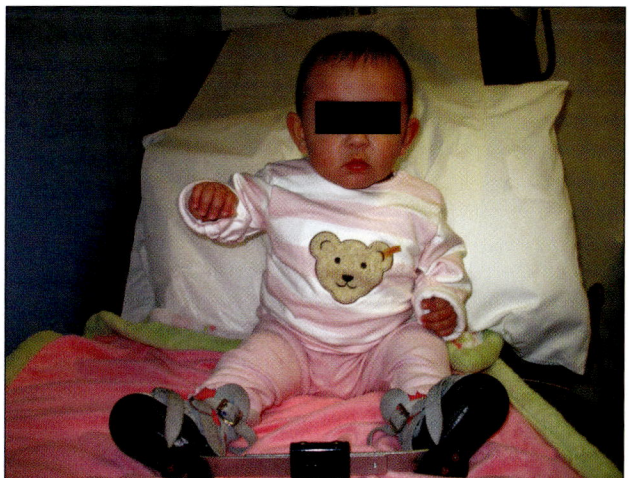

FIGURE 23

EVIDENCE

Alves C, Escalda C, Fernandes P, Tavares D, Neves MC. Ponseti method: does age at the beginning of treatment make a difference? Clin Orthop Relat Res. 2009;(467):1271–7.

In this retrospective review, 68 children with 102 idiopathic clubfeet were treated by the Ponseti method. Children were separated into two groups based on age at the onset of treatment. Patients younger than 6 months and those older than 6 months demonstrated equal rates of initial correction (100%), rates of relapses (8%), need for posteriomedial release (0%), and need for a split tibialis anterior transfer (5%) at a minimum of 30 months' follow-up. (Level II evidence [prognostic study])

Cooper DM, Dietz FR. Treatment of idiopathic clubfoot: a thirty-year follow-up note. J Bone Joint Surg [Am]. 1995;77:1477–89.

The authors presented a retrospective review of 45 patients with 71 feet treated with the Ponseti method for a clubfoot deformity at 30 years' follow-up. Using pain and functional limitation as outcomes, 78% of patients demonstrated good to excellent results. A within-group analysis showed that sedentary occupation and normal body mass index were variables associated with better outcomes. (Level IV evidence)

Dobbs MB, Gordon JE, Walton T, Schoenecker PL. Bleeding complications following percutaneous tendoachilles tenotomy in the treatment of clubfoot deformity. J Pediatr Orthop. 2004;24:353–7.

In this retrospective review, 134 consecutive infants underwent treatment of clubfoot deformity by the Ponseti method. A percutaneous tenotomy was performed in 91% of the clubfeet treated. Four patients had significant bleeding complications following the procedure. Three of those patients were presumed to have an injury to the peroneal artery, and one patient was presumed to have an injury to the lesser saphenous vein. (Level IV evidence)

Dobbs MB, Rudzki JR, Purcell DB, Walton T, Porter KR, Gurnett CA. Factors predictive of outcome after use of the Ponseti method for the treatment of idiopathic clubfeet. J Bone Joint Surg [Am]. 2004;86:22–7.

In this retrospective review, 51 consecutive patients were treated with the Ponseti method for clubfoot deformity. The parents of 21 patients were noncompliant with the use of orthotics, and this factor was most closely associated with recurrence of the deformity. Parental educational level was also associated with recurrence. The severity of the deformity, age of the patient, and parental income were not associated with recurrence of the deformity. (Level II evidence [prognostic study])

Laaveg SJ, Ponseti IV. Long-term results of treatment of congenital club foot. J Bone Joint Surg [Am]. 1980;62:23–31.

The authors presented a retrospective review of 70 patients with 104 clubfeet who were treated with the Ponseti method. At 10- to 27-year follow-up, all patients with unilateral clubfoot deformity demonstrated a corrected foot that was smaller and narrower, and the circumference of the leg on the normal side was larger. Limb lengths were equal. Fifty-three percent of the feet demonstrated no relapse and 47% had at least one recurrence. The rating of function was significantly greater in patients who did not require a split tibialis anterior transfer compared to those who did. Overall, 88.5% of feet had satisfactory functional results and 90% of patients were satisfied with both the appearance and function of the foot. (Level IV evidence)

Morcuende JA, Abbasi D, Dolan LA, Ponseti IV. Results of an accelerated Ponseti protocol for clubfoot. J Pediatr Orthop. 2005;25:623–6.

In this retrospective review of 230 patients with 319 clubfeet treated with the Ponseti method, patients were separated into two groups at the onset of treatment based on geographic considerations. Patients were assigned to either 5 or 7 days between manipulations and cast changes. Ninety percent of patients required five or fewer casts, and there was no difference between the two groups. There was also no difference between the two groups in the rate of Achilles tenotomy or additional surgery for correction of the deformity. Average time from onset of treatment to Achilles tenotomy was 16 days in the 5-day group and 24 days in the 7-day group. Recurrence of deformity in compliant patients was equal in the two groups. Noncompliance was associated with an 8.5-fold increased rate of deformity recurrence. (Level III evidence)

Morcuende JA, Dolan LA, Dietz FR, Ponseti IV. Radical reduction in the rate of extensive corrective surgery for clubfoot using the Ponseti method. Pediatrics. 2004; 113:376–80.

In this retrospective review, 157 patients with 256 clubfeet were treated with the Ponseti method followed by a foot abduction brace. Deformity correction was achieved in 98% of patients, and 90% of those patients required five or fewer casts. Four patients required an anterior tibial tendon transfer, and four other patients required extensive posteromedial releases. Eleven percent of patients had recurrence of the deformity. This was most closely associated with compliant use of the foot abduction brace. (Level IV evidence)

Richards BS, Faulks S, Rathjen KE, Karol LA, Johnston CE, Jones SA. A comparison of two non-operative methods of idiopathic clubfoot correction: the Ponseti method and the French functional (physiotherapy) method. J Bone Joint Surg [Am]. 2008;90: 2313–21.

The authors presented a prospective comparison of patients treated with the Ponseti method and the French functional method for clubfoot deformity. Patients with previously untreated clubfoot deformity under the age of 3 months were allowed to select their treatment after both options were explained to them. Patients were followed for a minimum of 2 years, and an average of 4.3 years. A good outcome was defined as a plantigrade foot with or without an Achilles tenotomy. Initial correction was achieved in 94.4% of patients treated with the Ponseti method, and 95% of patients treated with the physiotherapy method. Half of the patients who relapsed following the Ponseti method were salvaged nonoperatively. All patients who had recurrence of the deformity after the physiotherapy method required operative intervention. At final follow-up, 72% of patients treated with the Ponseti method and 67% of patients treated with the physiotherapy method had good results. This difference was not statistically significant. (Level II evidence)

Thacker MM, Scher DM, Sala DA, van Bosse HJ, Feldman DS, Lehman WB. Use of the foot abduction orthosis following Ponseti casts: is it essential? J Pediatr Orthop. 2005;25:225–8.

In this retrospective review, 30 consecutive patients with 44 idiopathic clubfeet were treated with the Ponseti method and placement in a foot abduction orthosis. Patients were separated into compliant and noncompliant groups based on parent history. Outcomes were assessed based on Dimeglio scores at the time of presentation, on initiation of treatment with the foot abduction orthosis, and at 6- and 9-month follow-up. At the time of application of the orthosis, there was no difference between the two groups. At final follow-up, the Dimeglio scores were significantly better in the compliant group compared to the noncompliant group. In addition, the compliant group demonstrated significant improvement in Dimeglio scores during treatment with the foot abduction orthosis. Noncompliant patients demonstrated worsening Dimeglio scores during attempted treatment with the foot abduction orthosis. (Level III evidence)

Resection of Talocalcaneal Tarsal Coalition and Fat Autograft Interposition

Constantine A. Demetracopoulos and David M. Scher

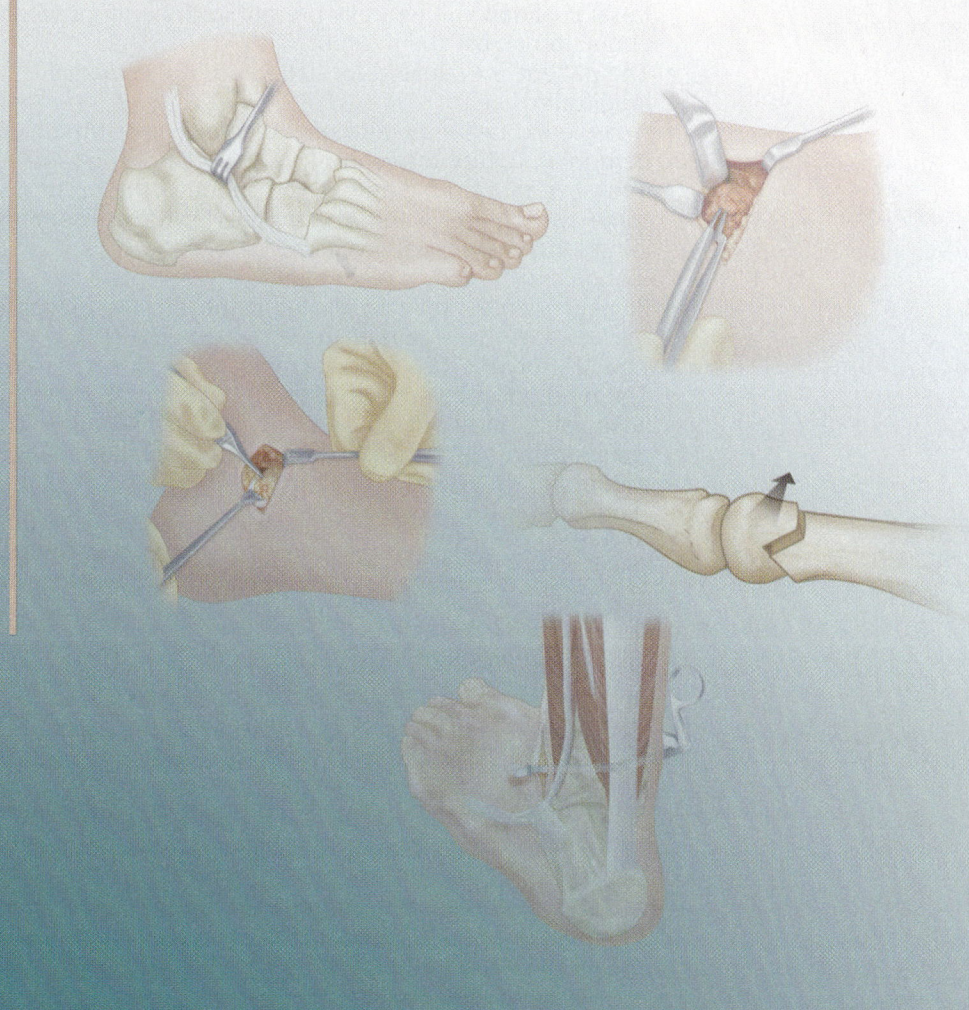

PITFALLS

- *Poor results are associated with resection of talocalcaneal coalitions that involve greater than 50% of the subtalar articular surface, and patient with severe hindfoot valgus.*
- *The presence of degenerative changes within the subtalar joint is a relative contraindication to resection of talocalcaneal coalitions.*

Treatment Options

- A trial of nonoperative treatment is indicated in all patients with a painful tarsal coalition. Nonoperative treatment includes activity modification, anti-inflammatory medication, and immobilization in a short-leg walking cast for 4–6 weeks.
- Asymptomatic coalitions do not require treatment.
- Interposition of a portion of the flexor hallucis longus tendon may substitute for fat autograft interposition in talocalcaneal coalitions.

INDICATIONS

- A persistently painful coalition that is not responsive to nonoperative treatments such as activity modification, anti-inflammatory medication, or immobilization in a short-leg walking cast for 4–6 weeks

EXAMINATION/IMAGING

- Gait
  - The patient is observed for an antalgic gait, characterized by a decreased stance phase on the affected extremity, and the position of the foot during stance phase is evaluated. Patients will often present with an out-toeing gait.
- Alignment
  - Hindfoot and midfoot alignment is examined. Patients with a tarsal coalition will typically present with hindfoot valgus and abduction across the midfoot.
  - The patient is evaluated for flattening of the medial longitudinal arch.
  - A single-leg heel rise will assess the flexibility of the flatfoot deformity. Failure to reconstitute the arch of the foot is indicative of a rigid hindfoot and suggests the presence of some abnormality within the subtalar or transverse tarsal joints, such as a tarsal coalition.
- Palpation
  - Point tenderness may be elicited plantar to the medial malleolus in the region of the sustentaculum tali.
- Range of motion
  - The hindfoot is inverted and everted while stabilizing the ankle joint, and compared to the contralateral side. Tarsal coalitions are associated with pain and limitation of subtalar motion.
- Radiographs
  - Anteroposterior (AP), lateral, and oblique views of the foot are obtained.
  - The lateral view of the foot (Fig. 1A) is evaluated for a continuous C-shaped line between the posterior aspect of the talar dome and the posterior facet of the subtalar joint (C-sign).
  - A Harris axial view may demonstrate a middle-facet talocalcaneal coalition (Fig. 1B), although commonly a computed tomography (CT) scan is necessary to adequately identify it.
  - Standing AP, lateral, and Saltzman hindfoot alignment views may be used to assess alignment. A Saltzman view can be useful to quantify hindfoot valgus.
- A CT scan is necessary to better visualize a suspected talocalcaneal coalition, and determine the portion of the subtalar joint that is involved (Fig. 2). The coronal images are the best for examining the subtalar joint.
- Magnetic resonance imaging may be helpful in cases in which the diagnosis is equivocal and a cartilaginous or fibrous coalition is present.

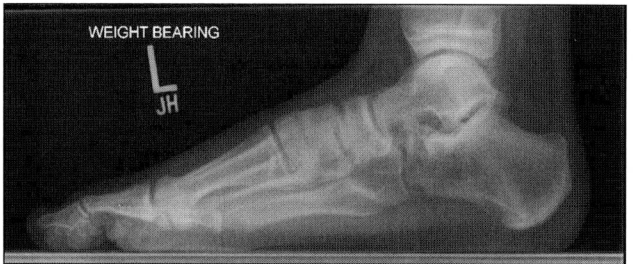 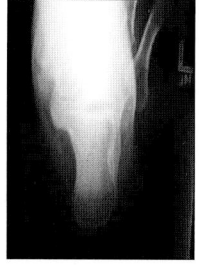

A

FIGURE 1

B

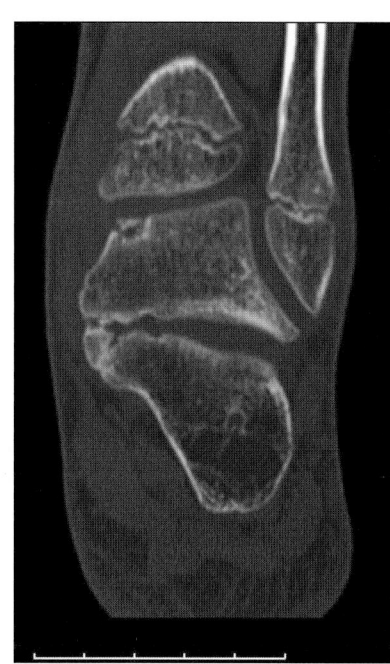

FIGURE 2

SURGICAL ANATOMY

- Coalitions may form as a result of failure of segmentation of the individual tarsal bones during fetal development.
- Talocalcaneal coalitions occur within the subtalar joint, commonly affecting the middle facet.
- The size of a talocalcaneal coalition is described with respect to the percentage of the subtalar joint that is coalesced.
- Coalitions may be osseous, cartilaginous, or fibrous.

POSITIONING

- The patient is placed supine on a radiolucent operating room table.
- The leg is allowed to assume an externally rotated position so that the medial aspect of the hindfoot is easily accessible.
  - A small bump may be placed on the contralateral hip to facilitate this position.
- A nonsterile tourniquet may be placed on the upper thigh.

PORTALS/EXPOSURES

- A horizontal incision is made along the medial aspect of the hindfoot centered over the sustentaculum tali. It should start at the anterior margin of the Achilles tendon and extend distally to the navicular tuberosity (Fig. 3). The skin and subcutaneous tissue are incised sharply.
- The posterior tibial tendon and the flexor digitorum longus (FDL) tendon are identified dorsally. The sheath of the FDL is opened along the length of the incision (Fig. 4A and 4B).
- The neurovascular bundle is identified posterior to the FDL tendon, and the Achilles tendon at the most proximal aspect of the incision.

PEARLS

- *Make the incision long enough to adequately visualize the subtalar joint. Prior to resecting the coalition, be sure to identify the anterior, middle, and posterior facets of the subtalar joint.*

PITFALLS

- *To prevent wound complications, do not undermine the tissue during the approach.*

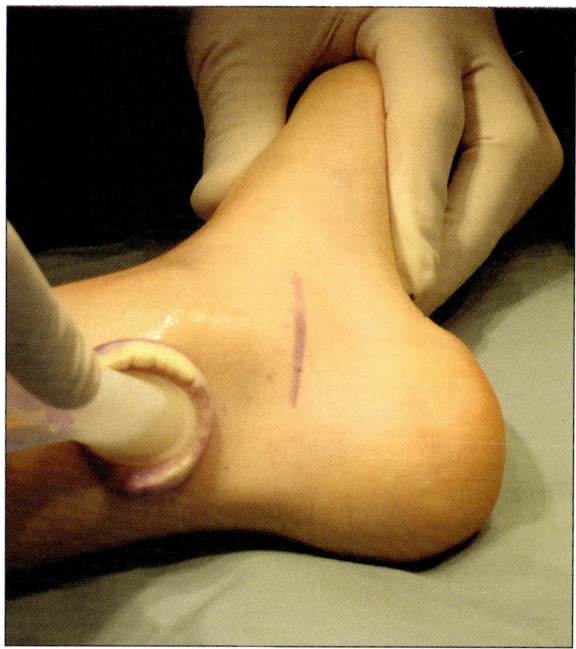

FIGURE 3

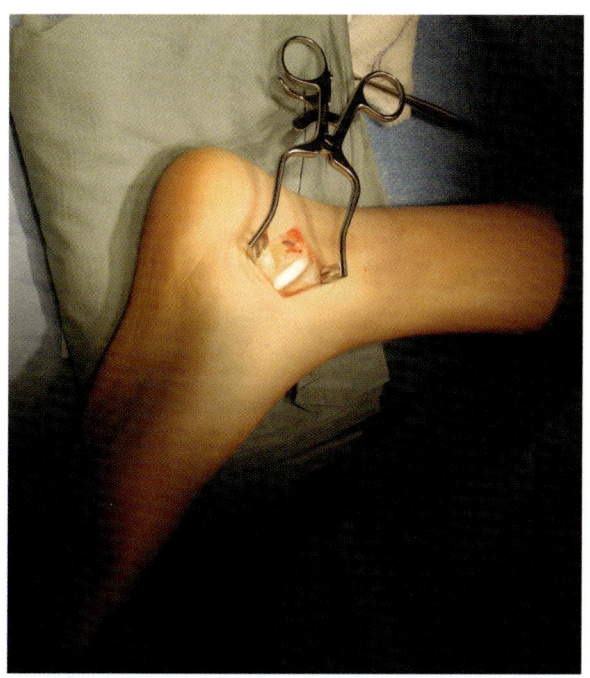

A
FIGURE 4

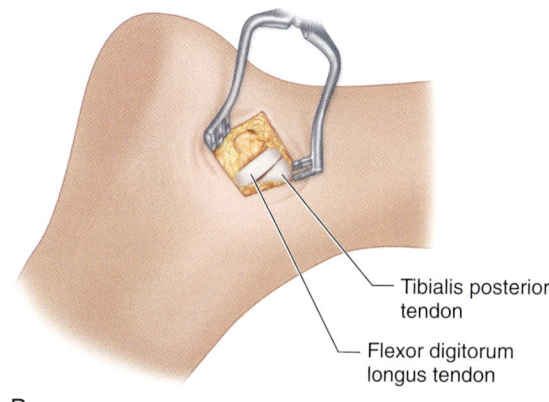

Tibialis posterior
tendon

Flexor digitorum
longus tendon

B

- The FDL tendon is retracted plantarly and the sustentaculum tali palpated (Fig. 5A and 5B). The coalition lies dorsal to the sustentaculum tali and deep to the medial portion of the sheath of the FDL tendon.
- The medial portion of the FDL tendon sheath and the underlying periosteum are incised at a point dorsal to the prominence of the sustentaculum tali (Fig. 6). This layer is developed so that it may be used later for closure.
- The normal cartilage of the subtalar joint is identified and the boundaries of the coalition are visualized.

PROCEDURE

STEP 1

- The FDL is retracted plantarly.
- Identification of the flexor hallucis longus posteriorly can help with identification of the posterior facet of the subtalar joint (Fig. 7A and 7B).

PEARLS

- *Pay close attention to the preoperative CT scan to estimate how far lateral to go in the resection of the talocalcaneal coalition.*

PITFALLS

- *During resection of the talocalcaneal coalition, pay careful attention to the level of the resection to avoid resecting bone from the body of the talus and calcaneus.*

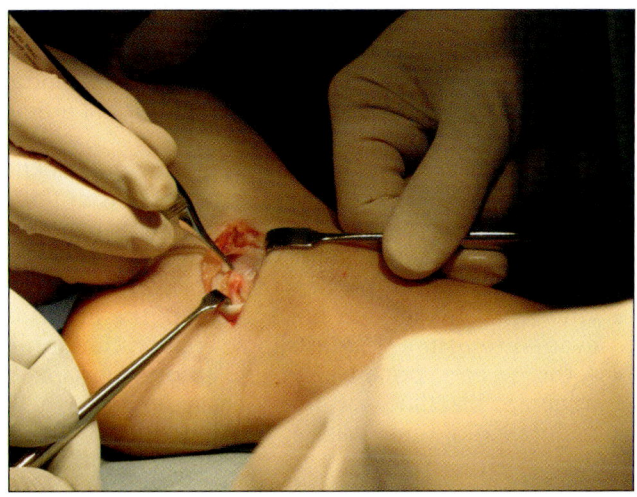

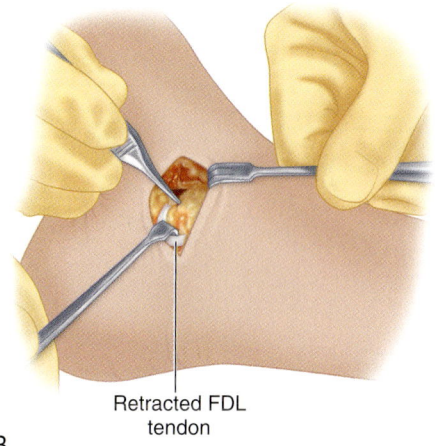

Retracted FDL
tendon

A

B

FIGURE 5

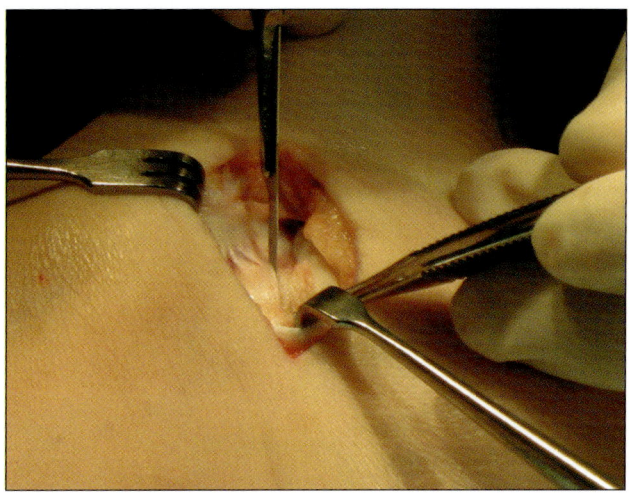

FIGURE 6

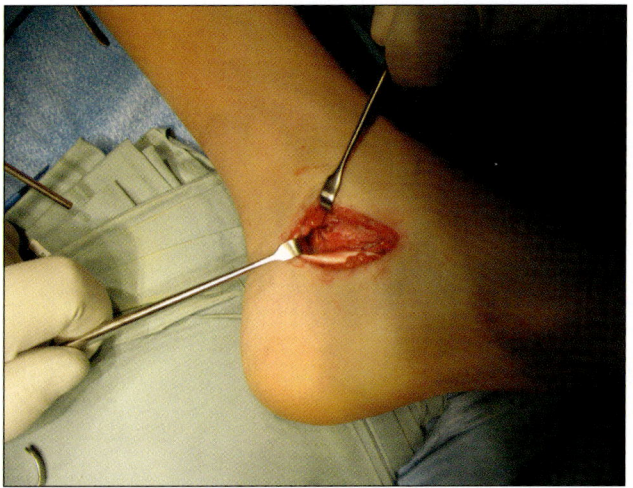

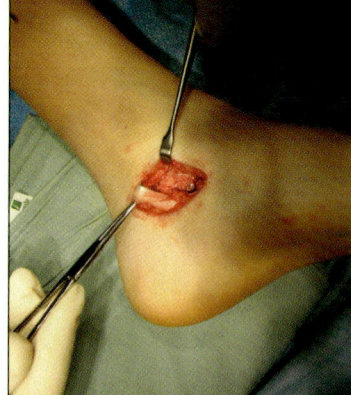

A

B

FIGURE 7

- Figure 8 shows the placement of needles where the native subtalar joint has been identified adjacent to the coalition.
- With the use of a high-speed burr, rongeurs, and curettes, the coalition that lies within the areas of normal articular cartilage is resected (Fig. 9).
  - The surgeon should resect from known to unknown areas to remain in the correct plane for resection of the coalition.
  - Resection is continued until normal articular cartilage is encountered deep within the wound.
  - Figure 10 shows a resected talocalcaneal coalition.
- Once the coalition has been resected, the foot is inverted and everted to assure there is supple motion through the joint.
- A thin layer of bone wax is applied over the area of resection to minimize bleeding and theoretically decrease the risk of recurrence of the coalition.

STEP 2

- Fat autograft interposition (preferred technique)
  - The neurovascular bundle is retracted anteriorly to expose the retrocalcaneal fat pad (Fig. 11).
  - A piece of fat 1 cm in diameter is excised from the area and placed within the area of the excised coalition (Fig. 12).
- FHL tendon interposition
  - The FHL tendon sheath is opened inferior to the sustentaculum tali.
  - The tendon of the FHL is split longitudinally, and the superior half of the tendon is placed in the coalition site.
  - The interphalangeal joint of the great toe is taken through a range of motion to assure that motion of the great toe is not restricted. If there is restricted motion, a longer split is created within the FHL tendon and the interphalangeal joint is re-examined distally.

PEARLS

- *Care must be taken to assure that an adequately sized fat graft is obtained for interposition.*

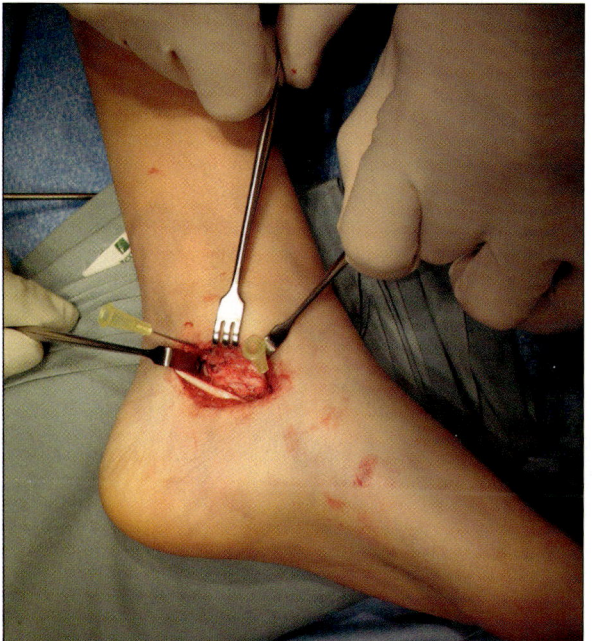

FIGURE 8

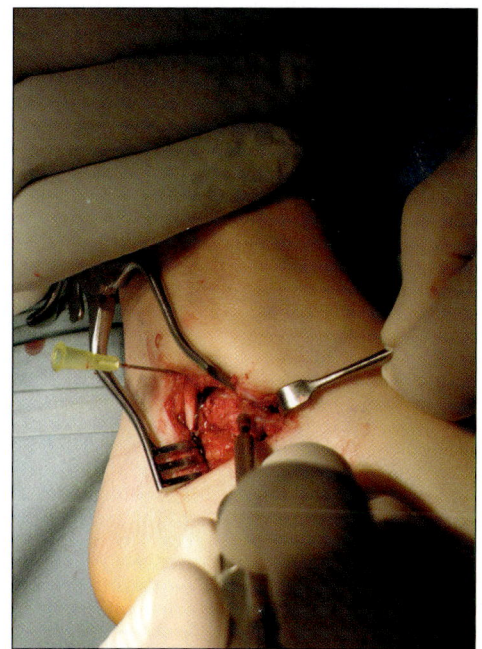

FIGURE 9

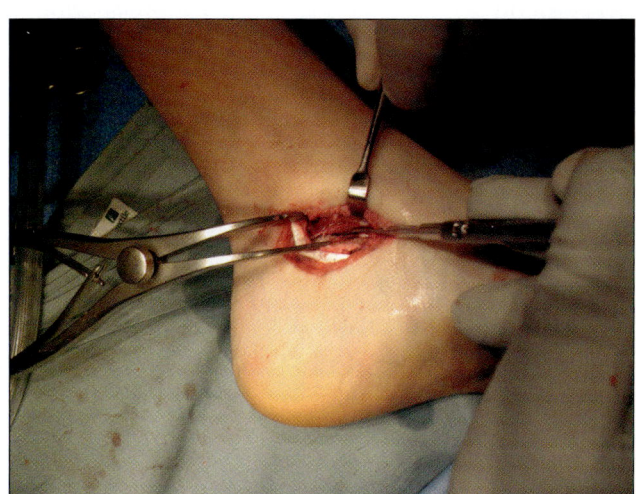

FIGURE 10

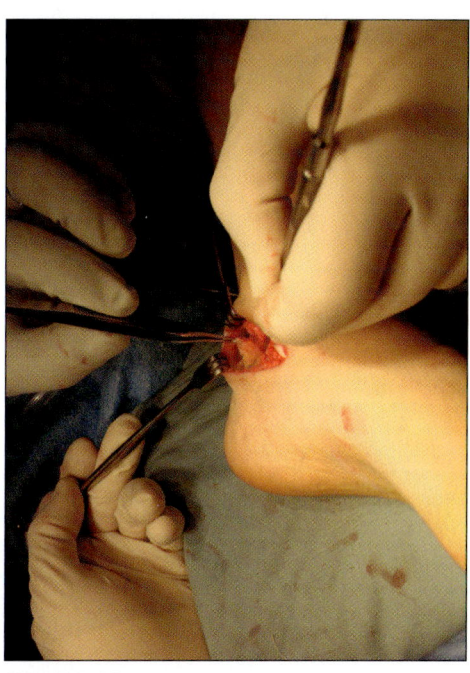

FIGURE 11

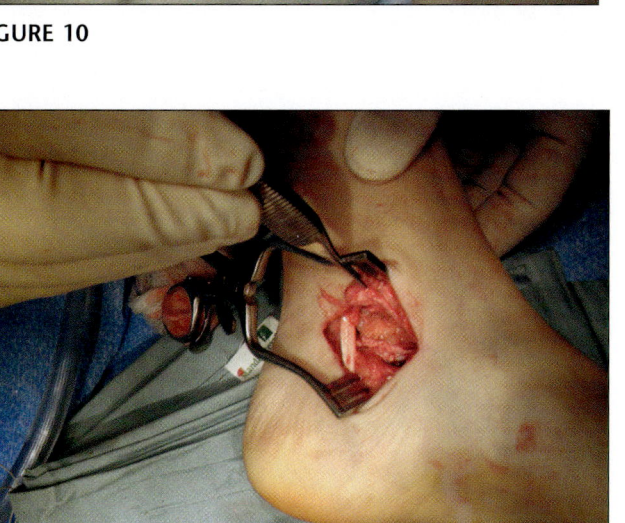

FIGURE 12

STEP 3

- If fat graft is used, the layer of the periosteum and FDL tendon sheath is repaired over the fat graft to secure it in place (Fig. 13).
- If the FHL tendon is used for interposition, the periosteum of the talus is sutured to the periosteum from the sustentaculum to prevent displacement of the tendon.
- The tourniquet is released, and adequate hemostasis assured.
- The subcutaneous tissue is closed with absorbable sutures, and the skin with an absorbable subcuticular suture or nonabsorbable nylon sutures.
- The extremity is placed in a short-leg cast or split. If a cast is used, it may be univalved or bivalved.

Complications

- Failure to resect adequate bone
- Injury to adjacent cartilage
- Poor wound healing
- Recurrence of coalition

POSTOPERATIVE CARE AND EXPECTED OUTCOMES

- The patient remains non–weight bearing in the cast or splint for 2–3 weeks.
- Progressive weight bearing is allowed following cast removal.
- Exercises focus on active, active-assisted, and passive range of motion of the subtalar joint.
- Greater than 85% of patients have good to excellent results.
- Poor results and persistent pain are more likely in coalitions constituting greater than 50% of the subtalar joint and in cases with concomitant severe hindfoot valgus.

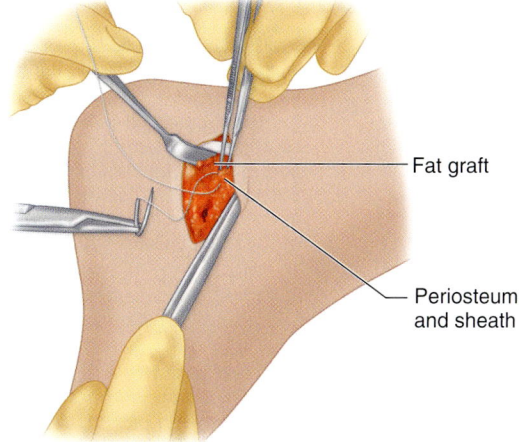

Fat graft

Periosteum
and sheath

FIGURE 13

EVIDENCE

Kumar SJ, Guille JT, Lee MS, Couto JC. Osseous and non-osseous coalition of the middle facet of the talocalcaneal joint. J Bone Joint Surg [Am]. 1992;74:529–35.

In this retrospective review, 16 patients (18 feet) underwent resection of a talocalcaneal coalition after failed conservative management. Three feet has resection without interposition, six had interposition of fat, and nine had interposition of a portion of the FHL tendon. Sixteen feet had good to excellent results at an average of 4 years postoperatively. Good to excellent results were defined as lack of clinical symptoms, little to no cortical irregularity at the resection site, and greater than 50% subtalar motion. (Level IV evidence)

Luhmann SJ, Schoenecker PL. Symptomatic talocalcaneal coalition resection: indications and results. J Pediatr Orthop. 1998;18:748–54.

In this retrospective review, 20 patients (25 feet) underwent operative intervention of a symptomatic talocalcaneal coalition. A statistically significant association was demonstrated between patients with a poor outcome and a talocalcaneal coalition measuring greater than 50% of the size of the posterior facet on preoperative CT. In addition, a poor outcome was associated with heel valgus greater than 21°. (Level IV evidence)

Olney BW, Asher MA. Excision of symptomatic coalition of the middle facet of the talocalcaneal joint. J Bone Joint Surg [Am]. 1987;69:539–44.

Nine patients with 10 symptomatic talocalcaneal coalitions underwent excision of the coalition and autogenous fat interposition. Eight feet demonstrated good to excellent results at an average of 42 months postoperatively. One foot required revision surgery for an incomplete excision at the time of the initial surgery. (Level IV evidence)

Raikin S, Cooperman DR, Thompson GH. Interposition of the split flexor hallucis longus tendon after resection of a coalition of the middle facet of the talocalcaneal joint. J Bone Joint Surg [Am]. 1999;81:11–9.

Ten patient with 14 talocalcaneal coalitions underwent resection of the coalition and interposition of a split portion of the FHL tendon after failed nonoperative management. At an average of 51 months postoperatively, 11 feet had excellent results according to their AOFAS Ankle-Hindfoot scores. No patients had significant morbidity from the use of a portion of the FHL. One patient had poor results that were attributed to the presence of degenerative changes in the posterior facet of the talocalcaneal joint. The authors made the recommendation that this procedure should be contraindicated in such patients. (Level IV/V evidence)

Sakellariou A, Sallomi D, Janzen DL, Munk PL, Claridge RJ, Kiri VA. Talocalcaneal coalition: diagnosis with the C-sign on lateral radiographs of the ankle. J Bone Joint Surg [Br]. 2000;82:574–8.

Twenty patient with a diagnosis of talocalcaneal coaltion confirmed by CT were compared to 22 controls. The C-sign, described as a C-shaped line on the lateral radiograph of patients with a talocalcaneal coalition, was examined for its sensitivity, specificity, and inter/intraobserver reliability. The C-shaped line is due to a blunting of the posterior and middle subtalar joint spaces. CT scans were used for comparision. The C-sign demonstrated a 98% sensitivity, a 98% specificity, a positive predictive value of 97%, and a negative predictive value of 98%. (Level II evidence)

Scranton PE Jr. Treatment of symptomatic talocalcaneal coalition. J Bone Joint Surg [Am]. 1987;69:533–9.

Fourteen patients with 23 symptomatic talocalcaneal coalitions were retrospectively reviewed after treatment. Five feet in three patients had successful nonoperative treatment with resolution of pain and return to full activity. Fourteen feet underwent resection of the coalition and fat interposition, and four feet underwent triple arthrodesis. Indications for resection of the coalition for the authors included size less than 50% of the width of the joint surface between the talus and calcaneus, absence of degenerative changes, and failure of conservative management. Thirteen of 23 feet demonstrated good results, defined as no functional limitation, no pain, and presence of subtalar motion. (Level IV evidence)

Stormont DM, Peterson HA. The relative incidence of tarsal coalition. Clin Orthop Relat Res. 1983;(181):28–36.

Forty-three patients and 60 tarsal coalitions were retrospectively reviewed. Calcaneonavicular coalition was found to be the most common type, occuring 53% of the time. Talocalcaneal coalition occurred 37% of the time. Sixty-eight percent of calcaneonavicular coalitions and 22% of talocalcaneal coalitions were bilateral. Pain was the most common presenting complaint. Five patients presented with a painless flatfoot. (Level IV evidence)

Wilde PH, Torode IP, Dickens DR, Cole WG. Resection for symptomatic talocalcaneal coalition. J Bone Joint Surg [Br]. 1994;76:797–801.

In this retrospective review, 17 patients (20 feet) with symptomatic talocalcaneal coalitions underwent resection. All 10 patients with heel valgus less than 16° and a coalition area measuring less than 50% of the area of the posterior facet of the calcaneus had excellent or good results. Fair or poor results were observed in 10 feet with heel valgus greater than 16° and a coalition area greater than 50% of the posterior facet of the calcaneus. (Level IV evidence)

Resection of Calcaneonavicular Coalition and Fat Autograft Interposition

Constantine A. Demetracopoulos and David M. Scher

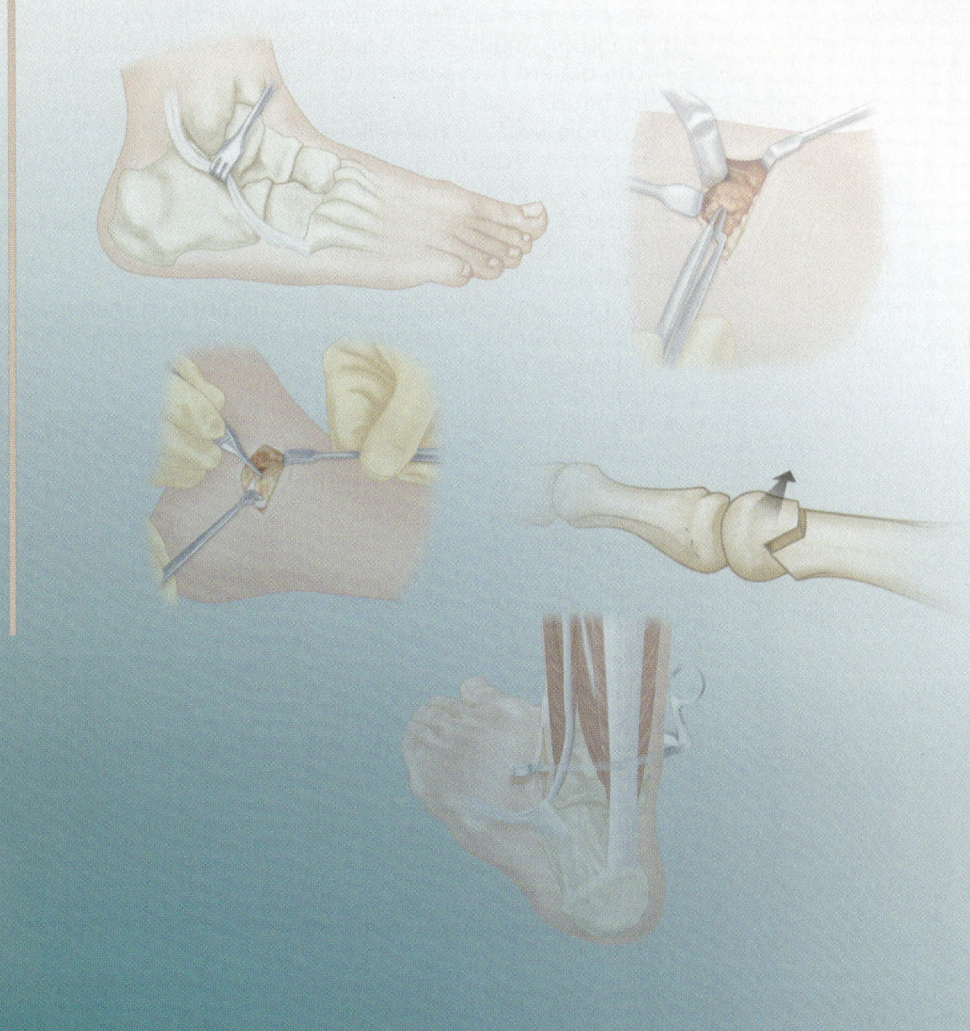

Treatment Options

• A trial of nonoperative treatment is indicated in all patients with a painful tarsal coalition. Nonoperative treatment includes activity modification, anti-inflammatory medication, and immobilization in a short-leg walking cast for 4–6 weeks.

• Asymptomatic coalitions do not require treatment.

• Interposition of the extensor digitorum brevis muscle may substitute for fat autograft interposition in calcaneonavicular coalitions.

INDICATIONS

■ A persistently painful coalition that is not responsive to nonoperative treatments such as activity modification, anti-inflammatory medication, and immobilization in a short-leg walking cast for 4–6 weeks

EXAMINATION/IMAGING

■ Gait
  • The patient is observed for an antalgic gait, characterized by a decreased stance phase on the affected extremity, and the position of the foot during stance phase is evaluated.
  • Patients will often present with an out-toeing gait.
■ Alignment
  • Hindfoot and midfoot alignment are examined. Patients with a calcaneonavicular coalition will typically present with hindfoot valgus and abduction across the midfoot.
  • The patient is evaluated for flattening of the medial longitudinal arch.
  • A single-leg heel rise will assess the flexibility of the flatfoot deformity. Failure to reconstitute the arch of the foot is indicative of a rigid hindfoot and suggests the presence of some abnormality within the subtalar or transverse tarsal joints, such as a tarsal coalition.
■ Palpation
  • In a calcaneonavicular coalition, point tenderness may be elicited directly over and distal to the anterior process of the calcaneus (Fig. 1).
■ Range of motion
  • The hindfoot is inverted and everted while stabilizing the ankle joint, and compared to the contralateral side. Tarsal coalitions are associated with pain and limitation of subtalar motion.
■ Radiographs
  • Anteroposterior (AP), lateral, and oblique views of the foot are obtained. Figure 2A shows an AP view of child with a calcaneonavicular coalition.
  • The oblique and lateral views of the foot are evaluated.
    ◆ The "anteater nose" sign is a prominent anterior process of the calcaneus seen on the lateral view (Fig. 2B).
    ◆ The oblique view is the best for visualization of a calcaneonavicular coalition. In Figure 2C, note the connection between the anterior process of the calcaneus and the lateral aspect of the navicular
  • Standing AP, lateral, and Saltzman hindfoot alignment views may be used to assess alignment.
■ CT scan is necessary evaluate for concomitant talocalcaneal coalitions.
■ Magnetic resonance imaging may be helpful in cases in which the diagnosis is equivocal and a cartilaginous or fibrous coalition is present.

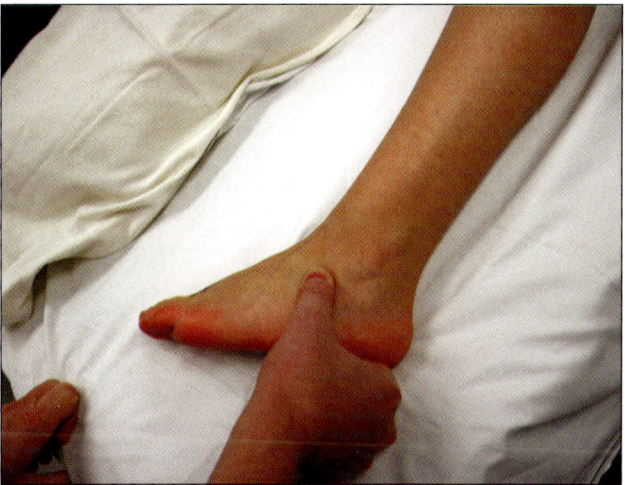

FIGURE 1

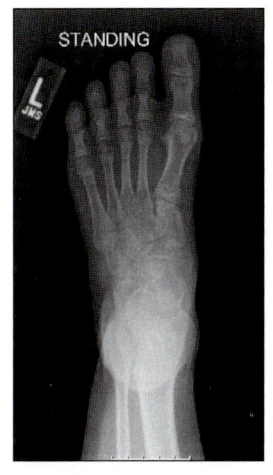

A

FIGURE 2

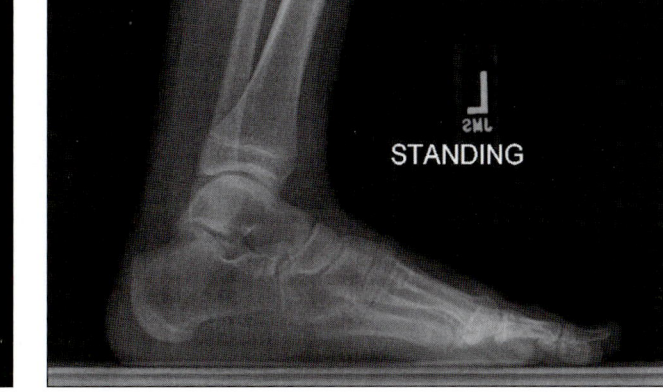

B

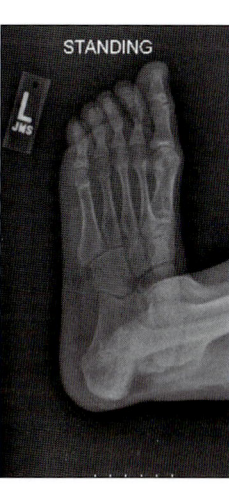

C

SURGICAL ANATOMY

- Coalitions may form as a result of failure of segmentation of the individual tarsal bones during fetal development.
- Calcaneonavicular coalitions occur between the anterior process of the calcaneus and the lateral-most aspect of the navicular.
- Coalitions may be osseous, cartilaginous, or fibrous.

POSITIONING

- The patient is placed supine on a radiolucent operating room table (Fig. 3).
- A bump is placed under the hip of the operative leg to internally rotate the extremity.
- A sterile tourniquet may be used on the upper thigh or an Esmarch tourniquet may be used at the level of the ankle.
- The extremity is prepped up to the buttocks to allow for harvesting of the fat autograft. The drapes are placed as proximal as possible to ensure that there is adequate visualization of the gluteal crease (Fig. 4).

PORTALS/EXPOSURES

- Landmarks are drawn on the skin (Fig. 5). The anterior process of the calcaneus, the cuboid, the fifth metatarsal, and the peroneal and extensor tendons, are marked. An elevator is used with fluoroscopy to find the correct level directly above the coalition.
- The incision is marked on the skin. It lies between the extensor and peroneal tendons (Fig. 6).
- An oblique incision is made along the lateral aspect of the foot overlying the anterior process of the calcaneus. The skin and subcutaneous tissue are incised sharply.
- The inferior extensor retinaculum is identified. It must be incised to expose the origin of the extensor digitorum brevis (EDB) (Fig. 7).
- The EDB is exposed and followed proximally to the sinus tarsi (Fig. 8).

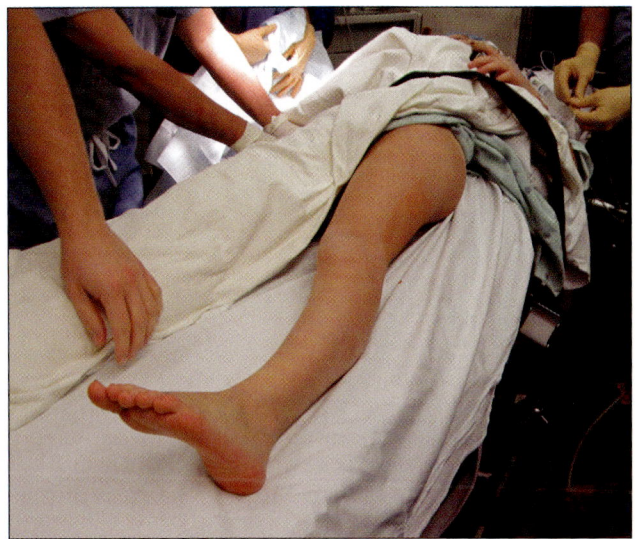

FIGURE 3

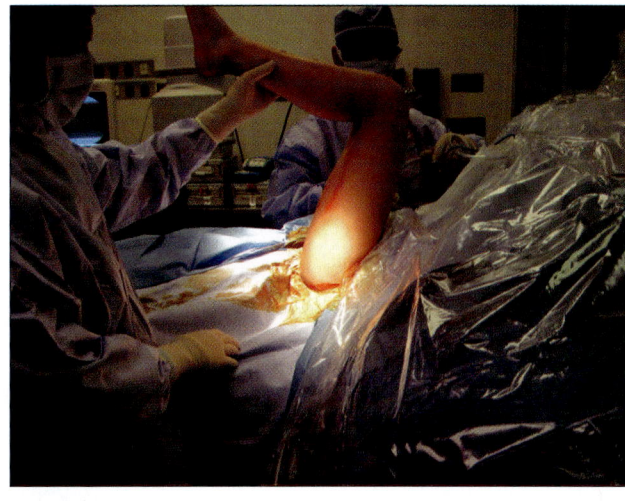

FIGURE 4

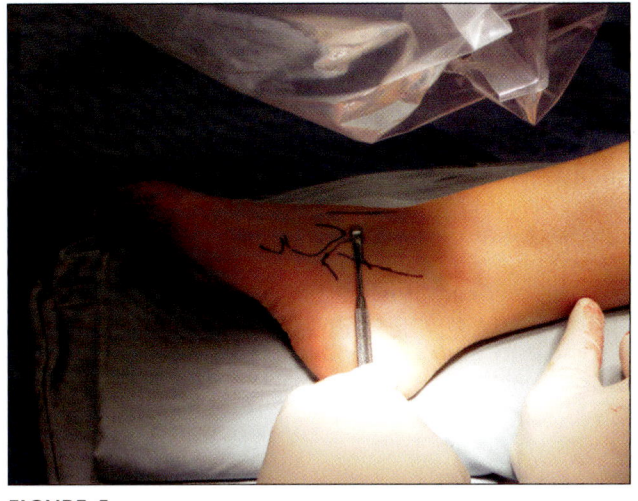

FIGURE 5

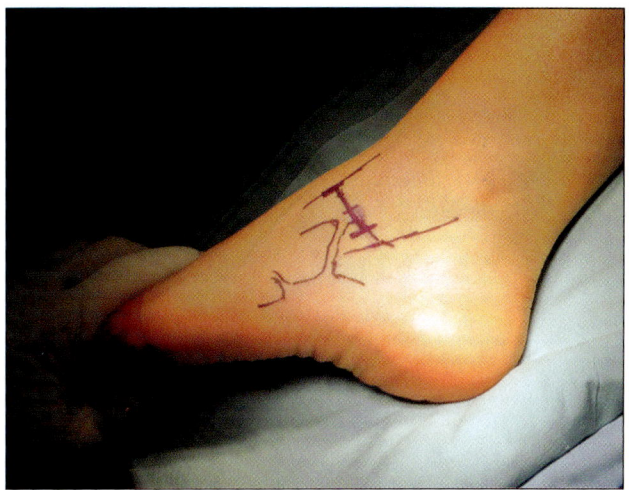

FIGURE 6

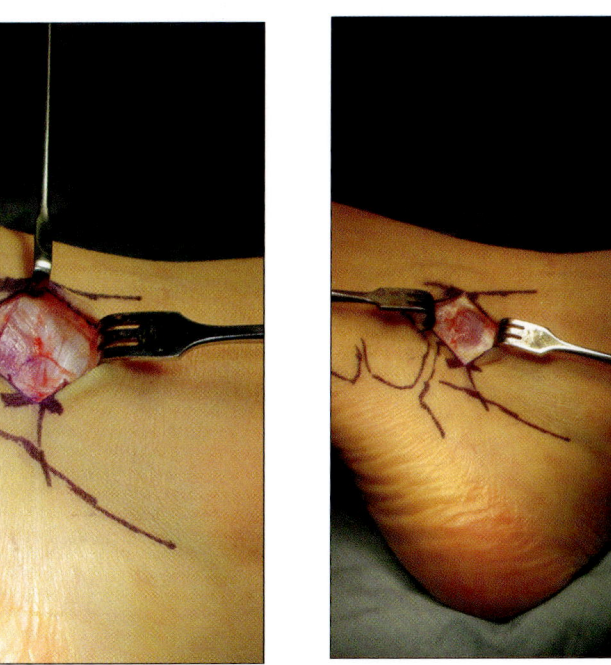

FIGURE 7

FIGURE 8

PEARLS

- *Once the anterior process of the calcaneus is exposed, place a needle within the coalition and confirm its location with an oblique fluoroscopic view (Fig. 10).*

PITFALLS

- *To prevent wound complications, do not undermine the tissue during the approach.*

- *Avoid extending the dissection into the calcaneocuboid joint.*

PEARLS

- *Pituitary or Kerrison rongeurs may be used to resect the most plantar portion of the calaneonavicular coalition.*

PITFALLS

- *The head of the talus is at risk of inadvertent damage while resecting the calcaneonavicular coalition. When performing the medial cut of the navicular, be cautious as the osteotome reaches the proximal and plantar aspect of the navicular, as the talar head is immediately proximal and medial to this location.*

- The distal aspect of the inferior extensor retinaculum and the fibrofatty tissue within the sinus tarsi are incised to expose the origin of the EDB.
- The origin of the EDB is incised and reflected distally to expose the anterior process of the calcaneus and the calcaneonavicular coalition (Fig. 9).

PROCEDURE

STEP 1

- The EDB is retracted distally.
- A small osteotome is used to remove a trapezoidal piece of bone (Fig. 11).
  - The first cut is made at the medial aspect of the anterior process of the calcaneus, just lateral to the coalition as identified fluoroscopically. The cut is angled 40–60° from the vertical and directed medially toward the lateral aspect of the navicular.
  - A second cut is made at the lateral-most aspect of the navicular directed to the same point as the first cut.
  - The piece of bone is removed, and resection of the remaining portions of the coalition is continued with rongeurs.
  - Enough bone must be removed so that a visible space is created between the calcaneus and the navicular (Fig. 12).
- Fluoroscopic views are used to confirm that the coalition has been adequately resected (Fig. 13). An adequate resection has been performed when, on the oblique radiograph, a line can be drawn along the lateral border of the talar neck that falls adjacent to the lateral-most aspect of the navicular and another line can be drawn along the medial aspect of the calcaneus that lies adjacent to the medial border of the cuboid.
- A thin layer of bone wax is applied over the area of resection to minimize bleeding and theoretically decrease the risk of recurrence of the coalition.

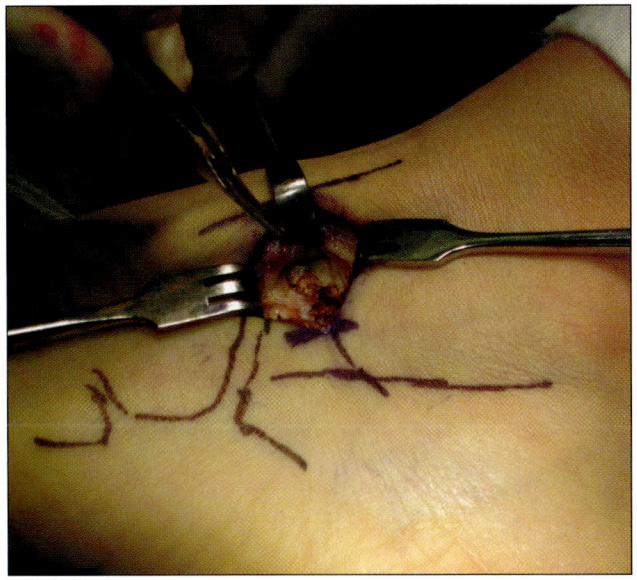

FIGURE 9

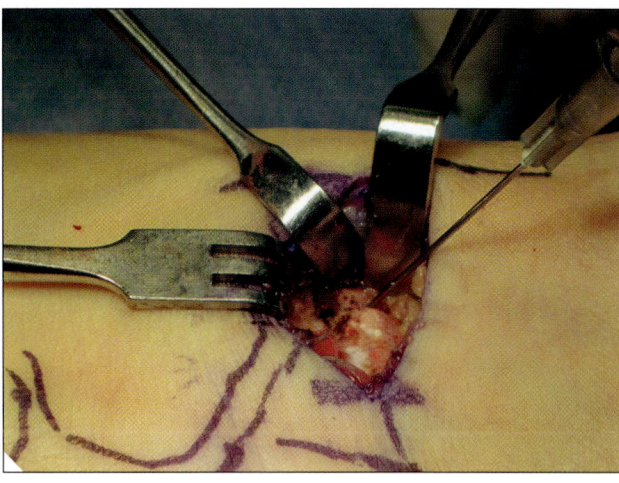

FIGURE 10

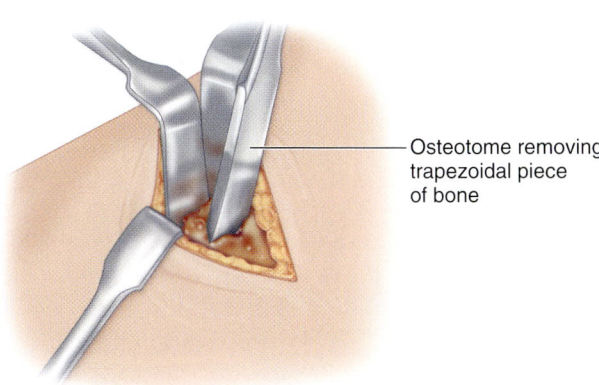

Osteotome removing
trapezoidal piece
of bone

FIGURE 11

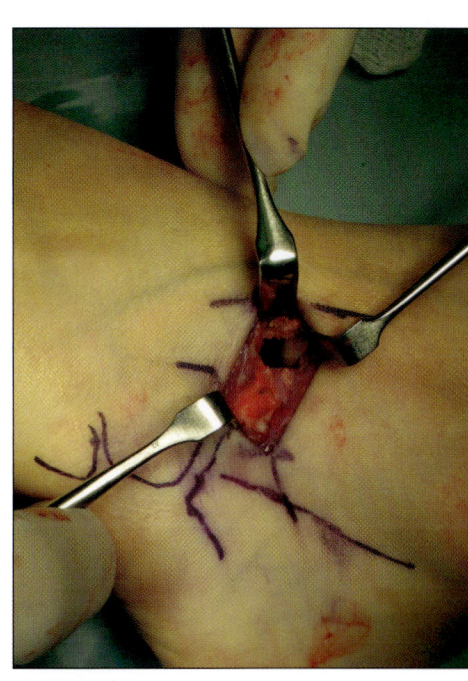

FIGURE 12

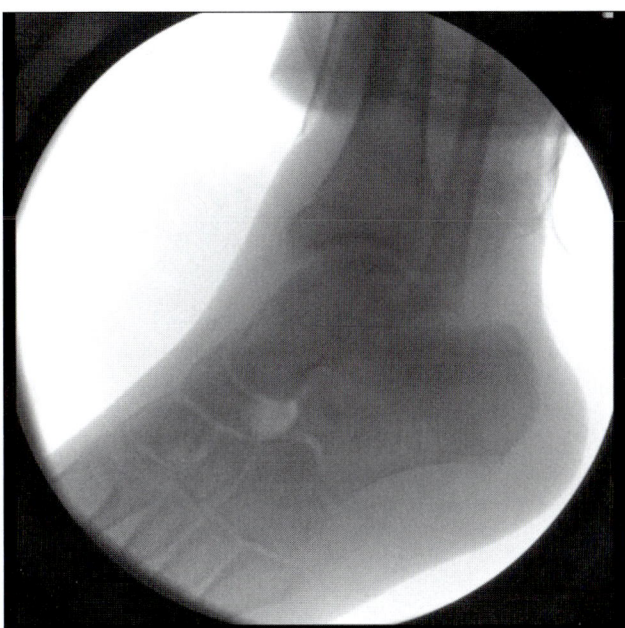

FIGURE 13

Controversies

• The EDB muscle belly may not be long enough to reach the plantar-most aspect of the space between the calcaneus and navicular following resection. In addition, detachment and transfer of the EDB can be more disfiguring, causing a depression along the dorsolateral foot where the muscle was previously lying. For these reasons, some authors advocate interposition of fat graft rather than the muscle belly.

STEP 2

■ Fat autograft interposition (preferred technique)
  • This can be performed either prior to or following resection of the coalition.
  • A transverse incision is made in the gluteal crease at the base of the buttocks of the operative leg (Fig. 14).
  • A piece of subcutaneous fat measuring approximately 2 cm in diameter is removed (Fig. 15).
    ◆ Note that, if the fat is harvested prior to the coalition resection, is should be stored in a specimen cup on a wet Raytec sponge (Fig. 16).
  • The fat is placed directly into the excised calcaneonavicular coalition (Fig. 17A and 17B).
■ Extensor digitorum brevis muscle interposition
  • Heavy absorbable sutures are placed through the proximal end of the EDB.
  • The ends of the sutures are passed through Keith needles.
  • The Keith needles are passed through the space and exit the medial side of the foot.
  • The sutures are passed through a piece of sterile felt and a button, and tied over the button. This will in effect draw the muscle into the gap between the anterior process of the calcaneus and the navicular.

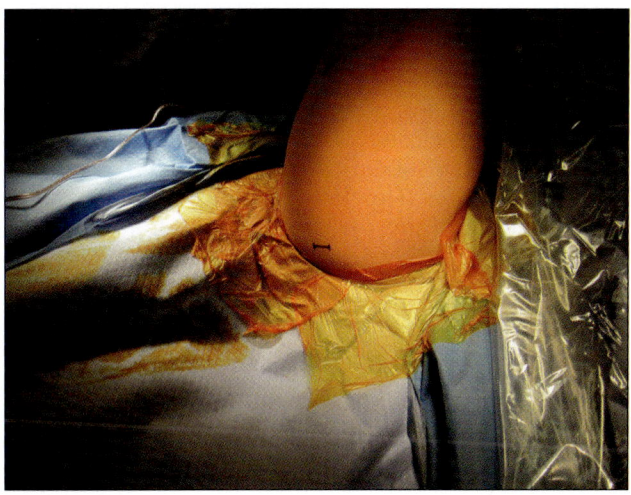

FIGURE 14

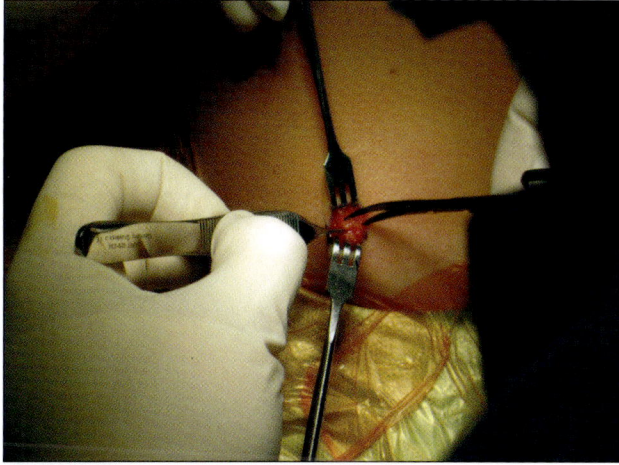

FIGURE 15

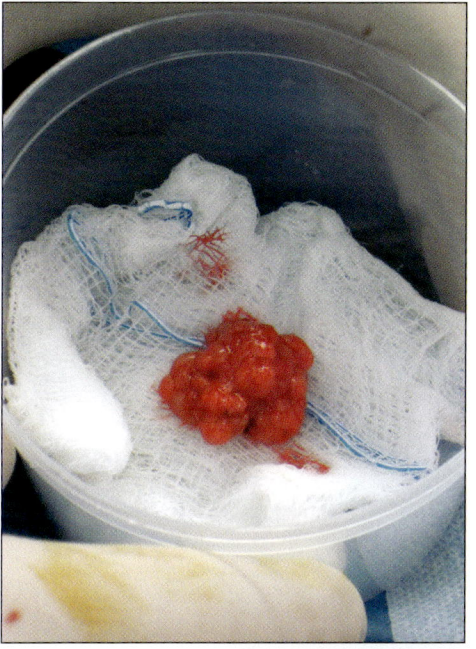

FIGURE 16

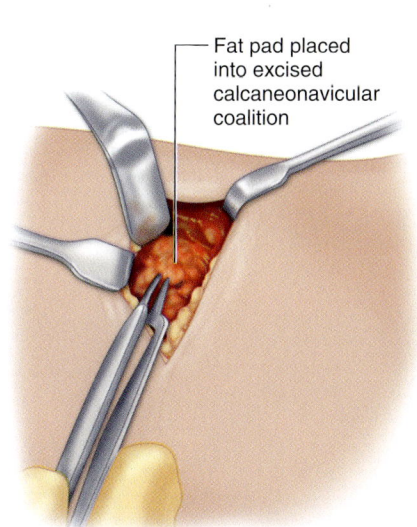

Fat pad placed
into excised
calcaneonavicular
coalition

FIGURE 17 A

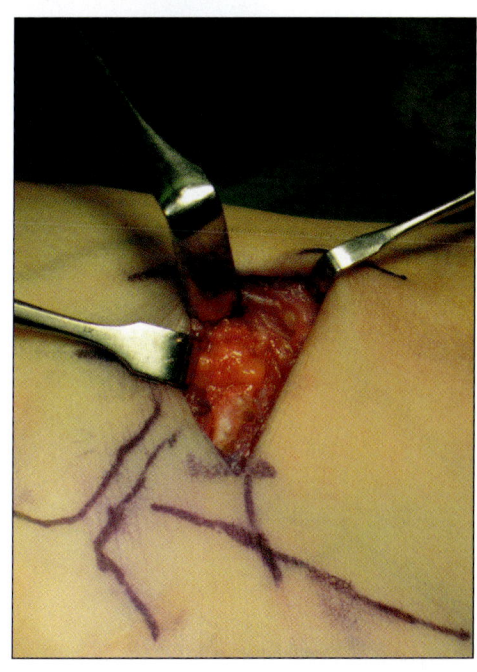

B

Step 3

- If fat graft is used, the EDB is repaired to its origin with absorbable suture (Fig. 18).
- The tourniquet is released, and adequate hemostasis assured.
- The subcutaneous tissue is closed with absorbable sutures, and the skin with an absorbable subcuticular suture or nonabsorbable nylon sutures (Fig. 19).
- The extremity is placed in a short-leg cast or split. If a cast is used, it may be univalved or bivalved.

POSTOPERATIVE CARE AND EXPECTED OUTCOMES

- The patient remains non–weight bearing in the cast or splint for 2–3 weeks.
- Progressive weight bearing is allowed following cast removal.
- Exercises focus on active, active-assisted, and passive range of motion of the subtalar joint.
- Greater than 90% of patients have good to excellent results.

Complications

- Failure to resect adequate bone
- Injury to adjacent cartilage
- Poor wound healing
- Recurrence of coalition

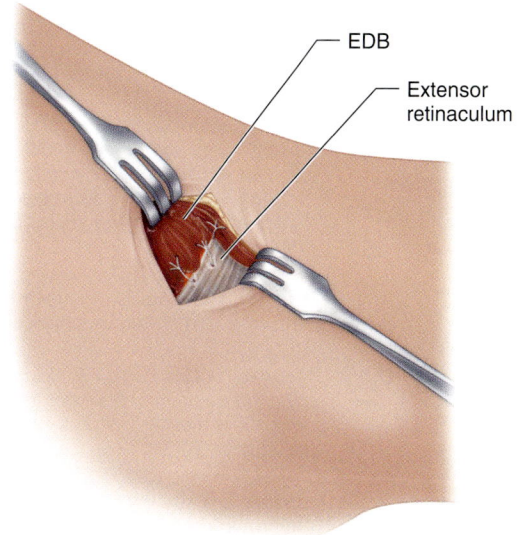

EDB

Extensor
retinaculum

FIGURE 18

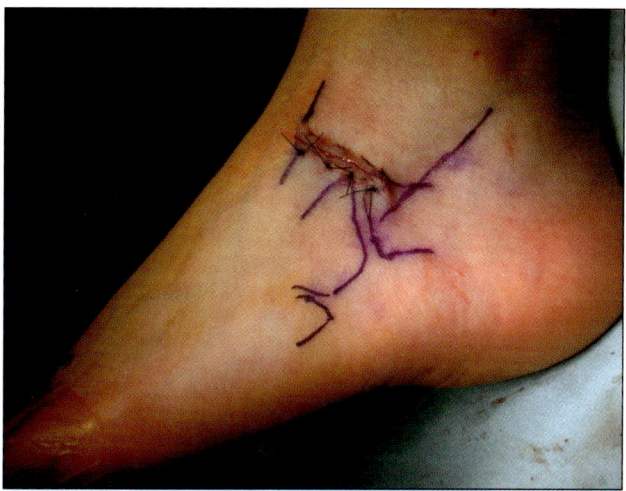

FIGURE 19

EVIDENCE

Gonzalez P, Kumar SJ. Calcaneonavicular coalition treated by resection and interposition of the extensor digitorum brevis muscle. J Bone Joint Surg [Am]. 1990;72:71–7.

A series of 48 patients who underwent calcaneonavicular excision and interposition of the extensor digitorum brevis muscle were evaluated at 2–23 years' follow-up. Seventy-seven percent of patients were asymptomatic with minimal cortical irregularity at the resection site, and could demonstrate greater than 50% subtalar motion. Results were best in cartilaginous coalitions in patients less than 16 years of age at the time of operation. (Level IV evidence)

Moyes ST, Crawfurd EJ, Aichroth PM. The interposition of extensor digitorum brevis in the resection of calcaneonavicular bars. J Pediatr Orthop. 1994;14:387–8.

Fourteen patients with 19 calcaneonavicular coalitions underwent resection of the coalition and interposition of the extensor digitorum brevis. Ninety percent of patients were asymptomatic without evidence of recurrence at an average of 3.4 years postoperatively. (Level IV evidence)

Mubarak SJ, Patel PN, Upasani VV, Moor MA, Wenger DR. Calcaneonavicular coalition: treatment by excision and fat graft. J Pediatr Orthop. 2009;29:418–26.

A retrospective review of 69 patients with 96 calcaneonavicular coalitions who underwent coalition resection and fat autograft interposition was performed at an average of 29 months postoperatively. Eighty-seven percent of patients returned to full activity, 74% had improved subtalar motion, and 5% of patients required revision surgery. In a cadaveric study, the authors were able to demonstrate that, in the case of EDB interposition, only 64% of the gap was covered, leaving a 1-cm gap on the plantar aspect of the coalition without tissue interposition. (Level IV evidence)

Oestreich AE, Mize WA, Crawford AH, Morgan RC Jr. The "anteater nose": a direct sign of calcaneonavicular coalition on the lateral radiograph. J Pediatr Orthop. 1987; 7:709–11.

The authors presented a retrospective review of patients with a diagnosis of calcaneonavicular coalition. Patients greater than 9 years of age with both oblique and lateral radiographs of the foot were included in the study. Twenty-one patients (30 feet) participated in the study. All 30 feet with the diagnosis of calcaneonavicular coalition demonstrated a "nose-like protrusion of the anterior superior calcaneus" that headed toward the middle region of the navicular. This was compared to 125 control feet without the diagnosis of tarsal coalition, which did not demonstrate this type of calcaneal morphology. (Level III evidence)

Stormont DM, Peterson HA. The relative incidence of tarsal coalition. Clin Orthop Relat Res. 1983;(181):28–36.

Forty-three patients and 60 tarsal coalitions were retrospectively reviewed. Calcaneonavicular coalition was found to be the most common type, occuring 53% of the time. Talocalcaneal coalition occurred 37% of the time. Sixty-eight percent of calcaneonavicular coalitions and 22% of talocalcaneal coalitions were bilateral. Pain was the most common presenting complaint. Five patients presented with a painless flatfoot. (Level IV evidence)

Varner KE, Michelson JD. Tarsal coalition in adults. Foot Ankle Int. 2000;21:669–72.

In this retrospective review of 32 feet in 27 adults with tarsal coalition, there were 18 subtalar coalitions, 14 calcaneonavicular coalitions, and 1 naviculocuneiform coalition. Seven of the 27 patients presented with a flatfoot; however, subtalar motion was decreased in 23 of 32 feet. Eleven feet were asymptomatic. Subtalar fusion was necessary for four feet. One patient underwent resection of the coalition. Most patient responded well to conservative management, which included activity modification, anti-inflammatory medication, and casting. (Level IV evidence)

Chevron Osteotomy for Adolescent Hallux Valgus

James A. Krcik, Jeremy S. Frank, and Lyle J. Micheli

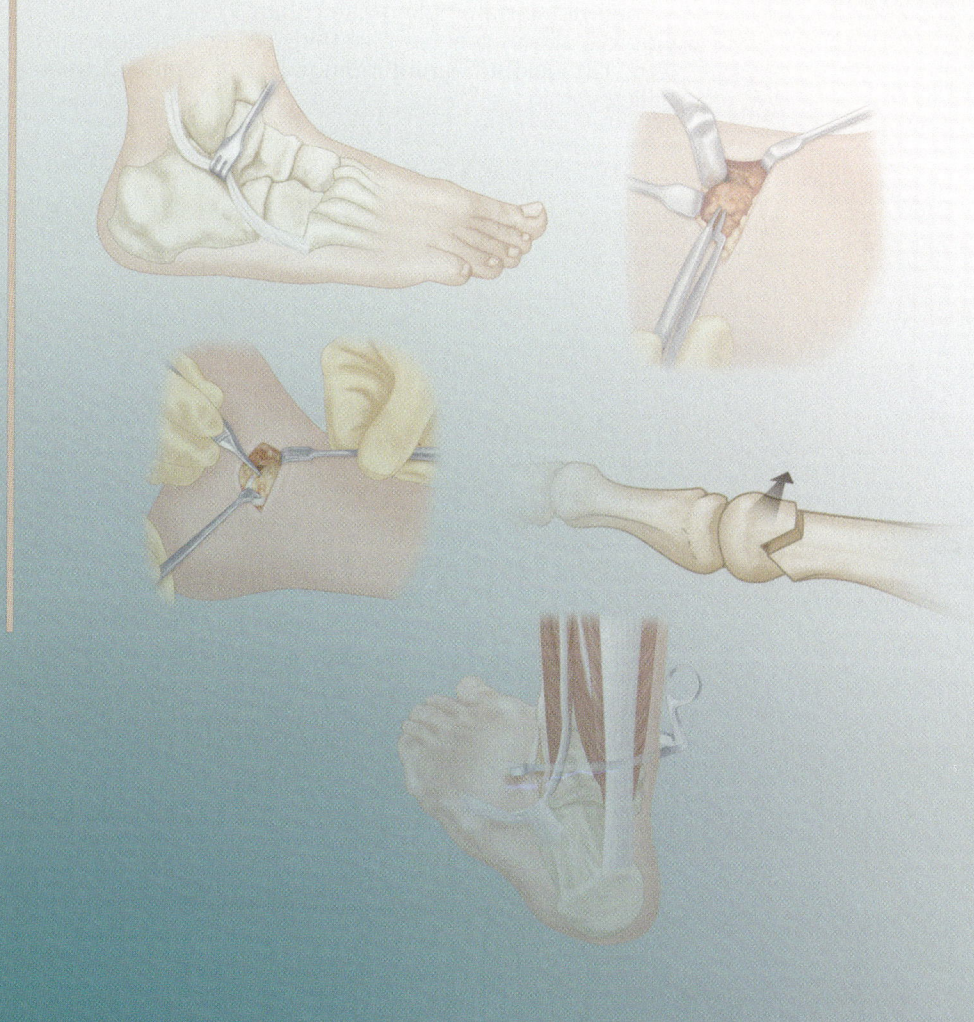

Treatment Options

• Nonoperative treatment with splints, pads, wide box shoes

INDICATIONS

■ Painful moderate hallux valgus (HV) that has failed nonoperative treatment
  • Mild HV: intermetatarsal angle less than 13°, HV angle less than 25°
■ Pain over medial eminence
■ No sesamoid subluxation
■ No pronation
■ Passively correctable

EXAMINATION/IMAGING

■ Anteroposterior, lateral, and oblique weight-bearing films of the foot are obtained and reviewed for hallux valgus.
  • Hallux valgus angle of greater than 15° but less than 35–40°
  • Intermetatarsal angle greater than 9° but less than 13°
■ Figure 1 shows preoperative (Fig. 1A) and postoperative (Fig. 1B) weight-bearing radiographs of a patient treated for hallux valgus.

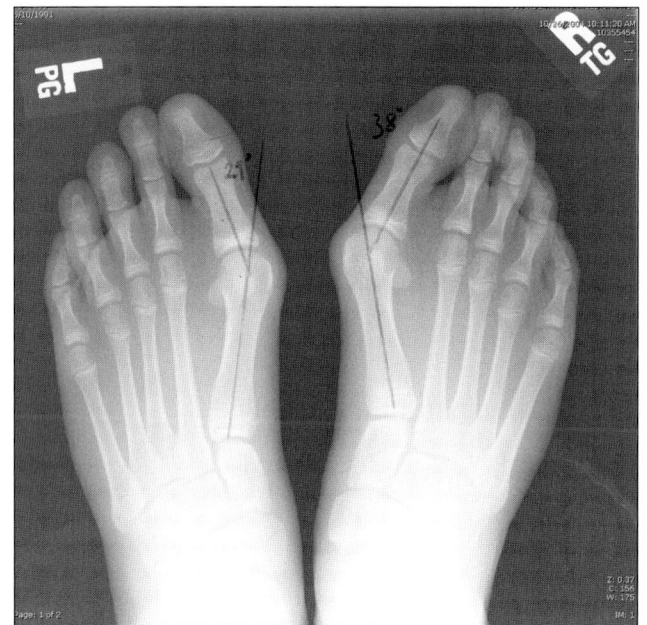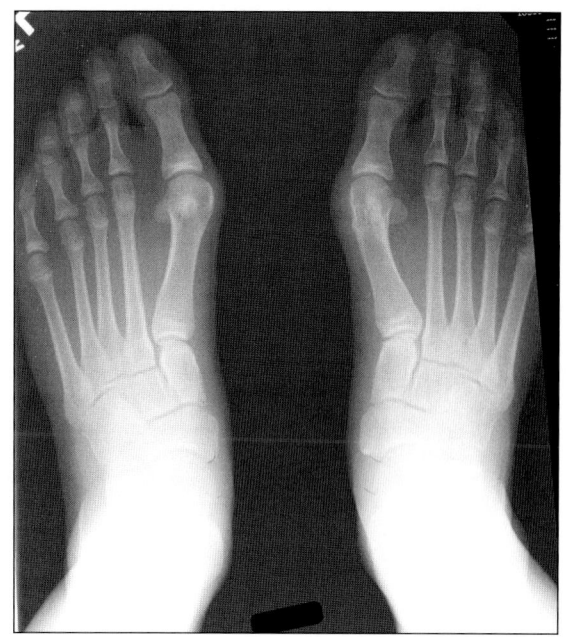

A B

FIGURE 1

- Figure 2 shows preoperative (Fig. 2A), intraoperative (Fig. 2B), and postoperative (Fig. 2C) radiographs.

SURGICAL ANATOMY

- Structures at risk include:
  - Dorsomedial sensory nerve and plantar medial nerve to great toe
  - Extensor tendon and nerve

POSITIONING

- The patient is placed supine on the operating room table.
- A bump is placed under the surgical side.

PORTALS/EXPOSURES

- Ankle block procedure
  - 0.5% Marcaine (15–30 ml) is injected:
    - Adjacent to the deep peroneal nerve (near the dorsalis pedis)
    - Adjacent to the posterior tibial nerve under the medial malleolus
  - 0.5% Marcaine (15 ml) is injected in a wheal anteriorly at the level of the ankle joint to anesthetize the branches of the superficial peroneal nerve and sural nerves.
- Approach
  - A longitudinal skin incision 4–7 cm long is made dorsomedial and centered over the medial eminence.
  - Dissection is performed down to the capsule.
    - Metzenbaum scissors are used to cut through subcutaneous tissue.
    - The capsule and metatarsal shaft are exposed with an elevator.
  - The bursa and subcutaneous tissues are dissected from the joint capsule.
    - The dorsomedial sensory nerve and plantar medial nerve to the great toe must be protected.

PITFALLS

- *Watch for the extensor tendon and nerve.*
- *When injecting 0.5% Marcaine, be sure you are not in a vessel.*

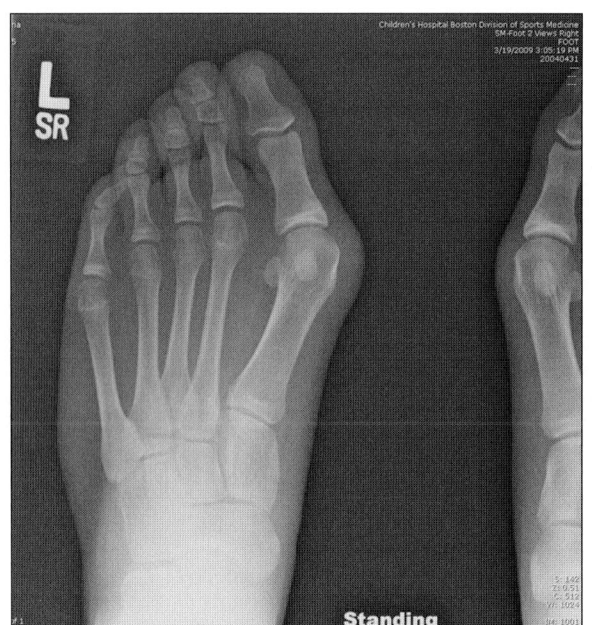

A

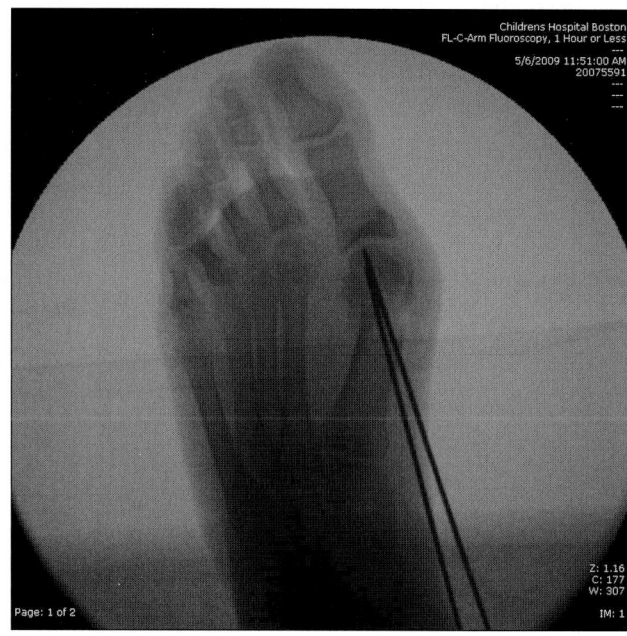

B

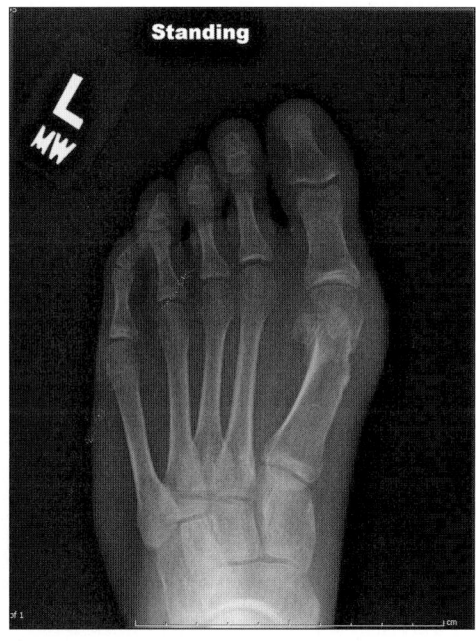

C

FIGURE 2

PROCEDURE

STEP 1

- A metatarsophalangeal (MTP) capsulotomy is performed.
  - An L-shaped capsular incision is made.
    - ◆ The horizontal limb is plantar medial adjacent to the medial margin of the medial (tibial) sesamoid.
    - ◆ The vertical limb is a few millimeters proximal to MTP joint line.
  - The capsule is dissected off from the medial eminence and proximally to the metaphyseal flare. A beaver blade is used for this.
- The lateral joint contracture is released by perforating the lateral capsule under direct vision.
- The area is exposed distally to the proximal phalanx.
- The MTP joint is exposed (Fig. 3) with an L-shaped flap.
  - This allows visualization of the sagittal groove of the medial eminence.
  - Any dorsal spurs are removed.

STEP 2

- Medial prominence resection can be performed using osteotomes or a micro-sagittal saw.
  - The medial eminence is removed starting at the sagittal groove.
    - ◆ The surgeon should avoid the medial sesamoid groove plantarly.
  - Resection continues parallel to medial border of the foot, not to the shaft of the first metatarsal.
  - The resection cut exits proximally at the junction of the head and neck.
- A chevron osteotomy (V-shaped, horizontal, apex distal) is performed at the head-neck level.
  - The center of the metatarsal head is marked.
  - The apex of the horizontal V-shaped osteotomy will be 2 cm distal to the center of the metatarsal head.
  - Using a V-shaped angle of 55°, the shaft is cut.
  - The cuts are kept so that the distal part slides lateral and slightly proximal, aiming at the fifth metatarsal [5MT] head.
  - If more correction is needed, the apex of the cut can be mde more proximal and the plantar cut shallower.
  - A 3/32-inch Kirschner wire (K-wire) is used to make a hole at the apex of the osteotomy, aiming toward the head of the 5MT.
  - Then separate plantar and dorsal cuts are made.
  - The plantar cut should angle more shallowly (Fig. 4).

STEP 3

- Realignment
  - A small towel clip is used to stabilize the metatarsal.
  - The distal fragment is displaced laterally by 4–5mm or ⅓ of the width of the metatarsal head.
- Fixation
  - Two smooth 0.045-inch K-wires are inserted from proximal to dorsal in the diaphysis.
  - The wires usually start at the base of the incision proximally, or just through the skin across the osteotomy, and exit through the head and plantarward.
  - Position of the K-wires is checked under fluoroscopy.
  - The wires are cut proximally and buried under the skin.
  - Fixation may also be done using:
    - ◆ 2.4-mm solid flat-head screws
    - ◆ Screws, bone pegs, or staples

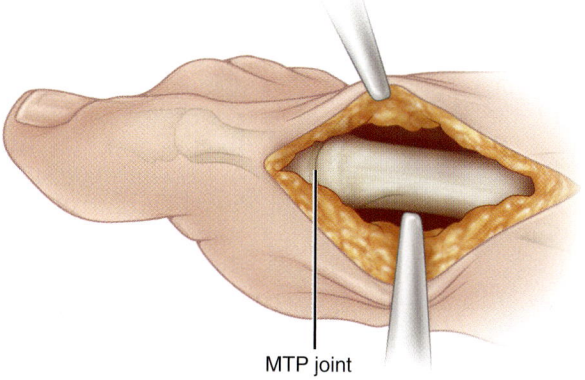

MTP joint

FIGURE 3

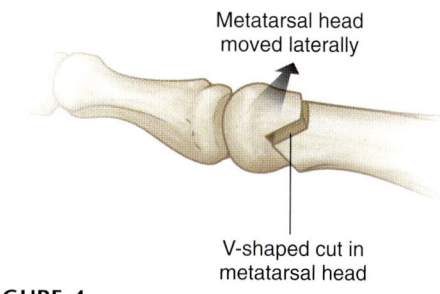

Metatarsal head
moved laterally

V-shaped cut in
metatarsal head

FIGURE 4

- The remaining prominence of the metaphysis is resected in a plane parallel to the medial border of the foot.
- The capsule is closed.
  - Redundant capsule is excised.
  - A medial capsulorrhaphy of the L-shaped capsulotomy is performed with 2-0 Vicryl mattress sutures. These should pull the toe over.
  - A "corner"-type stitch is used with a loop in the flap, and the knots tied proximally.
  - Plantar sutures are placed first, snapping and cutting until all three stitches are placed.
    - The surgeon should stay plantar with these sutures and make sure they do not flex the first toe.
    - The toe is held overcorrected during closure.
  - Plantar advancement allows sesamoid reduction.
- Figure 5 shows preoperative (Fig. 5A) and postoperative (Fig. 5B and 5C) radiographs of a patient following realignment and fixation.

POSTOPERATIVE CARE AND EXPECTED OUTCOMES

- The patient is placed in a splint.
- Crutches are used for 1 week, and heel walking is permitted at 2 weeks.
- Weight bearing in wide box shoe as tolerated is permitted at 3 weeks.
- A toe spacer and bunion splint are placed at 2 days postoperative. These are used for 6 weeks.
- Pin removal is scheduled at 6 weeks.
- After pin removal, crutches and a postoperative wide box shoe are used for 2 weeks. Radiographs are checked before discontinuing crutches.

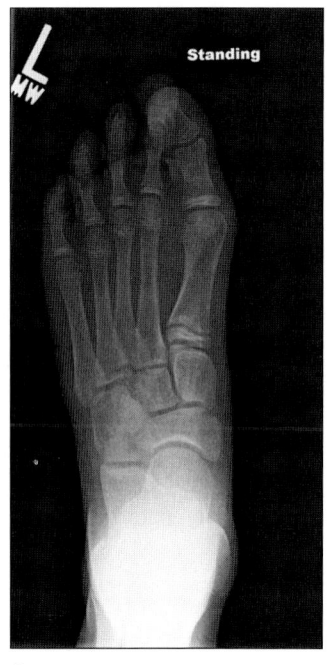

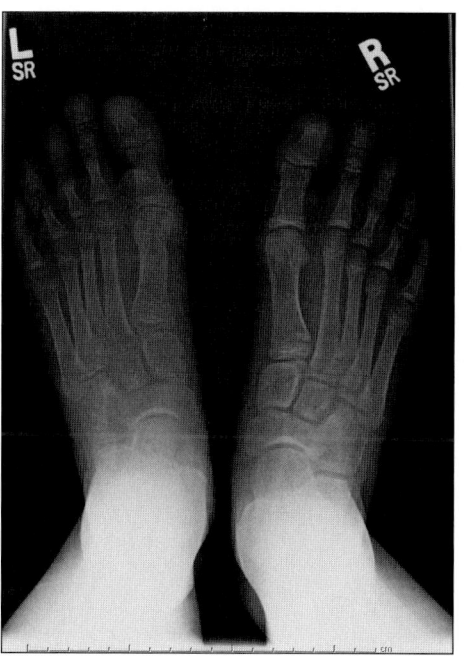

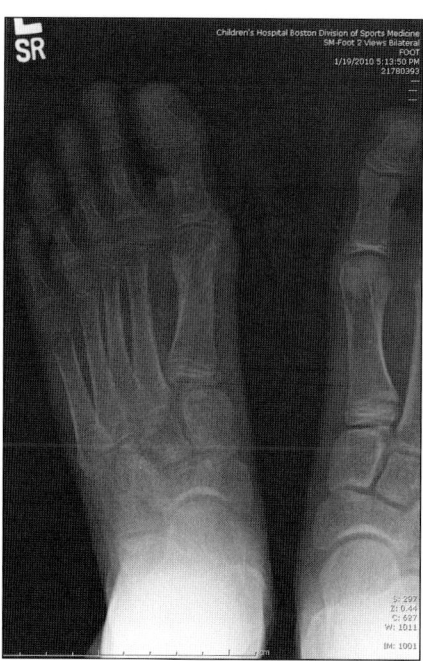

A

B

C

FIGURE 5

EVIDENCE

Austin DW, Leventen EO. A new osteotomy for hallux valgus: a horizontally directed "V" displacement osteotomy of the metatarsal head for hallux valgus and primus cavus. Clin Orthop Relat Res. 1981;(157):25–30.

A brief description of osteotomy cut similar to osteotomy cut described in this chapter.

Campbell JT. Hallux valgus: adult and juvenile. In Richardson EG (ed). Orthopaedic Knowledge Update: Foot and Ankle 3. Rosemont, IL: American Academy of Orthopaedic Surgeons, 2004:3–15.

Padanilam TG. Disorder of the first ray. In Richardson EG (ed). Orthopaedic Knowledge Update: Foot and Ankle 3. Rosemont, IL: American Academy of Orthopaedic Surgeons, 2004:17–25.

Zimmer T, et al. Treatment of hallux valgus in adolescents by the chevron osteotomy. Foot Ankle Int. 1989;9:190–3.

Article on 20 adolescents that underwent chevron osteotomy for painful hallux valgus. After an extended period of time (64 months), most expressed satisfaction to their surgery. Cosmetic improvement, pain relief, and improvement in shoe wear were noted in most of the patients. X-rays didn't correlate with clinical results. Overall, chevron osteotomy thought to be a good option for treating adolescent bunion.

Osteotomies of the Foot for Cavus Deformities

Scott J. Mubarak

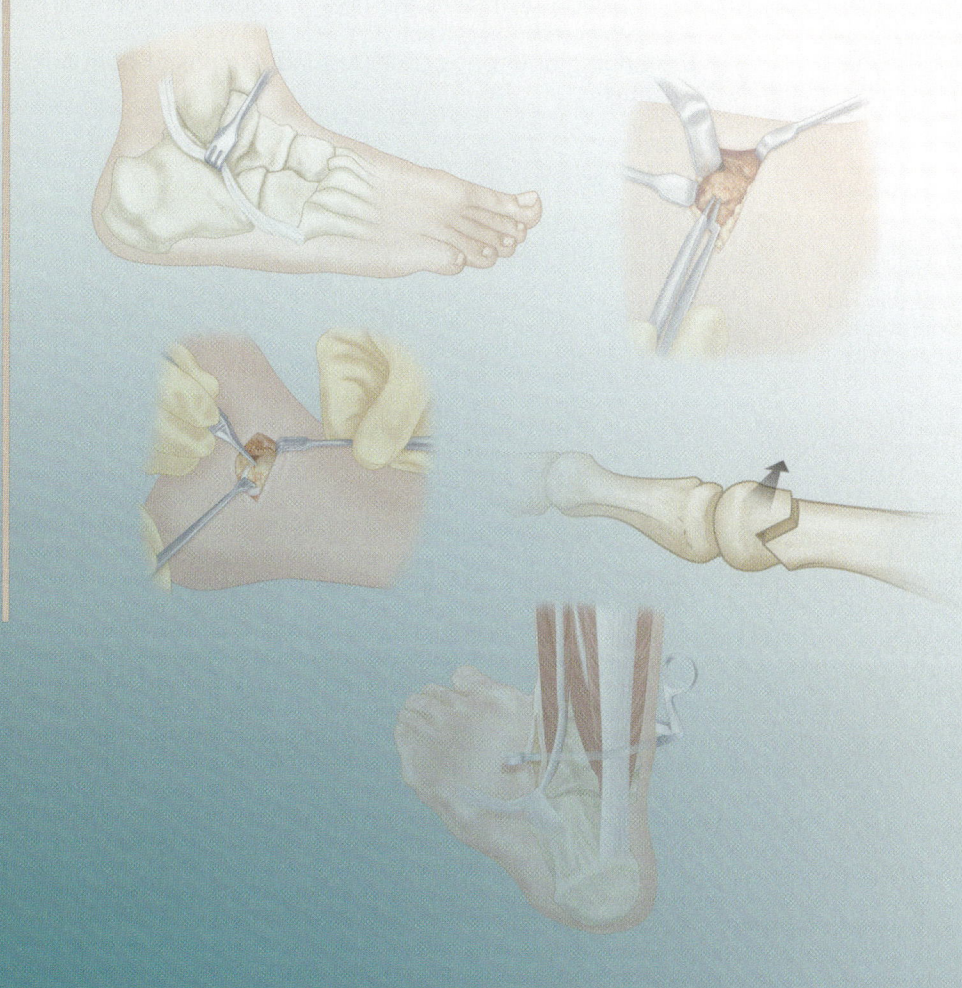

PITFALLS

- *All cavus foot deformities should be thoroughly worked up for a possible cause for the condition. If the cavus cause is neurologic (Fig. 2), after correcting the bony deformity, later follow-up with tendon transfer to the forefoot or toes is often needed.*

Controversies

- If the forefoot is flexible, orthotics and soft tissue procedures should be considered. Multiple plantar releases and tendon transfers can be used in the more supple feet. We prefer orthotics for the flexible feet and bony procedures if the feet are rigid.

Treatment Options

- Fusions: McElvenny and Caldwell (1958) described fusion of the first metatarsal, cuneiform, and navicular joints.

- Triple arthrodesis: Saltzman et al. (1999) detailed long-term follow-up at 25 and 40 years after a triple arthrodesis. This study found suboptimal results for triple arthrodesis as time went on and thus demonstrates the need for joint-sparing surgery in younger patients.

- Osteotomies across joints: Japas (1968) described his "V" osteotomy of the midfoot. Wilcox and Weiner presented their "Akron dome osteotomy" in 1985, and recently provided longer term follow-up (Weiner et al., 2008). These are salvage surgical options.

INDICATIONS

- Rigid cavus foot with plantar flexion of the first ray (Fig. 1A and 1B)
- Ankle/foot instability symptoms, including pain
- Painful metatarsal heads and callosities
- Ankle and foot sprains, and/or fractures

EXAMINATION/IMAGING

- All patients are assessed to evaluate the flexibility of the hindfoot varus using the kneeling test (Fig. 3A–C).
  - This technique is easier and more reliable than the Coleman block test. It allows the surgeon to tell if a sliding calcaneal osteotomy will be necessary to correct heel varus.
  - The patient's forefoot is hinded to check the calcaneus position relative to the tibia; if valgus, the forefoot only is corrected.
- Standing anteroposterior (AP) radiographs of both ankles are obtained.

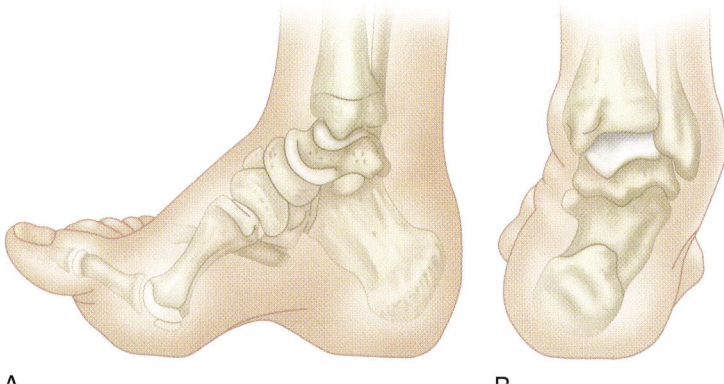

A

B

FIGURE 1

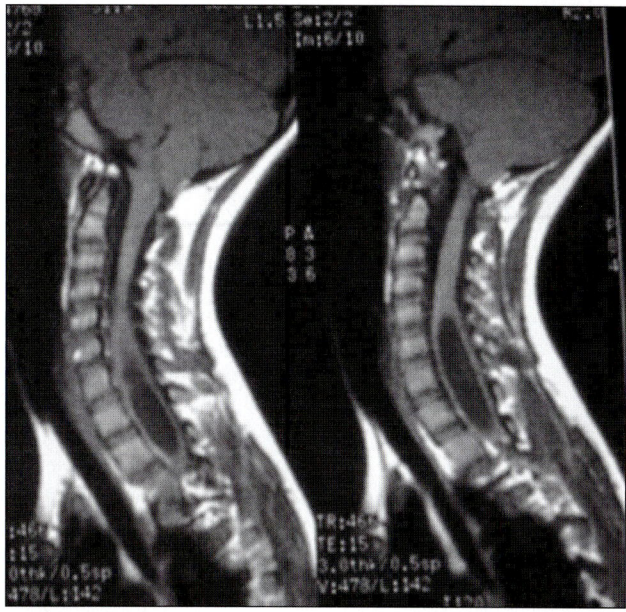

FIGURE 2

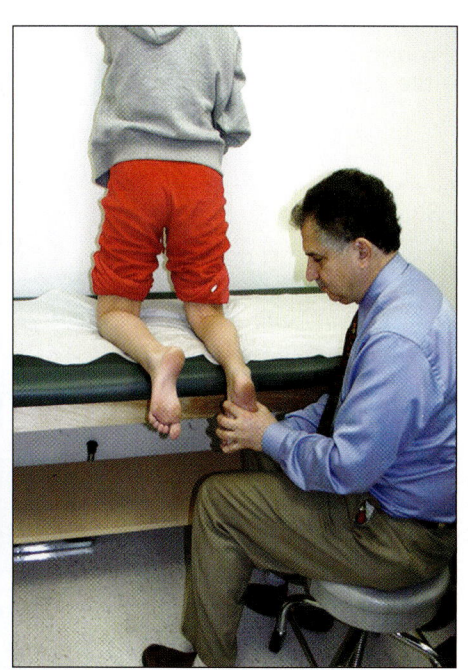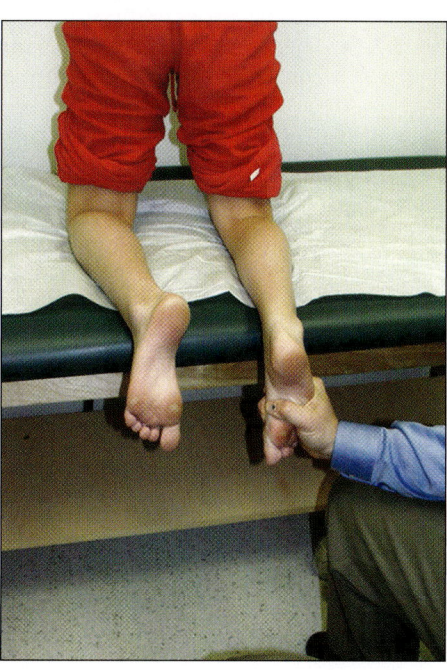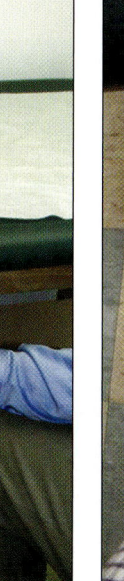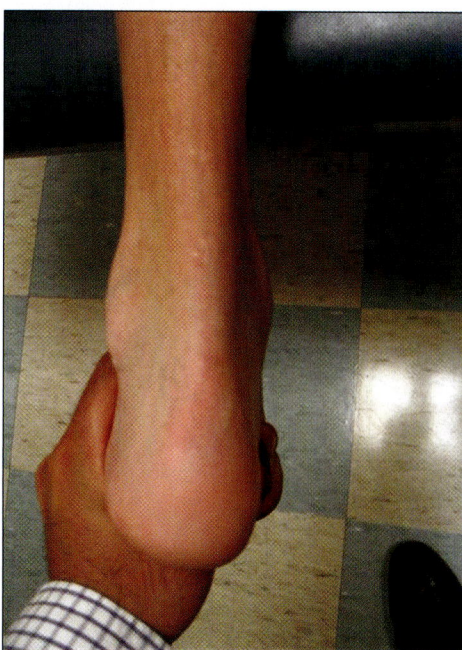

A

B

C

FIGURE 3

- Standing AP and lateral (Fig. 4) radiographs of both feet are examined, focusing of the apex of the deformity.
- Preoperative computed tomography scans with three-dimensional reconstruction may be considered to visualize the deformity.

SURGICAL ANATOMY

- The sural nerve is at risk when lengthening the gastrocnemius-soleus and on approach to the calcaneus and cuboid laterally.

POSITIONING

- The patient is placed supine with the foot at the end of the operating table so that surgeon can sit comfortably.

PROCEDURE

STEP 1: FIRST RAY OSTEOTOMIES

- A dorsal closing wedge osteotomy of the first metatarsal and opening wedge osteotomy of the medial cuneiform are performed.
- The first metatarsal and cuneiform are identified through a medial incision on the foot (Fig. 5).
- The anterior tibial tendon is partially dissected free of its attachment to the cuneiform in order to perform an osteotomy in the middle of this bone.
  - Using fluoroscopy, needles are placed to identify the midportion of the cuneiform and a location at least 1 cm distal to the physis of the first metatarsal (Figs. 6 and 7).
  - Careful attention is paid to not disturb the first metatarsal physis with either the osteotomy or physeal stripping on the lateral aspect of that bone.
- A dorsal closing wedge osteotomy is then performed on the first metatarsal (Fig. 8). A large 20–30° wedge is removed.
- Next, an opening wedge osteotomy of the medial cuneiform is performed based on the plantar surface (Fig. 9).
  - The wedge from the metatarsal will be inserted into the plantar aspect of the medial cuneiform later.
  - These osteotomies will be fixed with one or two Kirschner wires (K-wires) after completing the other osteotomies.

PEARLS

- *Partial decubitus may bring the hip joint capsule more directly into view and better define the iliac crest and originating muscles.*

Equipment

- Image intensifier in the room

PEARLS

- *Delay surgery until the patient's first metatarsal physis is closed to allow for a more proximal metatarsal cut (Fig. 10).*
- *Take a large wedge of about 30° from the first metatarsal.*

PITFALLS

- *Avoid injury to the first metatarsal growth plate with periosteal stripping.*

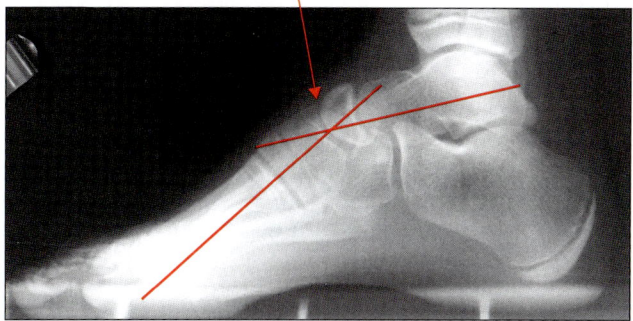

Focus on Apex of Deformity

FIGURE 4

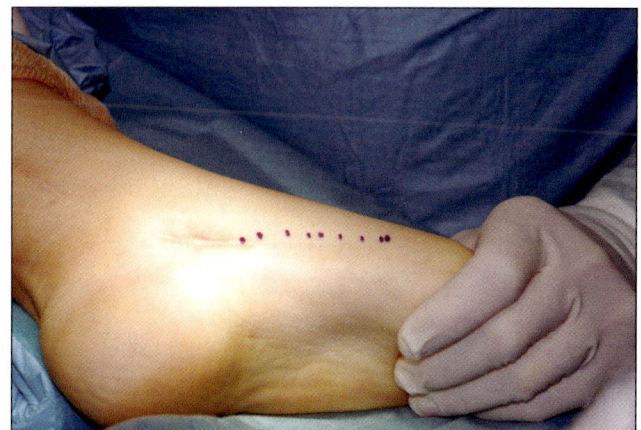

FIGURE 5

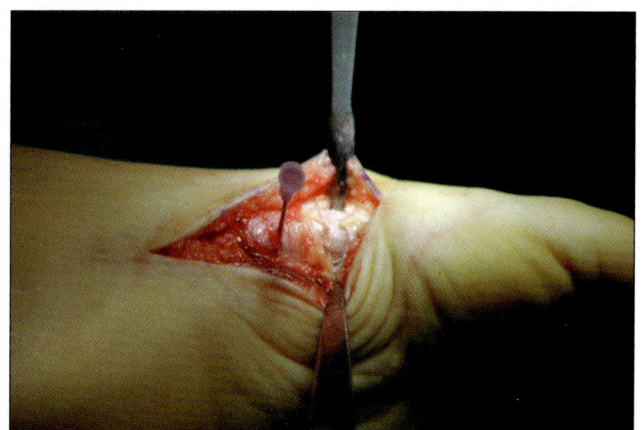

FIGURE 6

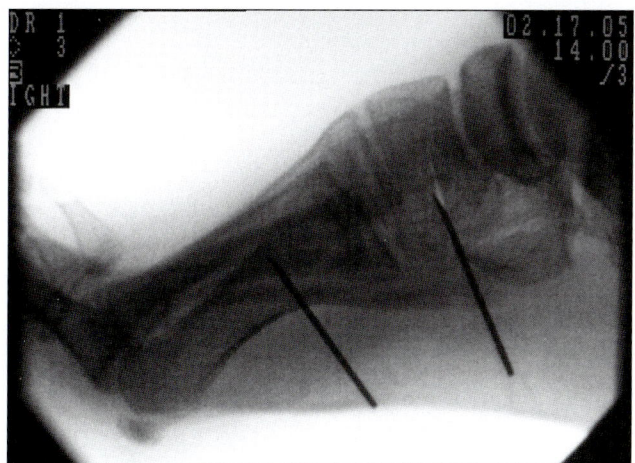

FIGURE 7

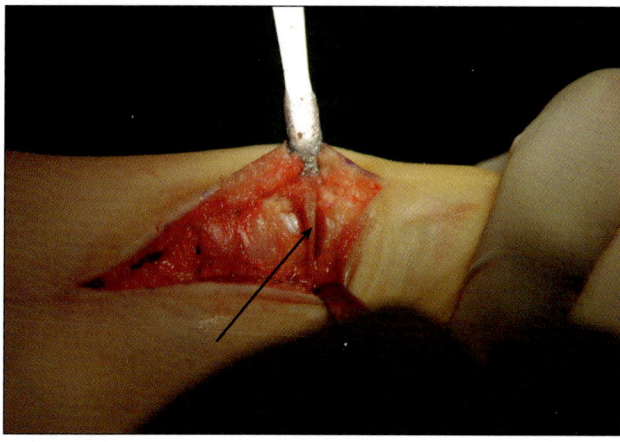

FIGURE 8

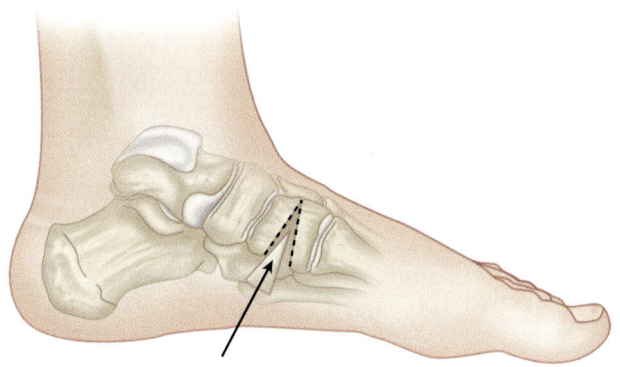

FIGURE 9

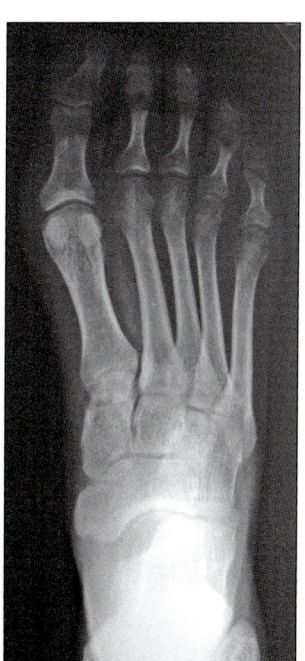

FIGURE 10

STEP 2: CUBOID CLOSING WEDGE OSTEOTOMY

- A cuboid closing wedge osteotomy corrects the forefoot varus and aids dorsiflexion of the forefoot. The removed wedge can be used as supplemental bone grafting for the cuneiform as necessary.
- The calcaneal-cuboid and cuboid–fifth metatarsal joints are identified.
- A cuboid lateral closing wedge about 5–10 mm in size is removed (Fig. 11).
- This osteotomy will be fixed with one K-wire.

STEP 3: METATARSAL OSTEOTOMIES

- If there is plantar prominence of the second and third metatarsal heads after the above osteotomies, dorsal closing wedge metatarsal osteotomies should be considered.
- A single incision was made over the dorsum of the foot between the second and third metatarsals (see Fig. 11).
- Closing abduction wedge osteotomies at the base of these metatarsals is performed.
- These are fixed individually also with intramedullary K-wires.

STEP 4: CALCANEAL OSTEOTOMY

- If there is fixed hindfoot deformity as determined preoperatively by the kneeling test (see Fig. 3), or if residual varus remains after the above osteotomies, this osteotomy is performed.
- The calcaneal osteotomy is a lateral displacement and closing wedge of the calcaneus.
- Figure 12 shows the lateral incision placement for approach to the calcaneus and cuboid.
- The lateral calcaneus is exposed just below the peroneals (Fig. 13)
- A saw is used to cut two thirds of the way through plus the anterior and posterior corners (Fig. 14). An osteotome is used to complete the cut.
- A Chandler retractor allows easy exposure to the calcaneus (Fig. 15).
- A lateral closing wedge osteotomy is performed using the saw (Fig. 16).
- If there is a calcaneus position of the os calcis, the osteotomy of this bone can be rotated into a more neutral position.

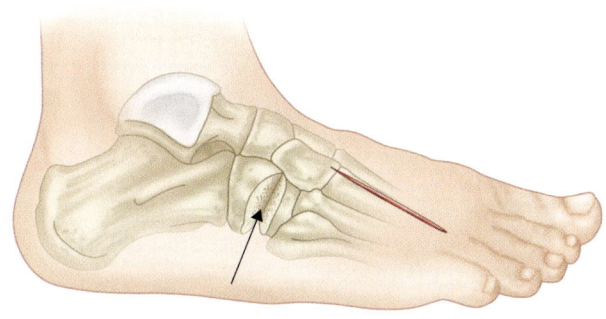

FIGURE 11

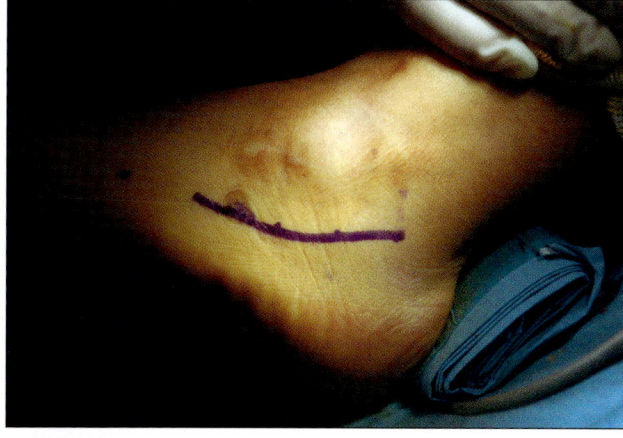

FIGURE 12

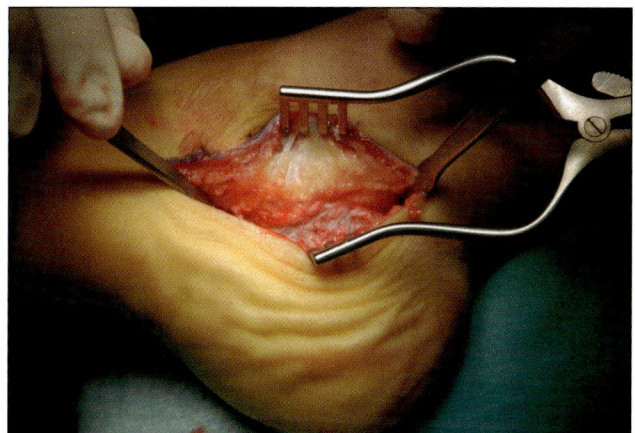

FIGURE 13

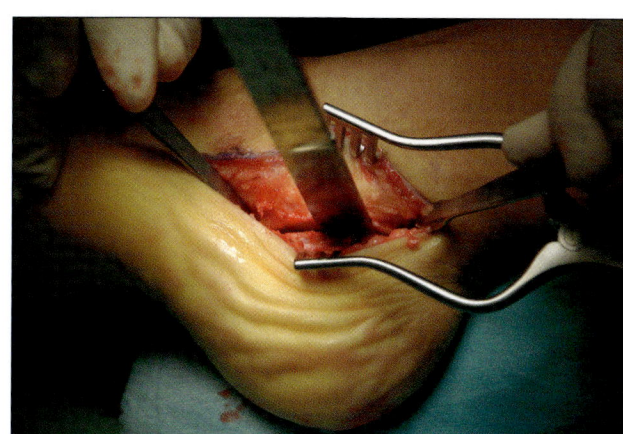

FIGURE 14

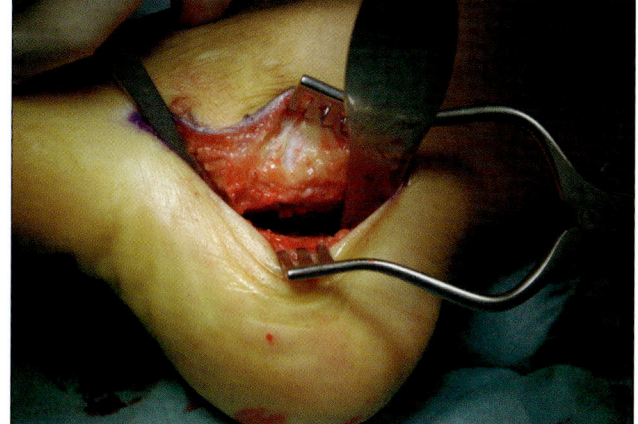

FIGURE 15

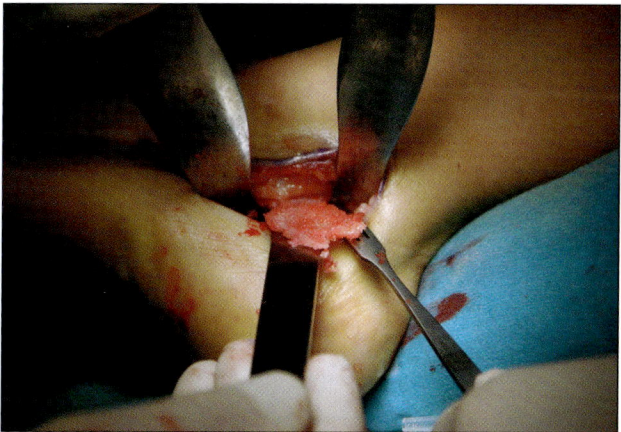

FIGURE 16

Step 5: K-Wire Fixation

- All of the osteotomy sites are then fixed with K-wires.
- Fixation starts with the first metatarsal, where pinning of the first ray and then the medial cuneiform is accomplished with the bone graft placed in the open wedge osteotomy of the cuneiform (Fig. 17).
- The pins are also readied in position in the cuboid and metatarsals for sequential pinning.
- After pinning of the forefoot, the calcaneus is positioned and also fixed with two K-wires entering through the heel in a plantar-to-dorsal direction (Fig. 18).

Step 6: Plantar Fasciotomies

- Fasciotomies of the superficial plantar fascia are also performed through a small percutaneous incision if the fascia is tight after the osteotomies are fixed.

Step 7: Peroneus Longus–to–Peroneus Brevis Transfer

- If the patient had neurologic involvement, such as Charcot-Marie-Tooth disease, this transfer is considered.
- The peroneus longus tendon is released just under the cuboid and reattached to the peroneus brevis to decrease the plantar pull of the first metatarsal and aid the abduction on the foot (Fig. 19).
  - This should be performed after the cuboid closing wedge.
  - The bones are pinned to set the new tendon length.

POSTOPERATIVE CARE AND EXPECTED OUTCOMES

- After the bones are fixed and wounds closed, the patient is placed in a below-the-knee cast, which is widely split.
- The univalved cast is closed at 1 week. The cast and pins are removed under oral light sedation at about 4 weeks in the clinic and radiographs are obtained.
- A new below-the-knee walking cast is applied for a second 4 weeks for a total of 8 weeks of immobilization.

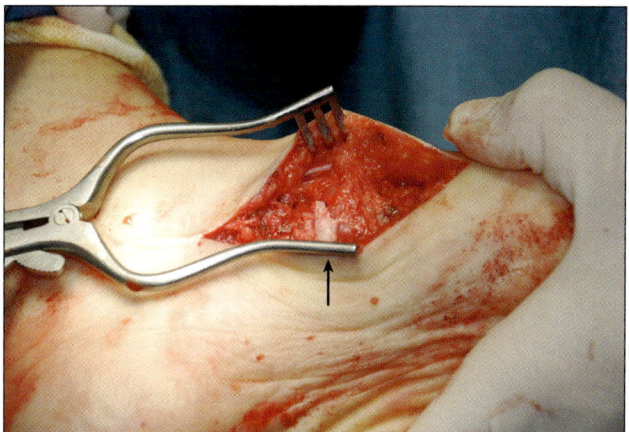

FIGURE 17

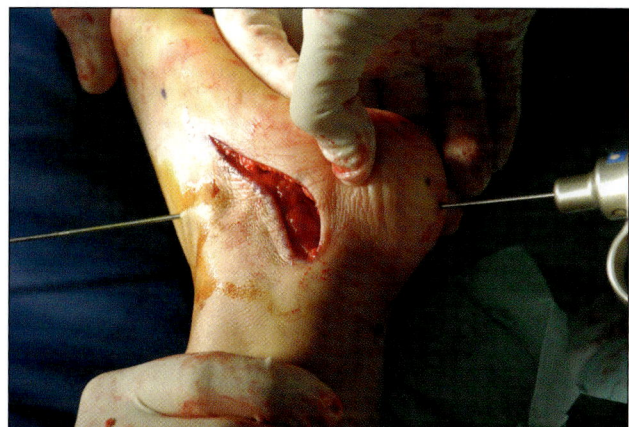

FIGURE 18

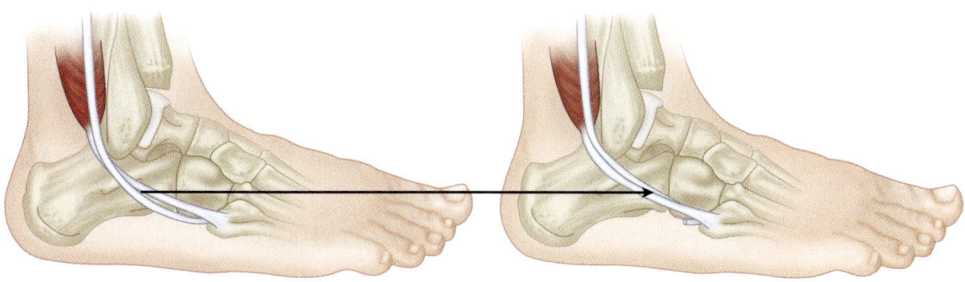

FIGURE 19

EVIDENCE

Coleman SS, Chesnut WJ. A simple test for hindfoot flexibiltiy in the cavovarus foot. Clin Orthop Relat Res. 1977;(133):60–2.

The authors described the standing test for supple versus rigid hindfoot varus. (Level IV evidence)

Dwyer FC. Osteotomy of the calcaneum for pes cavus. J Bone Joint Surg [Br]. 1959;41:80–6.

In this paper, the author described a lateral closing wedge calcaneal osteotomy to correct varus deformity. In 1963, he described a medial opening wedge calcaneal osteotomy to correct the "relapsed clubfoot." (Level IV evidence)

Giannini S, Ceccarelli F, Benedetti MG, et al. Surgical treatment of adult idiopathic cavus foot with plantar fasciotomy, naviculocuneiform arthrodesis, and cuboid osteotomy: a review of thirty-nine cases. J Bone Joint Surg [Am]. 2002;84(Suppl 2):62–9.

The authors decribed midfoot fusions to correct the cavus. (Level IV evidence)

Japas LM. Surgical treatment of pes cavus by tarsal V-osteotomy: preliminary report. J Bone Joint Surg [Am]. 1968;50:927–44.

The author described osteotomies across joints with his "V" osteotomy of the midfoot. (Level IV evidence)

Koutsogiannis L. Treatment of mobile flat foot by displacement osteotomy of the calcaneus. J Bone Joint Surg [Br]. 1971;53:96–100.

The author modified Dwyer's wedge osteotomy and described his results with a "displacement" osteotomy of the calcaneus. (Level IV evidence)

McElvenny RT, Caldwell GD. A new operation for correction of cavus foot; fusion of first metatarsocuneiform navicular joints. Clin Orthop. 1958;4(11):85–92.

The authors described fusion of the first metatarsal, cuneiform, and navicular joints. (Level IV evidence)

Mubarak SJ, Van Valin SE. Osteotomies of the foot for cavus deformities in children. J Pediatr Orthop. 2009;29:294–9.

The authors provided a description of the operation outlined here. (Level IV evidence)

Saltzman CL, Fehrle MJ, Cooper RR, et al. Triple arthrodesis: twenty-five and forty-four-year average follow-up of the same patients. J Bone Joint Surg [Am]. 1999;81:1391–402.

The authors detailed long-term follow-up at 25 and 40 years after a triple arthrodesis. This study found suboptimal results for triple arthrodesis as time went on and thus demonstrated the need for joint-sparing surgery in younger patients. (Level IV evidence)

Siffert RS, del Torto U. "Beak" triple arthrodesis for severe cavus deformity. Clin Orthop Relat Res. 1983;(181):64–7.

The authors described a triple arthrodesis to correct cavus. (Level IV evidence)

Weiner DS, Morscher M, Junko JT, et al. The Akron dome midfoot osteotomy as a salvage procedure for the treatment of rigid pes cavus: a retrospective review. J Pediatr Orthop. 2008;28:68–80.

The authors described osteotomies across joints with their "Akron dome osteotomy." (Level IV evidence)

Flexor Tenotomy for Congenital Curly Toe

Susan T. Mahan

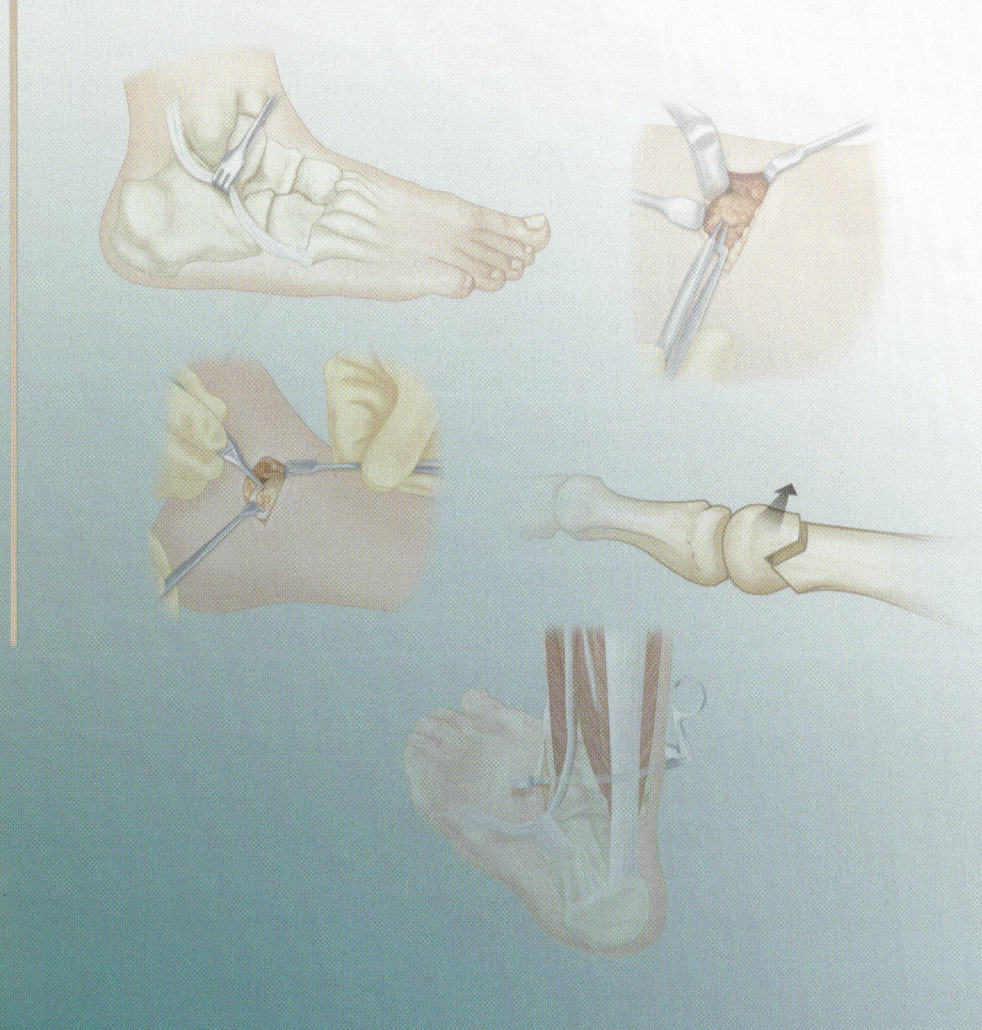

Treatment Options

• Flexor to extensor tendon transfer (originally described by Girdlestone) is an alternate procedure for correction of curly toe, but in a randomized double-blind prospective trial was found to have no difference in outcome. Others have found flexor-to-extensor transfer to have a higher morbidity than flexor tenotomy, including higher rates of postoperative stiffness.

INDICATIONS

■ Persistence of the congenital curly toe deformity later in childhood.

■ Symptoms, including skin breakdown, painful callosities, and shoewear issues, which are not amenable to nonoperative care.

■ Conservative measures, including taping and splinting, are generally not successful for symptomatic curly toe after age 6 years.

EXAMINATION/IMAGING

■ Curly toe is characterized by flexion at the proximal interphalangeal joint, varus deviation, and external rotation usually of the third or fourth toe. Flexing of the metatarsophalangeal joint should allow the distal deformities to be passively corrected.

■ The curly toe is usually the third or fourth toe (Fig. 1), which tucks under (and appears to lift up) the more medial toe.

SURGICAL ANATOMY

■ Figure 2 shows the relevant surgical anatomy for the release of a curly toe.

■ Digital branches of the plantar artery and digital neurovascular bundles run on the medial and lateral side of the toe, outside the tendon sheath.

■ The flexor digitorum brevis splits at the level of the metacarpal into two slips that then insert medially and laterally on the middle phalanx. The flexor digitorum longus inserts more distally on the base of the distal phalanx.

■ The incision should be over the proximal phalanx to readily access and release both flexor tendons.

POSITIONING

■ The patient is placed supine with a tourniquet on the operated limb.

■ The surgery may be performed with the surgeon seated facing the sole of the foot.

PORTALS/EXPOSURES

■ An oblique or transverse incision is made over the plantar aspect of the proximal phalanx.

■ The subcutaneous tissue is divided and the flexor sheath opened.

PROCEDURE

■ A small curved hemostat is placed around the three tendon slips (including the long and two short flexor tendons) and they are pulled out of the wound (Fig. 3).

■ The tendons are completely divided.

■ The interphalangeal joints are passively corrected to confirm correction of the deformity.

■ The incision is irrigated and closed with simple absorbable skin sutures.

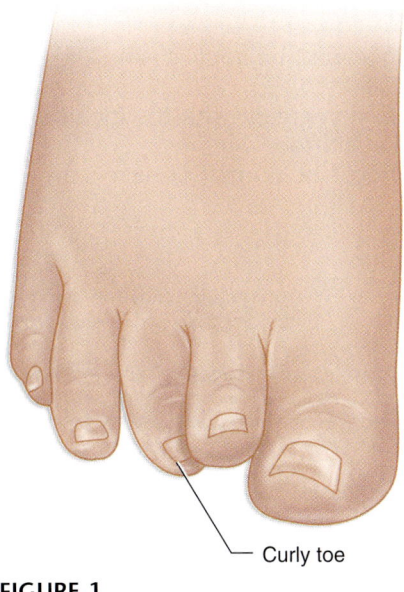

Curly toe

FIGURE 1

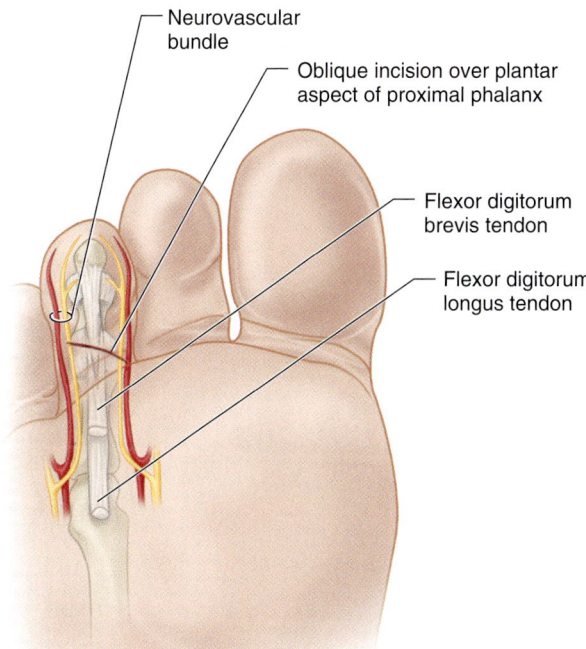

Neurovascular bundle

Oblique incision over plantar aspect of proximal phalanx

Flexor digitorum brevis tendon

Flexor digitorum longus tendon

FIGURE 2

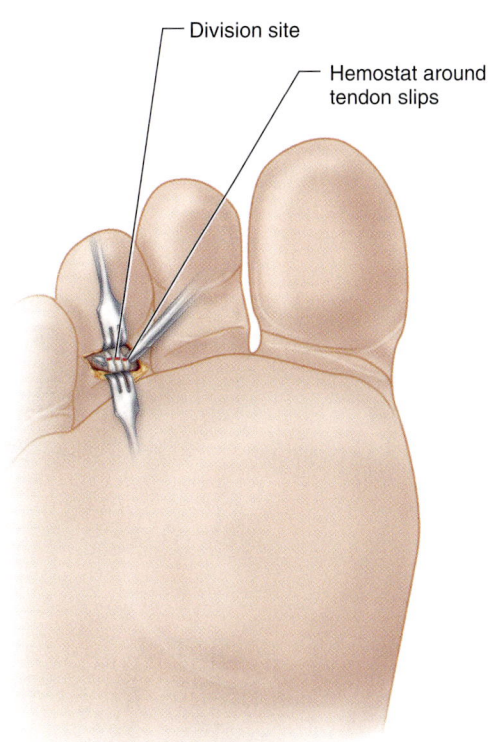

Division site

Hemostat around tendon slips

FIGURE 3

POSTOPERATIVE CARE AND EXPECTED OUTCOMES

- A soft dressing should be applied, and the patient may ambulate as tolerated.
- Crossing the flexion crease with the incision may lead to tethering and a stiff toe.
- Appearance should be normal or near-normal in 95% of feet.

EVIDENCE

Hamer AJ, Stanley D, Smith TWD. Surgery for curly toe deformity: a double-blind, randomised, prospective trial. J Bone Joint Surg [Br]. 1993;75:662–3.

This prospective, randomized, double-blinded clinical trial compared flexor tenotomy to flexor-to-extensor transfer for congenital curly toe. All patients in the trial were bilaterally affected and one foot received one procedure while the other foot received the other procedure. There was no difference between the two procedures, and all operated toes were satisfactory at follow-up. Flexor tenotomy was found to be satisfactory treatment for congenital curly toe, and the additional tendon transfer was not found to be necessary.

Pollard JP, Morrison PJM. Flexor tenotomy in the treatment of curly toes. Proc R Soc Med. 1975;68:14–5.

The authors presented a retrospective review of flexor tenotomy compared to flexor-to-extensor transfer for treatment of curly toes. Results of flexor-to-extensor transfer were found to be less satisfactory in both appearance and function. Fifty-eight percent of toes that underwent the tendon transfer were found to be stiff.

Ross ERS, Menelaus MB. Open flexor tenotomy for hammer toes and curly toes in childhood. J Bone Joint Surg [Br]. 1984;66:770–1.

This retrospective review with average 9.8-year follow-up found normal or nearly normal appearance in 95% of treated toes. Tethering from a flexion crease scar caused stiffness in those with poor results.

Tibialis Posterior Tendon Transfer

Travis Matheney and Michael Glotzbecker

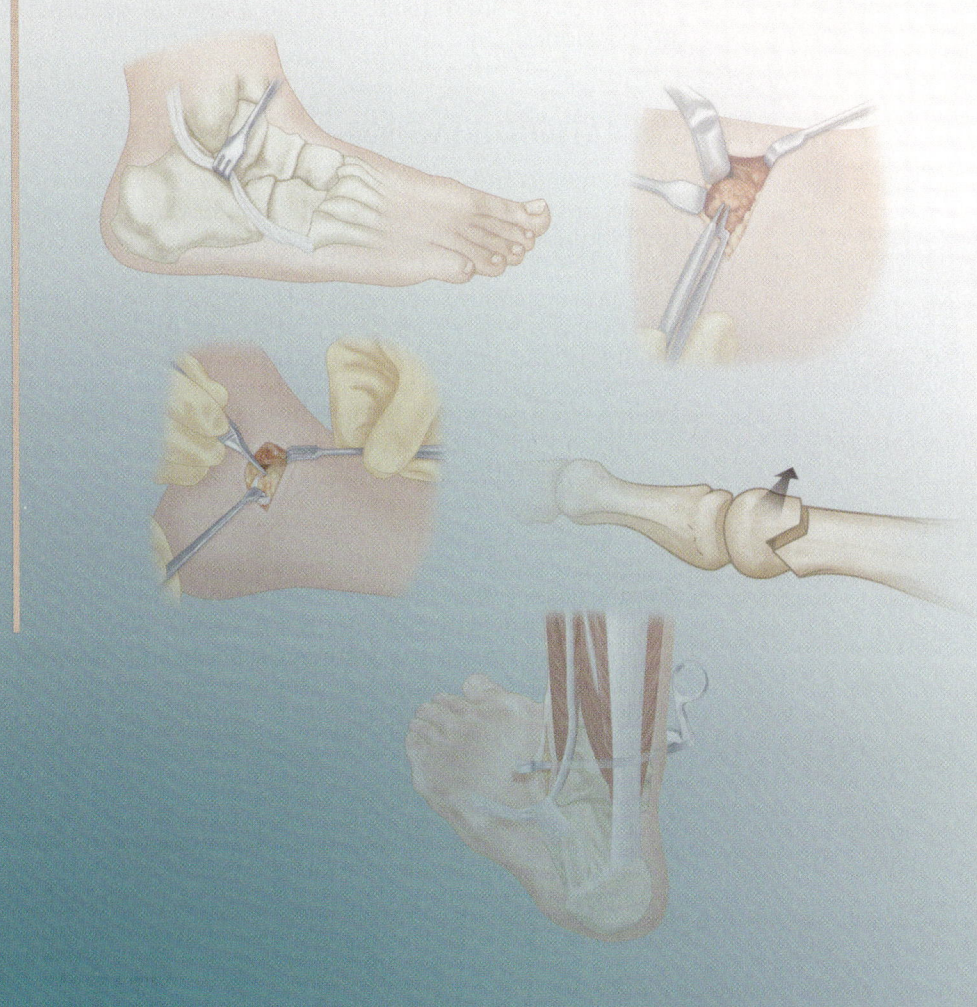

Controversies

- Whether to transfer to the entire tendon or perform a split transfer is debated. Proponents of splitting the transfer state that the results are very good and do not risk collapse of the hindfoot into valgus, one complication of transferring the entire tendon.

Treatment Options

- Prior to surgery, attempts can be made to improve range of motion with serial casting.
- An articulated ankle-foot orthosis or supramalleolar orthosis that can control the foot motion may be more desired by the patient and family.

INDICATIONS

- Spastic, flexible equinovarus-cavovarus foot deformity in the ambulatory child or adult with cerebral palsy or brain injury with "over-pull" of the tibialis posterior.
- Recurrence of clubfoot deformity.
- Patients with weak dorsiflexion secondary to neuromuscular disease.
- Lengthening and transfer of the tendon have both been described.
- Additionally, one may transfer all or half of the tendon.
- Consideration should be given to whether the foot and ankle have adequate motor units to power dorsiflexion and are struggling with the varus over-pull of the tibialis posterior, in which case a split transfer might be advised; or the patient would benefit more from assistance with dorsiflexion and transfer of the entire tendon due to a general weakness of dorsiflexion.

EXAMINATION/IMAGING

- The peroneus brevis may be relatively weaker, allowing the tibialis posterior to "over-pull" the midfoot into supination and the hindfoot into varus, especially during the swing phase of gait.
- The gastrocnemius-soleus must also be assessed for contracture.
- The goal is a balanced foot in both stance and gait.
- Hindfoot varus flexibility may be tested with the Coleman block test (Coleman and Chestnut, 1977).
- Preoperative plain films, including standing anteroposterior, lateral, and oblique views of both feet, should be obtained to confirm no fixed bony deformity.

SURGICAL ANATOMY

- The tibialis posterior has a broad insertion and is best found proximal to the first ray through the medial incision.
- When transferring to the peroneus brevis, care should be taken not to completely disrupt the lateral fascia protecting the peroneal tendons from subluxation over the lateral malleolus.

POSITIONING

- The patient is positioned supine with a small rolled blanket beneath the ipsilateral greater trochanter.
- A nonsterile tourniquet is applied to the proximal thigh, and the remainder of the leg is prepped in sterile manner.

PORTALS/EXPOSURES

- Three incisions are outlined in Figure 1.
- Three or four incisions are used, and incision placement depends on whether one is performing a whole-tendon or split-tendon transfer.

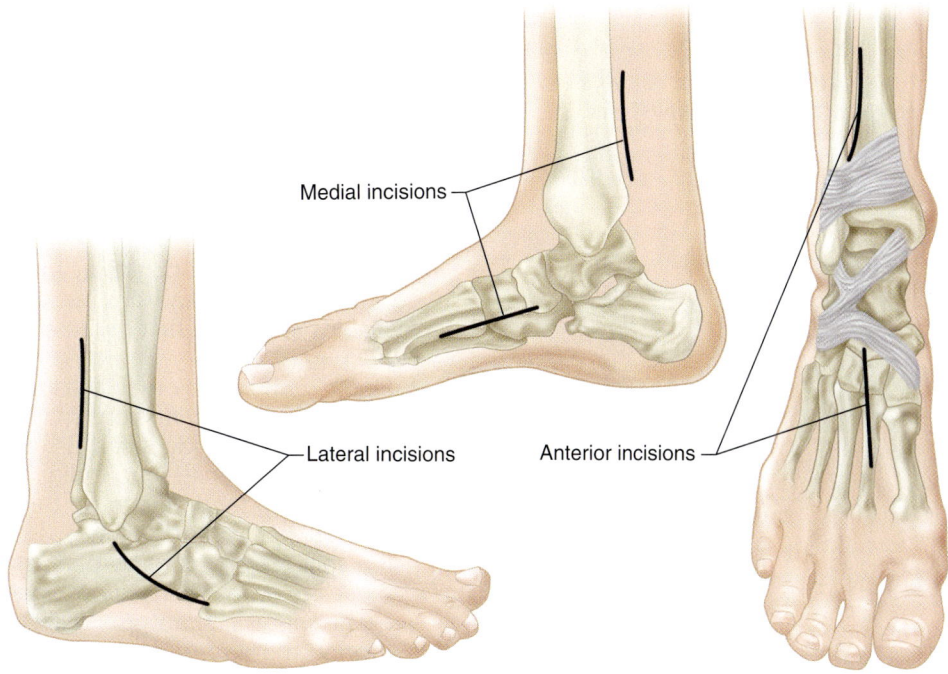

Medial incisions

Lateral incisions

Anterior incisions

FIGURE 1

PROCEDURE

STEP 1

- The tourniquet may be used at the surgeon's discretion. The procedure does not typically result in a particularly bloody field.
- If a gastrocnemius-soleus lengthening is required, this should be performed first and the wound closed before proceeding with the tendon transfer portion of the surgery.

STEP 2

- The tendon transfer begins at the medial side of the foot with an incision extending from just anterior to the tip of the medial malleolus along the first ray to the medial cuneiform (see Fig. 1).
  - Figure 2 shows the medial aspect of the foot with proximal and distal medial incisions marked.
- The tendon is first identified proximal to its fanlike insertion and the sheath is opened longitudinally.
  - If the entire tendon is to be transferred, it is harvested from its insertion as far distal as possible (Fig. 3).
  - If a split transfer is to be performed, the plantar half is sharply harvested from its insertion, again as far distal as possible.
    - ◆ The split is carried proximally and the foot is everted to bring more of the proximal tendon into view.
  - The tendon sheath *should not* be completely opened proximal to the tip of the malleolus to maintain a constraint for the remaining tendon.
  - A nonabsorbable suture is used to tag the free end of the tendon for a split transfer and a heavy absorbable suture is used for transferring the entire tendon.

STEP 3

- The second incision is made approximately 1 cm above the medial malleolus along the posterior border of the tibia.
- If the entire tendon is to be transferred, the surgeon may be able to eliminate this incision by making a larger window in the interosseous membrane (see Step 4) and pulling the transfer through.
- If utilizing this second incision, the tibialis posterior tendon sheath lies just beneath the deep fascia and immediately posterior to the lateral border of the tibia. The sheath is opened and the tendon is brought proximally into the wound.
- Figure 4 shows the right foot with a hemostat pulling the proximal tibialis posterior tendon into the wound from its distal release. Note that in this particular case an additional Z-lengthening of the Achilles tendon has already been performed.

STEP 4

- At this point the preparation is made to pass the free end of the tendon.
- To transfer the entire tendon, an anterior incision is made over the anterior muscle compartment lateral to the tibial crest (see Fig. 1).
  - The anterior compartment muscles and neurovascular bundle are carefully elevated off the interosseous membrane.
  - A 2-cm-wide × 4-cm-high window is made in the interosseous membrane (Fig. 5). The tibialis posterior lies directly behind the membrane. Care is taken not to plunge with the knife through this membrane to avoid injury to vascular structures posterior to it.
  - The free tibialis muscle and tendon are brought through the window and the medial incisions are closed.

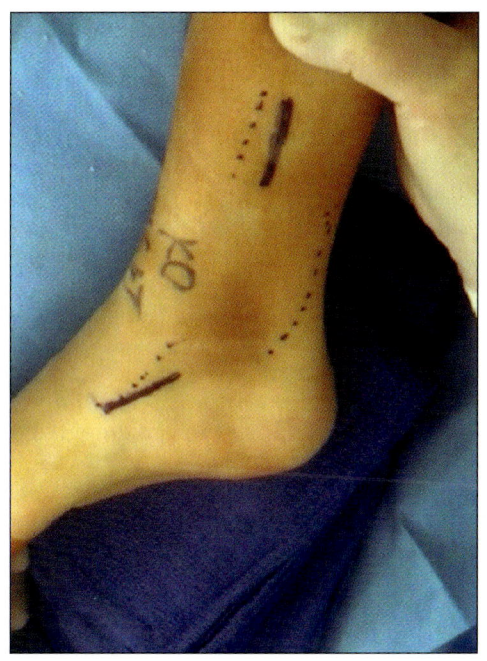

FIGURE 2

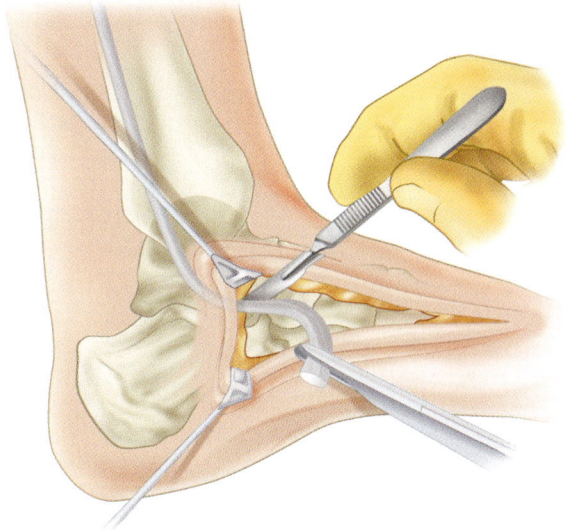

FIGURE 3

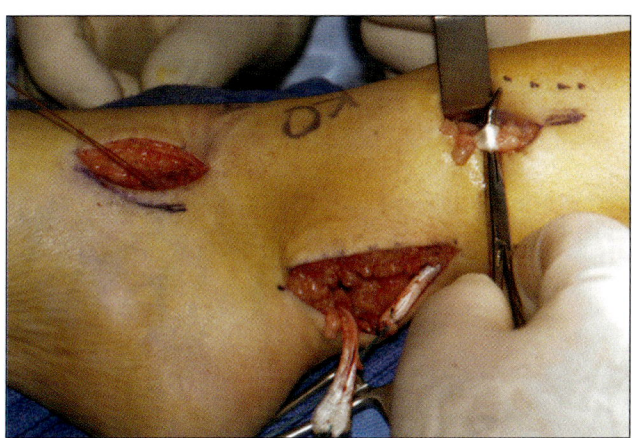

FIGURE 4

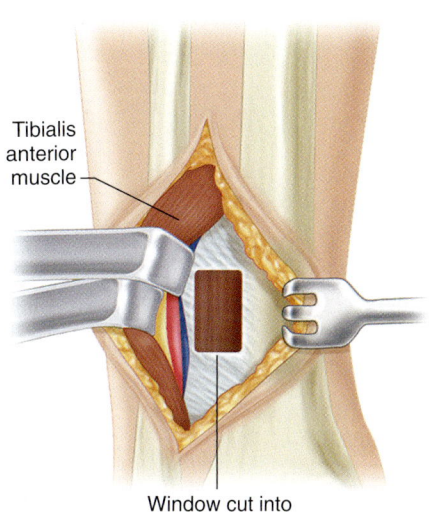

Tibialis anterior muscle

Window cut into interosseous membrane

FIGURE 5

- Figure 6 shows the medial foot with malleable tendon passer and transferred end of the tibialis posterior tendon attached and ready to pull through to the anterior wound (left side of picture).
■ For a split transfer, a third incision is made extending from the distal posterior fibula proximally 3 cm and the peroneus brevis is identified (see Fig. 1).
  - A tendon passer is used to pass the free end of the tendon from *medial* to *lateral,* being careful to stay in contact with the posterior tibia.
  - Figure 7 shows a cross section and the posterior aspect of the ankle. In the cross-sectional view, the *arrow* depicts the correct passage of the tendon along the posterior tibia. In the posterior view, the tendon passer is seen bringing the split end of the tendon through to the proximal lateral incision adjacent to the peroneus brevis.
  - After passage, the surgeon must confirm that the tendon is released enough proximally so as not to create an acute angle toward the lateral wound.

STEP 5

■ The final incision is now made to prepare the tendon transfer insertion site (see Fig. 1).
■ For whole-tendon transfer, an incision is made over the second (or middle) cuneiform.
  - The dorsal periosteum is carefully elevated. A 4.5-mm drill hole is created through the cuneiform and the free tendon is passed from the anterior wound with a tendon passer beneath the extensor retinaculum.
  - Figure 8 shows the anterior right foot depicting the tibialis whole tendon pulled through the interosseous window and passing beneath the extensor retinaculum to the distal, anterior incision over the second cuneiform.
  - Figure 9 shows the tibialias posterior about to be pulled through from the proximal to distal anterior wound using a malleable tendon passer.

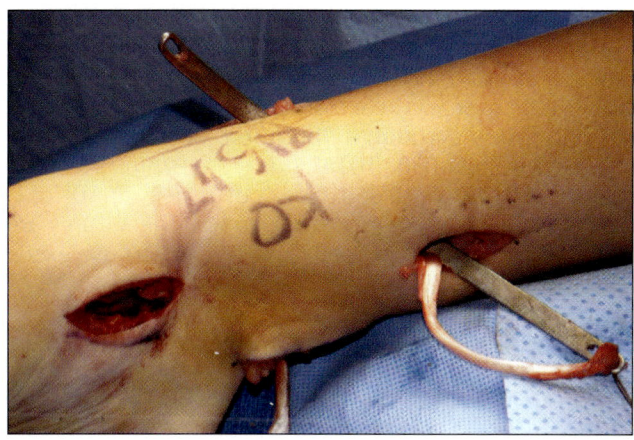

FIGURE 6

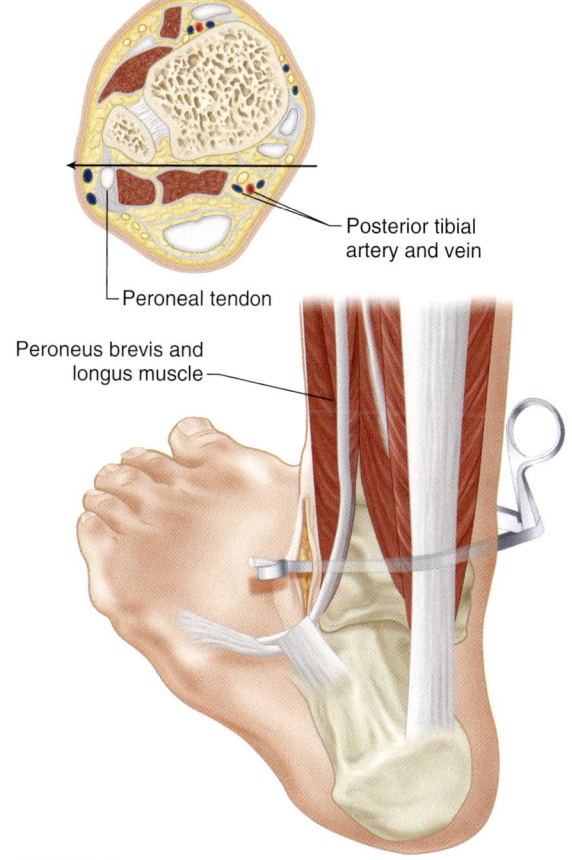

Posterior tibial artery and vein

Peroneal tendon

Peroneus brevis and longus muscle

FIGURE 7

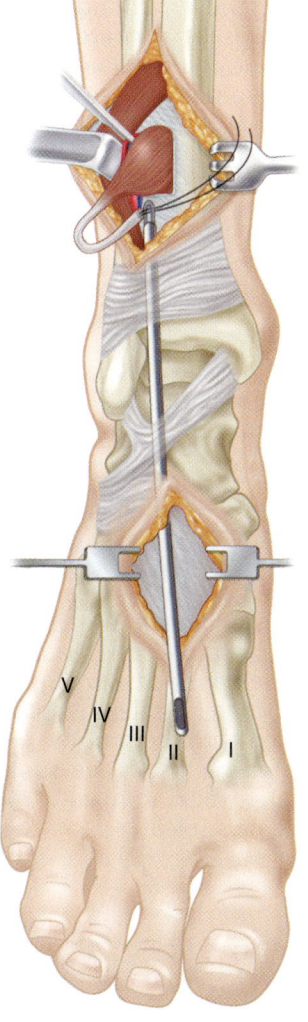

V
IV
III
II
I

FIGURE 8

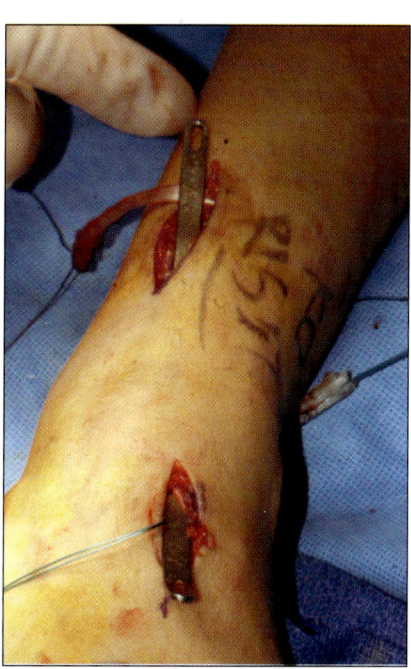

FIGURE 9

- The anterior wound is now closed. A straight Keith needle is used to pass the free tendon through the dorsal hole in the cuneiform and pull its two absorbable tagging stitches through the plantar skin, each stitch as a separate pass. The needles are passed through a "bumper" of sterile felt and then a sterile button (Fig. 10)
- The midfoot incision is closed. The foot is held in 10° of dorsiflexion and neutral subtalar motion as the sutures are tied down over the button. Care is taken not to use excessive force for the knot as it may result in pressure ulceration of the plantar skin.

- For the split-tendon transfer, a fourth incision is made extending from the base of the fifth metatarsal and extending along the course of the peroneal tendons to the tip of the lateral malleolus (see Fig. 1).
  - The sheath of the peroneus brevis is opened sharply. A tendon passer is used to pass the free tibialias posterior end behind the lateral malleolus, inside the sheath of the brevis and underneath the retinaculum holding the peroneal tendons in place.
  - Two or three longitudinal splits are made in the distal peroneus brevis and the free end of the tibialis posterior transfer is woven through them (Fig. 11).
  - The ankle is set at neutral subtalar position for varus and valgus, and the distal end of the tendon transfer is sutured to the insertion of the peroneus brevis. The interwoven areas are oversewn with nonabsorbable suture.
  - The remaining wound is closed with an assistant holding the foot in corrected position.

STEP 6

- The wounds are dressed and a short-leg cast is applied with the ankle in slight dorsiflexion and neutral hindfoot position.

POSTOPERATIVE CARE AND EXPECTED OUTCOMES

- Weight bearing is allowed or restricted based on surgeon preference.
- The cast is removed at 2 weeks and bivalved/re-lined for skin and wound check.
- The patient remains in a cast for 4–6 weeks total. If new braces are required as a result of a new position of the foot, the patient may be casted for this at the first postoperative visit and then returned to the previous cast until brace pickup, generally at the 4- to 6-week postoperative time point.
- If a gastrocnemius-soleus lengthening is performed in conjunction with the transfer, a knee immobilizer may be used full time for the first 2 weeks followed by nighttime wear for an additional 4 weeks to maintain the new length of the healing gastrocnemius-soleus.

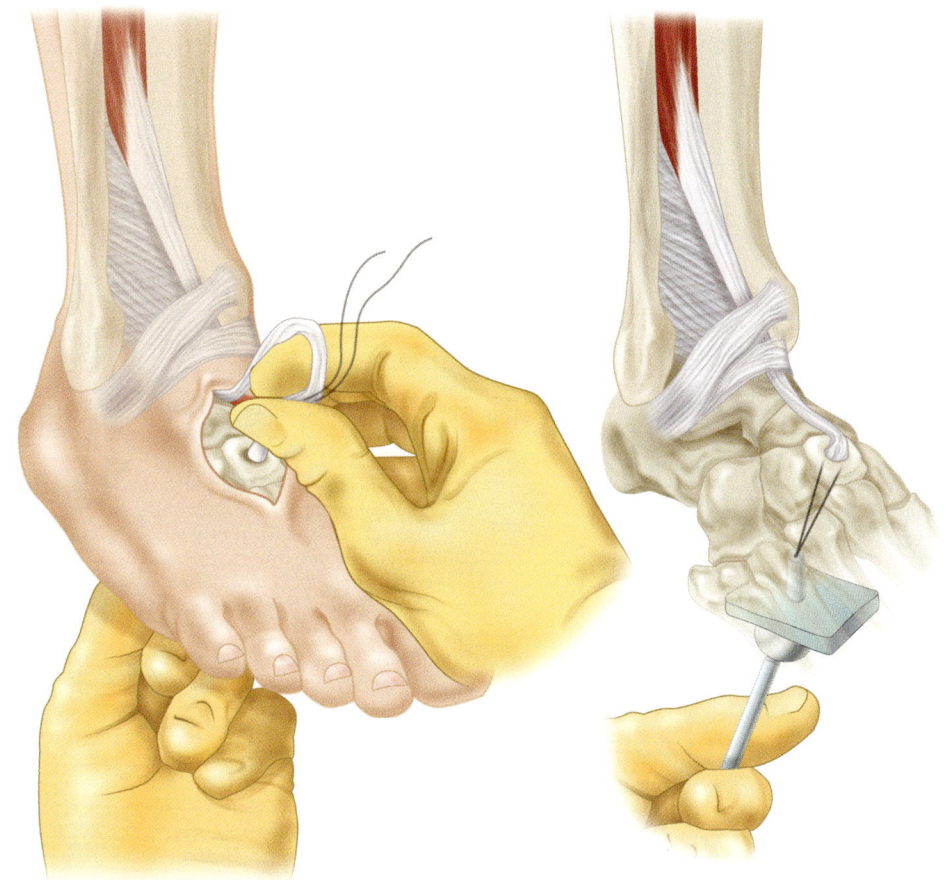

FIGURE 10

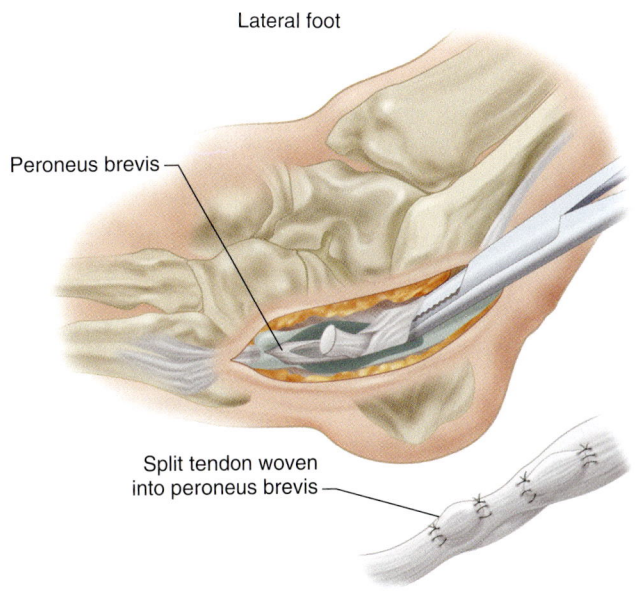

Lateral foot

Peroneus brevis

Split tendon woven
into peroneus brevis

FIGURE 11

EVIDENCE

Coleman SS, Chestnut WJ. A simple test for hindfoot flexibility in the cavovarus foot. Clin Orthop Relat Res. 1977;(123):60–2.

(Level V evidence)

Grzegorzewski A, Borowski A, Pruszczynski B, Wranicz A, Domzalski M, Snyder M. Split tibialis posterior transfer on peroneus brevis for equinovarus foot in CP children. Chir Narzadow Ruchu Ortop Pol. 2007;72:117–20.

The authors found that, in the ambulatory child with diplegia or hemiplegia and flexible equinovarus foot secondary to over-pull of the tibialis posterior, a split transfer to the peroneus brevis resulted in functional improvement in 89% at an average follow-up of 4.6 years. (Level IV evidence)

Miller GM, Hsu JD, Hofer MM, Rentfro R. Posterior tendon transfer: a review of the literature and analysis of 74 procedures. J Pediatr Orthop. 1982;2:363–70.

The authors performed a retrospective analysis of 74 tibialis posterior transfers using a single technique in patients with varied neuromuscular conditions and a minimum 2-year follow-up. Patients with Duchenne's muscular dystrophy with increased gait weakness were good candidates. The best candidate was the ambulatory child with cerebral palsy, but electromyographic gait analysis was highly recommended to confirm dysfunction of the tibialis posterior throughout all of the swing phase. (Level IV evidence)

Root L, Miller SR, Kirz P. Posterior tibial tendon transfer in patients with cerebral palsy. J Bone Joint Surg [Am]. 1987;69:1133–9.

The authors retrospectively reviewed the outcomes of 57 whole-tendon transfers through the interosseous membrane with an average of 9.3 years' follow-up. In order for the tendon transfer to be successful, the foot had to be passively correctable to at least a neutral position and the tendon had to be passed superficial to the extensor retinaculum and inserted into the lateral cuneiform bone. The authors noted that the heel cord should be lengthened before the tendon transfer. (Level IV evidence)

Split Transfer of the Tibialis Anterior Tendon

Travis Matheney

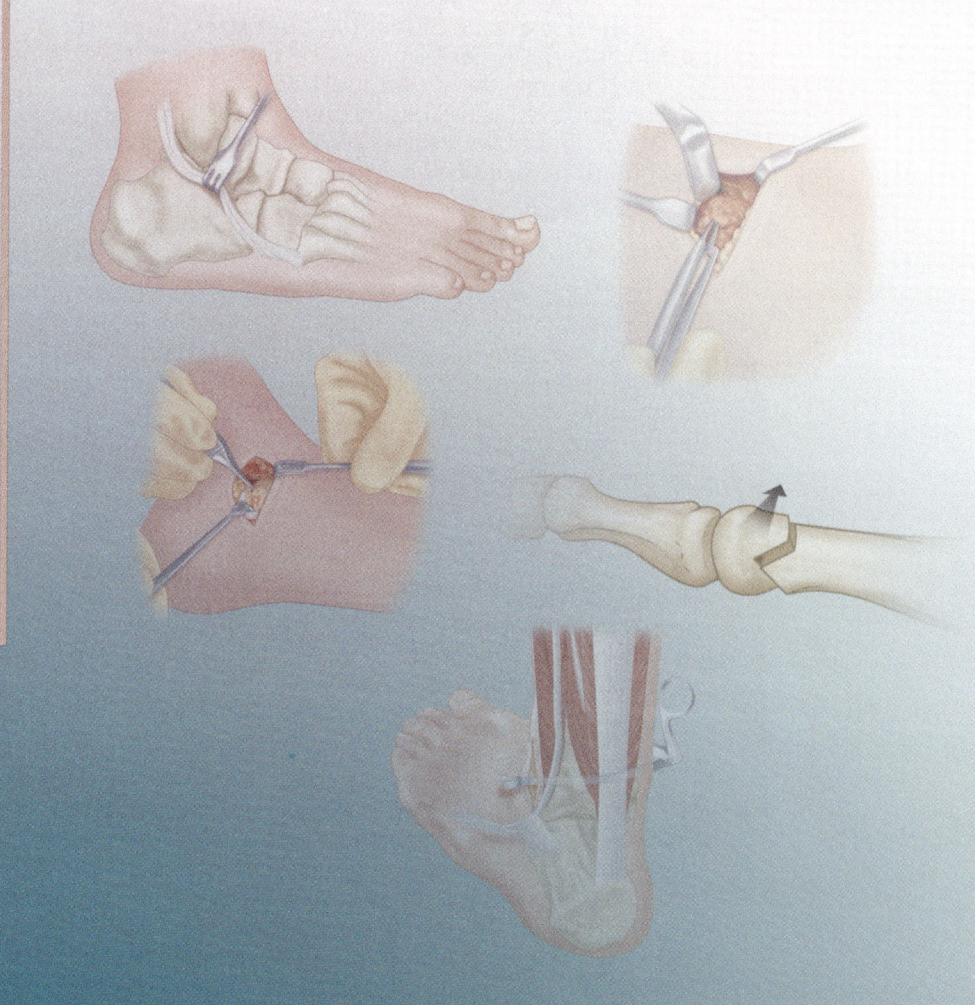

Treatment Options

- Prior to surgery, attempts can be made to improve range of motion with serial casting.
- An articulated ankle-foot orthosis that can control the foot motion may be more desired by the patient and family.

INDICATIONS

- Spastic, flexible equinovarus-cavovarus foot deformity in the ambulatory child or adult with cerebral palsy or brain injury
- Recurrent flexible clubfoot cavovarus deformity
- Weak peroneal muscles and relative "over-pull" of the tibialis anterior leading to foot supination and cavus deformity

EXAMINATION/IMAGING

- The peroneus longus may be relatively weaker, allowing the tibialis anterior to "over-pull" the midfoot into supination and cavus, especially during early stance and during the swing phase of gait.
- The gastrocnemius-soleus and tibialis posterior must also be assessed for contracture.
- The goal is a balanced foot in both stance and gait.
- Hindfoot varus flexibility may be tested with the Coleman block test (Coleman and Chestnut, 1977).
- Preoperative plain films, including standing anteroposterior, lateral, and oblique views of both feet, should be obtained to confirm no fixed bony deformity.

SURGICAL ANATOMY

- The tibialis anterior has a broad insertion and is best found proximal to the first ray through the medial incision.
- When transferring to the cuboid, care should be taken to protect sensory nerve braches from the superficial peroneal nerve.
- The surgeon should try to avoid injury to the short toe extensor muscle belly when exposing the cuboid.

POSITIONING

- The patient is positioned supine with a small rolled blanket beneath the ipsilateral greater trochanter.
- A nonsterile tourniquet is applied to the proximal thigh, and the remainder of the leg is prepped in sterile manner.

PORTALS/EXPOSURES

- Three incisions are outlined in Figure 1:
  - An incision is made along the medial foot distal to the medial malleolus dorsal to the glabrous plantar skin. This will allow access to the insertion of the tibialis anterior as well as the distal extent of the tibialis posterior and plantar fascia (if they are to be lengthened).
  - An incision is made in the distal and anterior lower leg just proximal to the extensor crease and lateral to the anterior tibial spine.
  - An oblique incision is made either in line with the peroneus longus tendon (if transferring to this tendon) or over the cuboid (if transferring to cuboid) in line with the normal skin creases.

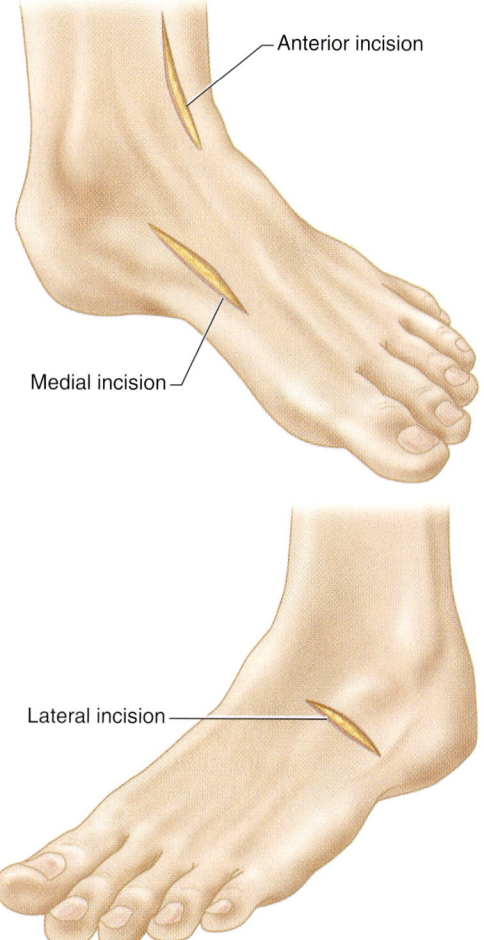

Anterior incision

Medial incision

Lateral incision

FIGURE 1

PEARLS

• *Care should be taken not to over-lengthen the gastrocnemius-soleus.*

PROCEDURE

STEP 1

■ The tourniquet may be used at the surgeon's discretion. The procedure does not typically result in a particularly bloody field.

■ If a gastrocnemius-soleus lengthening is required, this should be performed first and the wound closed before proceeding with the tendon transfer portion of the surgery.

STEP 2

■ The medial incision is made first. Superficial crossing veins are cauterized. If a tibialis posterior tendon or plantar fascia lengthening is to be performed, the surgeon should begin with these.

■ The tibialis anterior tendon is exposed proximal to the insertion and its sheath opened sharply for the distal 2–3 cm.

  • It is easier to find the tendon proximal to the fanlike insertion. The insertion should be carefully exposed as distal as possible.

  • The surgeon will need to harvest the lateral aspect of the tendon as far distal as possible to gain as a maximal amount of length for the transfer (Fig. 2).

■ The free end of the tendon is tagged with a nonabsorbable suture, being careful not to cause "bunching" of the end.

STEP 3

■ The proximal incision is then made. The proximal tibialis anterior is identified and its tendon sheath opened longitudinally.

■ A blunt, malleable tendon passer is passed antegrade through the sheath and the free tendon end is brought proximally into the anterior wound (Fig. 3).

STEP 4

■ The peroneus brevis is seen in the plantar aspect of the wound and the muscle of the short toe extensors in the dorsal aspect. Care must be taken when exposing the dorsal-lateral cuboid to stay *extra*-periosteal to maintain the most stout version of the lateral cuboid cortex.

■ Two drill holes are made in the cuboid with a drill bit large enough to match the diameter of the free end of the tendon for transfer. One hole is made proximal and dorsal, the other distal and plantar (Fig. 4). In Figure 4, the tendon is brought out of the proximal wand. On the left side is the forefoot.

■ A malleable, blunt tendon passer is used to pass the free tendon end beneath the extensor retinaculum toward the lateral incision (Fig. 5).

■ At this point, the lateral and anterior incisions are closed.

STEP 5

■ A 90° clamp may be gently passed through the cuboid drill holes to assure a smooth passage.

■ The free end of the tibialis anterior is passed antegrade through into the proximal hole and out through the distal hole.

■ The foot must be supported at *all* times from this point onward in 10° of dorsiflexion and slight eversion.

■ The tendon free end is sutured back onto itself. This may be augmented by either passing additional sutures through the surrounding periosteum and transferred tendon or placing suture anchors to augment the repair.

■ The lateral wound is closed and a sterile dressing placed.

STEP 6

■ A short-leg cast is applied with 10° of dorsiflexion and slight eversion.

PEARLS

• *Care must be taken not to be aggressive here as it is easy to break through the lateral cuboid bone bridge between drill holes.*

• *Ideally, there will be enough tendon to allow the free end of the tendon to be sutured back to itself once passed through the cuboid.*

• *Passage of the tendon can be assisted by first passing a stitch through the cuboid bone canal and then using this suture to "feed" the tagging suture attached to the tendon through the canal.*

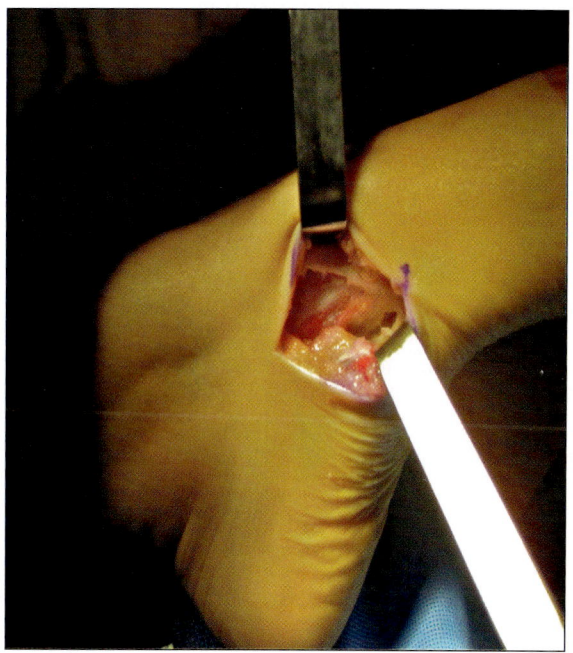

FIGURE 2

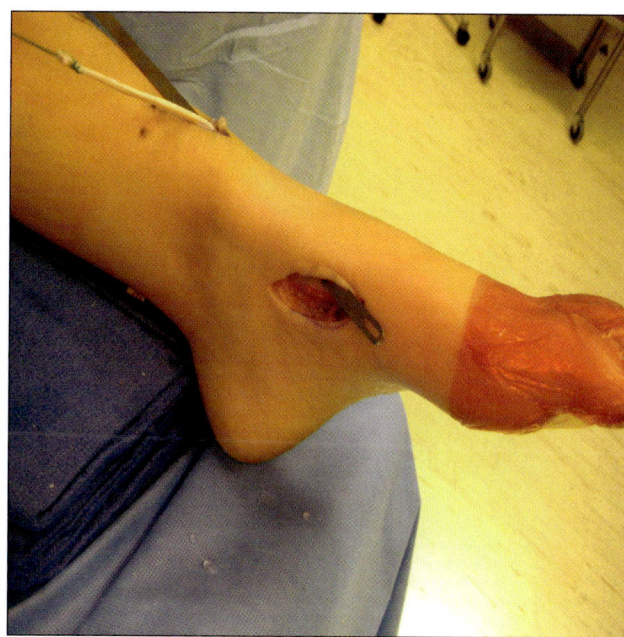

FIGURE 3

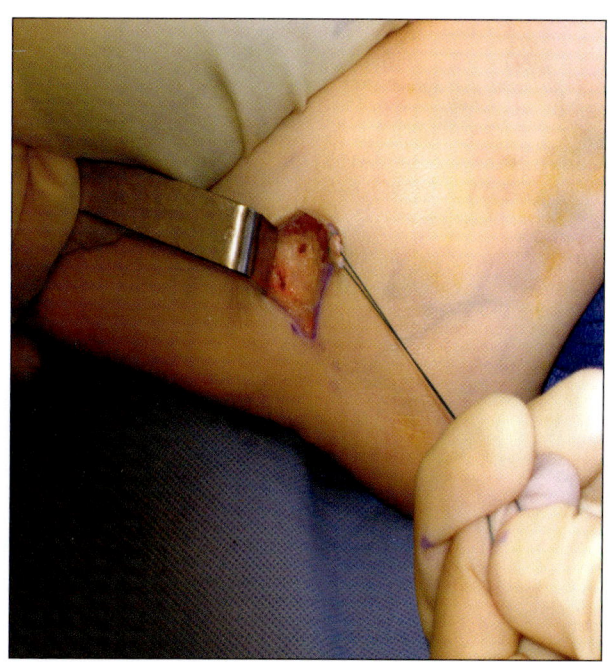

FIGURE 4

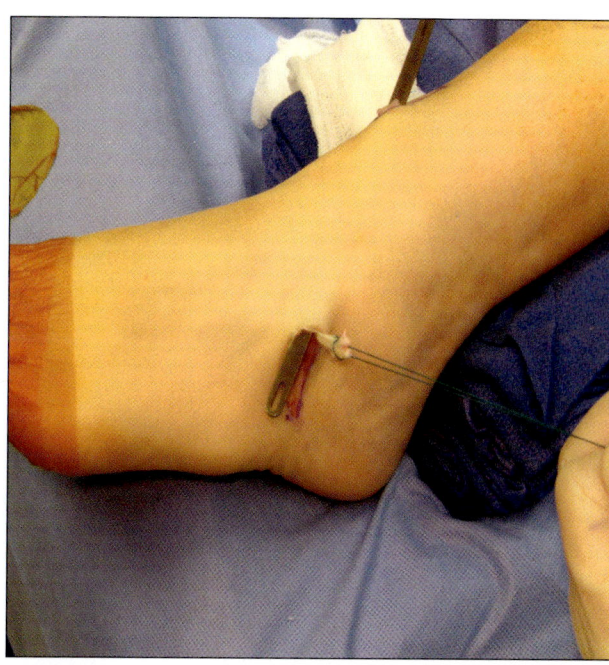

FIGURE 5

POSTOPERATIVE CARE AND EXPECTED OUTCOMES

- Weight bearing is allowed or restricted based on surgeon preference.
- The cast is removed at 2 weeks and bivalved/re-lined for skin and wound check.
- The patient remains in a cast for 4–6 weeks total. If new braces are required as a result of a new position of the foot, the patient may be casted for this at the first postoperative visit and then returned to the previous cast until brace pickup, generally at the 4- to 6-week postoperative time point.
- If a gastrocnemius-soleus lengthening is performed in conjunction with the transfer, a knee immobilizer may be used full time for the first 2 weeks followed by nighttime wear for an additional 4 weeks to maintain the new length of the healing gastrocnemius-soleus.

EVIDENCE

Coleman SS, Chestnut WJ. A simple test for hindfoot flexibility in the cavovarus foot. Clin Orthop Relat Res. 1977;(123):60–2.

(Level V evidence)

Farsetti P, Caterini R, Mancini F, Potenza V, Ippolito E. Anterior tibial tendon transfer in relapsing congenital club foot: long-term follow-up study of two series treated with a different protocol. J Pediatr Orthop. 2006;26:83–90.

The authors reviewed two separate series in which the entire tibialis anterior tendon was transferred to the third cuneiform and found that it corrected and stabilized relapsing clubfeet. (Level IV evidence)

Hosalkar H, Goebel J, Reddy S, Pandya NK, Keenan MA. Fixation techniques for split tibialis anterior transfer in spastic equinocavovarus feet. Clin Orthop Relat Res. 2008;(466):2500–6.

The authors, while also comparing two different methods of fixation of the tibialis anterior transfer, found that, in correctly selected patients, it improved ambulatory status and eliminated the need for bracing in 77% of patients. (Level IV evidence)

Calcaneal-Cuboid-Cuneiform Osteotomy for the Correction of Valgus Foot Deformities

Scott J. Mubarak

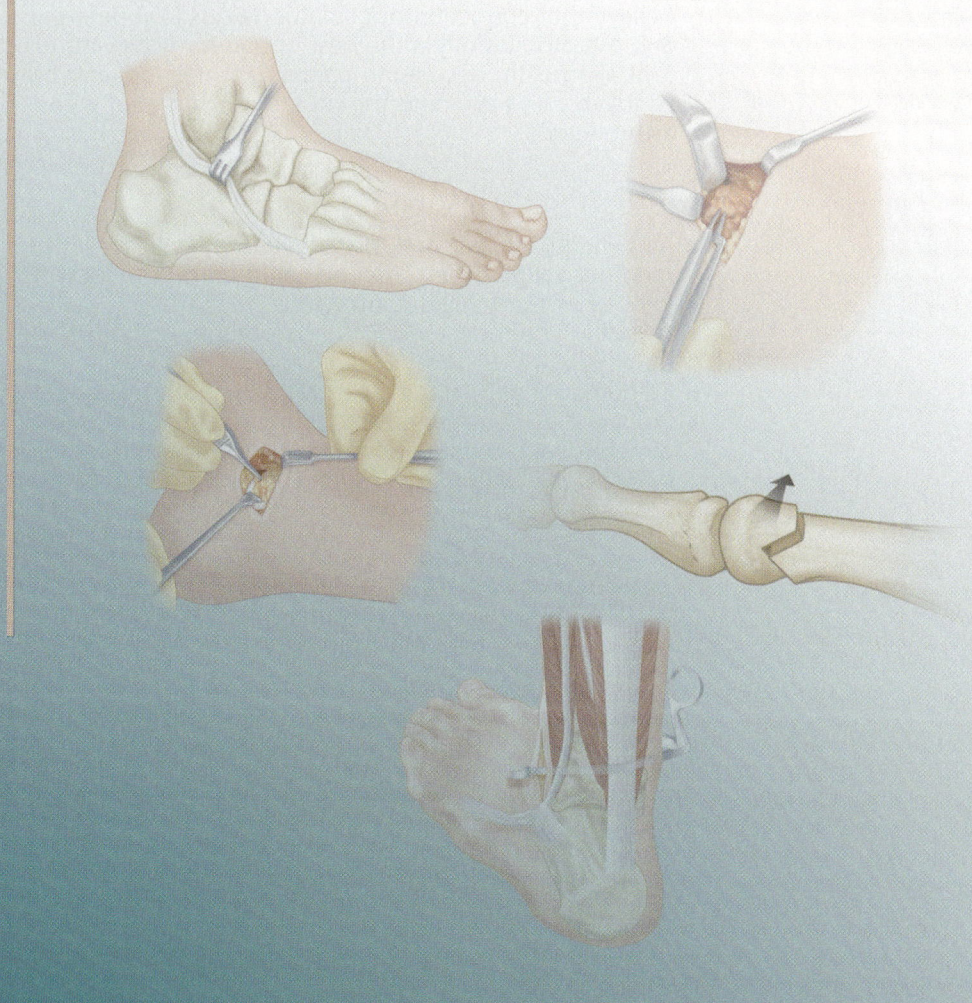

PITFALLS

- *Unrecognized hindfoot coalition—preoperative computerized tomography should be considered.*

INDICATIONS

- Valgus foot deformities are a relatively common problem in pediatric orthopedics. They may be seen in children with cerebral palsy, myelomeningocele, overcorrected clubfeet, and some syndromes. All patients have a severe valgus deformity, defined as greater than 15° of hindfoot valgus.
- Pain on ambulation, especially if asymmetric (Figs. 1 and 2)
- Rigid flatfeet (tarsal coalition) made "flexible" but deformity persists
- Shoe or brace problems
- Skin breakdown
- Our early results with a combination of calcaneal-cuboid-cuneiform (3-C) osteotomies to correct severe valgus foot deformity compare favorably with similar series that used arthrodesis or other techniques to correct the deformity. We believe that correction of pediatric valgus foot deformity with 3-C osteotomies offers the best option for achieving excellent foot alignment; decreasing pain and skin, shoe, and brace problems; and avoiding the problems associated with arthrodesis.

EXAMINATION/IMAGING

- All patients are assessed to evaluate the flexibility of the hindfoot valgus. The surgeon should be sure to lock the subtalar joint to assess Achilles contracture.
- Standing anteroposterior (AP) radiographs of both ankles are obtained.
- Standing AP and lateral radiographs of both feet are examined.
- Preoperative computed tomography scans with three-dimensional reconstruction may be considered to visualize the deformity.

Treatment Options

- Surgical options for the treatment of valgus foot deformity range from soft tissue procedures to triple arthrodesis.

- Dwyer first described a lateral closing wedge calcaneal osteotomy to correct varus deformity in 1958. In 1963, he described a medial opening wedge calcaneal osteotomy to correct the "relapsed clubfoot." In 1971, Koutsogiannis modified Dwyer's wedge osteotomy and described his results with a "displacement" osteotomy of the calcaneus.

- Evans described lengthening of the anterior calcaneus to correct valgus deformity in 1975. This technique with changes has been popularized by Mosca (1995), who also recommends cuneiform plantar-flexion osteotomy.

- Extra-articular subtalar arthrodesis, as initially described by Grice, was for many years the surgical procedure of choice for valgus foot deformity. Although Grice reported good results in 41 of 52 patients, others reported unsatisfactory results as high as 64%.

- Triple arthrodesis represents the final and most definitive surgical option for valgus foot deformity. It is unquestionably reliable in correcting deformity and maintaining normal foot position. In a review of 46 triple arthrodeses, Adelaar et al. (1976) reported degenerative changes in 39% of adjacent joints. Angus and Cowell (1986) reported degenerative changes in (39%) of 80 feet.

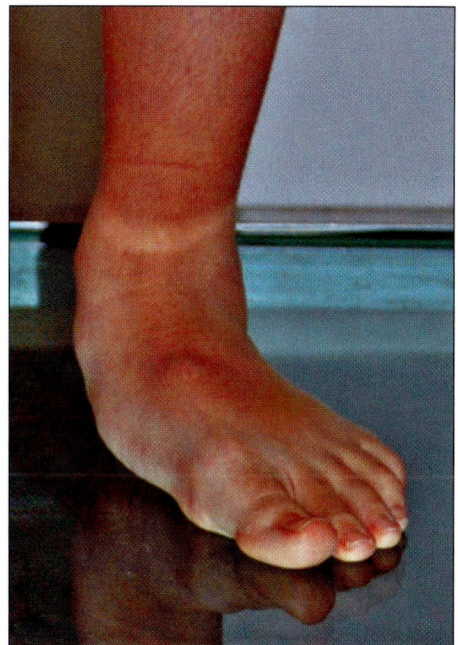

FIGURE 1

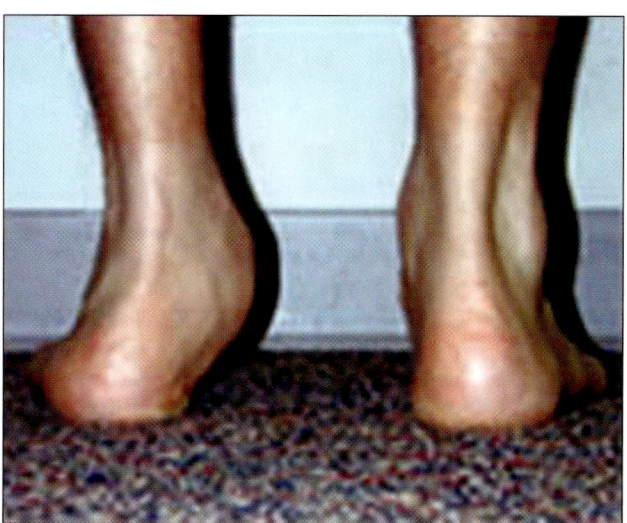

FIGURE 2

Instrumentation/ Implantation

• Chandler retractors

• Small power saw

• Lamina spreader

• Kerrison rongeur

SURGICAL ANATOMY

■ The sural nerve is at risk when lengthening the gastrocnemius-soleus and on approach to the calcaneus and cuboid laterally (Fig. 3).

POSITIONING

■ The patient is placed supine with the foot at the end of the operating table so that surgeon can sit comfortably (Fig. 4).

PORTALS/EXPOSURES

■ Lateral approach to the distal leg for tendon lengthening
■ Lateral approach to the calcaneus and cuboid
■ Medial approach for talonavicular and cuneiform

PROCEDURE

STEP 1

■ If indicated, an Achilles tendon or peroneus brevis lengthening, or both, is performed at the muscle-tendon junction through a posterolateral longitudinal incision in the distal one third of the leg (Fig. 5).
■ The peroneus is superficial and is retracted to expose the brevis, which is lengthened (Fig. 6).

STEP 2

■ The calcaneus is approached through a lateral incision.
■ The sural nerve is identified and retracted dorsally.
■ The peroneal tendons are reflected superiorly but left in their groove, exposing the lateral calcaneus (Fig. 7). The peroneal tendons and sural nerve are retracted superiorly, and Chandler retractors are placed to protect the medial structures.
■ Chandler retractors are placed around the calcaneus to protect the Achilles and peroneal tendons. The lateral cortex is cut with a saw or osteotome, and this cut is extended to the proximal and distal "corners" of the calcaneus, leaving only a narrow bridge of bone medially (Fig. 8). The image intensifier is used as necessary to find the appropriate location on the calcaneus.

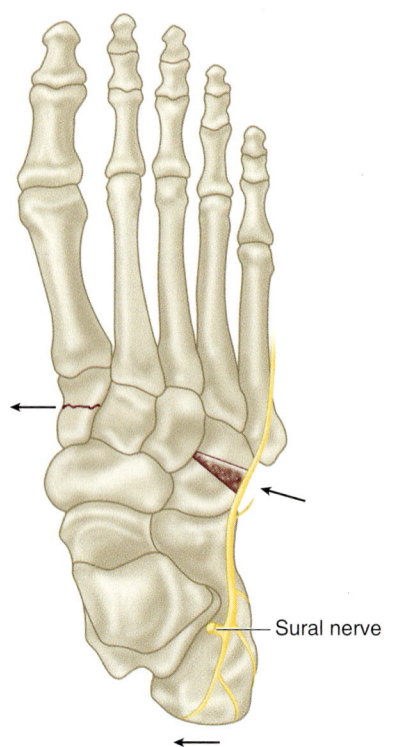

Sural nerve

FIGURE 3

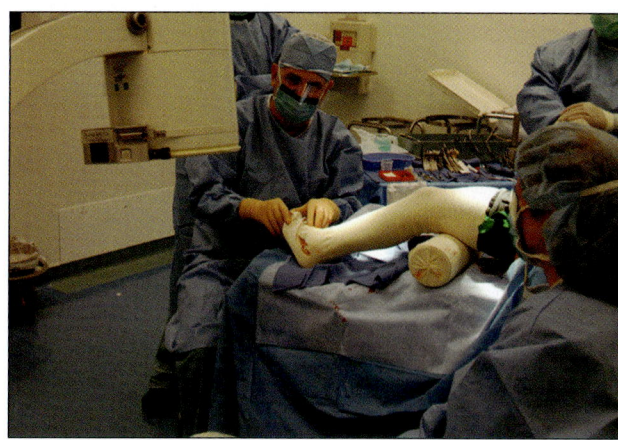

FIGURE 4

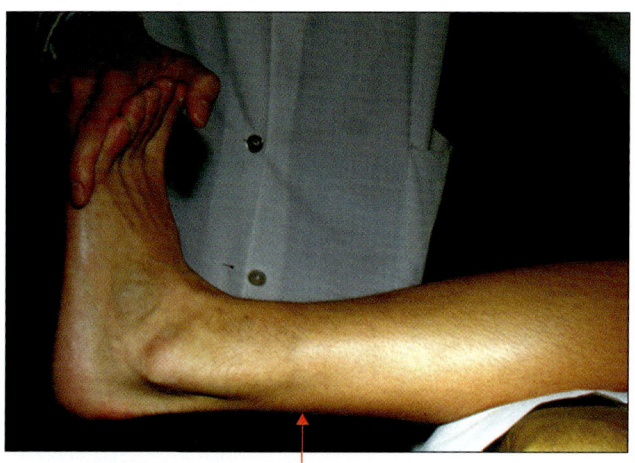

Step 1–Lateral Incision-Vulpius tendo-achilles recession
and peroneus brevis lengthening also at muscle tendon
junction

FIGURE 5

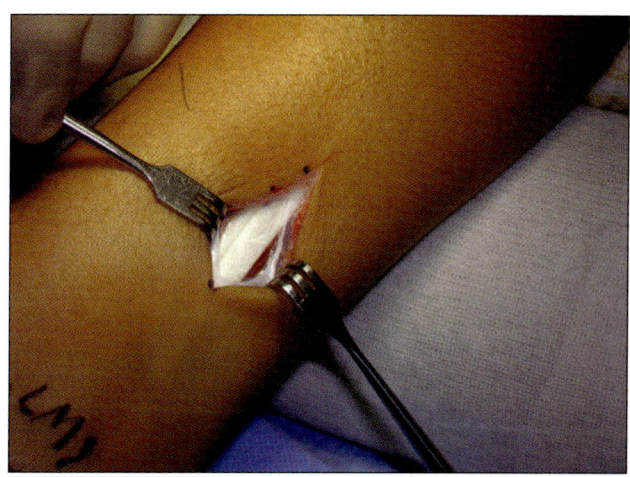

FIGURE 6

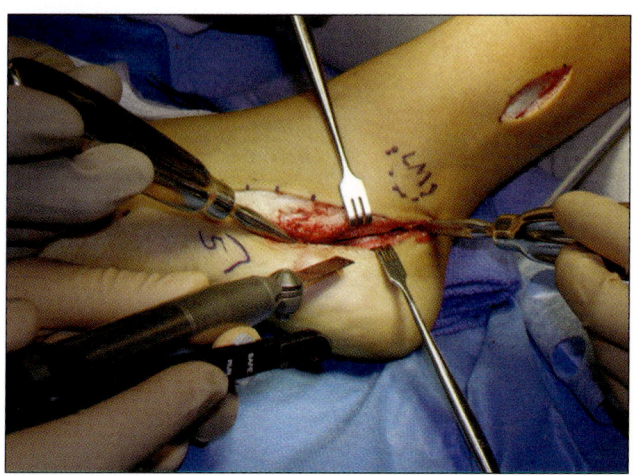

FIGURE 7

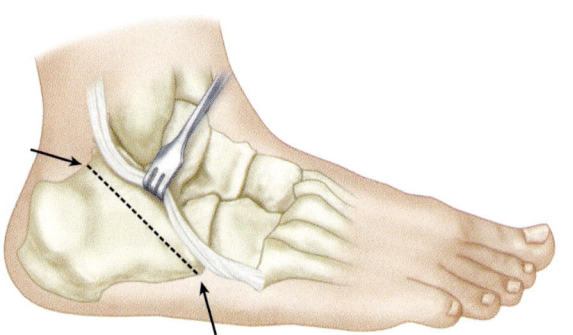

FIGURE 8

- A Chandler retractor is used to visualize the medial side (Fig. 9).
- The medial cortex can then be cut with an osteotome, and a Kerrison rongeur is then used to remove any sharp corners under direct vision (Fig. 10).
- The soft tissues are released medially until the tuberosity fragment of the calcaneus is freely mobile.
- Freeing of the periosteum and obtaining mobility of the tuberosity fragment are the most important components in achieving correction.
- The entire cut surface of the calcaneus should be visible with a well-placed Chandler retractor (Fig. 11) or lamina spreader (Fig. 12).
- A wedge (3–5 mm) of bone (Fig. 13A) is removed medially to allow closing wedge correction (Fig. 13B).

STEP 3

- The cuboid is exposed by using the distal portion of the incision and retracting the peroneal tendons plantarly.
- The calcaneal-cuboid and cuboid-metatarsal joints are identified in order to localized the midportion of the cuboid (Fig. 14).
- An osteotomy is made in the midportion of the cuboid.
- A smooth laminar spreader is placed within the cuboid to ensure that the osteotomy is complete and adequate to allow the opening wedge graft to be inserted.

PITFALLS

- *Care is taken to avoid opening the calcaneal-cuboid and cuboid-metatarsal joints.*

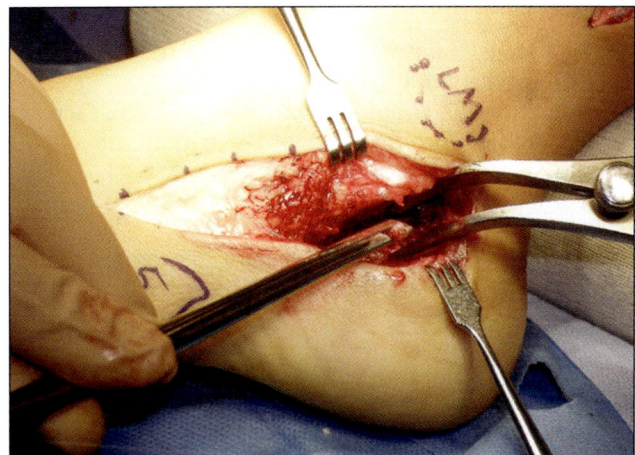

FIGURE 9

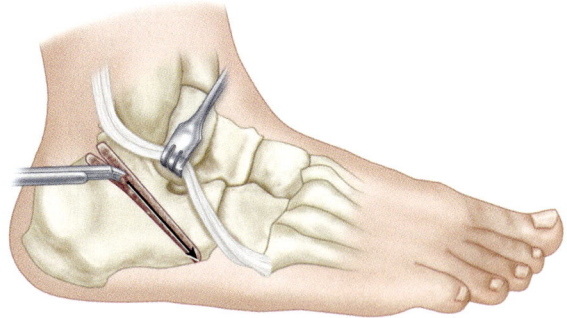

FIGURE 10

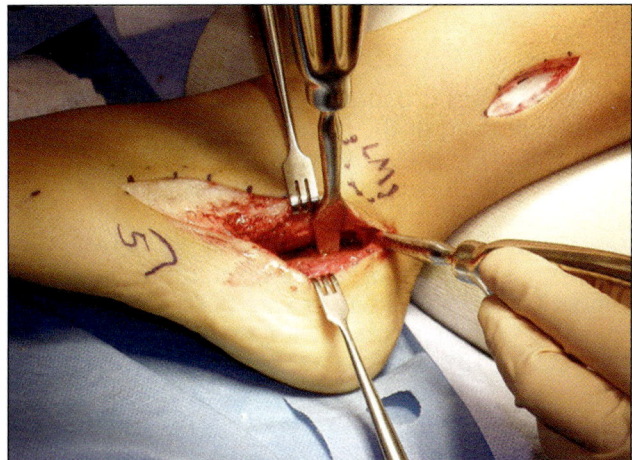

FIGURE 11

You should see the medial side well. Use a saw to perform a closing wedge osteotomy.

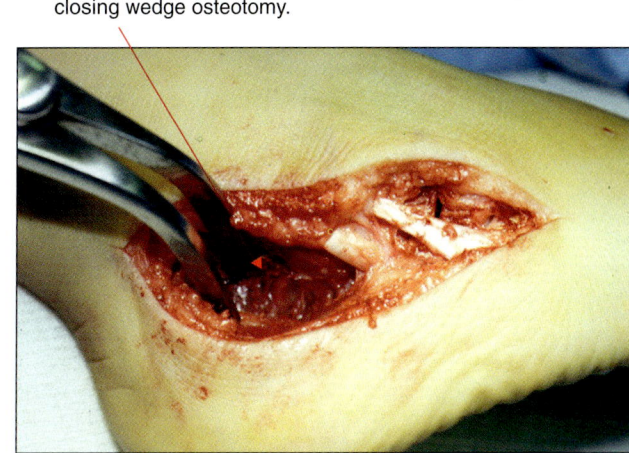

FIGURE 12

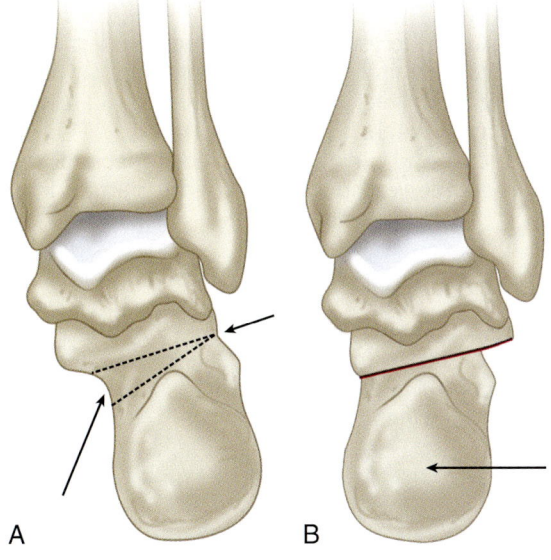

A   B

FIGURE 13

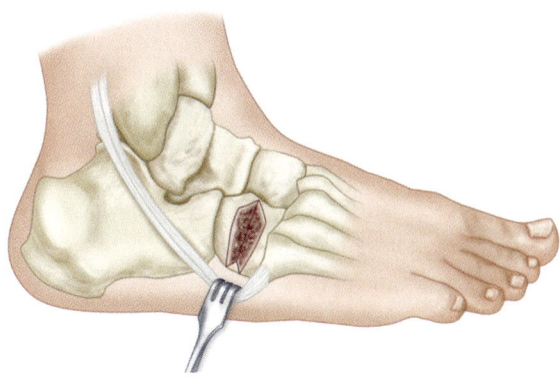

FIGURE 14

STEP 4

- A medial incision is then made from the navicular to the first metatarsal and the medial cuneiform is exposed.
- The anterior tibial tendon is released from the plantar surface of the cuneiform. The joints on either side of the cuboid are identified so that osteotomy can be performed in the midportion. The image intensifier is used as necessary to find the appropriate location.
- If there is subluxation of the talonavicular joint, a medial reefing can be performed if deemed appropriate. The talonavicular joint is opened and the capsule advanced to tighten this ligament (Fig. 15).
- A Chandler retractor is placed on the lateral aspect of the cuneiform
- A closing wedge of bone is removed from the plantar surface in the central third of the cuneiform (Fig. 16).
  - This osteotomy allows plantar flexion and pronation of the forefoot, re-creating a longitudinal arch.
  - The wedge will be used laterally for the opening wedge in the cuboid.

STEP 5

- Fixation of the osteotomies is performed.
- Pins are readied for pinning of the forefoot.
- The removed cuneiform wedge is inserted into the cuboid (see Fig. 16). Additional graft, if needed, can be obtained from the calcaneus.
- The forefoot is placed in a pronated and slightly adducted position, and the cuneiform is closed in a plantar direction and pinned by using a 0.062-inch Kirschner wire (K-wire) (Fig. 17).
- The cuboid graft is pinned into place with a percutaneous 0.062-inch K-wire (Fig. 18).
- Lastly, the calcaneus is held in a medially displaced, corrected position and percutaneously pinned with two 0.062-inch K-wires (Fig. 19).

POSTOPERATIVE CARE AND EXPECTED OUTCOMES

- The pins are left out through the skin, bent 90°, and protected with felt (Fig. 20).
- After routine closure, the foot is placed into a well-molded below-the-knee cast, which is widely split to allow swelling.
- This cast is closed at 1 week, and the patient remains non–weight bearing for 4 weeks.
- At 4 weeks, the cast and pins are removed under oral sedation.
- A new below-the-knee walking cast is used for an additional 4 weeks.

Complications

- Hypergranulation of wounds that responded to application of silver nitrate.
- Delayed union of the cuneiform that may require prolonged casting or open bone grafting.
  - Consequently, we now prefer to perform osteotomy of the cuneiform only after it has developed a "mature" ossific center. Generally, this is in children older than 6 years.

PITFALLS

- *Avoid delayed union of the cuneiform by perform osteotomy of the cuneiform only after it has developed a "mature" ossific center. Generally, this is in children older than 6 years.*

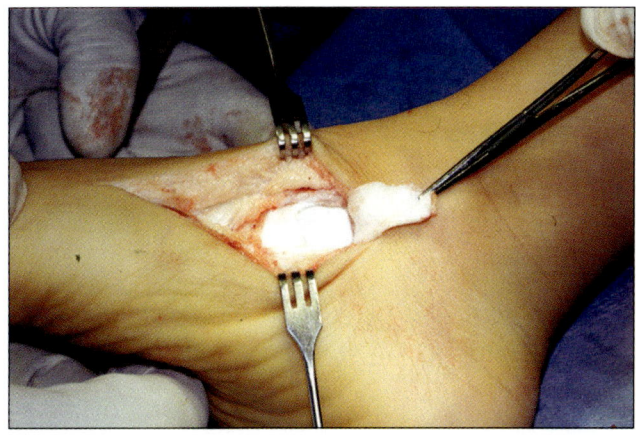

FIGURE 15

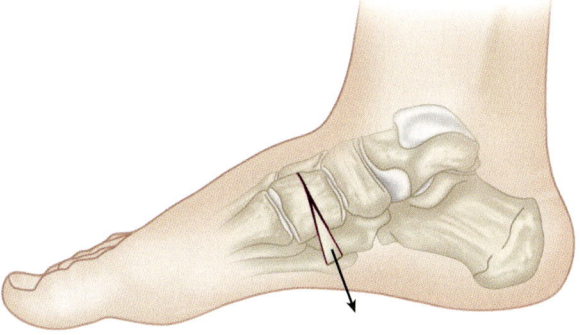

FIGURE 16

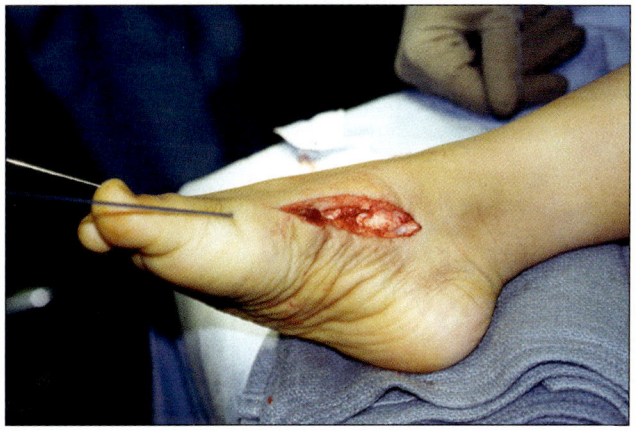

FIGURE 17

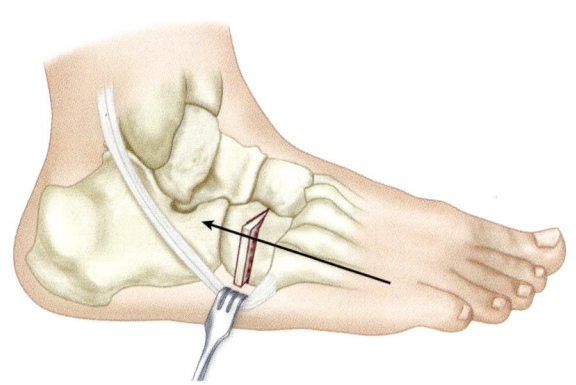

FIGURE 18

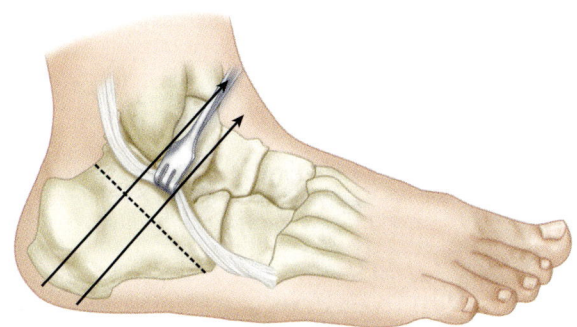

FIGURE 19

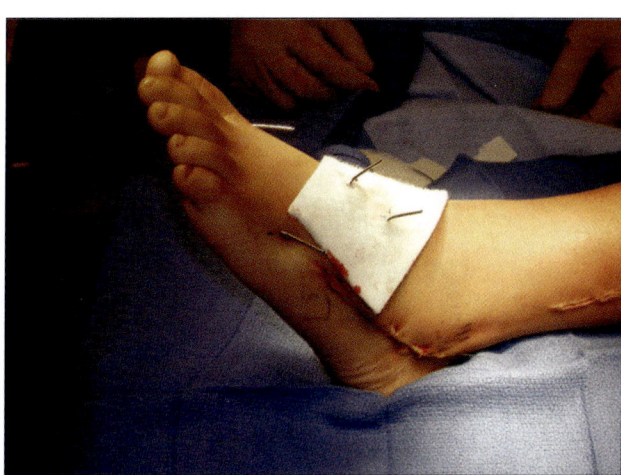

FIGURE 20

EVIDENCE

Adelarr RS, Dannelly EA, Meunier PA, Stelling FH, Goldner JL, Colvard DF. A long term study of triple arthrodesis in children. Orthop Clin North Am. 1976;7:895–908.

In a review of 46 triple arthrodeses, the authors reported degenerative changes in 39% of adjacent joints. (Level IV evidence)

Angus PD, Cowell HR. Triple arthrodesis: a critical long-term review. J Bone Joint Surg [Br]. 1986;68:260–5.

The authors reported degenerative changes in 39% of 80 feet. (Level IV evidence)

Dwyer FC. The treatment of relapsed club foot by the insertion of a wedge into the calcaneum. J Bone Joint Surg [Br]. 1963;45:67–75.

The author first described a lateral closing wedge calcaneal osteotomy to correct varus deformity in 1958. In 1963, he described a medial opening wedge calcaneal osteotomy to correct the "relapsed clubfoot." (Level IV evidence)

Evans D. Calcaneo-valgus deformity. J Bone Joint Surg [Br]. 1975;57:270–8.

The author described lengthening of the anterior calcaneus to correct valgus deformity. (Level IV evidence)

Koutsogiannis E. Treatment of mobile flat foot by displacement osteotomy of the calcaneus. J Bone Joint Surg [Br]. 1971;53:96–100.

The author modified Dwyer's wedge osteotomy and described his results with a "displacement" osteotomy of the calcaneus. (Level IV evidence)

McHale KA, Lenhart MK. Treatment of residual clubfoot deformity—the "bean shaped" foot—by opening wedge medial cuneiform osteotomy and closing wedge cuboid osteotomy. J Pediatr Orthop. 1991;11:374–81.

The authors presented a procedure for double osteotomy to correct forefoot adduction. (Level IV evidence)

Mosca VS. Calcaneal lengthening for valgus deformity of the hind-foot. J Bone Joint Surg [Am]. 1995;77:500–12.

This technique, with changes, has been popularized by the author, who also recommended cuneiform plantar-flexion osteotomy. (Level IV evidence)

Scott SM, James PC, Stevens PM. Grice subtalar arthrodesis followed to skeletal maturity. J Pediatr Orthop. 1988;8:176–83.

Extra-articular subtalar arthrodesis, as initially described by Grice, was for many years the surgical procedure of choice for valgus foot deformity. Although Grice reported good results in 41 of 52 patients, these authors reported unsatisfactory results as high as 64%. (Level IV evidence)

Vedantam R, Capelli AC, Schoenecker PL. Subtalar arthrodesis for the correction of planovalgus foot in children with neuromuscular disorders. J Pediatr Orthop. 1998; 18:294–8.

The authors discussed stabilizing the subtalar joint using synthetic devices to prevent valgus collapse. (Level IV evidence)

SPINE

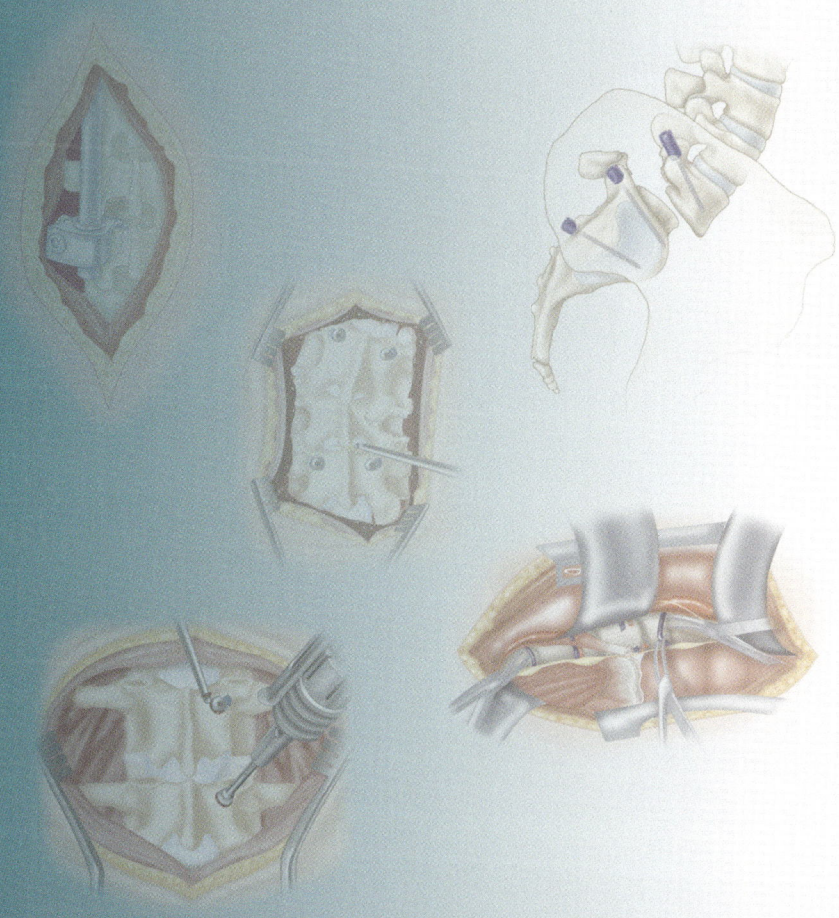

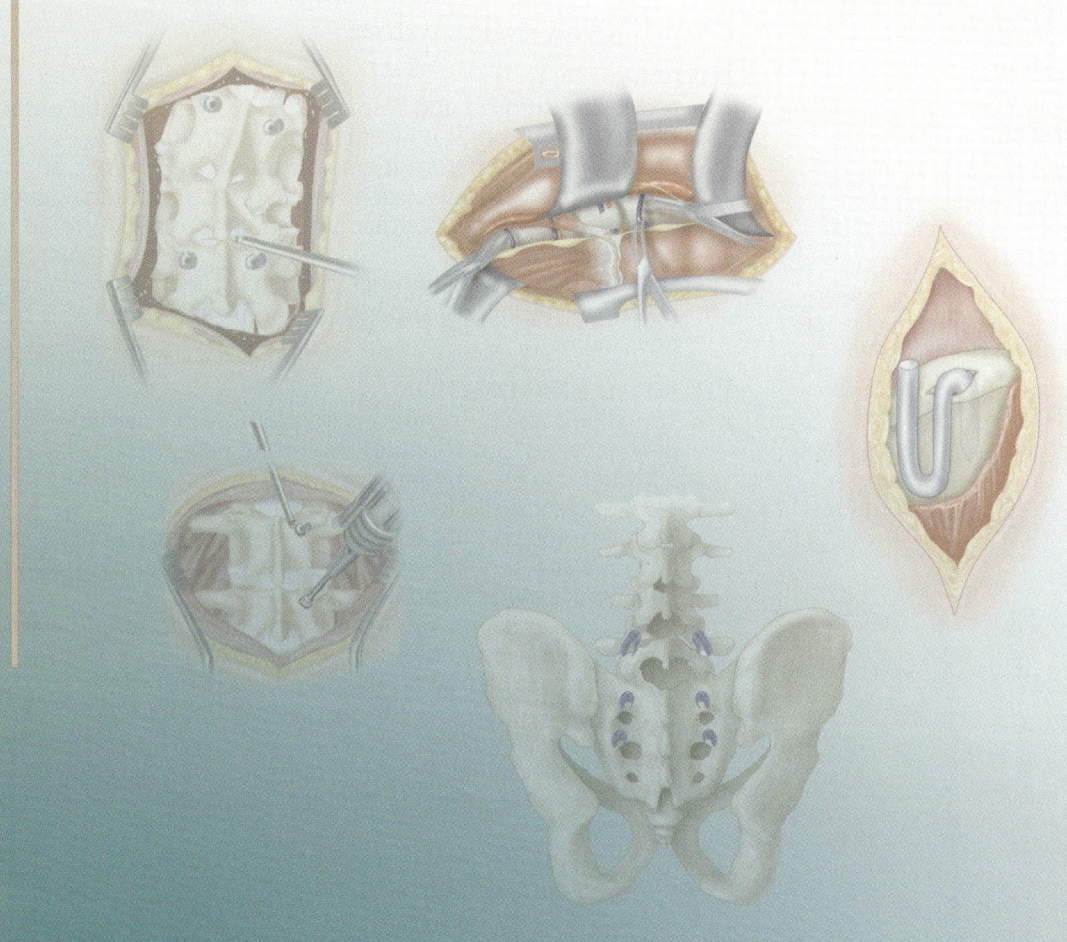

Vertical Expandable Prosthetic Titanium Rib (VEPTR) Expansion Thoracoplasty

Robert M. Campbell, Jr.

Controversies

- VEPTR treatment can treat chest wall instability past skeletal maturity, but FDA compassionate exemption is needed.
- VEPTR treatment in children under age 6 months is not recommended because the devices are too bulky.
- Bisphosphonates may strengthen ribs for VEPTR use.
- In cases of absent proximal rib, rib autografts with a longitudinally osteotomized clavicle can provide a "first rib" for VEPTR attachment.

INDICATIONS

- Food and Drug Administration (FDA)–approved indications for VEPTR procedures (Campbell, 2005):
  - Presence of thoracic insufficiency syndrome (Campbell et al., 2003a)
  - Skeletally immature patient
  - Anatomic diagnosis
    - Absent ribs
    - Constrictive chest wall syndrome, including fused ribs and scoliosis
    - Hypoplastic thorax
    - Scoliosis of congenital or neurogenic origin without rib anomaly

EXAMINATION/IMAGING

HISTORY

- A detailed surgical and respiratory history should be obtained in children with thoracic insufficiency syndrome.
- Onset of clinical deformity, past surgical treatments, and associated morbidities, such as renal, gastrointestinal, central nervous system, and cardiac system abnormalities, must be documented.
- Past episodes of pneumonia, bronchitis, and asthma attacks or needs for respiratory support during illness should also be documented.

PHYSICAL EXAMINATION

- The child's ability to respond to pulmonary challenge, such as play activities and running, should be noted. Difficulty in such activities can be a helpful early warning of impending respiratory insufficiency/thoracic insufficiency.
- Both the lips and fingertips are examined for any signs of cyanosis and the fingertips for evidence of clubbing, suggesting long-term clinical hypoxia.
- If the patient is on oxygen, or dependent on more invasive respiratory support, the degree of respiratory insufficiency should be defined by the assisted ventilator ratings (AVRs) (Campbell and Smith, 2007):
  - +0: no assistance, on room air
  - +1: supplemental oxygen required
  - +2: nighttime ventilation/continuous positive airway pressure (CPAP)
  - +3: part time ventilation/CPAP
  - +4: full-time ventilator support
- Respiratory rate is assessed.
  - Normal respiratory rate at birth is 40–80 breaths per minute; that up to age 5 years, 20–40 breaths per minute; and 15–25 breaths per minutes is normal from age 6 to 12 years. Adult values, 15–20 breaths per minute, are reached after 15 years of age (Hoekelman, 1987).
  - Respiratory rate at rest above these values suggest occult respiratory insufficiency.
- The chest is assessed for clinical deformity and the circumference measured at the nipple line and compared to normal values for age to discern percentile of normal (Jones, 1988).
  - The thumb excursion test is performed to clinically measure the ability of each side of the chest to contribute to respiration by rib cage expansion.
  - The examiner's hands are placed around the base of the thorax with the thumbs posteriorly pointing upward at equal distances from the spine (Fig. 1).

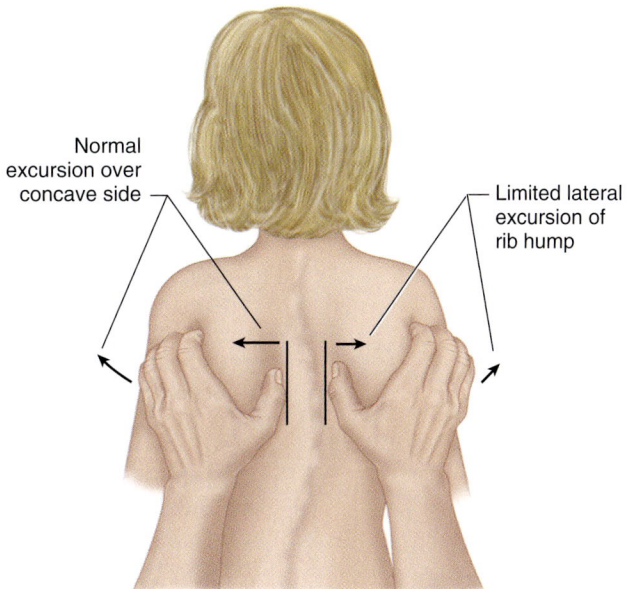

Normal excursion over concave side

Limited lateral excursion of rib hump

FIGURE 1

- With respiration, the thumbs move away from the spine symmetrically because of the anterior lateral motion of the chest wall.
- Each hemithorax is graded separately:
  - Greater than 1 cm of excursion of each thumb away from the spine during inspiration is graded as +3, and considered normal.
  - 0.5–1 cm of excursion is graded +2.
  - Motion up to 0.5 cm is graded as +1.
  - Complete absence of motion is graded +0.
- The concave fused-rib hemithorax often has a +0 thumb excursion test, and if there is significant rib hump deformity of the convex hemithorax, it will also be stiff and also have a +0 thumb excursion test.
- Assess for a marionette sign: the patient's head bobs synchronously with respiration.
  - This represents a form of secondary thoracic insufficiency syndrome in which the diaphragm, in effect, is doing a pushup against body weight because the "collapsing torso" deformities, such as lumbar kyphosis in myelomeningocele, or severe pelvic obliquity, raise abdominal pressure on the diaphragm by abnormal proximity to the pelvis (Fig. 2) (Campbell and Smith, 2007; Campbell et al., 2003b).

IMAGING STUDIES

- Weight-bearing anteroposterior (AP) and lateral radiographs of the entire spine, including the chest and pelvis on the same radiograph, are obtained.
  - The AP radiograph is analyzed for Cobb's angle, the interpedicular line ratio, the height of the thoracic spine in centimeters, and the space available for the lung.
  - The height of the thorax is determined by the radiographic height of the patient's thoracic spine, and this distance is divided by the normal thoracic spinal height for age, deriving a percentage of normal.
  - The lateral radiograph defines a loss of sagittal depth of the thorax, due to either pectus excavatum or thoracic spinal lordosis.
  - The AP and lateral radiographs enable identification of the volume depletion deformities (VDDs) of the thorax in the coronal and sagittal planes of the thorax.

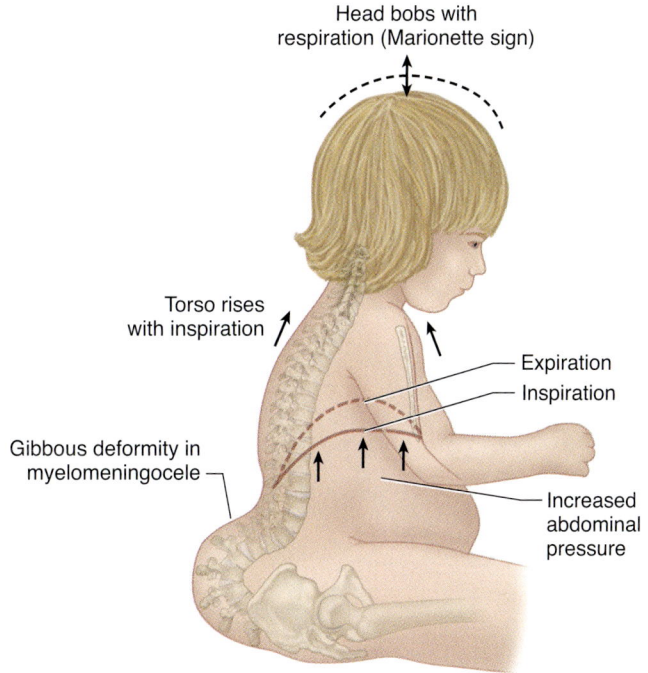

FIGURE 2

- Computed tomography (CT) scans of the entire chest and lumbar spine are performed at 5-mm intervals, unenhanced, with the scanner set for pediatric dosage to minimize radiation exposure (Campbell and Hell-Vocke, 2003; DiMeglio and Bonnel, 1990; Gollogly et al., 2004a; Gollogly et al., 2004b; Paterson et al., 2001). Usually type I, type II, and type III VDDs have a diminished thoracic volume on CT scan in the coronal plane reconstructions (Fig. 3) (Openshaw et al., 1984).
  - In type I and type II VDDs, windswept deformity of the chest is also common, with severe reduction in transverse volume of the convex hemithorax. Its severity can be defined by measurements of spinal rotation, the posterior hemithorax symmetry ratio, and the thoracic rotation of the CT "scan cut" at the level of maximum deformity.
    - CT lung scan volumes can be computed. Full-chest CT scans may be taken at yearly follow-up if percent normal lung volumes are being followed to detect progressive thoracic volume loss.
    - A more limited CT scan, localized at the level of maximum deformity, may also be followed yearly if CT lung volumes are not thought to be necessary.
  - Both ventilation-perfusion lung scans and 3-mm-cut CT scans with airway reconstruction can define airway compression deformity, if necessary.
- Magnetic resonance imaging (MRI) studies of the entire spinal cord are obtained to rule out spinal cord abnormalities.
- Either ultrasound or fluoroscopy of the diaphragm can be performed to document diaphragmatic function, but dynamic MRI study of the lungs will show great detail of diaphragm and chest wall function (Campbell et al., 2008a).
- When there is question of early cor pulmonale, echocardiograms are performed to detect tricuspid valve regurgitation.

PULMONARY FUNCTION STUDIES

- Routine spirometry pulmonary function studies are feasible for children age 5 years or older, and infant pulmonary function tests can be performed in younger patients, if available.
- When there is spinal deformity present, the overall height of the patient is usually decreased, and care must be taken to use arm span instead of height for normalization of pulmonary function test results.
- Pulse oximetry studies are also useful to detect significant amounts of hypoxia. An increase in AVR suggests progressive clinical respiratory insufficiency, and this is a strong indication for treatment.
- Comparison of past pulmonary function tests to current ones would be helpful in determining any deterioration of vital capacity as determined by decreasing percent normal vital capacity.

Treatment Options

- Posterior spine fusion: consider if nearing skeletal maturity
- Chest wall defects can be treated with Surgisis™ or Vicryl patches (Smith and Campbell, 2006)
- Hemivertebrectomy: for very limited area of congenital malformation
- Convex hemiarthrodesis/ hemiepiphysiodesis: limited area of congenital malformation
- Growing rods: flexible spine/ absence of rib fusion/correctable intercostal narrowing on bending radiographs

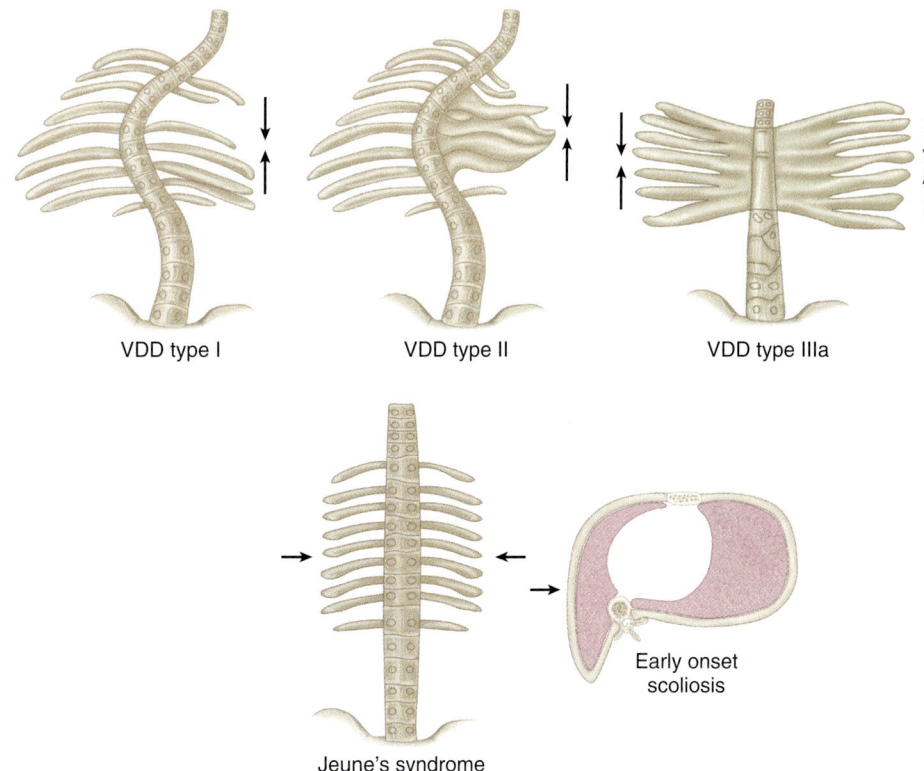

VDD type I   VDD type II   VDD type IIIa

Jeune's syndrome

Early onset
scoliosis

VDD type IIIb

FIGURE 3

Equipment

- Upper and lower extremities are monitored by both somatosensory evoked potentials and motor evoked potentials.
- Place a pulse oximeter transducer on the upper operative extremity to monitor the neurovascular bundle within the operative field.
- Central and arterial lines are placed.
- Prophylactic IV antibiotics are given.

Controversies

- Beanbag support can be used, but it is difficult to contour it around small children to allow adequate operative exposure.
- The prone position allows the best access to the spine and chest, but in very severe scoliosis cases the lateral decubitus position helps in spine correction.

SURGICAL ANATOMY

- Instability of the chest wall is documented on radiographs and CT scans, and degree of paradoxical chest wall motion over the bony defect is confirmed on physical examination (Campbell and Smith, 2003).
  - The goal of VEPTR surgery is to brace the unstable defect with multiple VEPTRs or use VEPTRs to stabilize ribs transported into the area of defect.
  - Care must be taken not to damage the lung when the skin incision is over the rib cage defect, and generally there is a large spine defect in the area of the chest wall defect, so care must be taken not to violate the dura in the exposure.
  - The exposure should cautiously approach the defect area, first proximally, then distally.
- Rib fusion is documented on radiographs and CT scans, and confirmed on physical examination by absence of movement with respiration on the thumb excursion test.
  - Even if gross bony synostosis is not present, longitudinal hemithorax constriction may be present from intercostal muscle scarring, evident on supine lateral bending radiographs when the affected intercostal spaces do not widen while bending into the convex side.
- Widespread dysraphism of the posterior elements is common, and the medial edge of the scapula may lie within the spinal canal itself through the defect, best seen on CT scan transverse sections.
  - A standard thoracotomy approach would place the spinal cord at risk when this abnormality is present, so the scapula should be cautiously retracted posteriorly and the rhomboid muscles sectioned directly off the edge of the scapula to avoid dural injury.
- Anomalous insertion of the diaphragm proximally may be seen on radiographs, as evidenced by decreasing volume available for the lung, or the diaphragm may be flail when its border inserts into soft tissue only when ribs are absent distally.
  - Both of these anomalies may require reconstruction during the VEPTR procedure.
- The brachial plexus may be difficult to locate, but the common insertion of the middle and posterior scalene muscles is a reliable landmark, with the brachial plexus found just anterior to it in the exposure.
- Stable rib attachment sites for device placement are evaluated on radiographs.
  - Rib thickness, attachment to spine, and orientation are assessed.

POSITIONING

- The prone position is now most commonly used (Fig. 4).
  - For the prone position, longitudinal soft rolls are placed under each side of the chest.
  - A transverse roll is placed under the pelvis.
  - The patient is immobilized by wide cloth tape padded with hand towels across the buttocks.
- The lateral decubitus position is used in cases of severe scoliosis, with the concave side up, to help correct deformity.

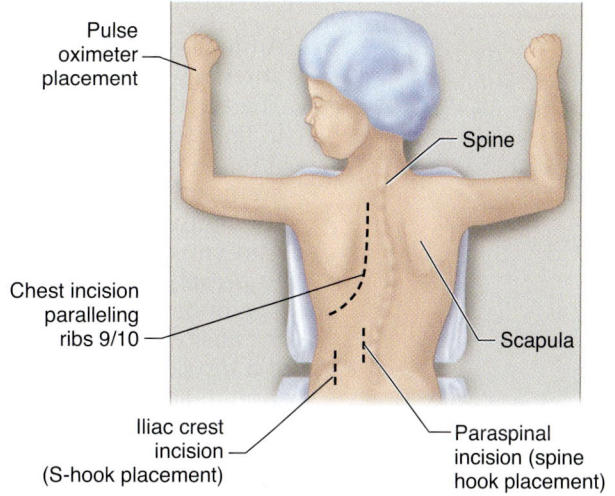

Pulse oximeter placement

Spine

Chest incision paralleling ribs 9/10

Scapula

Iliac crest incision (S-hook placement)

Paraspinal incision (spine hook placement)

FIGURE 4

PEARLS

- *Exposure can be improved by inserting a large retractor under the scapula and attaching the end of the handle to an ether screen through the drapes.*

- *Tilting the table can provide easier exposure.*

PORTALS/EXPOSURES

- A modified curvilinear thoracotomy incision is used, extending anteriorly between the ninth and tenth ribs.
- The trapezius, latissimus, and rhomboid muscles are sectioned in line with the skin incision.
- After complete exposure of the rib cage, the paraspinal muscles are next reflected by cautery, lateral to medial, up to the tips of the transverse processes of the spine.
- Care must be taken not to excessively expose the spine in order to prevent inadvertent fusion.
- The underlying chest wall deformity is then assessed for instability, fusion, and best sites for device attachment.
- If a distal attachment for a hybrid device is needed, a separate longitudinal paraspinous skin incision, 5 cm long, is then made 1 cm lateral to the midline at the level of the proximal lumbar spine (Fig. 5).
- A flap over the fascia is elevated medially to expose the midline of the spine. Cautery is used to longitudinally section the apophysis of the two posterior spinous processes at the correct interspace, and a Cobb elevator is used to strip the spine laterally. L2-3 is the most common interspace used.
- The ligamentum flavum is then resected. Gel foam is placed over the exposed dura.
- If posterior elements are lacking, an S-hook over the central iliac crest may be used for hybrid attachment (Fig. 6).
- A 5-cm longitudinal incision is made over the top of the central iliac crest. The apophysis is exposed by gentle use of a Cobb elevator.
- A 1-cm incision is made transversely by scalpel in the apophysis, with adequate cartilage below to cushion the S-hook over the crest. A Creigo retractor is inserted into the apophyseal incision to elevate the inner periosteum of the iliac crest and to probe correct position just lateral to the sacroiliac joint.

VEPTR EXPANSION THORACOPLASTY

- VEPTR expansion thoracoplasty is a general category of surgical procedures that can expand the volume-constricted thorax when there is three-dimensional deformity of the thorax due to spine deformity, as well as primary rib cage deformity.
- Multiple types of expansion thoracoplasties address each type of VDD of the thorax.
- All the procedures have in common the ability to enlarge the constricted area of the hemithorax with the goals of restoring thoracic volume, stability, and symmetry, with correction of spinal deformity without fusion, in order to allow growth of the thorax afterward.
- In contrast to classic spine fusion, in which the instrumentation "drives" the deformity correction, in VEPTR surgery the thorax first undergoes acute surgical reconstruction to increase volume and correct deformity, then the VEPTR devices are added to stabilize the reconstruction.
- The VEPTR device is made by Synthes Spine Company of West Chester, PA, and is available as a Humanitarian Use Device under an FDA Humanitarian Device Exemption, with Institutional Review Board approval required for the use of the device at each institution.

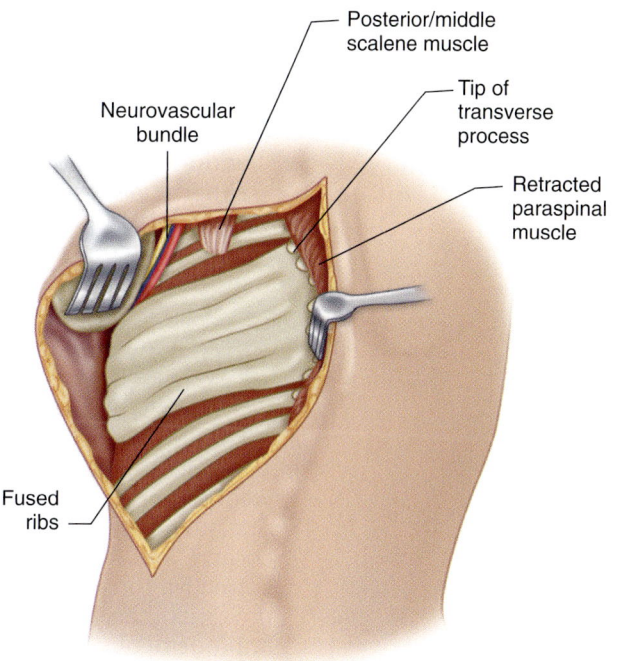

Posterior/middle scalene muscle

Tip of transverse process

Neurovascular bundle

Retracted paraspinal muscle

Fused ribs

Chest exposure

FIGURE 5

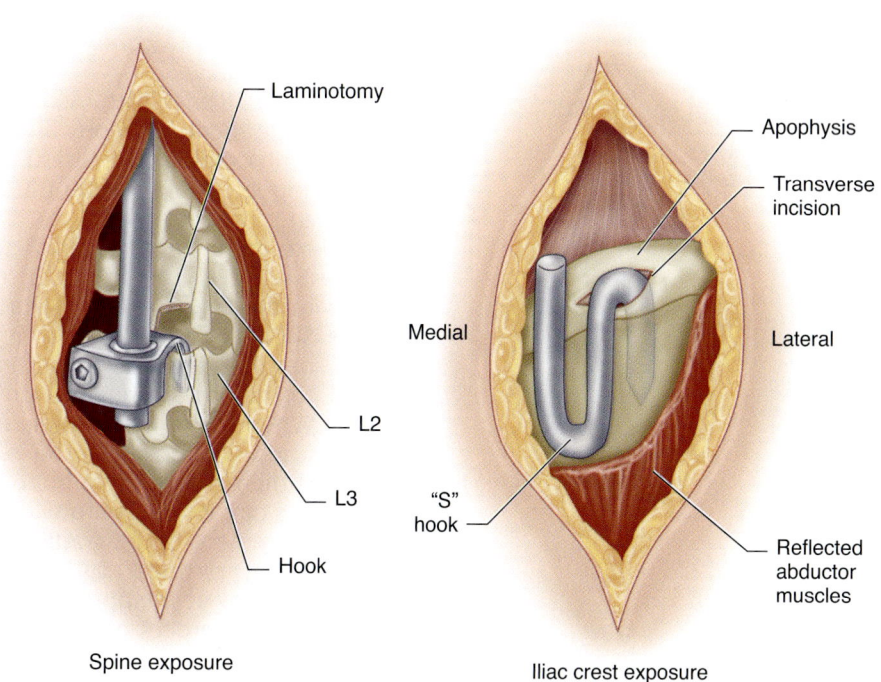

Laminotomy

L2

L3

Hook

Spine exposure

Apophysis

Transverse incision

Medial

Lateral

"S" hook

Reflected abductor muscles

Iliac crest exposure

FIGURE 6

- The first step in VEPTR treatment is to classify the thoracic VDD so that the proper VEPTR surgical strategy is chosen.
  - The VEPTR expansion thoracoplasty strategy for each VDD of the thorax is different.
  - In mixed types of VDD, VEPTR surgical treatment should address each individual segment of thoracic deformity with either appropriate longitudinal or lateral expansion of the constricted thorax.
  - The most common VDD of the thorax is unilateral constriction of the thorax in fused ribs and scoliosis.

PROCEDURE: VDD TYPE II, FUSED RIBS AND SCOLIOSIS

STEP 1

- The VEPTR expansion thoracoplasty for this VDD is an opening wedge thoracostomy.
- After the exposure is completed, the superior rib cradle site is chosen. The rib should be thick enough to support the corrective forces, attached solidly to the spine, and no more proximal than the second rib to avoid brachial plexus impingement.
- A 1-cm incision is made by cautery in the intercostal muscle, immediately beneath the rib of attachment.
- A Freer elevator is then inserted, pushing through the intercostal muscle to the lower edge of the rib, stripping the combined pleura/periosteum layer off from the rib anteriorly.
- A second portal is then placed by cautery above the rib of attachment. A second Freer elevator is inserted in this portal, pointing distally to strip off the periosteum of the rib anteriorly.
  - The two Freer elevators should touch in the "chopstick" maneuver, to confirm that a continuous soft tissue tunnel has been made.
- The VEPTR trial instrument is then inserted into the portals to enlarge them superiorly and inferiorly.
- The rib cradle cap is inserted by forceps into the superior portal, facing laterally, to avoid the great vessels and the esophagus, then turned distally.
- Next, the superior rib cradle is inserted into the inferior portal, just lateral to the tip of the transverse process, and is mated with the cradle cap and attached with a cradle cap lock (Fig. 7).
  - Superior cradle insertion is similar when the attachment rib has fibrous adhesions instead of intercostal muscles linking it to the ribs above and below.
  - When the superior cradle needs to be placed within a mass of fused ribs, however, the inferior portal for the superior cradle is then created by a bone burr, creating a slot 5 mm × 1.5 cm, and a 5-mm wide superior portal is cut by burr for placement of the cradle cap.
- The VDD of fused ribs commonly requires a transverse osteotomy at the apex of the constricted hemithorax from the transverse processes of the spine to the rib costochondral junction. This is termed an opening wedge thoracostomy, and is performed with a Kerrison ronguer.
  - A no. 4 Penfield elevator is threaded underneath the line of bone resection to protect the lung.
  - Sometimes an adjacent line of fibrosis between ribs just above or below the middle of the bone plate is identified, and this can also be used as the cleavage point for the opening wedge thoracostomy.

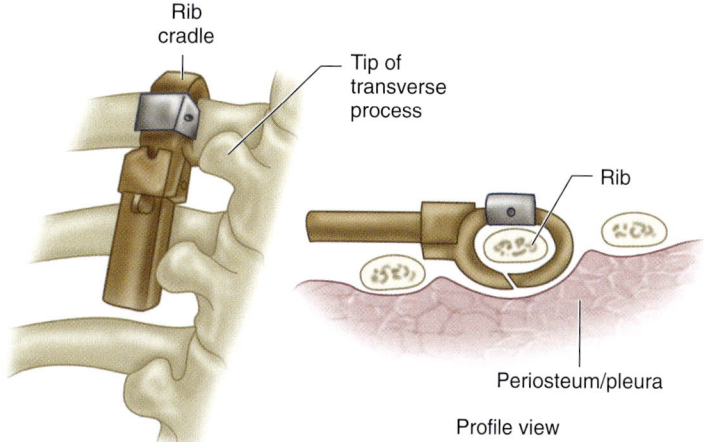

FIGURE 7

- If there is solid bone extending medially from the tip of the transverse process down to the spine at the posterior point of the thoracostomy, then it is resected with a ronguer under direct vision, carefully pulling the final fragment of bone away from the spine with a curved curette to avoid canal violation.
- AO bone spreaders are then inserted into the thoracostomy interval and used to widen it. The Synthes rib spreaders are next inserted to hold the hemithorax out to corrected length. When the proximal fused ribs are oriented in the horizontal orientation, then correction is considered to be adequate.
- The pleura is carefully stripped proximally and distally by a Kidner, often with only minimal tearing.

Step 2: Rib-to-Rib VEPTR

- A rib-to-rib device only is used medially in a patient younger than 18 months.
- Synthes rib distractors hold the opening wedge thoracostomy open to the corrected position, then the distance from the bottom of the implanted rib cradle to the inferior rib of attachment is measured.
- The correct-length VEPTR rib sleeve and inferior cradle are then attached to the previously placed rib cradle and extended down to a stable rib near the inferior margin of the thorax, commonly the ninth or tenth rib, and the rib cradle is locked into place.
- The device is tensioned by 5 mm of distraction, then a distraction lock is added (Fig. 8).
- The rib-to-rib medial device can be converted to a hybrid VEPTR for better spine control once the patient is 18 months of age.

Step 3: Hybrid Device Implantation

- In children older than age 18 months, with adequate spinal canal width, a hybrid VEPTR device is used medially.
- The size of hybrid lumbar extension rib sleeve needed is determined by measuring from the bottom of the rib of attachment encircled by the superior rib cradle down to the end plate of T12. (This can usually be estimated by palpating the 12th rib clinically.) The distance in centimeters should correspond to the number inscribed on the rib sleeve and the hybrid lumbar extension.
- The hybrid device is assembled and locked with a distraction lock.
- To estimate the proper length, the device is then placed into the field with the rib sleeve engaged into the implanted superior cradle proximally and the spinal rod marked by a skin marker pen approximately 1.5 cm below the bottom of the spinal hook. The Synthes rib distractors should be in place to provide the corrected hemithorax length.
- The hybrid is removed from the field and the rod cut smoothly by a tabletop rod cutter.
  - Avoid using a bolt cutter because the resulting sharp edges may cut through the overlying soft tissues.
  - The end of the rod is bent into slight lordosis and valgus by a French bender so that the rod will line up with the axis of the spine after implantation and conform to the lordosis of the lumbar spine.
- Hybrid devices are always inserted in a proximal-to-distal direction to avoid penetrating the chest and causing cardiopulmonary injury.
  - A subfascial canal is created for safe passage of the sized lumbar hybrid extension by a long Kelly clamp, threaded from the proximal incision through the paraspinal muscles, into the distal incision, with care taken not to violate the chest and the pericardium.

PEARLS

- At least 1 cm of bone should be encircled by the superior rib cradle.

- If the rib chosen is too slender, then two ribs are encircled with an extended cradle cap added to the construct in order to encircle it.

PITFALLS

- If the opening wedge thoracostomy interval is quite large, a segment of distal ribs may be osteotomized apart inferiorly, then rotated upward and tied by nonabsorbable suture to the VEPTRs to brace the defect.

- Alternatively, additional longitudinal rib-to-rib VEPTR devices may be implanted as needed with care to place them well below the neurovascular bundle superiorly.

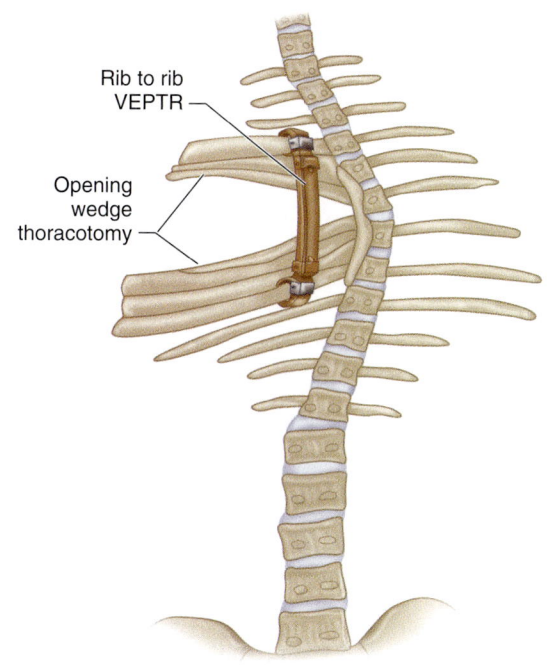

Rib to rib
VEPTR

Opening
wedge
thoracotomy

FIGURE 8

- A #20 chest tube is then attached to the clamp, and the tube pulled upward into the proximal incision. The distal end of the rod of the hybrid is then placed into the chest tube, and the device carefully guided through the muscle by the chest tube into the distal incision.
- The tube is removed, and the rod threaded into the hook, and then upward into the superior cradle. A distraction lock engages the superior cradle to the rib sleeve.

■ To perform the initial tensioning of the device, a Synthes C-ring is attached to the rod just above the hook, and a VEPTR distractor used to distract the device upward from the hook by the C-ring. The hook is then tightened. The C-ring is removed from the field. The Synthes rib distractor is then removed from the thoracostomy.

■ If there is adequate distraction from the hybrid device, then the proximal ribs should remain horizontal, and the combined corrected opening wedge thoracostomy and rib defect interval should be maintained.

■ An additional rib-to-rib VEPTR is then placed 3–4 cm anterior, much like a picket fence, to provide expansion for the thorax and stability for the underlying lung (Fig. 9). Proximally this additional device should be placed well below the neurovascular bundle to avoid compression.

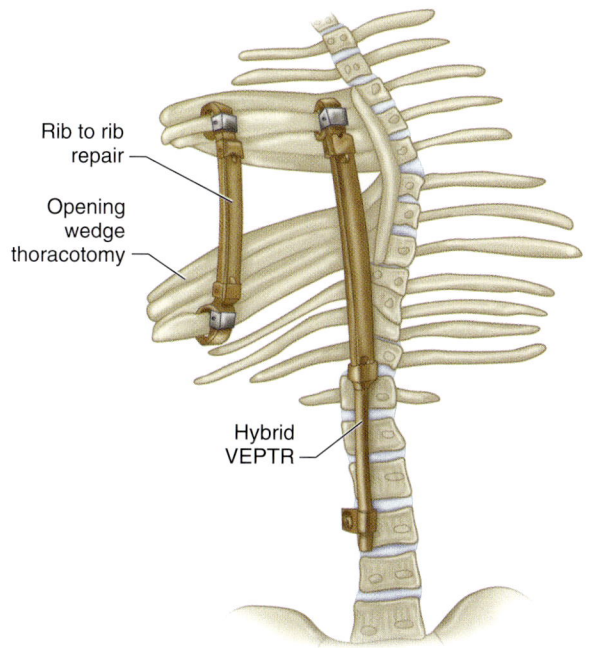

Rib to rib
repair

Opening
wedge
thoracotomy

Hybrid
VEPTR

FIGURE 9

- If there is scoliosis extending into the lumbar spine, or if there is considerable pelvic obliquity, or lumbar posterior elements are absent, such as in myelomeningocele, then the hybrid should extend down to the iliac crest for fixation with attachment by a S-hook (Fig. 10A–D).
  - This is termed an "Eiffel Tower" construct, because the force vectors from iliac crests to proximal ribs have an inferior upward and central orientation (Campbell et al., 2008b). The S-hook attachment to mid–iliac crest is termed *iliac crest pedestal fixation.* This construct is also a powerful means to address pelvic obliquity.
  - The hybrid shaft is threaded through a subfascial canal distally via chest tube, much like the hybrid insertion to the spine, and attached to the S-hook by a 5-mm/6-mm domino. The device is tensioned to optimal load without excessive force.
  - If space permits, a second device, rib to rib, is added laterally in the posterior axillary line to load share.
- The goal of all types of VEPTR expansion thoracoplasties is to correct the thoracic deformity with maximum expansion longitudinally and laterally of the constricted hemithorax in unilateral disease, or to increase thoracic volume and symmetry in bilateral disease in a staged fashion.
  - The contralateral procedure is performed 3–4 months after the first procedure.
  - The thorax should be equilibrated as much as possible in all planes, increasing space available for lung on the concave side to 100%, with symmetrical hemithorax width on radiograph, and symmetrical hemithorax volumes in the transverse plane on the CT scan.
  - Spondylothoracic dysplasia is treated with bilateral wedge osteotomies in staged procedures (Campbell, Smith, and Taichi, 2004).

STEP 4: CLOSURE

- The scapula is first brought distally to the approximate anatomic position, and the pulse oximeter reading on the "up" arm and somatosensory evoked potentials are checked for signs of acute thoracic outlet syndrome.
  - Patients with very anomalous proximal ribs, distracted into the area of the brachial plexus by VEPTR expansion thoracoplasty, are at risk for this syndrome, and the early signs are decrease in ulnar nerve tracings and diminished pulse oximeter signal.
  - Usually relaxation of the position of the scapula, allowing a more proximal position, resolves this problem.
  - If continued alterations in pulse oximeter and/or spinal cord monitoring are encountered, even with relaxation of the closure, it may be necessary to resect the anterolateral portion of the first and second ribs, lateral to the devices, in order to provide clearance for the brachial plexus in the reconstructed thorax.
- The distal incisions over either the spine or the iliac crest are closed in layers.
  - Over the spine, a bone block of autograft, usually from rib resection, is placed from the superior lamina to the top of the hook, anchoring it with a single-level fusion.
  - To hold the hook in place until the bone block fuses, a #1 Prolene suture is wrapped around the shank of the hook and underneath the posterior spinous process at that level.
  - In closure of the iliac crest incision, the released abductor muscles are pulled over the S-hook to provide coverage and sutured in place.

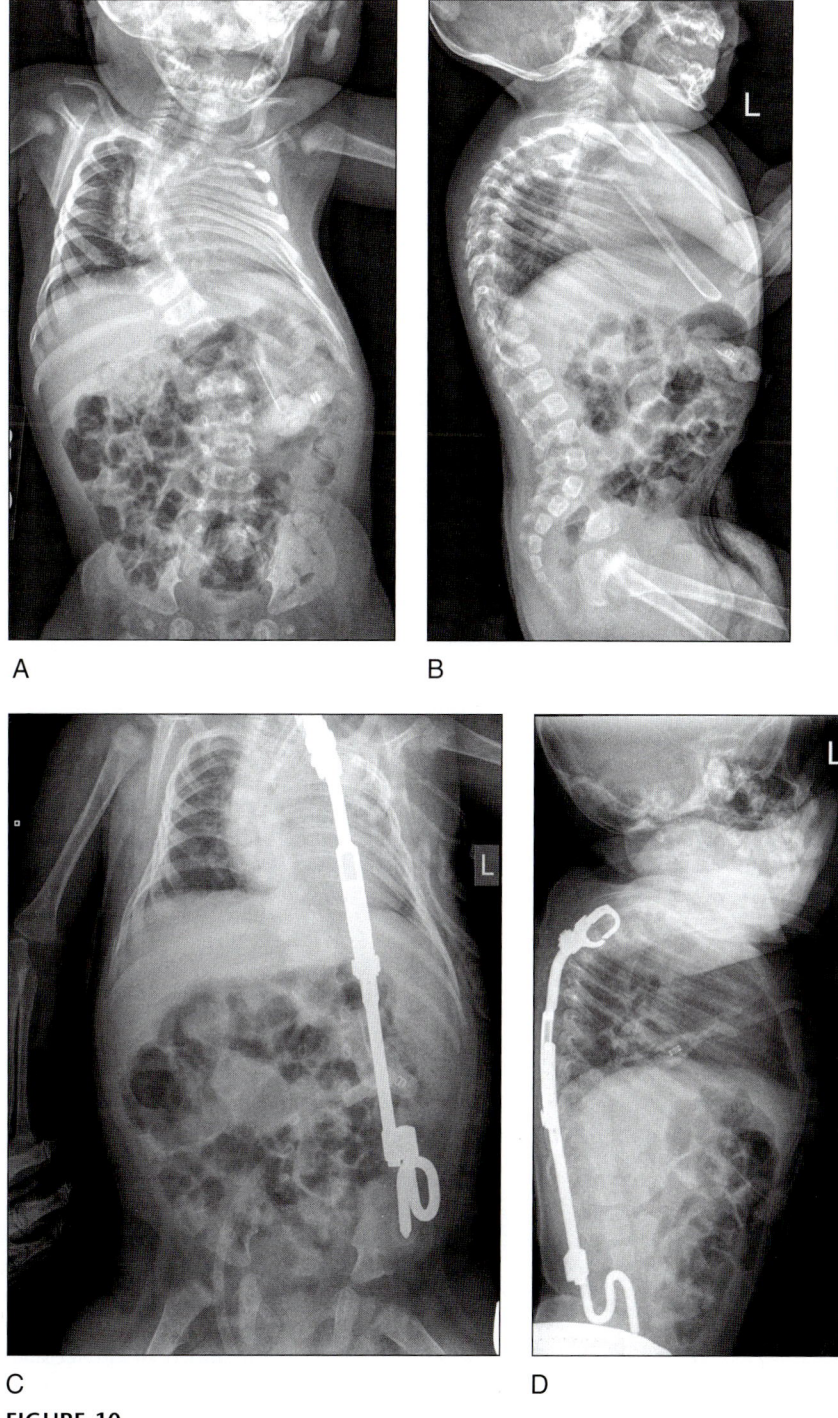

A

B

C

D

FIGURE 10

- Two subcutaneous Jackson Pratt (JP) drains are used in the thoracostomy incision. When there is substantial defect in the pleura (>4 cm), it is repaired with Surgisis by Cook Medical with an addition of a chest tube.

POSTOPERATIVE CARE AND EXPECTED OUTCOMES

- Patients are usually left intubated 24–72 hours.
- VEPTR thoracic reconstruction acutely alters pulmonary function mechanics to a much greater extent than a standard thoracotomy, so immediate extubation is often not well tolerated.
- The hematocrit is checked daily for 3 days. Although blood loss usually averages 50 ml, continual oozing underneath the large flaps results in a 50% risk for postoperative transfusion.
  - Generally, a hematocrit of 30% or greater is optimal for oxygen-carrying capacity for these patients. Fluid management should be on the restrictive side to prevent acute pulmonary edema.
- Once weaned off the ventilator, the patient can be transferred to the surgical ward.
- Jackson Pratt drains are removed when their individual drainage decreases to 20 ml or less over a 24-hour period.
- Chest tubes are removed once their drainage equals 1 ml/kg of patient weight over 24 hours.
  - If the patient goes into respiratory distress after drains and chest tubes are removed, the surgeon should consider checking for acute reaccumulation of the pleural effusion with compression of the lung
  - Temporary chest tube drainage can address this through placement of an anterior pigtail chest tube.
- Vigorous pulmonary toilet, including chest percussion, is needed postoperatively.
- The patients are mobilized as soon as possible.
- Specific detailed postoperative care is available in other publications.

COMPLICATIONS

- VEPTR surgeries have the tendency for complications inherent to all repetitive surgery approaches, with growing rod technique being the most equivalent (Klemme et al., 1997; Tello, 1994).
- Each surgical incision, whether for the primary implantation, expansion, or replacement of a VEPTR, is a new opportunity for skin slough, infection, or other operative complication.
- The long duration of VEPTR treatment also increases risk of migration of devices.
  - The most common VEPTR complication is an asymptomatic upward migration of the superior cradle of the device into the rib of attachment over time. It is not due to breakage of the rib or erosion, but rather a remodeling process of the rib reacting from the stress of the distraction forces of the device.
  - Within a few months of implantation, the rib of attachment begins to thicken, extending bone beneath the rib cradle, strengthening the interface between the device and the rib.

- As the years go by, the device appears to gradually "move" upward to lie centrally in the middle of the thickened rib. This is probably due to remodeling of the rib from constant upward pressure of the rib cradle, much like the way braces induce gradual movement of teeth through the bone of the jaw over time.
- Eventually the device begins to emerge through the upper edge of the rib, and may completely dislodge, but often either clinical prominence or radiographic appearance will identify the problem early, and allow reattachment during a scheduled VEPTR expansion surgery.
- Even if there is complete dislodgement, there are often minimal symptoms, because the device is covered by the thick muscle of the trapezius.
- As a rule, the longer a patient has an implanted device, the higher the likelihood of migration. To factor in the time component of VEPTR migration, a migration index, representing the risk per year of complete migration per patient, was derived based on the number of complete migrations per patient divided by years since implantation.
- Infection in VEPTR patients is often associated with skin slough. Many of these patients have comorbidities, such as myelomeningocele or syndromes, that probably make them prone to surgical infection.
- VEPTR breakage is rare, with most incidents occurring with earlier design devices.
- VEPTR patients have complex, rare spine and chest wall deformities, with a significant incidence of spinal cord abnormalities, and a high rate of neurologic injury should be expected from the large corrections in spinal deformity from VEPTR techniques, but neurologic injury from VEPTR surgery is rare, usually transient, and, unlike spinal surgery, is unique in that the upper extremities are more involved than the lower extremities.
  - Upper brachial plexopathy has been seen in five early San Antonio VEPTR patients, all resolving spontaneously except one patient who has small residual dyesthesias. The probable basis for brachioplexopathy in VEPTR patients is the compression of the brachial plexus by expansion thoracoplasty elevation of malformed, fused ribs, documented in one patient on MRI. Improved monitoring of procedures has decreased the incidence of this complication.
  - There have been three lower extremity neurologic injuries in our experience in San Antonio.
    - One was a monoplegia after a dural tear from a spinal canal violation with a ronguer. This almost completely resolved a year after surgery.
    - Another was a delayed paraplegia in a patient with sharp, angular congenital kyphosis. There were normal somatosensory evoked potentials and wake-up test during surgery, but delayed paraplegia was evident when the patient awoke from respiratory support sedation several days postimplantation. Removal of the device did not improve neurologic status and the paraplegia is permanent.
    - The third "injury" was a poorly communicative patient with a ventriculoperitoneal shunt who presented several days

post–VEPTR expansion procedure with refusal to walk. Neurologic examination was equivocal. Shunt malfunction was present, and during revision the VEPTR was shortened. The patient began to walk again postoperatively, but it is unclear whether the shunt malfunction or VEPTR surgery was the basis for the change in ambulatory status.

PREVENTION OF COMPLICATIONS

- To prevent neurologic injury during VEPTR implantation, the preoperative CT scan should be checked carefully for areas of dysraphic spine within the area of approach.
- There is also risk of lumbar spine dysraphism of the posterior spinal elements in patients with extensive congenital scoliosis. A large Cobb elevator should be used in stripping the paraspinal muscles to minimize the risk of violating the canal during exposure.
- To avoid premature device migration, an extra-periosteal soft tissue–sparing technique should be used when performing cradle insertion or opening wedge thoracostomies, avoiding the stripping of rib periosteum, because of the subsequent risk of devascularization.
- To avoid distal migration of a rib-to-rib device, be sure the device is well aligned to the osseous ribs of attachment. Usually the standard superior rib cradle and the inferior rib cradle of the rib-to-rib VEPTR are in neutral position, but if the inferior osseous rib of attachment is oriented differently from the superior rib, then the VEPTR may not fit well around the inferior rib. A 30° angled right-handed or left-handed inferior VEPTR cradle may be used to better fit the inferior cradle around the rib in such a situation.
- In placement of lumbar hooks, it is important not to violate the cortex of the lamina of attachment because this weakens its ability to withstand the distraction forces. If the interspace is too small for the hook, then a superior laminotomy of the interspace is performed.
- It is important to place the hybrid lumbar extension in the lumbar spine below any areas of junctional kyphosis seen on the lateral weight-bearing radiograph, with the VEPTR hook placed at least two levels below this to prevent accentuating the kyphosis.

Equipment

- Spinal cord monitoring is used for all procedures, primary implants, replacements, and expansion.
- Prophylactic IV antibiotics are given and maintained for 2 days.

TREATMENT OF COMPLICATIONS

- Superior migration of a rib cradle is treated by accessing the cradle, usually at time of expansion surgery, through a limited incision of the proximal portion of the thoracotomy incision, and reimplanting it into the rib of attachment, which is usually reformed, or a more distal rib.
  - Curved curettes are extremely useful for shaving the hypertrophied rib down to acceptable size for reimplantation of the rib cradle.
  - Inferior cradle migration is treated in a similar fashion.
- For infection, débridement without removal of devices is generally performed, with irrigation by a dilute Betadine solution. The skin edges are then loosely approximated with Prolene sutures, leaving a 5-mm gap in the wound, allowing it to close by second intention. The patient is maintained on 4–6 weeks of IV antibiotics, with culture results determining the specific antibiotic. Sometimes it is helpful to add a Wound Vac overlying the device to help it with healing.
- Recurrent infections require removal of the rib sleeve and the lumbar hybrid extension or the inferior rib cradle, and the patient is maintained on 6 weeks of antibiotics. When sedimentation rate/C-reactive protein levels have normalized, and the wound is healed, then reinsertion of the device can be considered.
- Skin slough is treated by débridement and mobilization of flaps. Primary closure is possible, but loose approximation with Prolene suture is preferred.
- In patients with long-standing VEPTR devices, dense soft tissue scarring sometimes occurs over devices and recurrent skin slough becomes a problem. For these patients, soft tissue expanders are placed laterally to mobilize skin, the scar is resected, and then the new skin is transferred posteriorly over the devices with the assistance of a plastic surgeon.

VEPTR EXPANSION

- The VEPTR device should be expanded on schedule twice a year.
- More frequent expansions, every 3–4 months, over a year or two may be justified with severe deformity not totally responsive to the initial thoracoplasty.
- Delay in expansion risks recurrent deformity that may not be responsive to aggressive device expansion later.

POSITIONING

- The patient is usually placed in a prone position.
- Drape should extend well beyond the expected incision sites in case a VEPTR dislodgement occurs proximally or distally so that re-seatment can be performed through separate incisions without redraping.

PORTALS/EXPOSURES

- Each individual device is accessed by a 3-cm incision.
- If the distraction lock is exposed through the prior thoracotomy incision, a Freer elevator is inserted proximally along the top of the device and used to elevate the overlying muscle.
  - Cautery is inserted into the soft tissue tunnel created by the Freer elevator, and used to release the muscle deeply on each side of the device, so that a thick muscle flap is mobilized with the free edge at the skin incision.
  - The same approach is used distally.
- If there is no prior incision over the distraction lock access point, a new skin incision is made paralleling the device.
  - The muscle incision is next made by cautery *along the side of the device,* then the cautery is turned sideways to release the muscle flap off the device.
  - The full-thickness muscle flap is reflected by a Freer elevator, then the distraction locks of the device are removed, and the expansion procedure performed.

PROCEDURE

STEP 1

- The distraction lock is removed with either the notched wedge instrument or the lock removal forceps.
- The distraction pliers are inserted and the VEPTR is expanded until the reactive force increases substantially (Fig. 11). Generally this occurs at 1 cm of expansion.
  - The medial device is always expanded first. The adjacent lateral devices are then expanded approximately half that distance.
  - For bilateral devices, the concave hemithorax is expanded first, then the convex side.
- A distraction dead bolt peg is placed distally in the VEPTR to hold the device out to length, and the distraction pliers are removed from the field to gain room for lock insertion.
- The distraction lock is then inserted with a distraction lock holder.
  - If there is an early large increase in reactive force, the surgeon should first distract a few millimeters, lock the distraction pliers for 3 minutes to allow dissipation of force, then expand another 2–3 mm, until a full 5 mm of distraction is obtained. Then the device can be locked in place with a new distraction lock.

STEP 2

- The mobilized muscle flaps are closed without tension over the locks in a multiple-layer closure with absorbable suture.
- Soft dressings are applied
- A single AP radiograph is taken in the operating room to check device position.

POSTOPERATIVE CARE AND EXPECTED OUTCOMES

- Ambulation is permitted the day of surgery.
- Showers are permitted 7 days postoperative.
- Full activity is encouraged 3 weeks after surgery.
- Complications include infection, skin slough, and device dislodgement.

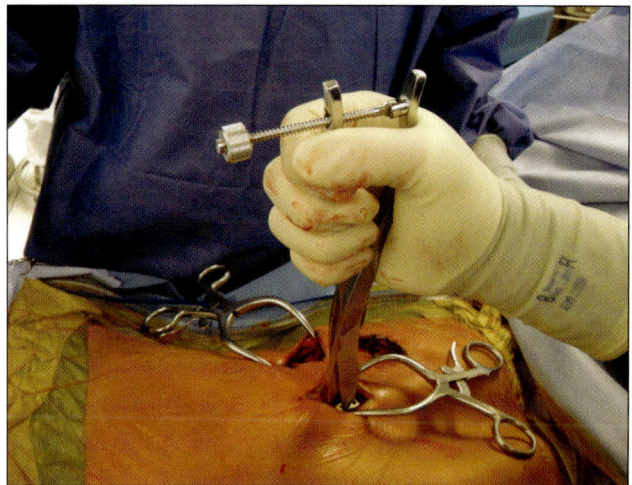

FIGURE 11

VEPTR REPLACEMENT

- Inherent VEPTR device expansion capability is somewhat limited in the very small sizes of device to 4–5 cm, but progressively increases with longer devices.
- Once the device has been completely expanded, change-out of the central rib sleeve portion and the inferior rib cradle/hybrid shaft is needed. This is usually accomplished through limited-access skip incisions.

POSITIONING

- The patient is usually placed in a prone position.
- Spinal cord monitoring and somatosensory and motor evoked potentials are used for all replacement procedures.

PORTALS/EXPOSURES

- A central incision of 3 cm is made at the distraction point, then another a small incision over the superior cradle, and then a third incision over the lumbar hook or the inferior cradle (Fig. 12).

PROCEDURE

STEP 1

- In a rib-to-rib VEPTR, the two distraction locks are removed, and also the rib cradle cap lock distally.
  - The distal rib cradle is rotated out of the way by forceps, but left in situ.
  - The inferior rib cradle is pulled outward to disengage it from the inferior rib of attachment.
  - The inferior rib cradle is slid distally out of the rib sleeve through the inferior incision.
  - The same maneuver is performed with the rib sleeve through the central incision.
- In a hybrid VEPTR, the lumbar extension shaft is released from the hook and slid out proximally through the central incision.
  - The replacement VEPTR is sized to be the same length as the completely expanded VEPTR that it replaces.

STEP 2

- In a rib-to-rib VEPTR, the new rib sleeve is slid up from the central incision to engage the imbedded superior rib cradle, and locked with a new distraction lock proximally.
  - The inferior rib cradle is threaded from the distal incision proximally to engage the rib sleeve, and the "shoehorn" instrument is used to key it into the distal attachment site around the rib.
  - The rib cradle is rotated back to engage the rib cradle and locked with a new cradle cap lock cap.
- In hybrid VEPTR replacements, the new lumbar extension is threaded into the rib sleeve, from the distal incision over the retained spinal hook, then slid back into the hook and the hook screw is tightened.
- The new device is then tensioned, much as is done during an expansion procedure, by distraction pliers.

PEARLS

- *Drape wide, since additional exposure may be needed if the limited-access incisions do not permit adequate exposure to perform the planned replacement.*

Equipment

- Prophylactic IV antibiotics are given and maintained for 2–3 days.

PEARLS

- *Meticulous soft tissue technique is used to prevent skin slough*

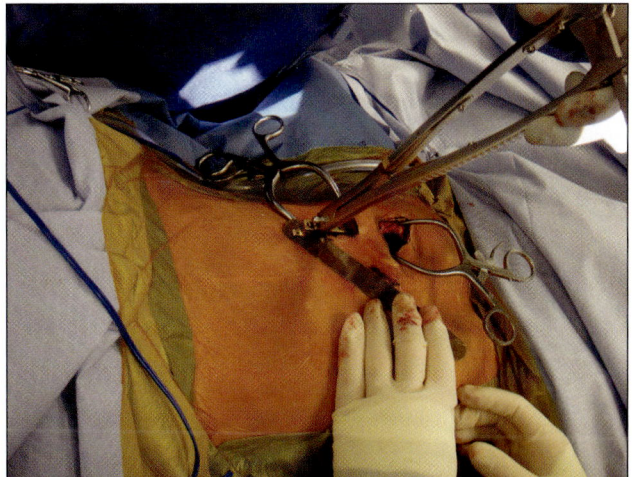

FIGURE 12

STEP 3

- Closure is in multiple layers with absorbable sutures over a # 7 JP round drain.
- Soft dressings are used to cover wounds.

POSTOPERATIVE CARE AND EXPECTED OUTCOMES

- Drains are removed when drainage is 20 ml or less over a 24-hour period.
- Chest tubes are removed when drainage is less than 1 ml/kg per 24 hours.
- Patients are usually able to ambulate within 24–48 hours postprocedure.
- Operative severity for replacement procedures is subjectively about 50% of an implantation procedure.
- Complications include infection, skin slough, upper/lower extremity neurologic injury, and device dislodgement.
- Subsequent expansion procedures are scheduled 6 months later, since replacement counts as a VEPTR expansion.

VEPTR PROCEDURE FOR EARLY-ONSET SCOLIOSIS

- The type IIb VDD associated with early-onset scoliosis is from the transverse constriction of the chest due to the windswept deformity from spine rotation into the convex hemithorax.
- The coronal plane type II VDD hemithorax constriction is identified by the area of multiple persistent intercostal space narrowing of the concave hemithorax in the bending radiographs.

CONTROVERSIES

- VEPTR expansion thoracoplasty treatment of early-onset scoliosis remains controversial.
- Some argue that the presence of a VEPTR on the chest wall will eventually stiffen the chest, adversely affecting respiration, but since the chest wall is already irreversibly stiff preoperatively, it seems unlikely that the VEPTR will affect matters one way or the other. It is assumed that growing rods do not stiffen the chest wall because of their central placement, but often the rods extend over the ribs on the concave side of the curve.
- Open concave VEPTR thoracostomy, open concave VEPTR thoracostomy with convex percutaneous rib-to-pelvis VEPTR, and bilateral percutaneous rib-to-pelvis VEPTR are all now used for early-onset scoliosis, without a clear-cut advantage of one method over another.
  - We prefer open concave VEPTR thoracostomy when the concave hemithorax is stiff preoperatively, and the intercostal spaces remain narrow on bending radiographs.
  - Supple intercostal spaces and a concave hemithorax that is mobile with respiration would argue for the bilateral percutaneous rib-to-pelvis VEPTRs.
  - Smith (personal communication) cautions about sagittal alignment issues with the percutaneous bilateral technique, and recommends it only for nonambulatory patients.
- These issues await clarification through a prospective clinical trial comparing VEPTR treatments, as well as comparing them to growing rod treatment.

Equipment

- Prophylactic IV antibiotics are given and maintained for 3–5 days.

POSITIONING

- The patient is placed in a prone position.
- Spinal cord monitoring is used.

PORTALS/EXPOSURES

- Exposures are the same as those used for fused ribs and scoliosis patients.
- Unilateral VEPTR procedures usually include one or two opening wedge thoracostomies through intercostal muscles at the apex of constricted hemithorax, using intercostal muscle lysis rather than transverse rib osteotomy of the concave hemithorax, based on persistent intercostal space narrowing on supine lateral bending radiographs.
- A second percutaneous convex VEPTR hybrid in the manner of Smith may be added for severe scoliosis, with exposure proximally involving using the top one-third of the traditional opening wedge thoracoctomy incision, with the distal iliac crest incision the same as used for the fused ribs and scoliosis exposure.

PROCEDURE

- The apex of the curve is often distal to the area of rib cage constriction.
  - The superior distraction point, where the superior cradle is attached, should be at the proximal end of the curve.
  - Care must be taken to not place it in the compensatory curve above the structural curve since the distraction force will just increase the compensatory curve without correction of the true curve.
- The superior cradle is placed in the usual fashion.
- Once the area of intercostal muscle narrowing is identified, then the central narrow intercostal muscle interval is released by cautery, with a right-angle clamp under the muscle to protect the underlying pleura.
- The pleura is mobilized by a Kidner, two to three ribs above and below the interval.
- Another opening wedge thoracostomy can be made two ribs above or below the initial release, if the area of constriction is widespread. The ribs are distracted apart by the Synthes rib spreader to lengthen the constricted hemithorax.

- A unilateral rib-to-spine VEPTR hybrid is then placed. A second rib-to-rib VEPTR device is often added to load share (Fig. 13A–D).
- Other constructs that can be used are bilateral rib-to-spine VEPTR hybrids, a unilateral rib-to-pelvis via "S" hook VEPTR hybrid, or bilateral rib-to-pelvis via "S" hook VEPTR hybrids.

POSTOPERATIVE CARE AND EXPECTED OUTCOMES

- Ambulation is permitted the day of surgery.
- Showers are permitted 7 days postoperative.
- Full activity is encouraged 3 weeks after surgery.
- Complications include infection, skin slough, and device dislodgement.

PEARLS

- *Treatment for infection is débridement and antibiotics.*
  - *Device removal is considered in only severe infections with frank abscess.*
  - *Often the superior rib cradle can be left in situ in these cases, simplifying reimplantation of the device later once infection has cleared.*

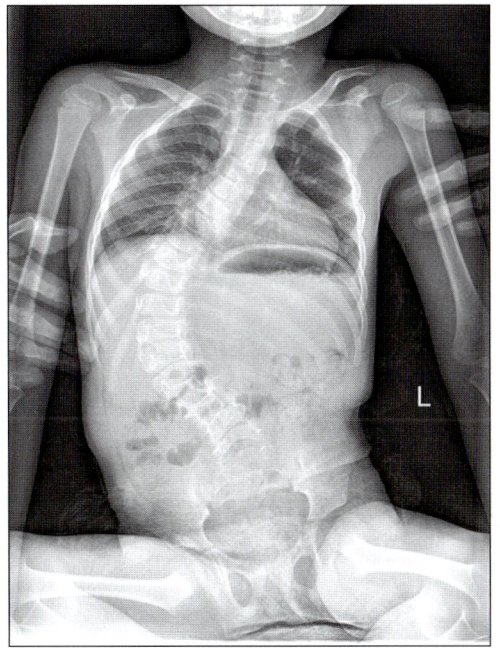

A

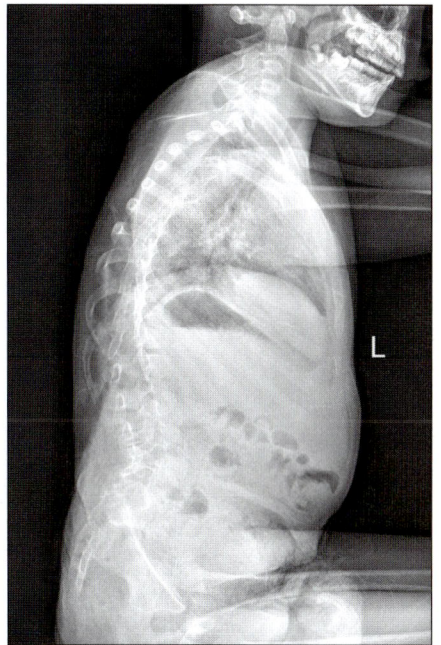

B

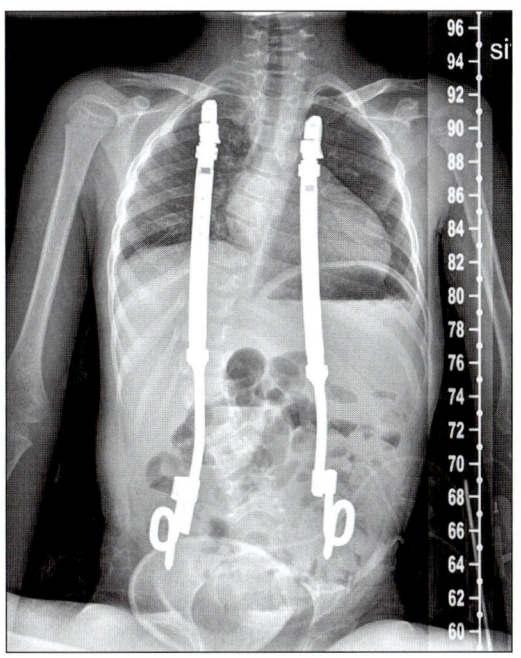

C

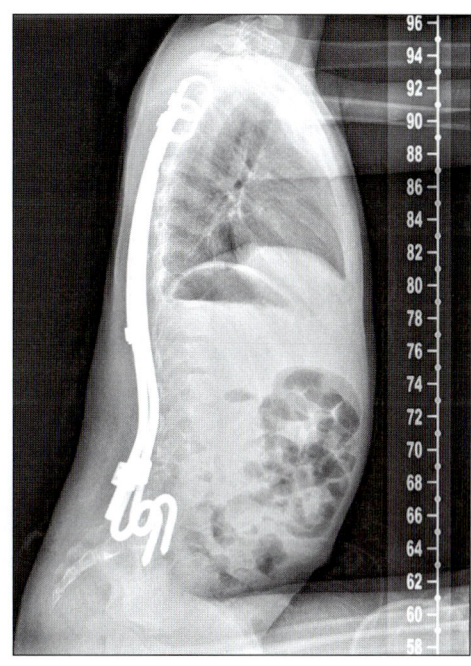

D

FIGURE 13

EVIDENCE

Campbell RM. Operative strategies for thoracic insufficiency syndrome by vertical expandable prosthetic titanium rib expansion thoracoplasty. Oper Tech Orthop. 2005;15:315–25.

Campbell RM, Adcox B, Smith MD, Simmons JW III, Cofer BR, Inscore SC, Grohman C. The effect of mid-thoracic VEPTR opening wedge thoracostomy on cervical-thoracic congenital scoliosis. Spine. 2007;32:2171–7.

Campbell RM Jr, Aubrey A, Smith MD, Simmons JW, Joshi A, Inscore S, Cofer B, Doski J. The characterization of the thoracic biomechanics of respiration in thoracic insufficiency syndrome by dynamic lung MRI: a preliminary report. Presented at the International Congress of Early Onset Scoliosis, Montreal, Canada, 2008a.

Campbell RM, Hell-Vocke AK. Growth of the thoracic spine in congenital scoliosis after expansion thoracoplasty. J Bone Joint Surg [Am]. 2003;85:409–20.

Campbell RM, Smith MD. Reconstruction of the thorax in patients with absent ribs and flail chest physiology using vertical expandable prosthetic titanium ribs (VEPTR). Poster presentation, American Association of Pediatric Surgeons Annual Meeting, 2003.

Campbell RM Jr, Smith MD. Thoracic insufficiency syndrome and exotic scoliosis. J Bone Joint Surg [Am]. 2007;89(Suppl 1):108–22.

Campbell RM Jr, Smith MD, Hell-Vocke AK. Expansion thoracoplasty: the surgical technique of opening-wedge thoracostomy. Surgical technique. J Bone Joint Surg [Am]. 2004;86(Suppl 1):51–64.

Campbell RM Jr, Smith MD, Mayes TC, Mangos JA, Willey-Courand DB, Kose N, Pinero RF, Alder ME, Duong HL, Surber JL. The characteristics of thoracic insufficiency syndrome associated with fused ribs and scoliosis. J Bone Joint Surg [Am]. 2003a; 85:399–408.

Campbell RM Jr, Smith MD, Mayes TC, Mangos JA, Willey-Courand DB, Kose N, Pinero RF, Alder ME, Duong HL, Surber J. The effect of opening wedge thoracostomy on thoracic insufficiency syndrome associated with fused ribs and congenital scoliosis. J Bone Joint Surg [Am]. 2003b;85:1615–24.

Campbell RM, Smith MD, Simmons JW III, Cofer BR, Inscore SC, Grohman C. The treatment of secondary thoracic insufficiency syndrome of myelomeningocele by a hybrid VEPTR "Eiffel Tower" construct with S-hook iliac crest pedestal fixation. Presented at IMAST, 2007, Bahamas; and Poster Exhibit, American Association of Orthopaedic Surgeons Annual Meeting, San Francisco, 2008b.

Campbell RM, Smith MD, Taichi IO, et al. The treatment of thoracic insufficiency syndrome associated with spondylocostal dysostosis and spondylothoracic dyplasia. Presented at the Scoliosis Research Society meeting, Buenos Aires, 2004.

DiMeglio A, Bonnel F. Le Rachis en Croissance. Paris: Springer, 1990.

Donnelley LF, Emery KH, Brody AS, Laor T, Gylys-Morin VM, Anton CG, Thomas SR, Frush DP. Minimizing radiation dose for pediatric body applications of single-detector helical CT: strategies at a large children's hospital. AJR Am J Roentgenol. 2001; 176:303–6.

Gollogly S, Smith JT, Campbell RM. Determining lung volume with three dimensional reconstructions of CT scan data: a pilot study to evaluate the effects of expansion thoracoplasty on children with severe spinal deformities. J Pediatr Orthop. 2004a; 24:323–8.

Gollogly S, Smith JT, White SK, Firth S, White K. The volume of lung parenchyma as a function of age: a review of 1050 normal CT scans of the chest with three-dimensional volumetric reconstruction of the pulmonary system. Spine. 2004b;29:2061–6.

Hoekelman RA. In Hoelkelman RA, Blatman S, Friedman SB, Nelson NM, Seidel HM (eds). Primary Pediatric Care. St. Louis: Mosby, 1987.

Jones KL (ed). Smith's Hereditary Malformations. Philadelphia: WB Saunders, 1988:694.

Klemme W, Denis D, Winter R, Lonstein J, Koop S. Spinal instrumentation without fusion. J Pediatr Orthop. 1997;17:734–42.

Openshaw P, Edwards S, Helms P. Changes in rib cage geometry during childhood. Thorax. 1984;39:624–7.

Paterson A, Frush DP, Donnelly LF. Helical CT of the body: are settings adjusted for pediatric patients? AJR Am Roentgenol. 2001;176:297–301.

Smith MD, Campbell RM Jr. Use of a bioabsorbable patch for reconstruction of large thoracic cage defects in growing children. J Pediatr Surg 2006;41:46–9.

Tello J. Subcutaneous rods and scoliosis. Orthop Clin North Am. 1994;167:87–95.

Hemivertebra Resection

Daniel J. Hedequist

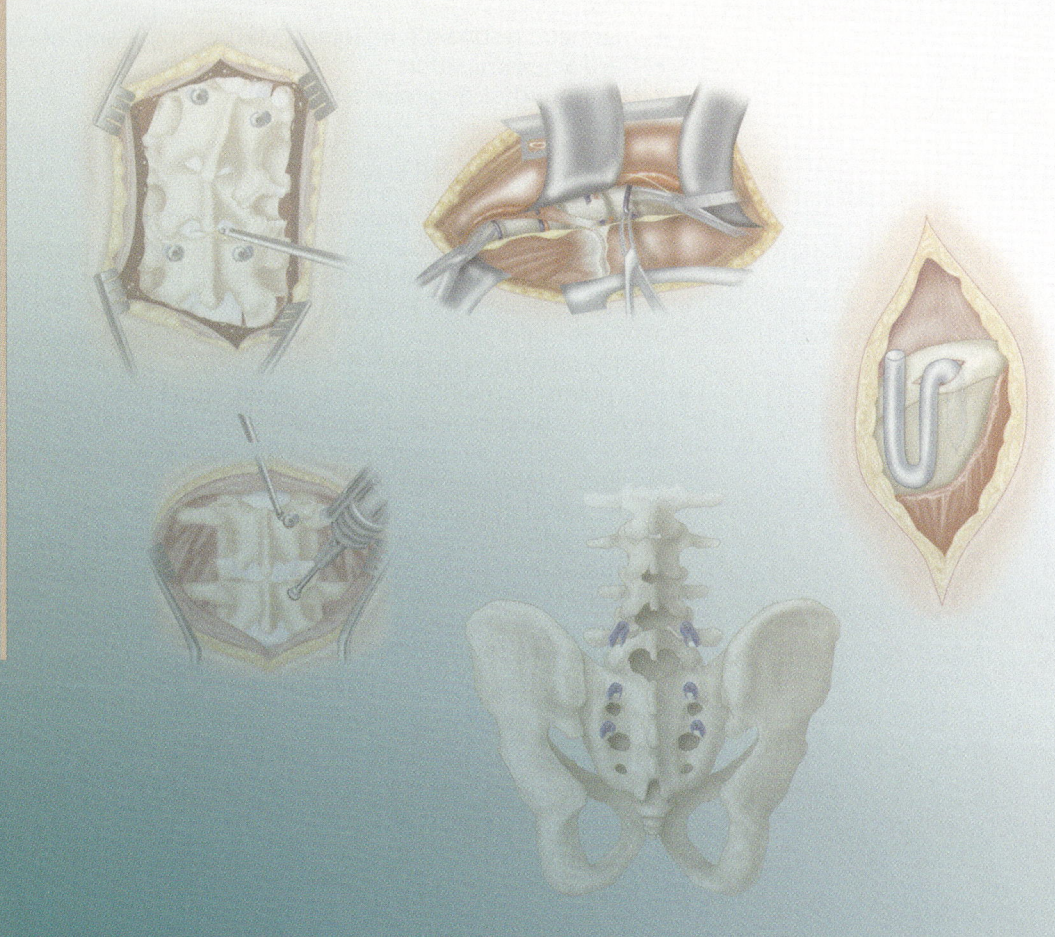

Controversies

- Age
- Curve size
- Location

Treatment Options

- Combined anterior/posterior hemivertebra excision
- Posterior-only hemivertebra excision
- Anterior-only hemivertebra excision
- In situ anterior/posterior fusion
- Convex hemiepiphysiodesis

INDICATIONS

- Progressive scoliosis secondary to a hemivertebra
- Progressive spinal imbalance secondary to a hemivertebra

EXAMINATION/IMAGING

- Standing posteroanterior (PA) and lateral 36-inch spine radiographs are obtained. Figure 1 shows standing radiographs of a patient with a thoracolumbar hemivertebra in PA (Fig. 1A) and lateral (Fig. 1B) views.
- Three-dimensional computed tomography (CT) scan will reveal the posterior elements (Fig. 2A) and the partial anterior fusion (Fig. 2B).
- Screening examinations should be done for additional morbidities:
  - Magnetic resonance imaging (MRI) of spine and brainstem
  - Cardiac examination
  - Ultrasound of genitourinary system

SURGICAL ANATOMY

- The relevant surgical anatomy for hemivertebra excision relies on a thorough understanding of the posterior spinal elements as well as the anatomy of the hemivertebra posterior elements.
- The preoperative CT scan is of utmost importance in order to assess for bifid midline structures and the relationship of the hemilamina compared to the levels above and below.
- Key points to resection are as follows: visualization down the corresponding pedicle and its relationship to the nerve roots above and below, the dura near the medial wall, and the epidural venous plexus.
- Understanding the anterior anatomy and whether or not the hemivertebra is segmented or partially segmented helps with complete resection anteriorly.

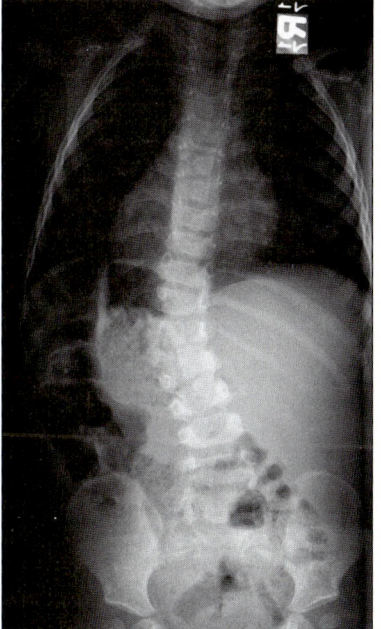 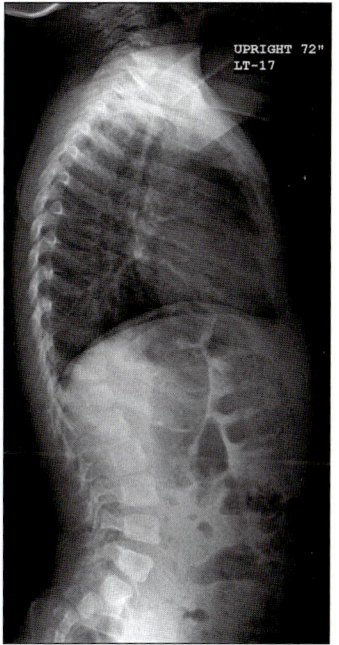

A   B

FIGURE 1

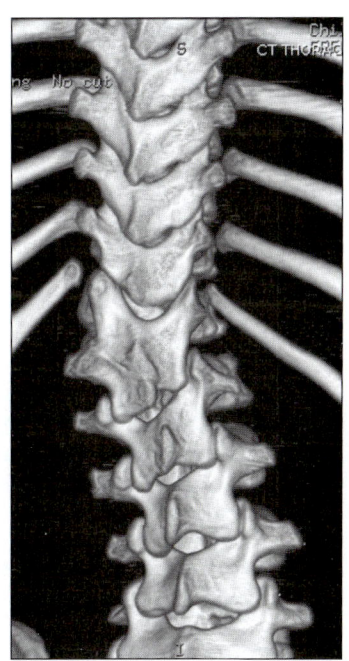 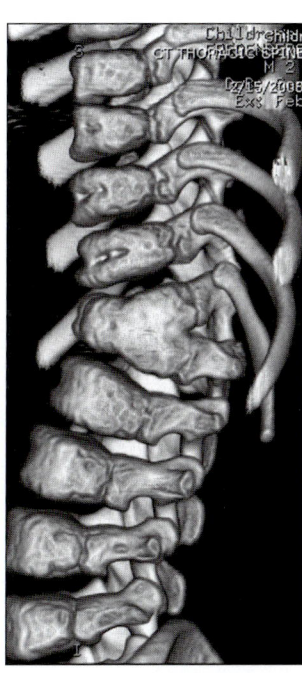

A 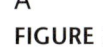   B

FIGURE 2

Equipment

- Radiolucent operating table
- Motor and sensory evoked potential monitoring

Instrumentation/ Implantation

- Fluoroscopic confirmation of pedicle screws
- Triggered electromyography for screw stimulation.
- Titanium implants in patients requiring further MRI

POSITIONING

- The patient is placed in the prone position on a radiolucent spinal frame.
- Padding is placed on the chest and iliac crests, taking care to keep the abdomen free to facilitate venous return (Fig. 3).
- The convex side needs to be elevated by 10–20° in order to allow bleeding and the dura to fall away from the operated resection site.
- The patient must have appropriate somatosensory and motor evoked potential monitoring in place.

PORTALS/EXPOSURES

- Standard posterior element exposure is done.
- A hypotensive anesthetic may be used, keeping the mean arterial pressure between 65 and 70 mm Hg, in order to help avoid excessive bleeding. Judicious use of electrocautery is done to keep the surgical field dry.
- Wide dissection is performed bilaterally to the tips of the transverse processes. The posterior element anatomy on the preoperative CT scans must be studied and understood for two main reasons.
  - The anatomy of the hemilamina in relationship to the levels above and below must be understood to confirm being at the correct level.
  - The surgeon must also be aware of any bifid structures in order to avoid unwanted penetration into the spinal canal.
- Once the transverse processes are completely exposed, it is helpful to use fluoroscopy or radiographs to confirm the position. It is helpful to mark the pedicle as there is usually a recognizable hemivertebra pedicle and a pedicle above and below the hemivertbra on the convex side.

PROCEDURE

STEP 1

- Placement of implant anchors is paramount prior to resecting the hemivertebra. The pedicle anatomy of the patient may be studied on the preoperative imaging studies.
- In general, the pedicles above and below the hemivertebra are usually large enough to accept screw placement. Screws may be placed in the standard technique into the vertebrae above and below the hemivertebra on both the convex and concave sides.
  - In children less than 8 years of age, we use a 4.5-mm rod system, and in those age 8 or greater, we use a 5.5-mm rod system.
  - Implants should be titanium if the child has any existing spinal dysraphism or cardiac anomalies that may potentially require an MRI in the future.
- Screw placement is then confirmed via both fluoroscopy (Fig. 4) and triggered electromyography (Fig. 5).
- We also will use a downgoing supralaminar hook on the vertebra above and an upgoing infralaminar hook on the vertebra below in order to increase stability; these are placed in the standard fashion after screw placement.

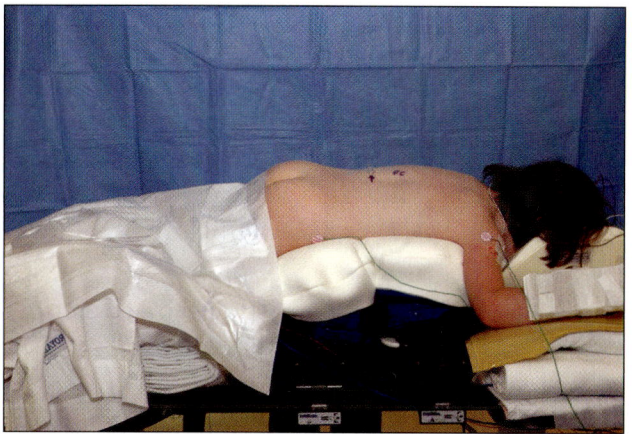

FIGURE 3

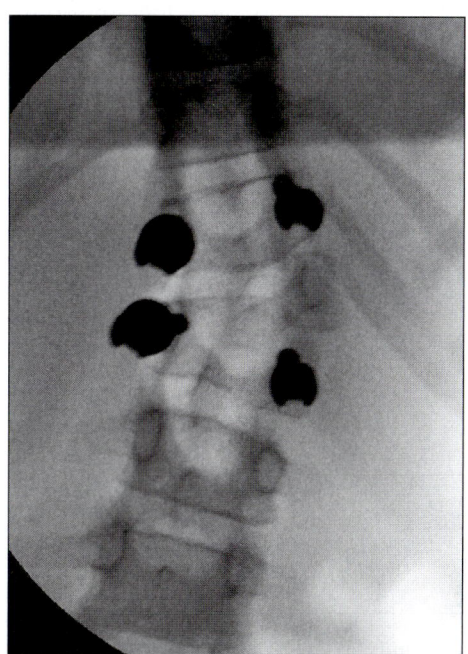

FIGURE 4

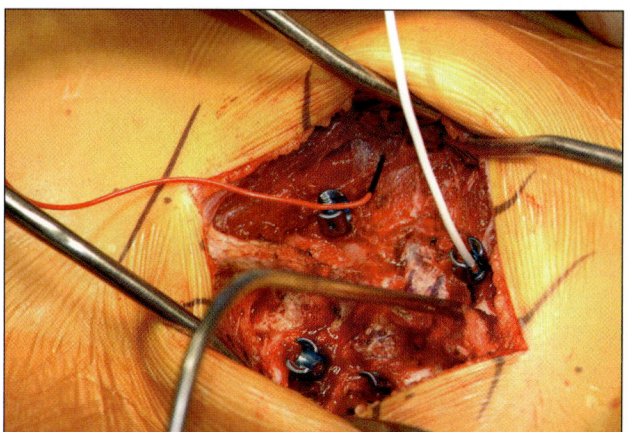

FIGURE 5

STEP 2

- Resection of the hemivertebra first begins with hemilamina resection. This can be done with Kerrison rongeurs (Fig. 6A and 6B) and starts with removal of the ligamentum flavum cephalad and caudad to the hemivertebra. Resection starts in the midline and then moves laterally out toward the corresponding facet. The transverse process then needs to be removed as well, making sure that care is taken not to damage the corresponding exiting nerve roots.

- Pedicle resection first starts by placing retractors extraperiosteally down the lateral side of the pedicle and against the anterolateral body to protect visceral structures. Figure 7 shows placement of a Cobb elevator down the anterolateral side of the hemivertebra, protecting visceral structures. We then start with a high-speed diamond-tipped burr, going down the pedicle and burring first the cancellous channel of the pedicle. The walls may then be burred down or a curette may be used to help collapse them down into the tract. A nerve root retractor acts as a protector against damage to the medial dura.

- A few important points merit mention as dissection continues down the pedicle toward the body.
  - The medial wall of the pedicle and down where the pedicle meets the body need the venous epidural plexus cleared off to aid in visualization and prevent unwanted bleeding. This is done by carefully using a bipolar cautery to prophylactically cauterize these vessels.
  - A headlamp is essential for visualization.
  - The nerve root above and below the hemipedicle must be protected and visualized during resection.

- Resection then continues down the pedicle and into the hemibody. Visualization continues to be paramount, and once again prophylactic cautery is important, as is the judicious use of gel foam and fibrin-soaked patties to help protect the medial dura. The visceral structure need to be continually protected by retraction. Figure 8 shows a clear view of the hemibody after pedicle resection, with an anterolateral retractor protecting visceral structures.

- Removal of the disks above and below can be difficult as they are frequently adherent to the bodies above and below. We aim for complete removal of the disks above and below as well as the hemivertebra all the way over to the concave side.

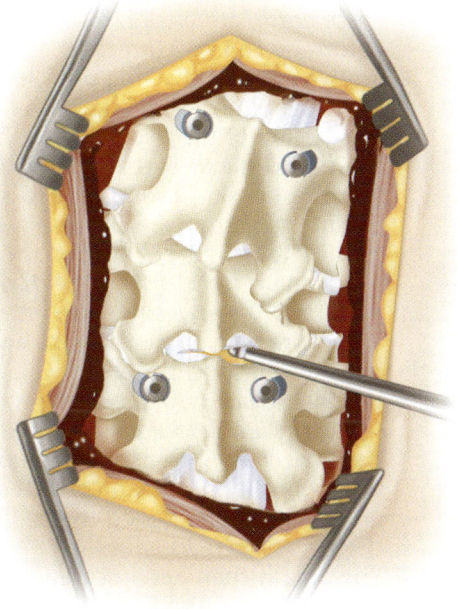

A

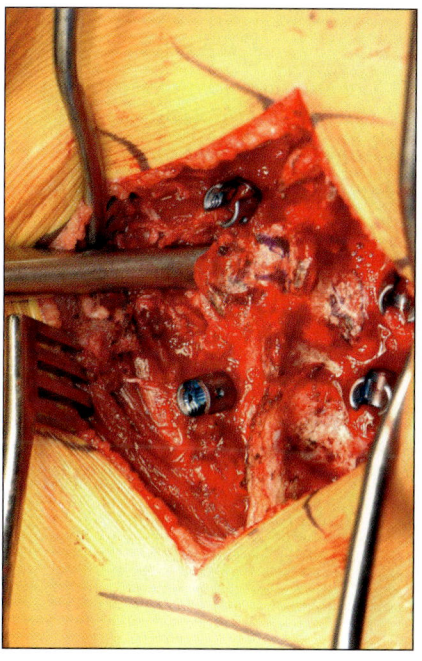

B

FIGURE 6

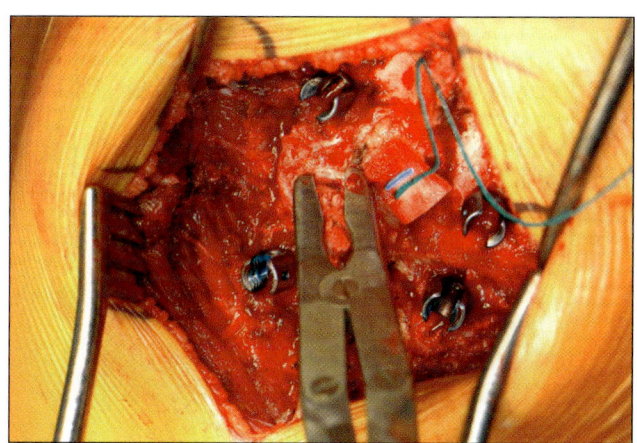

FIGURE 7

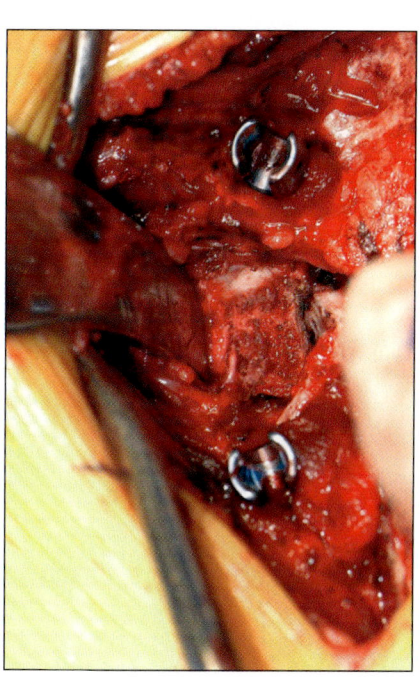

FIGURE 8

STEP 3

- Once complete wedge resection is performed (Fig. 9), the deformity can be corrected.
- We have found that the pedicles of small children are not strong enough to withstand the compressive forces required for the closure of the excision site. Thus, we place a rod between the supralaminar and infralaminar hooks and compress down the excision site, taking care to keep an eye on the dura and exiting nerve roots.
  - The site is usually closed down easily and completely if an adequate resection has been performed.
  - Figure 10 shows a wedge resection closed down after compression of the laminar hooks. Note that the pedicle screws have all become level, indicating complete correction.
- We then place two additional rods connecting the pedicle screws in order to add stability to the construct (Fig. 11). We then check an intraoperative fluoroscopic view to confirm that the deformity has been corrected to the desired amount. A crosslink is then applied to the two rods that are connected to the pedicle screws.
- The area is then decorticated, and abundant allograft as well as autograft from the hemivertebra is applied.
- Wound closure is performed in the standard manner.
- Figure 12 shows postoperative standing PA (Fig. 12A) and lateral (Fig. 12B) radiographs.

POSTOPERATIVE CARE AND EXPECTED OUTCOMES

- Most patients will be in the hospital for approximately 5 days; a postoperative intensive care unit stay is not required.
- In general, bracing is used for younger children who may be less reliable; this is done for 6 weeks.
- We generally obtain radiographs at the first visit at 4–6 weeks from the operation and then obtain radiographs and a CT scan at 3 months to assess the fusion.
- Patients may return to all nonsports activities at 3 months depending on the fusion appearance via CT scanning. Return to sports at 6 months is allowed. Long-term follow-up for these patients is required.

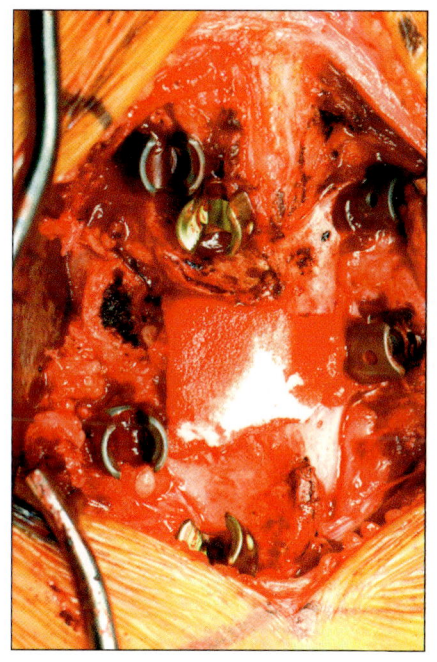

FIGURE 9

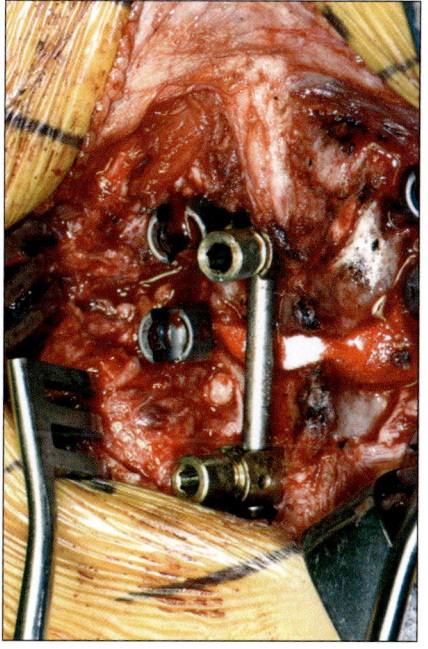

FIGURE 10

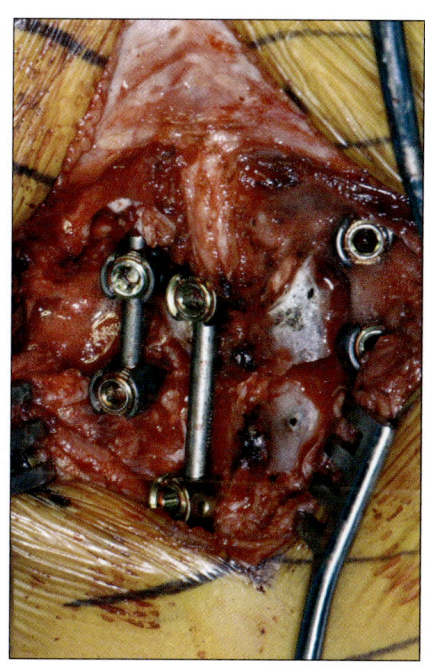

FIGURE 11

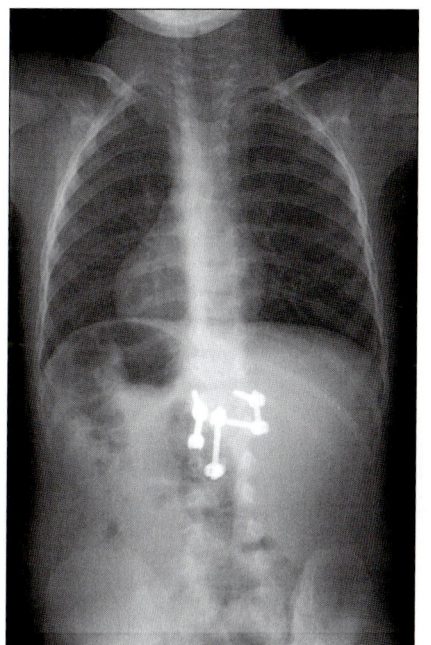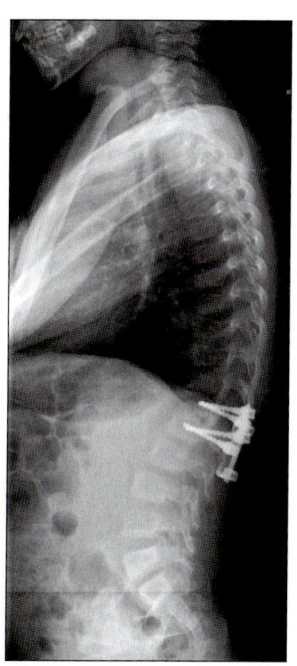

A

B

FIGURE 12

EVIDENCE

Hedequist DJ, Hall JE, Emans JB. Hemivertebra excision in children via simultaneous anterior and posterior exposures. J Pediatr Orthop. 2005;25:60–3.

Hedequist DJ, Hall JE, Emans JB. The safety and efficacy of spinal instrumentation in children with congenital spine deformities. Spine. 2004;29:2081–6; discussion, 2087.

Ruf M, Harms J. Pedicle screws in 1- and 2-year-old children: technique, complications, and effect on further growth. Spine. 2002;27:E460–6.

Ruf M, Harms J. Posterior hemivertebra resection with transpedicular instrumentation: early correction in children aged 1 to 6 years. Spine. 2003;28:2132–8.

Posterior Surgical Treatment for Scheuermann's Kyphosis

Daniel J. Hedequist

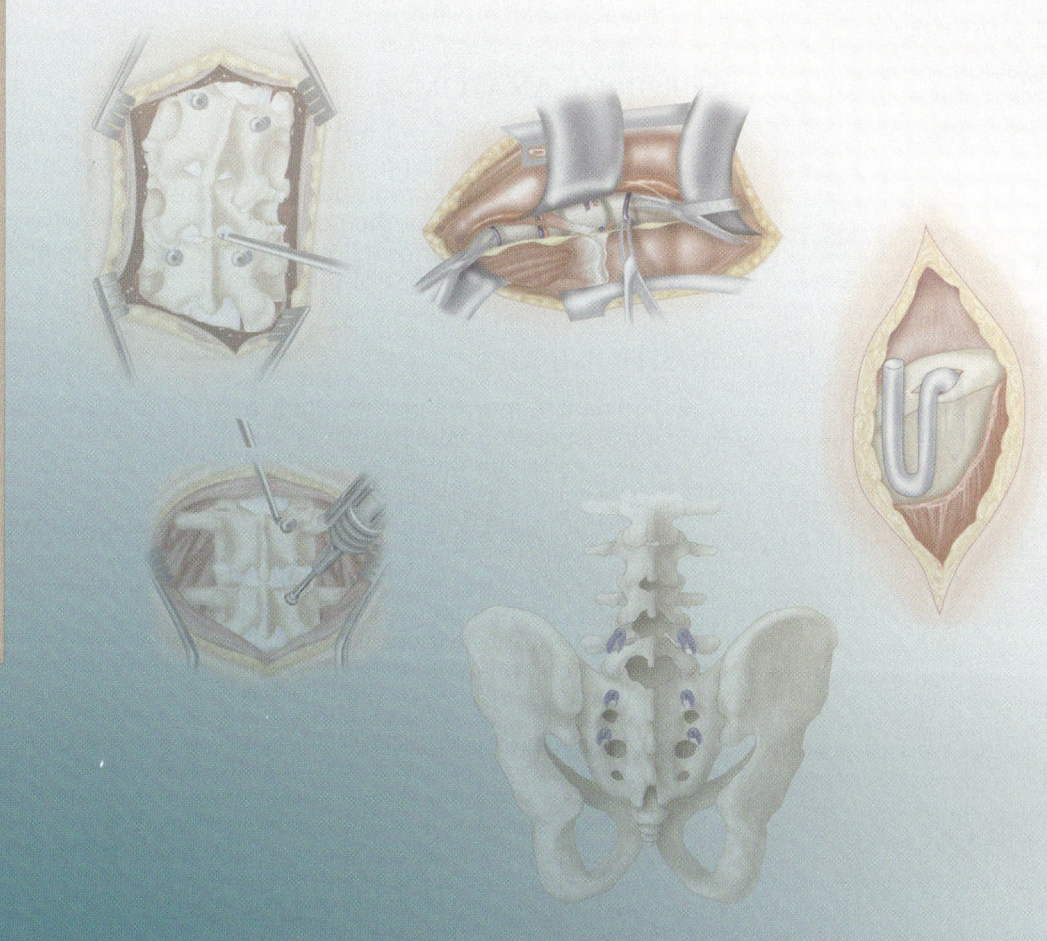

PITFALLS

- *Patient misperceptions*
- *Curves amendable to bracing*
- *Medical comorbidities*

Controversies

- Need for anterior release and fusion

Treatment Options

- Open/thoracoscopic anterior release and fusion with posterior fusion and instrumentation

PEARLS

- *A Mayfield headrest in order to control access to the cervicothoracic junction*
- *Armrests placed to facilitate surgeon access to the cervicothoracic junction*

PITFALLS

- *Poor proximal thoracic spine access secondary to head position*
- *Poor proximal access secondary to inadequate draping*

Equipment

- Motor and sensory evoked potential monitoring
- Radiolucent operating frame to confirm location and screw placement

PEARLS

- *Mean arterial pressure 65–70 mm Hg*
- *Judicious electrocautery*
- *Preservation of junctional interspinous ligaments*

PITFALLS

- *Inadequate exposure at proximal and distal ends*
- *Excessive soft tissue remaining on spine*

INDICATIONS

- Progressive kyphosis greater than 75°
- Intractable back pain
- Objectionable appearance to the patient
- Neurologic signs or symptoms

EXAMINATION/IMAGING

- Standing posteroanterior (PA) and lateral 36-inch radiographs are obtained. Figure 1 shows standing radiographs of a patient with kyphosis in PA (Fig. 1A) and lateral (Fig. 1B) views.
- A lateral radiograph in hyperextesion with a bolster under the kyphotic apex is also obtained.
- Magnetic resonance imaging is done to assess for any possible thoracic disk herniations.

SURGICAL ANATOMY

- Posterior-only treatment for Scheuermann's kyphosis requires an understanding of the posterior anatomic structures of the spine as well as the variations in pedicle anatomy.
- Intimate knowledge of the posterior structures allows for the surgeon to easily perform Ponte osteotomies (foramina to foramina) over the apex of the curve.

POSITIONING

- The patient may be placed prone on a standard radiolucent spinal operating frame.
  - The abdomen must be kept free, and bolsters are placed at the chest and iliac crest regions.
  - The arms are flexed at the elbows and placed forward with the axilla remaining free of any compression.
  - The head needs to be placed in a standard headrest with access at the cervicothoracic junction.
- The patient must have appropriate somatosensory and motor evoked potential monitoring in place.

PORTALS/EXPOSURES

- The exposure of the thoracic and lumbar spine entails standard techniques.
- Hypotensive anesthesia is useful, taking care to keep the mean arterial pressures in the 65- to 70-mm Hg range.
- Subperiosteal dissection is necessary in order to obtain adequate bone for fusion as well as clear anatomic landmarks for pedicle screw placement.
- Exposure is done with Cobb elevators and electrocautery, taking care to expose out to the tips of the spinous processes.

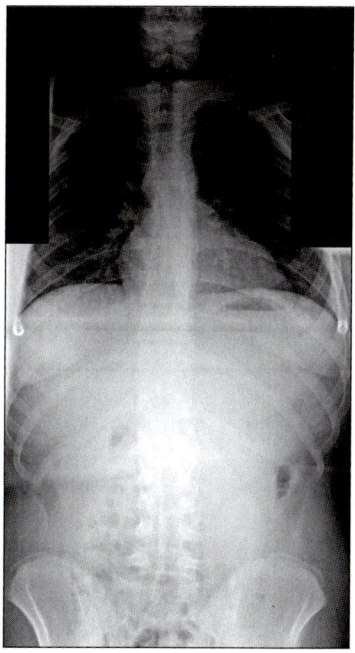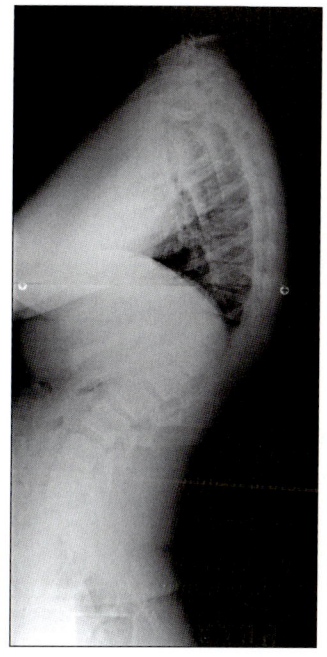

A   B

FIGURE 1

Instrumentation/ Implantation

- Fixed screw placement in thoracic spine
- Reduction screws at bottom and top of construct
- $\frac{1}{4}$-inch rod diameter system

PROCEDURE

STEP 1

- Pedicle screw placement begins distally in the lumbar spine, taking care to include the lumbar vertebra that is centered over the sacral spine in the lateral view.
- The use of fixed or variable screws will lead to reliable results in correcting kyphosis. The use of reduction screws at the distal levels may help capture the rods more easily, and may aid in rod capture proximally as well.
- Standard lumbar screw placement is performed, taking care to place as large a diameter of screw as possible, with the length of screws typically ranging from 40 to 50 mm.
- Thoracic screw placement is done after facetectomies at each corresponding level.
  - A freehand technique can be easily employed at each level. This is done by using a burr to create a starting point that can be referenced for each level. A cancellous blush should be seen, and a curved-tipped thoracic gearshift should be used to gain access to the first 20 mm of the pedicle.
  - This is followed by probing to make sure that the gearshift is contained and then switching the gearshift around so that the point is directed medially and down into the body. The hole is then probed and, if contained, a tap is then used followed by probing and then placement of an appropriate length and diameter of screw.
- Once the screws have been placed, we use fluoroscopic confirmation in both the AP and lateral planes to make sure the cascade of screws and length of screws have been placed appropriately.
- Triggered electromyography is used to test screw placement. We use a triggered response of 6 mA or lower as a threshold for screw removal and reprobing. The screw is then put back in if probing confirms adequate position.

STEP 2

- The most important step for adequate correction of kyphosis is the posterior osteotomies. The osteotomies are best referred to as "Ponte" osteotomies and include wide release from foramina to foramina. Frequently the midline has been ossified in Scheuermann's kyphosis and the osteotomies need to take place over the apical regions of the deformity.
- The osteotomy begins first with a complete facetectomy. Once this has been performed, the next step is resection of the ligamentum flavum. In kyphosis, the dura has fallen away from the apical dorsal element and is covered by epidural fat, making resection of the ligamentum inherently safe.
  - Figure 2 shows the start of posterior element resection; the midline is the beginning point, with a rongeur used after facetectomies have been performed.
  - Moving from the midline out toward the foramina, ligamentum resection laterally to the lateral recess is performed with a larger Kerrison rongeur (Fig. 3). This resection entails removing the superior facet surface of the level below (the inferior facet of the level above has been removed by facetectomy).
  - Resection should be done from foramina to foramina and usually will leave a 1 cm gap which will close down (Fig. 4).

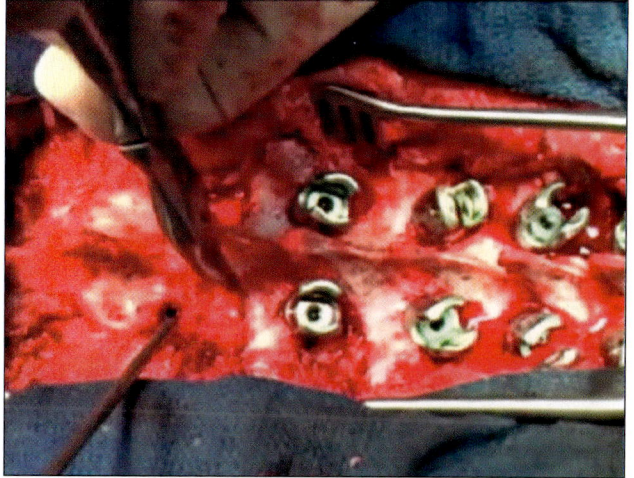

FIGURE 2

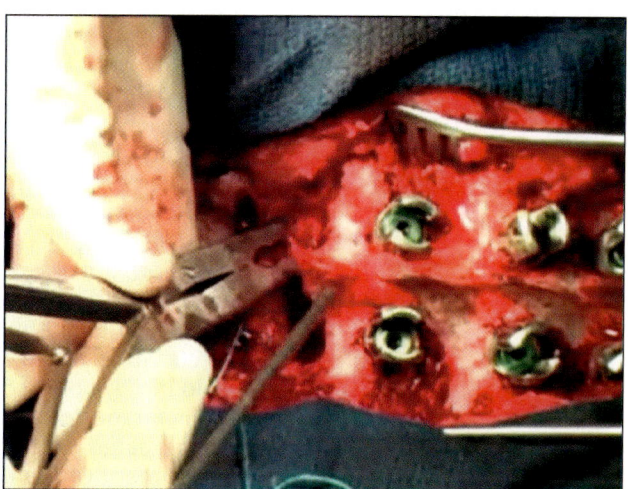

FIGURE 3

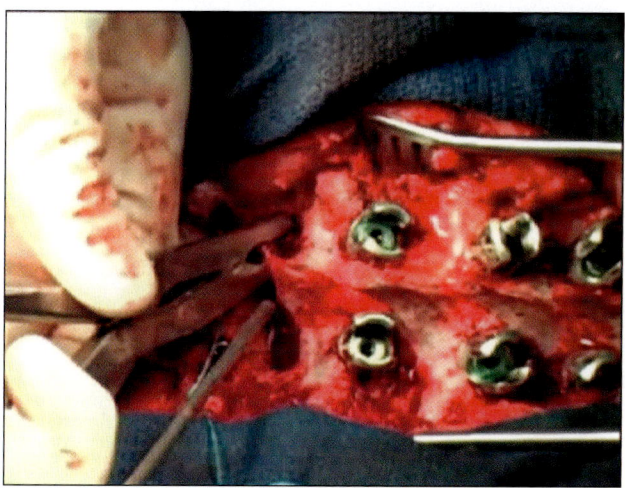

FIGURE 4

- A key point is to make sure complete resection has been performed out laterally. We also make sure that the ligamentum flavum and undersurface of the superior lamina have been resected in order to prevent compression onto the dura with deformity correction. The resection should be able to be freely move with a laminar spreader if the osteotomy is complete (Fig. 5).
- A gel foam sponge can then be placed over the resection site and continued osteotomies to the other levels may be performed. Figure 6 is an intraoperative photo taken after apical resections; gel foam is placed at each resection site (*arrows*).

STEP 3

- Once the pedicle screws have been placed and the Ponte osteotomies performed, the deformity may then be partly corrected.
- One of three different correction maneuvers may be used in order to fix the deformity: cantilever correction, temporary use of a Harrington compression rod, or segmental bilateral compression of screws.
  - Regardless of the method of correction, the rod system to be used should be a ¼-inch rigid rod.
  - During correction of the deformity, the mean arterial pressure should stay elevated and never drop below 65 mm Hg, and motor evoked potentials should be frequently run to assure the spinal cord signals remain healthy.
  - The surgeon also needs to be careful not to overcorrect the deformity as the incidence of junctional deformities increases with overcorrection.
- Cantilever correction may be performed by prebending two rods to the desirable sagittal contour. The rods are then captured proximally to the anchors and then crosslinked in order to load share. The rods are then pushed down (cantilevered) to the more distal anchor points and are captured. Stiff ¼-inch rods that are precontoured will then hold the spine in the desired alignment.
  - Disadvantages of a cantilever maneuver are the tremendous forces created on the proximal anchors and the rapid change in alignment of the spine, which can cause a relative ischemic state in the spinal cord.
  - In general, this mode of correction, if used, is best in smaller deformities.
- A Harrington compression rod works by compressing towards the apex of the deformity. This is done on a segmental basis with gradual correction of the deformity. Compression can be done slowly until the desired amount of correction is seen. Figure 7 shows a lateral view of the spine prior to placement of compression rods.
  - A threaded Harrington compression rod is placed into the pedicle screw anchors on one side, with set screws loosely capturing the rod (Fig. 8). Nuts are placed either rostral to the screws above the apex or caudal to the screws below the apex.

PEARLS

- *Harrington compression rod is optimal for gradual correction and load sharing.*
- *Mean arterial blood pressure should stay above 65 mm Hg.*
- *Radiograph after correction should confirm disk spaces opening up anteriorly.*

PITFALLS

- *Inadequate closure of osteotomy sites*

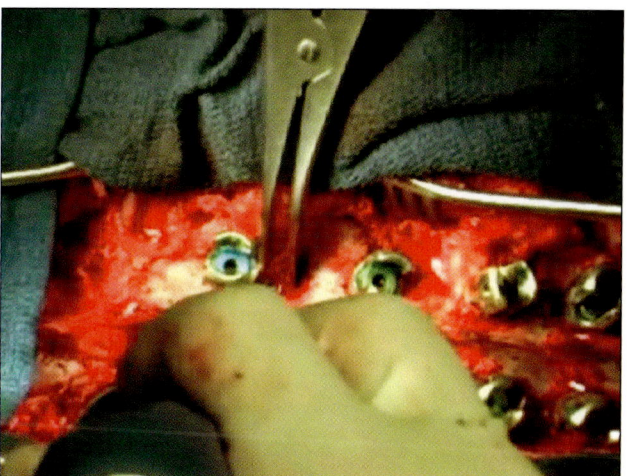

FIGURE 5

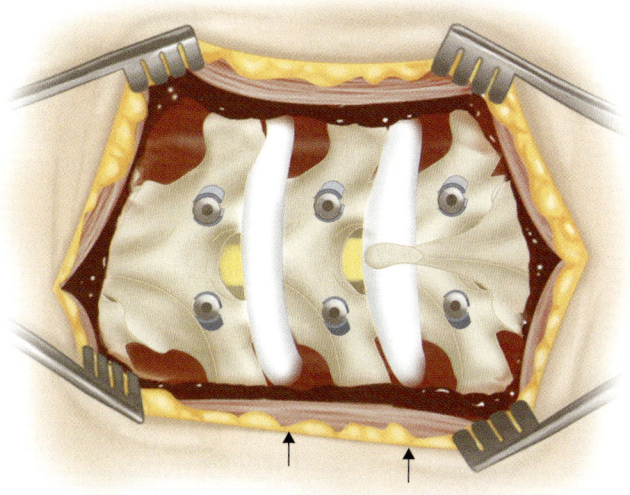

FIGURE 6

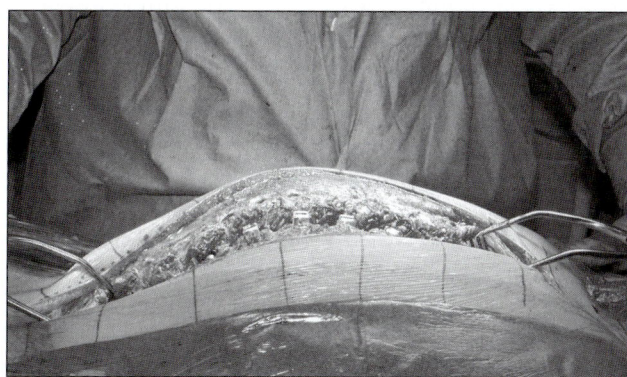

FIGURE 7

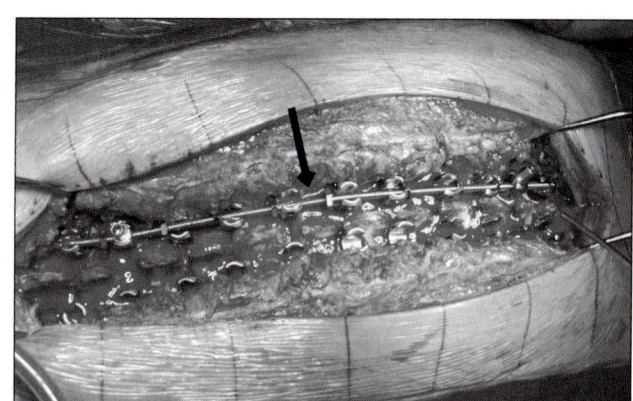

FIGURE 8

- Harrington wrenches are then used to compress the nuts towards the apex (Fig. 9), frequently switching compression from nut to nut in order to gain correction. Multiple wrenches can be used at one time on either side of the apex.
- The osteotomy sites should close down with compression. The clinical appearance of the spine will change, and a radiograph may be taken when the desired amount of correction has been reached to confirm that disk spaces are opening up anteriorly.
- Scoliosis may be created on the compressed side. If this starts to happen, then a second compression rod may be added to the other side; however, this is rarely needed.
- Once the deformity has been corrected, a solid ¼-inch rod is then bent into the appropriate contour and captured into place on the contralateral side. The Harrington compression rod is then removed and replaced by a second ¼-inch solid rod, and then crosslinks are applied.
- Segmental compression may also be performed on solid rods. Two ¼-inch rods may be overcontoured and sequentially captured into place; this alone will improve some of the deformity. Bilateral compression devices are then placed at each level with compression toward the apex of the kyphosis. This takes two or three separate rounds of compression at each level in order to gain correction. This is an effective way of correcting the deformity; however, it is time consuming and compression at each level needs to be undertaken two or three times.
- Figure 10 shows postoperative standing PA (Fig. 10A) and lateral (Fig. 10B) radiographs.

STEP 4

- Following instrumentation and correction, the spine needs to be abundantly decorticated and the arthrodesis site filled with either autologous graft or allograft.
- A deep subfascial drain should be applied and the tissues closed in the appropriate manner.

POSTOPERATIVE CARE AND EXPECTED OUTCOMES

- The patients in general are admitted to the hospital for 5–7 days. There is a need for more acute nursing care in the first 24–48 hours. There need to be frequent neurologic checks, and the blood pressure and hematocrit should be closely monitored.
- The patient can be mobilized starting on postoperative day 2, and should have the drains removed on day 3 during the dressing change. These wounds need to be monitored closely given that the associated increase in body mass index in these patients may predispose them to wound drainage.
- The patient is discharged on oral pain medications and needs follow-up at 1 month.
- The patient may begin a physical therapy program at 1 month postoperatively and then may begin doing sporting activities at 3 months postoperatively. Patients can be followed clinically and radiographically every 6 months for 2 years and then yearly for 5 years.

PITFALLS

- *Surgical treatment of kyphosis is associated with a higher risk of neurologic compromise, even in the postoperative period.*

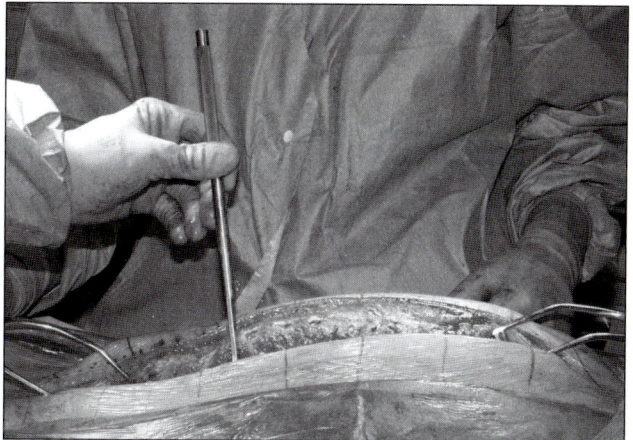

FIGURE 9

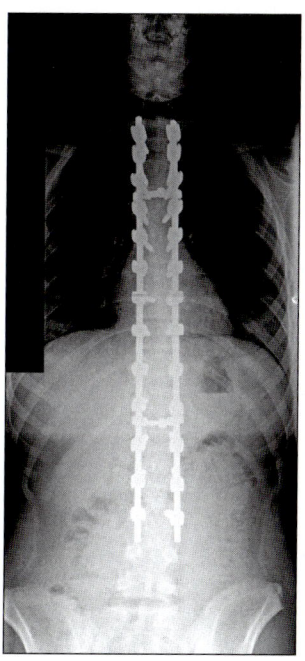

A

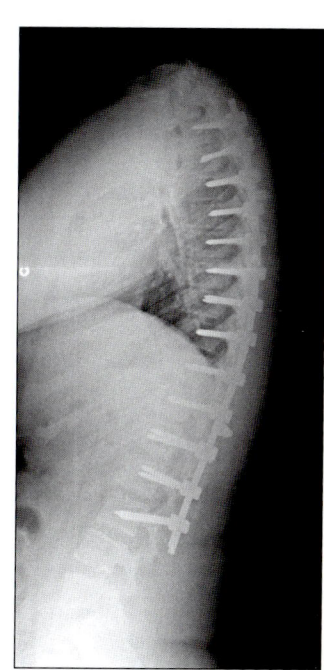

B

FIGURE 10

EVIDENCE

Cheh G, Lenke LG, et al. Loss of spinal cord monitoring signals in children during thoracic kyphosis correction with spinal osteotomy: why does it occur and what should you do? Spine. 2008;33:1093–9.

Geck MJ, Macagno A, et al. The Ponte procedure: posterior only treatment of Scheuermann's kyphosis using segmental posterior shortening and pedicle screw instrumentation. J Spinal Disord Tech. 2007;20:586–93.

Lee SS, Lenke LG, et al. Comparison of Scheuermann kyphosis correction by posterior-only thoracic pedicle screw fixation versus combined anterior/posterior fusion. Spine. 2006;31:2316–21.

Lonner BS, Newton P, et al. Operative management of Scheuermann's kyphosis in 78 patients: radiographic outcomes, complications, and technique. Spine. 2007;32:2644–52.

Petcharaporn M, Pawelek J, et al. The relationship between thoracic hyperkyphosis and the Scoliosis Research Society outcomes instrument. Spine. 2007;32:2226–31.

Scoliosis Correction

Daniel J. Hedequist

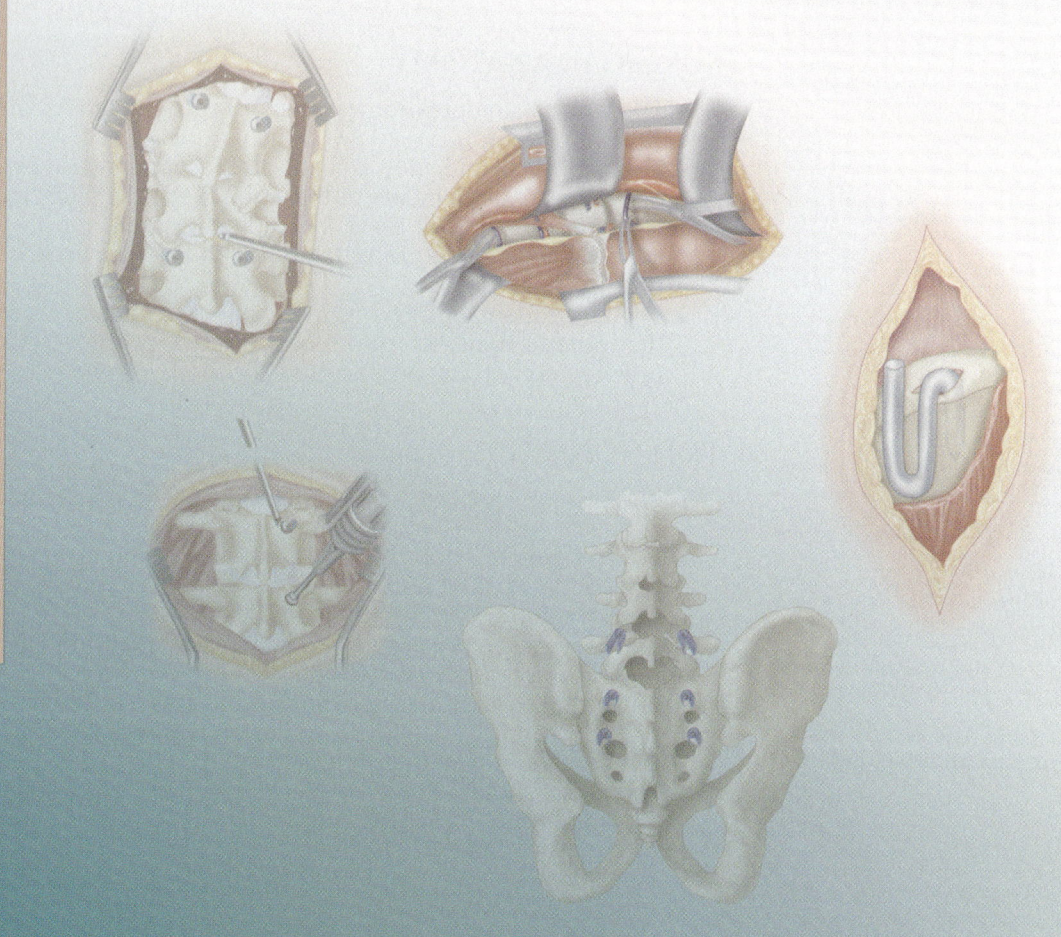

Treatment Options

- Posterior instrumented spinal fusion
- Anterior instrumented spinal fusion (open or thoracoscopic)
- Anterior release with posterior instrumented fusion

INDICATIONS

- Thoracic curves greater than 50°
- Thoracolumbar or lumbar curves greater than 40°
- Significant deformity
- Intractable pain (rarely)

EXAMINATION/IMAGING

- Standing 36-inch posteroanterior (PA) (Fig. 1) and lateral spine radiographs are obtained.
- Side-bending radiographs, such as the supine radiographs in Figure 2A and 2B, are also obtained.
- Magnetic resonance imaging for atypical curve patterns or neurologic findings

SURGICAL ANATOMY

- The surgical anatomy for a posterior instrumented fusion is straightforward.
- The midline skin incision is followed by subperiosteal exposure of the posterior elements of the spine. Regardless of the location, this starts at the spinous processes and moves laterally over the laminae and facet joints out to the transverse processes.
- The facet orientation moves from the horizontal facets of the the thoracic spine, which are not elevated, to the vertically oriented and prominent facets of the lumbar spine.

POSITIONING

- The patient is placed supine on a radiolucent spinal frame (Fig. 3).
- Bolsters are placed at the level of the chest and at the level of the iliac crests. The abdomen remains free in order to facilitate venous return.
- The shoulders are placed in a slightly abducted position with the arms bent 90° on armboards, taking care to pad the ulnar nerve; the axilla should remain free of pressure. The hips are placed in approximately 20° of flexion with the knees flexed and legs slightly elevated on pillows.
- Somatosensory and motor evoked potential leads are placed accordingly.

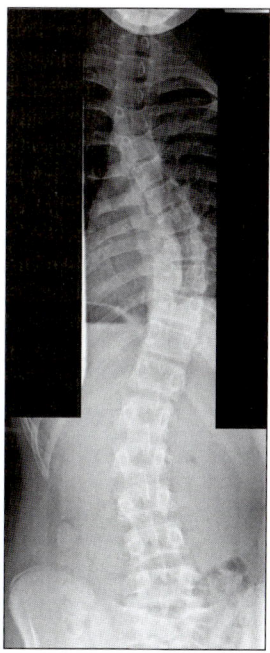

FIGURE 1

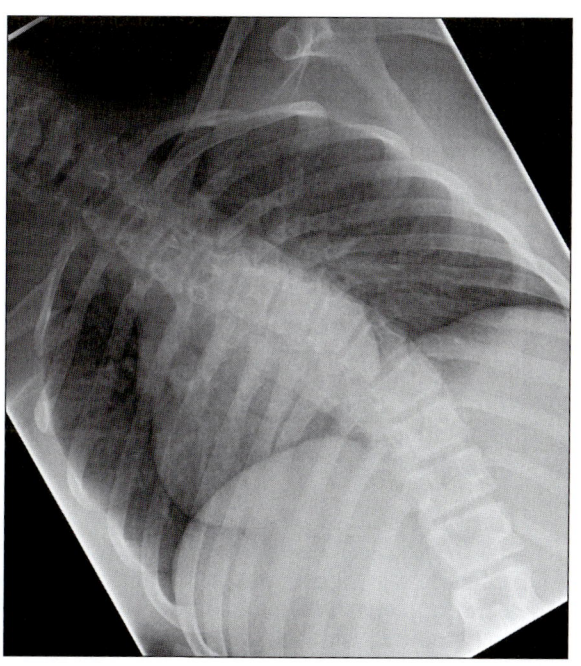

FIGURE 2 A

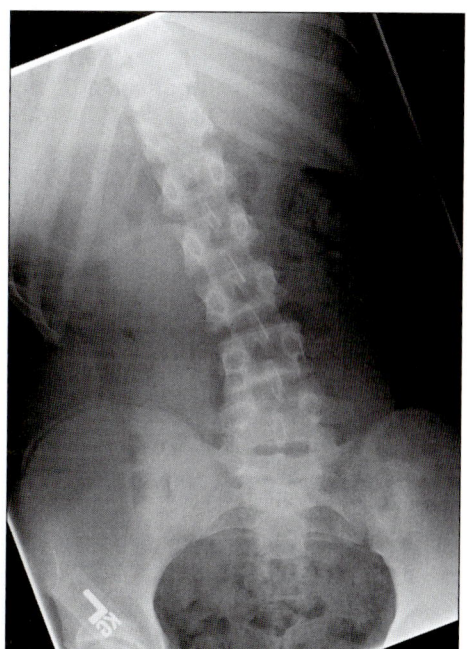

B

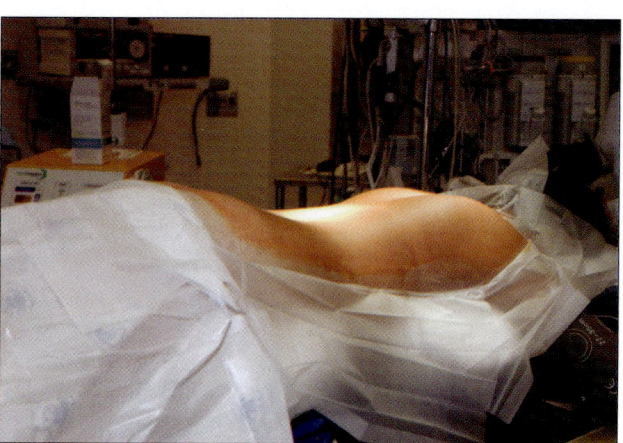

FIGURE 3

PORTALS/EXPOSURES

- A standard midline incision is made, with subperiosteal dissection of the paraspinal muscles off of the bony spine (Fig. 4).
- Cobb elevators, judicious use of electrocautery, and cell saver recycling suction apparatus are useful.
- Hypotensive anesthesia during exposure may facilitate a dry field with mean arterial pressures ranging from 65 to 70 mm Hg. Packing of areas with sponges after exposure helps facilitate the hemostasis.
- Relaxation of self-retaining retractors in areas of the wound that are not being operated on helps avoid muscle injury.

PROCEDURE

STEP 1

- After a thorough subperiosteal dissection of the posterior spine to the tips of the transverse processes, the next step is placement of pedicle screws.
- Screw placement is preferred at every level on both sides of the lumbar spine. Lumbar screws may be place by first perfoming a thorough facetectomy of the vertically oriented lumbar facet. The facet should be taken completely and leveled to be continous with the transverse process as this will facilitate screw placement.
  - The starting point for all lumbar screws is at the bisection of a line drawn horizontally from the transverse process with a line drawn vertically from the lateral border of the pars interarticularis. A burr is used to find the starting point, which will usually be a blush of cancellous blood.
  - A hand-held awl can then be used to gain access to the pedicle. The awl should be placed down 20 mm and then the pilot hole should be probed to assure that there is circumferential bony containment and a floor of bone. The awl can then be placed futher down, with most adolescents accepting at least a 40-mm length for pedicle screws.
  - The hole is then reprobed and, if the correct location is felt, then the pilot hole is tapped with a tap 0.5 mm smaller in diameter than the desired screw.
  - In the lumbar spine, given the variable angulation of pedicles, it is recommended that a variable-head screw be placed in order to facilitate ease of rod capture.
- Pedicle screw placement in the thoracic spine has become more commonplace. The pedicle anatomy and trajectory have been well studied and the key to pedicle screw placement is a stepwise technique.
  - The starting points for thoracic screws have been well studied and published. As a general rule, the medial lateral starting point should never be more medial than the middle of the facet joint. A large facetectomy should allow for visualization of the medial and lateral borders of the facet (Fig. 5) and is essential to screw placement.
  - Once a thorough and large facetectomy has been done, the starting hole may be created using a high-speed burr to find the cancellous blush (Fig. 6A and 6B).
  - An awl with a curved tip is then placed down to 20 mm. If confirmed to be in the correct location, then the awl is placed in the pilot hole with the curve then pointed medially and placed into the vertebral body to a depth of 30–35 mm (Fig. 7). The pilot hole is then reprobed and measurement of the pedicle depth is taken off of the probe (Fig. 8). If fully contained, then the hole is tapped with a tap 0.5 mm smaller than the standard screw (Fig. 9).

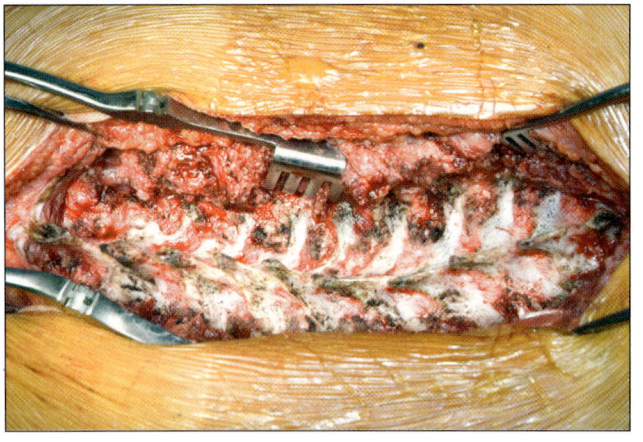

FIGURE 4

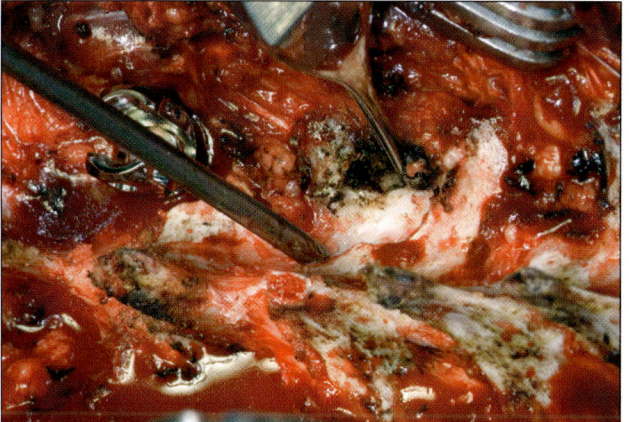

FIGURE 5

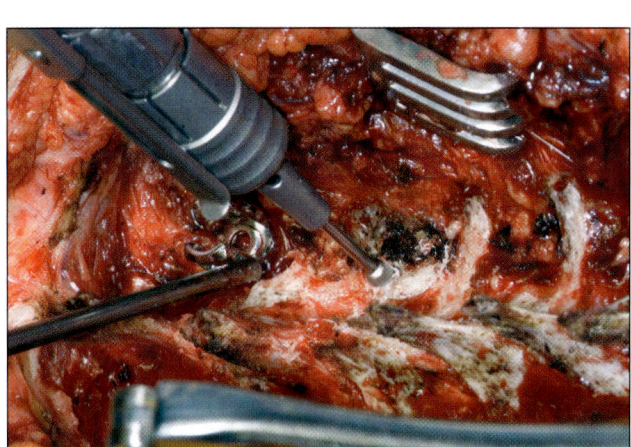

A

FIGURE 6

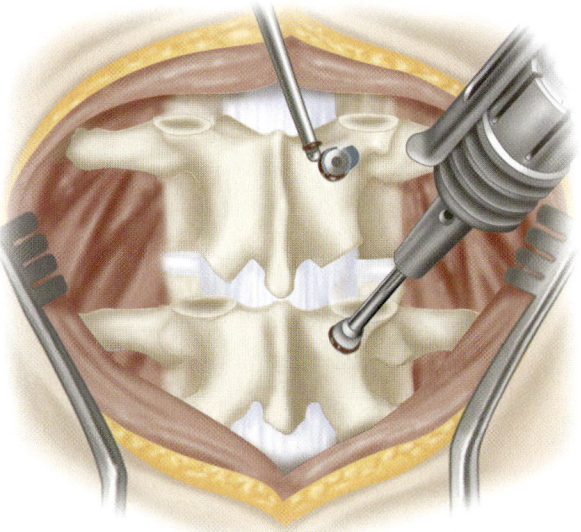

B

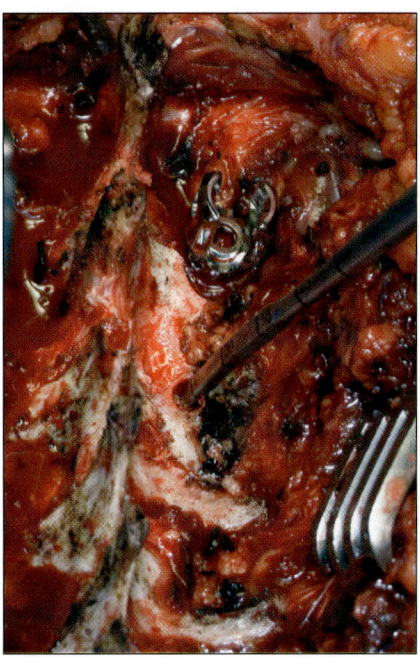

FIGURE 7

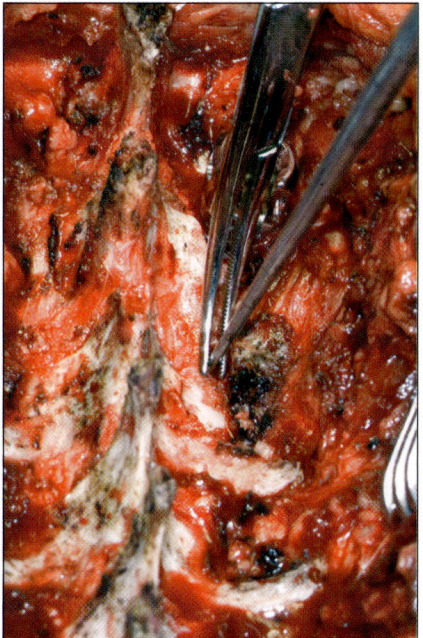

FIGURE 8

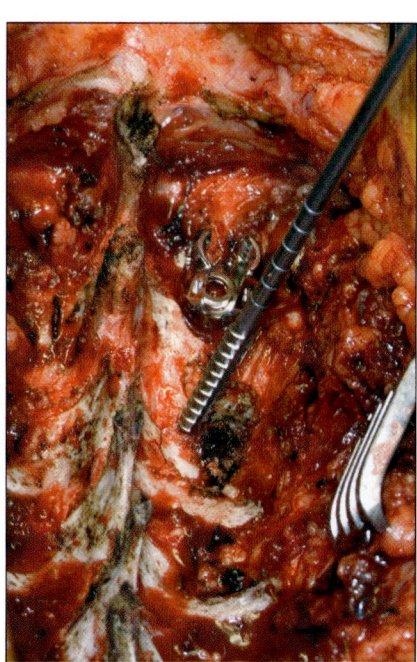

FIGURE 9

- In general, fixed-angle screws are thought to give more correction of Cobb's angle and the rotational deformity. Variable-angle screws, however, do afford significant correction and make rod capture easier.
- After concave screws have been placed, the convex screws are placed (Fig. 10). If significant rotation exists, then concave screws should be placed at each level to allow for derotation. Patients with only moderate rotation can have screws placed starting at T12, and then skipping two levels and placing a screw, and so forth.
- The top of a construct should have two consecutive screws and the bottom of a construct should have two consecutive screws.

■ Once screws have been placed, there are two essential steps remaining for safe screw confirmation.
- The first is obtaining radiographs on the table in both the anteroposterior (AP) and lateral planes. This can be done either with plain films or with fluoroscopy. All of the screws should have a continous cascade. Any screw that crosses the midline on the AP radiograph should be concerning for a medial violation. Any screw placed at a level where the medial border of the pedicle can be seen in its entirety is worrisome for lateral perforation. Screws that appear worrisome should be removed and the hole reprobed with replacement of the screw if probing confirms a correct location.
- The next step in evaluating screw placement is triggered electromyography (Fig. 11). The screw heads are stimulated with an electrical probe and a recording is done. Screws contained completely by bone should require large amounts of stimulation to obtain a distal response. Any screw that is stimulated and has a response less than 6 mA or a response that is significantly different from the other screws should be removed and the hole reprobed to confim no medial perforation.

STEP 2

■ The next step in correction of the deformity is rod capture and curve correction.
- In general, stiffer rods help improve curve correction and to help maintain sagittal balance. The rods should be contoured in order to try to match the desired sagittal plane alignment.
- In general, most deformities are corrected by first applying the concave rod. Deformities with associated hyperkyphosis need to be corrected using a cantilever-compression method on the convexity of the curve. This aids in "shortening" the deformity and likely is safer from a neurologic standpoint.

■ Rod capture for a standard curve would start by capturing the proximal screws and then sequentially capturing each distal level. Rod capture may be aided by apical reduction screws, which help translate the spine over to the rod (Fig. 12).
- Once rod capture has been performed on the concave side, the set screws are left loose and a derotation manuever is generally applied to bring the rod into the correct sagittal plane (Fig. 13A and 13B). At this point the deformity may be fully corrected, and the proximal and distal vertebrae may be balanced by selective compression and/or distraction.

PEARLS

- *Coronal plane bending to help achieve further deformity correction*
- *Maintenance of arterial blood pressure during correction maneuvers*
- *Convex compression for curves associated with hyperkyphosis*

PITFALLS

- *Unrecognized undercorrection due to poor radiographic confirmation*
- *Primary distraction manuevers*

Instrumentation/ Implantation

- Derotation devices applied on convex screws aid in deformity correction.

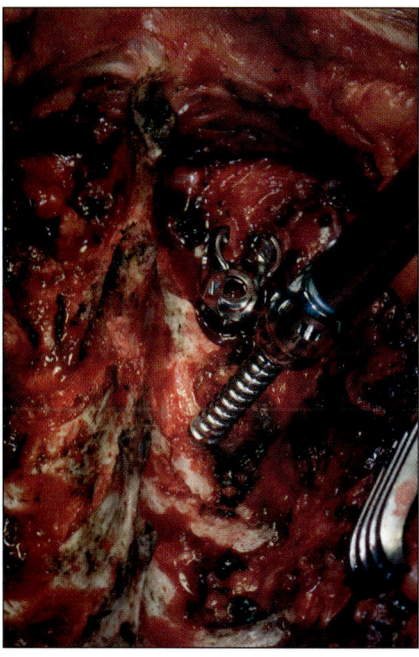

FIGURE 10

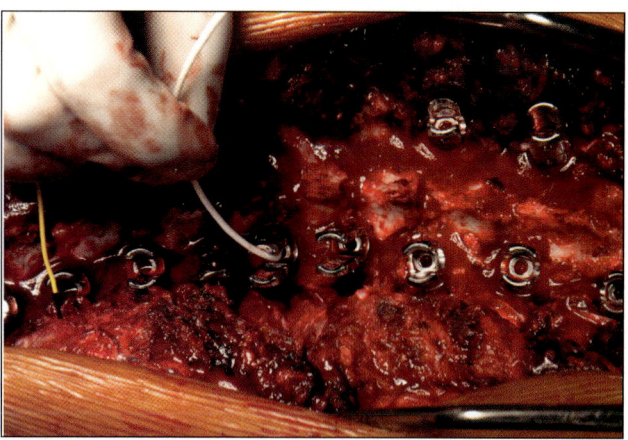

FIGURE 11

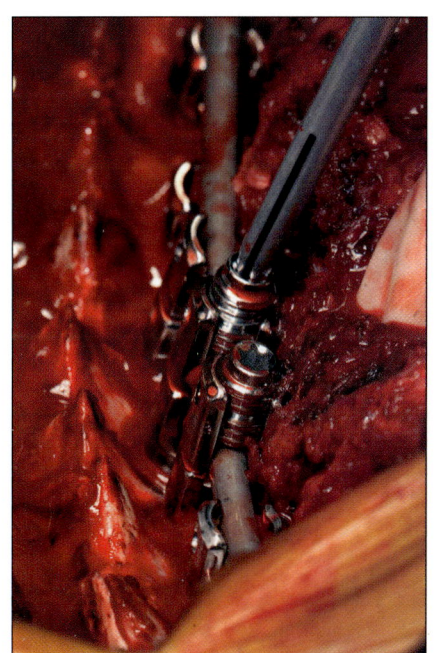

FIGURE 12

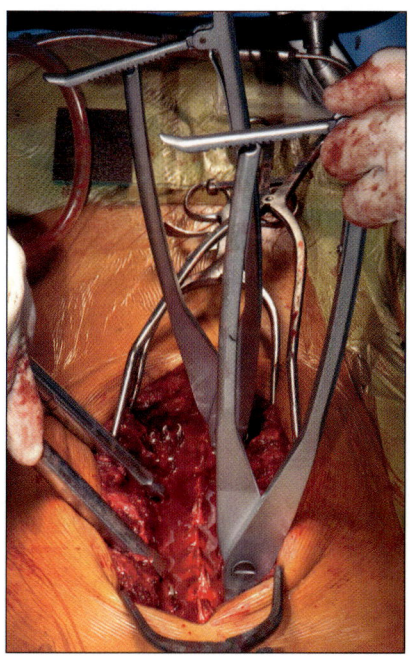

A

FIGURE 13

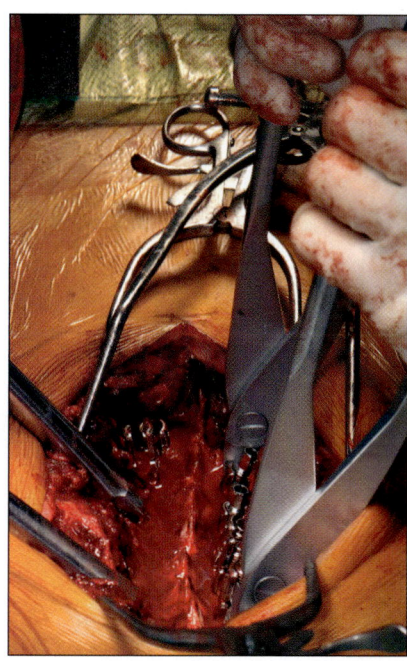

B

- The use of coronal plane benders has improved curve correction as the segmental fixation on the spine allows for improved purchase and control (Fig. 14). Coronal plane benders are generally used after rod rotation in order to gain some correction of the curve or balance of the lowest instrumented vertebra.
- Figure 15 shows curve correction after placement of the concave working rod. Rod capture of the second rod may be facilitated by placing a reduction screw at the base anchor site of the convex side of the curvature (Fig. 16).
■ Patients with a significant rib deformity may have an improved cosmetic result with the help of convex vertebral body derotation techniques (Fig. 17). Multiple devices are available to help with this depending on the implant system being used.
  - Derotation forces are applied to the screws during rod capture in order to diminish the rib deformity and improve Cobb's angle correction.
  - In general, the concave rod is captured as the devices derotate on the screws (Fig. 18).

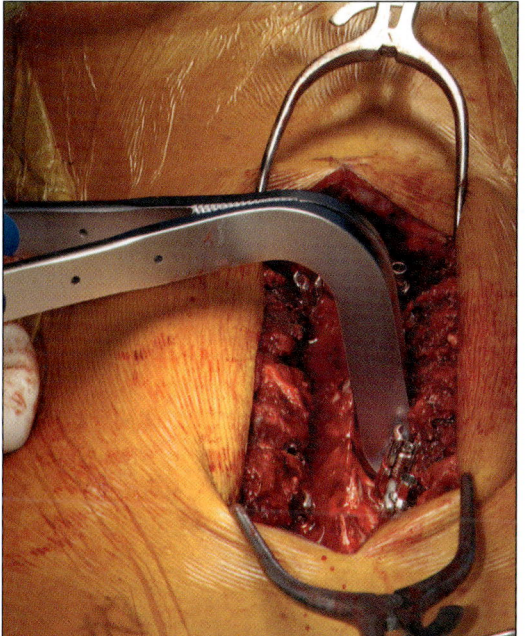

FIGURE 14

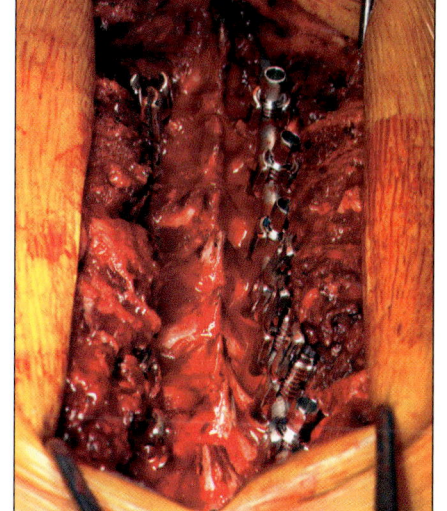

FIGURE 15

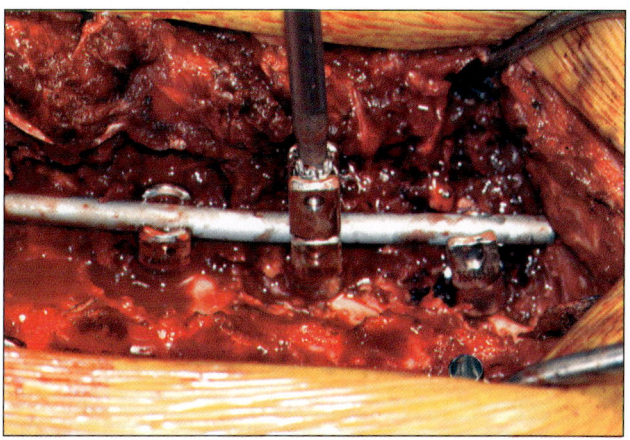

FIGURE 16

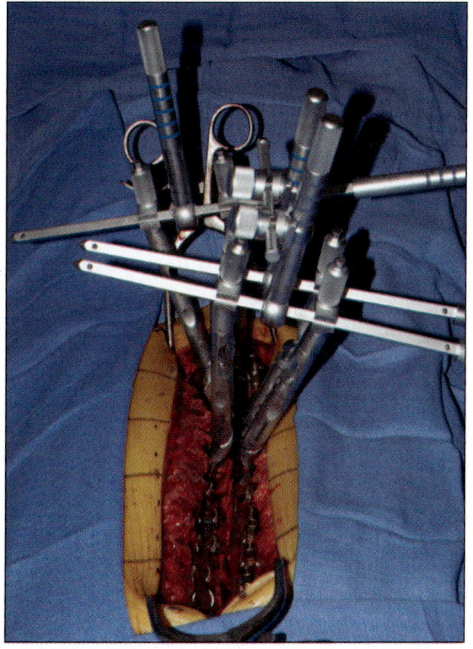
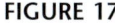

FIGURE 17

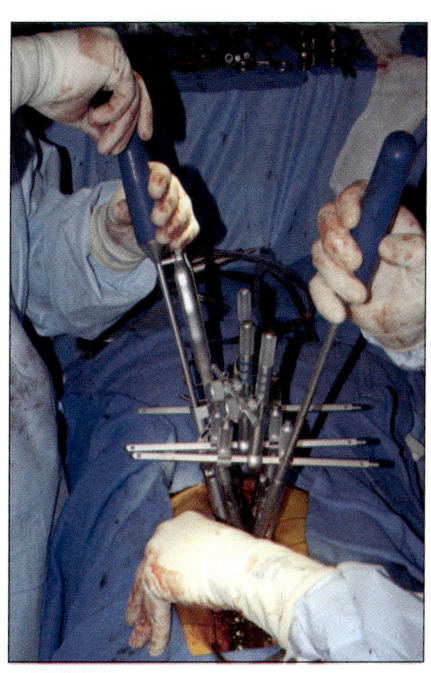

FIGURE 18

- Final position of the derotators should be horizontal after rod capture and derotation has been performed (Fig. 19).
  - Once the deformity is considered to be adequately corrected, either fluoroscopy or a full-length radiograph needs to be obtained in order to confirm adequate balance of the upper and lower instrumented vertebral bodies. If the radiographs confirm adequate correction, then all set screws need to be broken off and accounted for in the final count. Even with segmental pedicle fixation, crosslinks need to be applied near both ends of the instrumentation to improve torsional stability of the construct.

Step 3

- Once the deformity has been corrected, the spine must be adequately decorticated in order to allow for a large surface area for arthrodesis. This needs to be done as a stepwise technique at each level using either gouges or a high-speed irrigated burr.
- Once thorough decortication has been done, the field needs to be copiously irrigated out and the retractors released. Any paraspinal muscle that appears damaged or ischemic needs to be removed. Abundant corticocancellous allograft should then be applied at each level.
- The use of drains should be considered deep to the fascia as this allows for hematoma drainage during the first few days in order to permit the deep fascial layer to heal. The fascial layer needs to be closed in a watertight fashion with absorbable suture. The subcutaneous tissues and skin need to be closed accordingly.
- In Figure 20, standing postoperative PA (Fig. 20A) and lateral (Fig. 20B) radiographs show excellent correction of a thoracic curvature and nonoperative treatment of the lumbar curve.

POSTOPERATIVE CARE AND EXPECTED OUTCOMES

- Most patients can be sent to the standard floor with acute nursing for the first 24 hours. The hematocrit is checked on postoperative days 1 and 2 and, if a patient needs a transfusion, autologous blood is usually given.
- Mobilization is begun on day 2, and the patient is switched to oral pain medication on approximately day 3. The dressing change and drain removal is done on the morning of day 3.
- Patients do not require any postoperative bracing and are discharged usually on day 6 with sufficient oral pain medication. All patients require a dry wound prior to discharge. Routine PA and lateral radiographs are taken prior to discharge as well.
- At our institution, we see the patient back at 1 month postoperatively, when a standing PA and lateral spine series is obtained to assure that fixation remains solid. We then begin a physical therapy program focusing on periscapular and neck strengthening and mobilization.
- The patients are then seen back at 3 months, at which time they are released back to sports and physical education classes. Follow-up is every 6 months for the first 2 years and then yearly for the next 5 years.

PEARLS

- *Débridement of nonviable paraspinal musculature*
- *Thorough decortication to allow for increased surface area*
- *Subfascial drain placement*

Controversies

- Allograft versus local autograft versus iliac crest autograft

PEARLS

- *Meticulous wound monitoring*
- *Abundant pain medication for discharge*
- *Physical therapy at 1 month postoperatively*

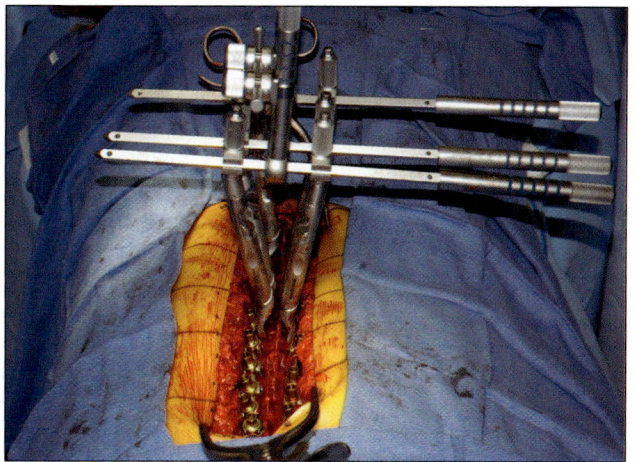

FIGURE 19

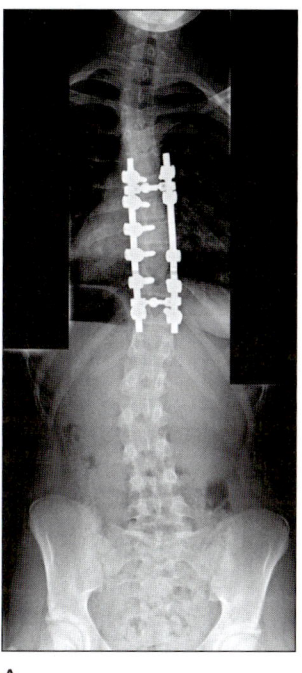

A

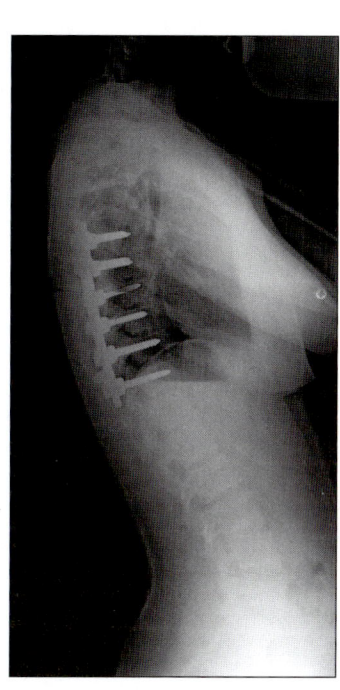

B

FIGURE 20

EVIDENCE

Kim YJ, Lenke LG, et al. Evaluation of pedicle screw placement in the deformed spine using intraoperative plain radiographs: a comparison with computerized tomography. Spine. 2005;30:2084–8.

Kim YJ, Lenke LG, et al. Free hand pedicle screw placement in the thoracic spine: is it safe? Spine. 2004;29:333–42.

Lenke LG, Betz RR, et al. Adolescent idiopathic scoliosis: a new classification to determine extent of spinal arthrodesis. J Bone Joint Surg [Am]. 2001;83:1169–81.

Raynor BL, Lenke LG, et al. Can triggered electromyography thresholds predict safe thoracic pedicle screw placement? Spine. 2002;27:2030–5.

Anterior Spinal Instrumentation and Fusion for Lumbar and Thoracolumbar Idiopathic Scoliosis

Lawrence I. Karlin

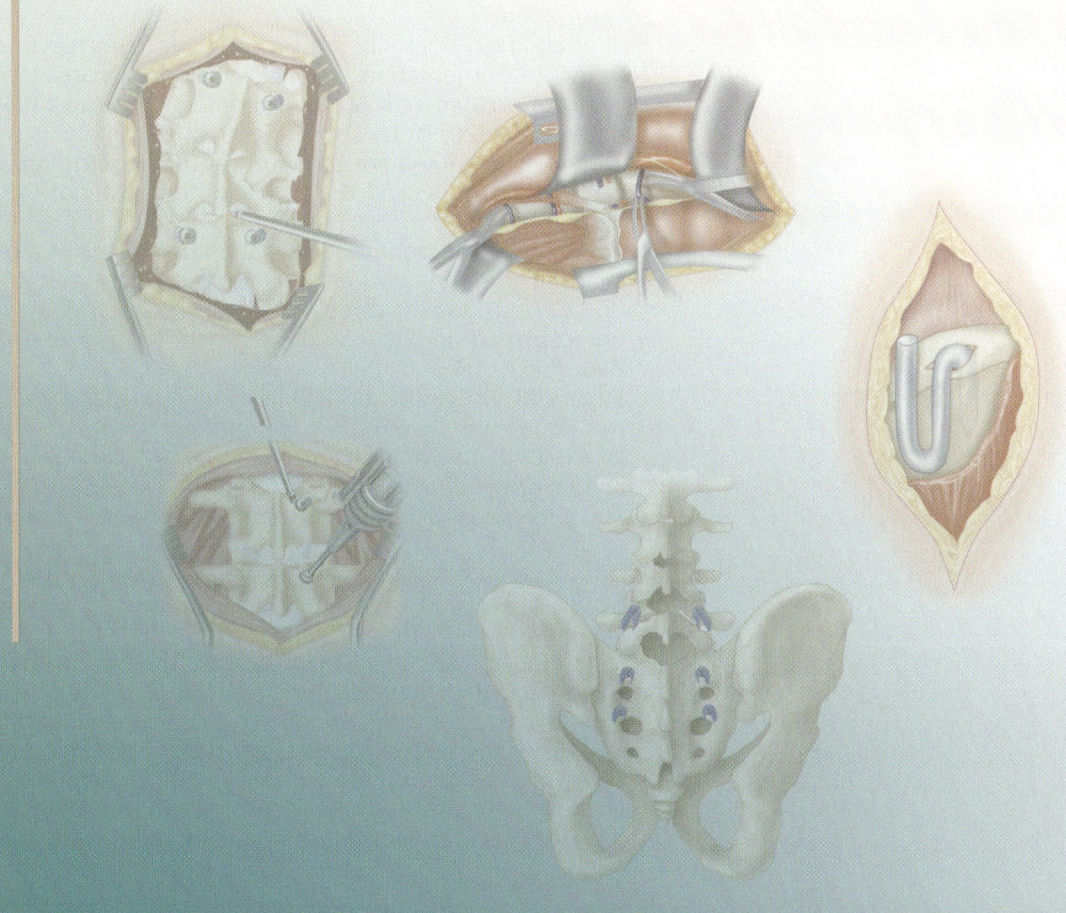

INDICATIONS

- Structural idiopathic lumbar or thoracolumbar scoliosis (TL/L) (Lenke 5) that has failed conservative treatment and/or has progressed to a degree associated with progression in adulthood.
- Selective treatment of TL/L scoliosis with associated thoracic curvatures.
  - Criteria for selective TL/L scoliosis instrumentation:
    - Thoracic curve of 50° or less
    - TL/L : T Cobb ratio ≥ 1.25
    - Thoracic curvature corrects to 20° or less on supine band radiographs
- Instrumentation level selection may vary. There are several acceptable methods to select the levels to be instrumented.
  - The standard technique is to include the entire Cobb measurement.
  - Hall et al. (1997) described a technique for short-segment selective instrumentation. In their initial discussion, structural curvatures greater than 60° and thoracic curvatures that did not correct to 20° or less on the corrective radiographs were excluded. The criteria are based on both the standing posteroanterior (PA) and the supine anteroposterior (AP) bend radiographs.
    - Standing PA radiograph: Select the apex. If this is a disk space, include the two cephalad and caudal vertebral bodies (four bodies, three disks). If a vertebral body, include one cephalad and one caudal segment (three vertebrae and two disks).
    - Supine AP active bend: Include those interspaces that do not "reverse."
    - When levels between the two views differ, choose the longer of the constructs.
    - This technique will often save one or even two motion segments.
    - An example of the short-segment technique is shown in Figure 1. The end vertebrae are T11 and L3. On the standing PA view (Fig. 1A), the apex is the T12-L1 disk. The levels are two above and two below: T11-L2. On the supine bend view, the thoracic curvature is flexible (Fig. 1C). The T10-11 and L2-3 disks reverse, and can be excluded (Fig. 1D). Here the method spares two motion segments. The curvature has been reversed, and there is spontaneous improvement of the thoracic deformity and excellent balance (Fig. 1E). Normal sagittal alignment is maintained (Fig. 1F).

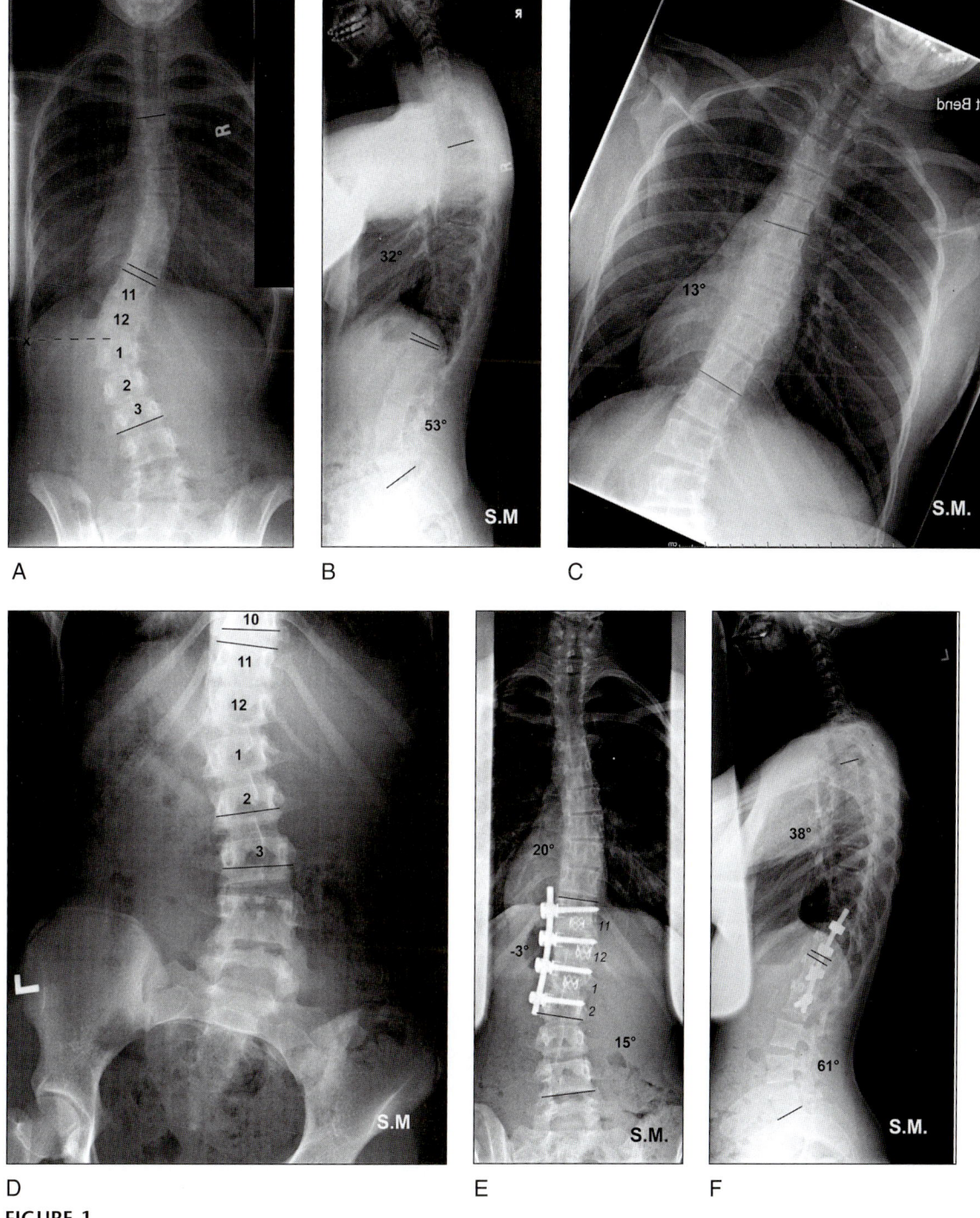

FIGURE 1

- The end instrumented vertebrae are often short of the Cobb terminals. In order to avoid imbalance, the deformity must be overcorrected by about 10°. This will frequently create an adjacent wedged disk space.
  - In Figure 2A and 2B, use of the short-segment technique with the overcorrection required to balance the spine produced subjacent disk wedging.
  - In Figure 3A–D, the lowest end vertebra (LEV) and lowest instrumented vertebra (LIV) coincide. There is no subjacent disk wedging. Note that the preoperative thoracolumbar kyphosis has been corrected by a single rod with structural interbody graft.
  - In Figure 4A and 4B, the LIV is clearly short of the LEV, but there is only mild subjacent disk wedging.

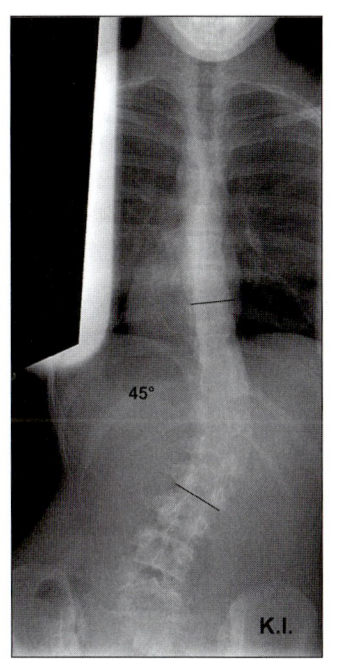

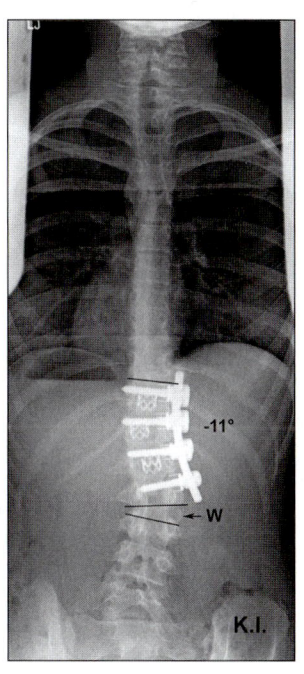

A

B

FIGURE 2

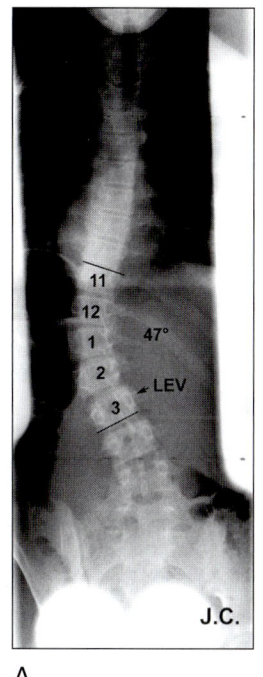

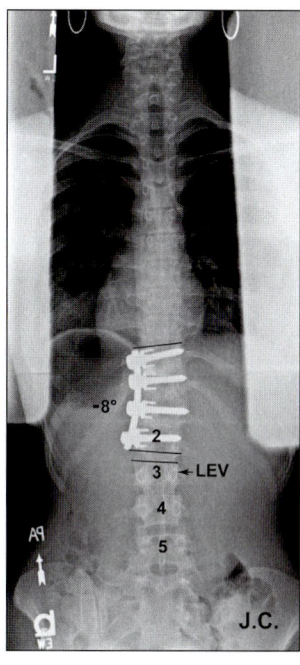

A

B

FIGURE 4

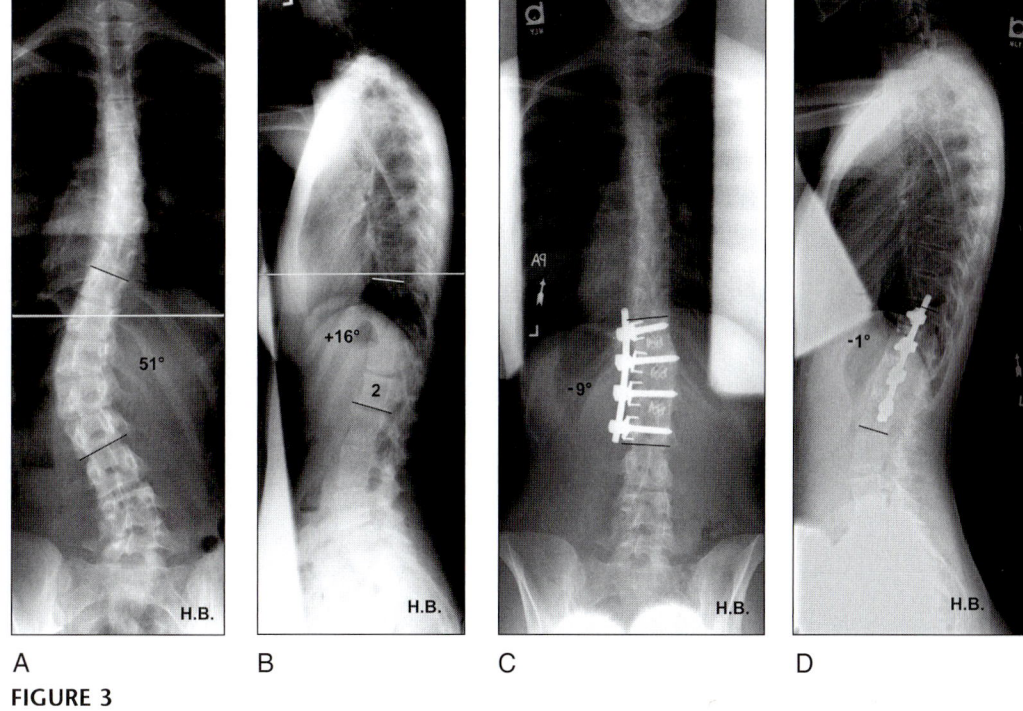

A

B

C

D

FIGURE 3

Controversies

- Comparable results may be obtained with posterior pedicle screw constructs. In the patient in (Fig. 6A–D, the excellent correction required a five-segment construct. A similar result might have been obtained with a posterior pedicle screw constuct.

- The relative benefit of sparing a motion segment at the expense of subjacent disk wedging is not known; there is uncertaintly about the benefit of the short-segment overcorrection technique versus the Cobb method.

Treatment Options

- Posterior spinal instrumentation and fusion with pedicle screw constructs may produce similar results, but will often require a longer construct.

- Either single-rod or dual-rod instrumentation may be used. In the patient in Figure 5A–D, the dual-rod system required no structural graft to maintain the sagittal alignment. We have not been able to obtain the same amount of coronal plane correction (overcorrection) with the present dual-rod systems.

PITFALLS

- *When a selective lumbar procedure is performed in individuals with large structural thoracic curvatures, unacceptable thoracic deformities or trunk imbalance may result.*

- *If there is significant growth remaining, residual thoracic scoliosis may progress.*

- *When using the short-segment overcorrection technique and ending short of the lowest end vertebrae, subjacent disk wedging will occur.*

- *Due to the kyphosing tendency of anterior instumentation, thoracolumbar kyphosis is a relative contraindication.*

EXAMINATION/IMAGING

- Thorough history and physical examination must be performed to establish true idiopathic diagnosis.
- The surgeon should note trunk decompensation, waist asymmetry, and relative paraspinal prominences of thoracic and thoracolumbar and/or lumbar curvatures.
- Radiographic imaging should include standing PA and lateral views of the entire spine and supine right and left bends of the thoracic and lumbar curvatures (see Fig. 1).

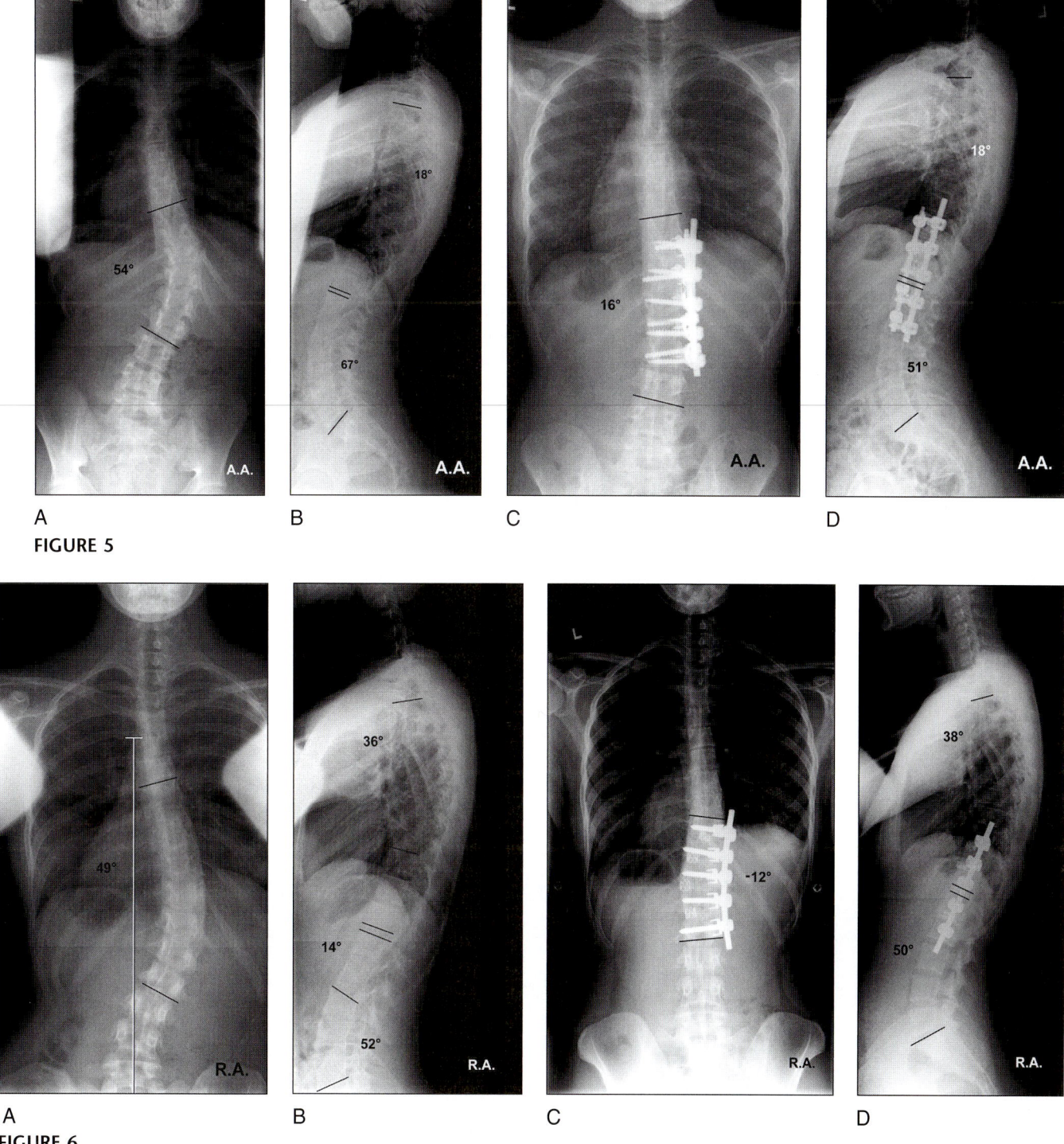

A
B
C
D

FIGURE 5

A
B
C
D

FIGURE 6

SURGICAL ANATOMY

■ Figure 7 shows the anatomic considerations for the chest and abdominal wall.

- Once they leave the ribs and costal cartilage, the intercostal neurovascular bundles pass obliquely across the abdominal wall in the interval between the internal oblique and transversalis muscles. The 10th bundle is directed to the level of the umbilicus, the 9th several centimeters above, the 11th between the umbilicus and pubis, and the 12th toward the inguinal area.

- The musculophrenic branch of the internal mammary artery and its vein lie behind the costal arch between ribs 7–10 and anastomose with the intercostal vessels. It must be cauterized or ligated when the arch is divided.

- Intercostal nerves 7–12 innervate the rectus muscle, penetrating it at its lateral border. Incisions along this semilunar line will denervate the muscle.

■ In this left-sided approach the aorta will lie anterior to the vertebral column (Fig. 8). The left diaphragmatic crus inserts on the first and second lumbar vertebral body and may shield the segmental vessels. The sympathetic chain lies over the vertebral column just anterior to the psoas.

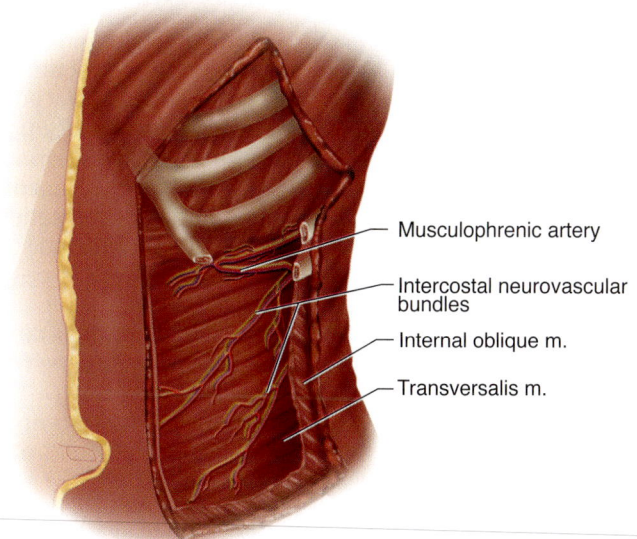

Musculophrenic artery

Intercostal neurovascular bundles

Internal oblique m.

Transversalis m.

FIGURE 7

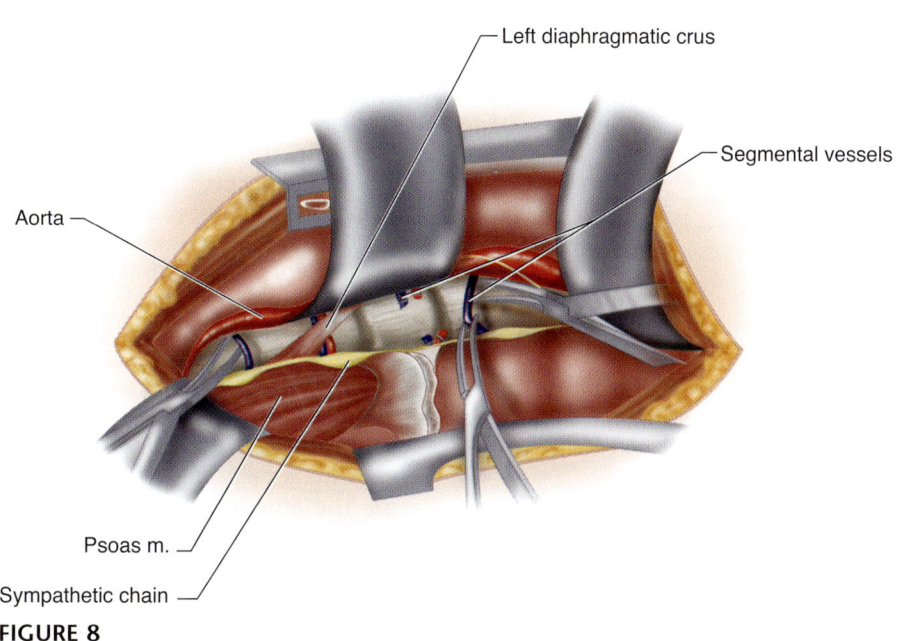

Left diaphragmatic crus

Segmental vessels

Aorta

Psoas m.

Sympathetic chain

FIGURE 8

PEARLS

- *Use a table that will work with you to promote spontaneous deformity. This can be a flat table that will allow the released deformity to collapse or a more conventional table with kidney rests and angle adjustments that can be lowered to aid in the correction. It is best, whenever possible, to have the instrumentation stabilize the correction rather than work against the inertia of the spinal curvature to obtain the correction.*

PITFALLS

- *Expose adequate body surface to allow extension of the approach should it be necessary to include additional segments.*

PEARLS

- *Carefully split the costal cartilage to expose the musculophrenic vessels, develop the peritoneal/transversalis plane, and expedite an anatomic closure.*

- *Exposure to the level of the pedicle helps orient the surgeon to the position of the spinal canal.*

PITFALLS

- *Do not coagulate vessels at the neuroforamina, the location of the vertically directed spinal cord anastamosing vessels.*

- *Beware of the obliquely oriented segmental nerves in the transversalis–internal oblique interval.*

- *The rectus innervation occurs at its lateral margin; incisions through the abdominal musculature should be lateral to this area.*

Controversies

- Segmental vessel ligation can be performed provisionally, allowing time for neurophysiologic monitoring changes to develop.

- Subperiosteal dissection increases the blood loss. We believe it improves the arthrodesis rate.

POSITIONING

- Proper positioning facilitates the exposure and can aid in the deformity correction.
- The patient is placed in the lateral decubitus position with the scoliotic convexity upward and appropriate padding is applied.
- Either a conventional or flat radiolucent table may be used.
  - The flat radiolucent table shown in Figure 9 permits biplanar imaging. The patient is placed in the lateral decubitus position with bolsters holding the pelvis. The upper torso is taped. A roll is positioned several fingerbreadths below the axilla.
  - A conventional table permits better support via kidney rests and may first be flexed to facilitate the approach and then lowered to allow the spine to fall into a corrected position prior to instrumentation manipulation.
- Neurophysiologic monitoring is routinely used.

PORTALS/EXPOSURES

- Rib resection permits a reliable chest entry and provides autogenous bone graft. The appropriate rib should be choosen based on the levels to be exposed.
  - Entry level selection: A horizontal line is drawn from the curve apex (see *dashed line* in Fig. 1A). The rib on the convexity of the deformity that is intersected at the lateral-most portion of the standing PA radiograph is selected. In general, the 9th rib is used when exposure of the T11-12 level is required, and the 10th rib for the T12-L1 level.
- An incision is made directly over the midpoint of the appropriate rib, extending proximally to the midaxillary line and distally as needed. The anterior border of the latissimus dorsi is developed and the dissection is taken beneath this structure (Fig. 10). In general, the incision will extend to the level of the umbilicus for exposures to the third lumbar vertebra.
- The rib periosteum is incised and the rib exposed in a subperiosteal manner (Fig. 11). The muscle fiber direction makes it easier to dissect posterior to anterior over the superior border, and anterior to posterior over the inferior border, where care is taken to avoid the neurovascular bundle.
- The anterior rib is separated at its costal cartilage junction and then resected posteriorly while avoiding injury to the neurovascular bundle (Fig. 12).
- The medial cartilage remnant is now split longitudinally and left in place as a landmark for closure (Fig. 13). Deep to the cartilage will be the musculophrenic vessels, which now must be coagulated. When incising the abdominal wall musculature, the segmental vessels and nerves traveling obliquely in the interval between the internal oblique and transversalis muscles must be avoided. The motor supply of the rectus (intercostal nerves 7–12) enters at its lateral margin; the incision must pass lateral to this border.

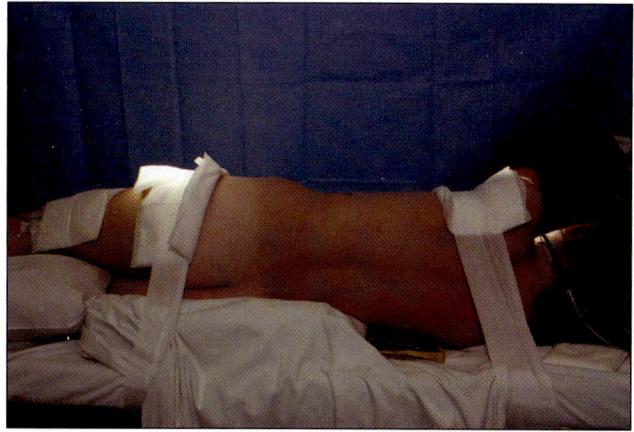

FIGURE 9

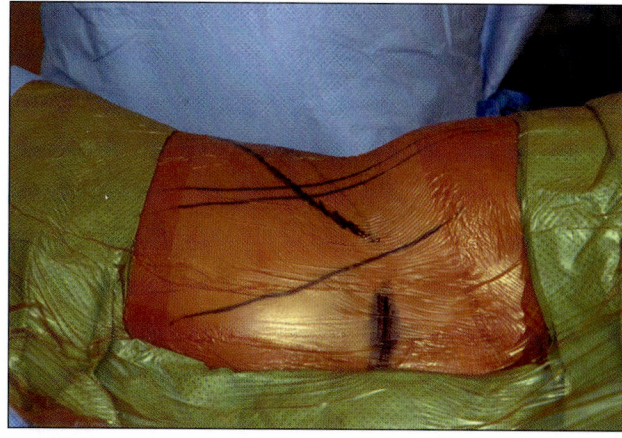

FIGURE 10

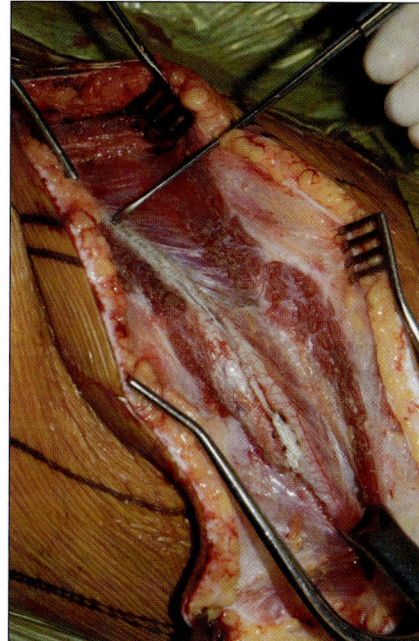

FIGURE 11

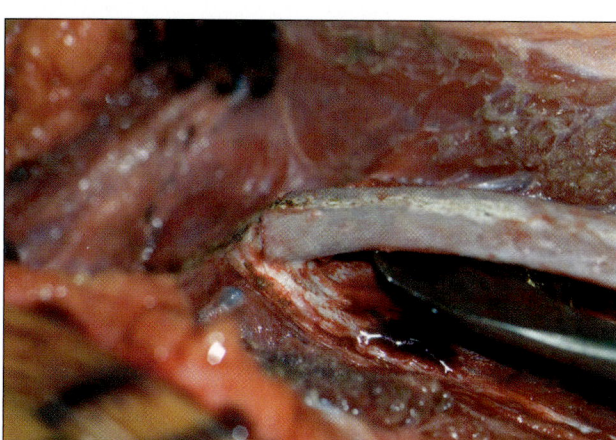

FIGURE 12

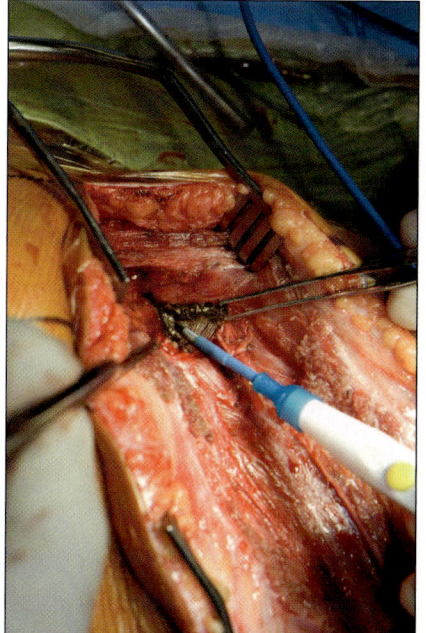

FIGURE 13

- The fatty tissue overlying the peritoneum is dissected free and the leading edge on the abdominal musculature undersurface is identified (Fig. 14). The peritoneum is reflected off the musculature, and the abdominal-layer incision is safely extended distally as needed.
- The chest cavity is entered by incising the rib bed and the lung is gently packed with a moist lap pad (Fig. 15).
- The peritoneum is swept off the undersurface of the diaphragm and the diaphragm incised (Figs. 16 and 17). It may be helpful to first plot out the cut, taking care to leave a 1- to 2-cm cuff. Cuts much closer to the centrum endanger the superior and inferior diaphragmatic arteries and the motor branch of the phrenic nerve; too small a cuff complicates the repair.
- Below the diaphragm, the peritoneum is swept off the spine and psoas.
- The parietal pleura is incised to the disk superior to the upper instrumented vertebrae.
- The surgeon must orient himself or herself to the spinal anatomy and, specifically, the intervertebral vessels by identifying the intervertebral disks (Fig. 18) The disks are more prominent than the vertebral bodies; they are the mountains and the bodies are the valleys. The diaphragmatic crurae also serve as landmarks; the left inserts over the anterolateral bodies and disks of the first two lumbar vertebrae and the right over the first three.
- Below the diaphragm, the spine is cloaked by the psoas. The anterior investing fascia is incised and then the psoas is reflected posteriorly (Fig. 19). To avoid injury to the segmental vessels, the dissection plane must first be developed at the disk level. The genitofemoral nerve is usually within the muscle but exits at lumbar level 3 or 4. It must be protected.

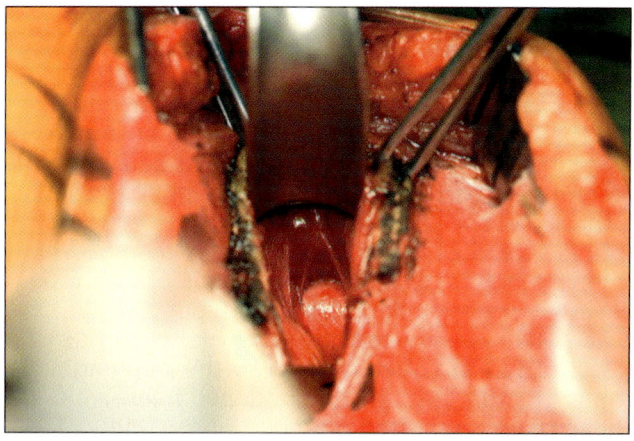

FIGURE 14

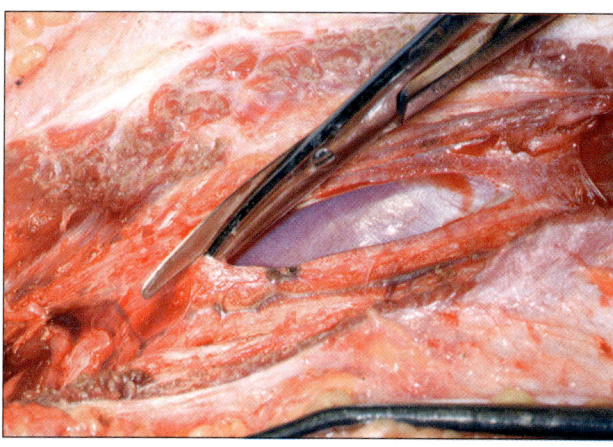

FIGURE 15

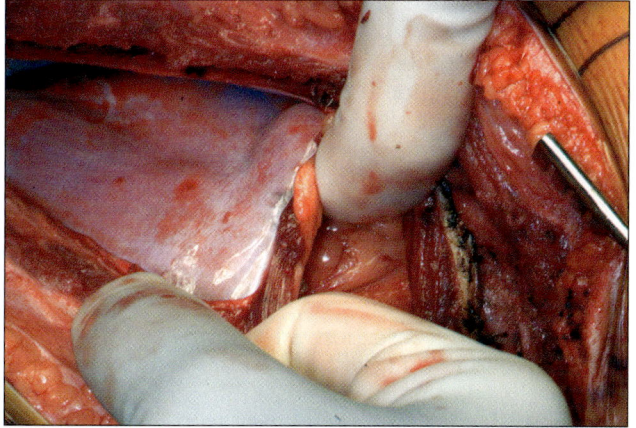

FIGURE 16

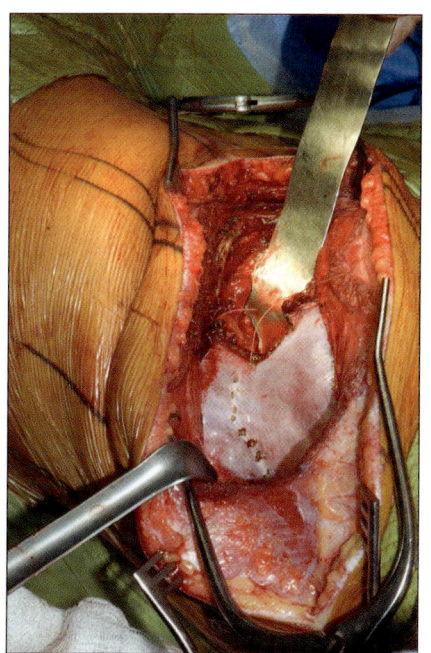

FIGURE 17

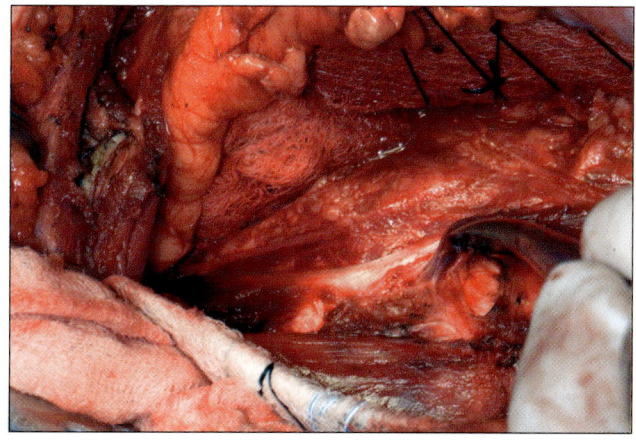

FIGURE 18

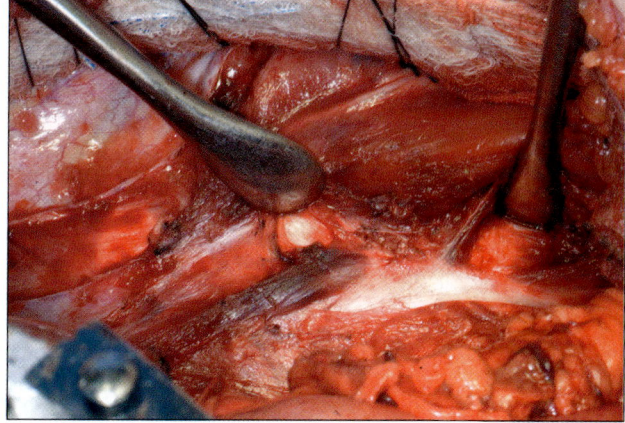

FIGURE 19

■ The segmental vessels overlying the levels of instrumentation are ligated and divided (Fig. 20).

- First the vessels are dissected off the underlying vertebral body, exposing at least a 1 cm length. Ligatures are now placed, and the vessels cut between ties, leaving an ample stump. Dissection near the neuroforamina must be avoided as vessels entering here participate in the anastomotic network supplying the spinal cord. Dissection beneath the vessels often produces venous bleeding. This is usually the nutrient vessel to the vertebral body. Complete the division of the segmental vessels and then address the vertebral body bleeding with either cautery or bone wax. The segmental vessels to T12 and L1 are often covered by the diaphragmatic crus, and that structure must first be dissected free.

■ The sympathetic chain is reflected posteriorly. Now, the periosteum of the vertebral bodies is incised and anterior and posterior periosteal and annulus fibrosis flaps are developed. The anterior flap is taken beyond the vertebral midline and the posterior flap to the base of the pedicle (Figs. 21–23). Exposing the pedicle base helps orient the subsequent instrumentation. The rib heads should be removed if they interfere with complete disk removal or instrumentation. In general, below T10 the ribs articulate with a single vertebral facet and do not insert on the adjacent rib. The staple to be used is placed at that level against the body to see if the rib compromises the staple.

PROCEDURE

STEP 1: INTERVERTEBRAL DISK EXCISION AND SPINAL DESTABILIZATION

■ A meticulous, complete disk resection will destabilize the spine, allowing better correction and less stress on the instrumentation anchors, and well-dissected and exposed end plates provide a superior environment for fusion. A clear view of the anatomy permits the surgeon to properly orient the instrumentation.

■ The annulus is removed widely with a scalpel (Fig. 24) and the nucleus pulposis with a rongeur (Fig. 25).

PEARLS

- *Initiating diskectomies at the apex of the curvature allows the spine to "flatten out," making access to the end disks easier.*

- *Spreading the disk space with a laminar spreader helps define the interval between the annulus and PLL and expedites the dissection.*

Controversies

- PLL removal, I believe, is not necessary for this procedure; there is no compelling evidence that this enhances correction, but it does add the risk of neurologic injury and additional blood loss.

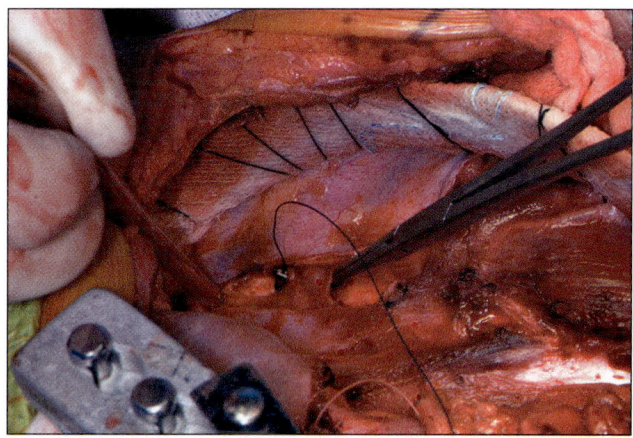

FIGURE 20

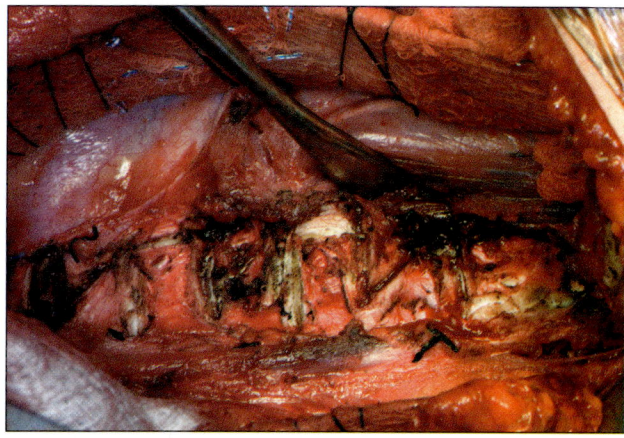

FIGURE 21

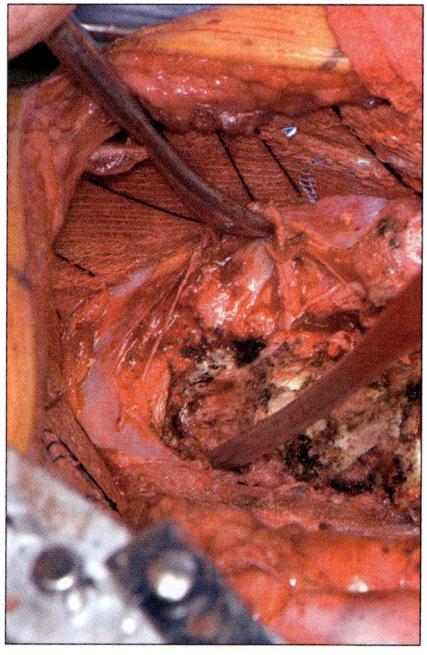

FIGURE 22

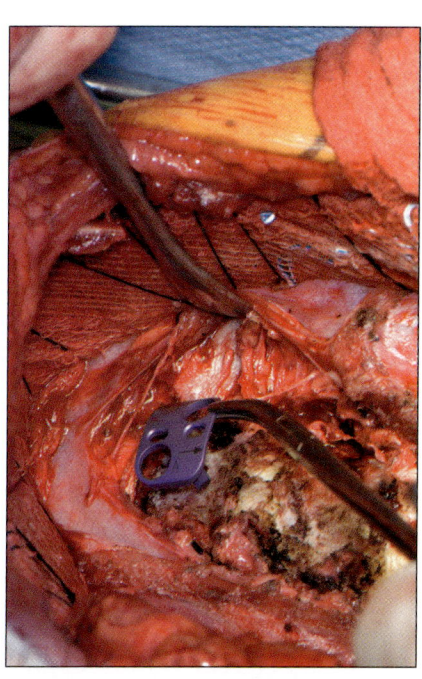

FIGURE 23

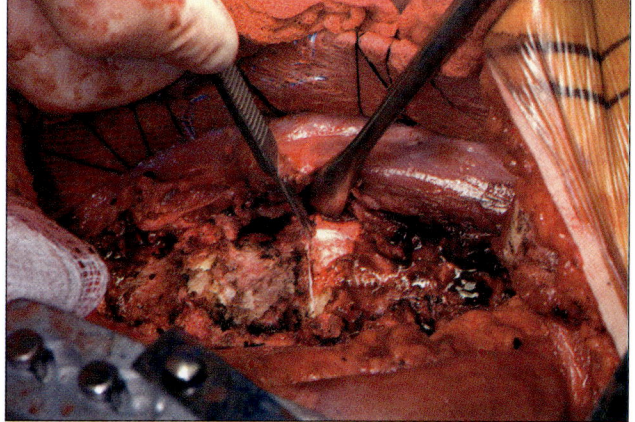

FIGURE 24

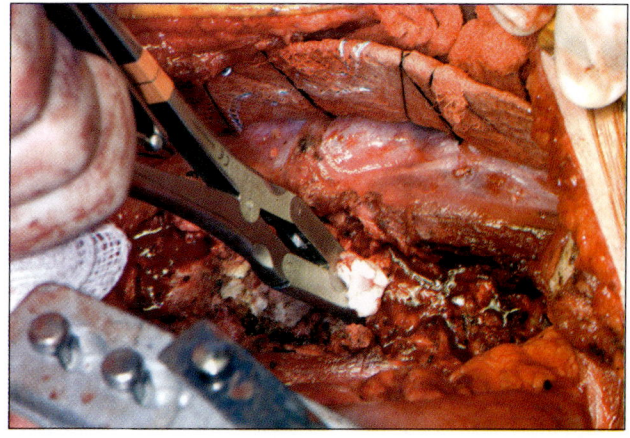

FIGURE 25

- The interval between the vertebral body and the cartilagenous end plate is developed with a Cobb elevator and dissection continues toward the spinal canal. The end plate is detached by rotating the Cobb elevator or by using a cutting action of the curette. The plane is easily established in the skeletally immature individual, but is more difficult in the adult. Alternatively, it is removed with a chisel, referencing the flat edge against the vertebral body–end plate junction. Any remaining end plate is removed with curettes (Fig. 26).
- The remaining posterior rim of annulus is removed to the level of the posterior longitudinal ligament (Fig. 27). Removing the posterior annulus and end plate to the level of the posterior longitudinal ligament (PLL) will give an excellent release and aids in orientation; the canal location is revealed and this helps to properly direct the instrumentation. The interval between the PLL and annulus in skeletally immature individuals is nicely demonstrated when the posterolateral corner of the annulus is removed and the interspace placed on stretch by a lamina spreader. A pituitary rongeur can now be placed against the PLL, removing the posterior soft tissues (Fig. 28).
- The concave annulus can be further thinned with a rongeur or curette until the concave side can be distracted with a laminar spreader.
- A hemostatic agent is temporarily placed in the disk space.

STEP 2: INSTRUMENTATION AND BONE GRAFTING

- Either a single screw–single rod or double screw–double rod system may be used. The dual-rod configuration is superior in stiffness and less likely to be kyphogenic. Adding structural anterior support such as titanium cages or a diaphyseal ring allograft to the single-rod system obviates much of the mechanical difference. The single screw–single rod system utilizes a larger 6.35-mm rod and 6.5- to 7.5-mm screw. It seems to have greater reduction strength and in my experience is a better choice when performing the overcorrection technique.
- The vertebral staples are placed.
  - The staples, and the screws, must be placed to describe a gentle curve; a sudden deviation of one relative to its neighbor will make it difficult to capture the rod and place unnecessary stresses on the anchors.
  - The proper orientation will occur if the anchors are placed at consistent points in each vertebra. It is prudent to rehearse the instrumentation placement by marking out the entry points before impaction (Fig. 29). The proper-size staple for each level must be determined.
- The vertebral screws are inserted.
  - The screw holes, usually initiated by the staple impacter (Fig. 30), are deepened to the far cortex which is breeched with a straight awl (Fig. 31). The depth is estimated before using the awl by visualizing the adjacent interspace.
  - It is imperative that the trajectory be parallel to the end plate and directed so as not to enter the neuroforamen or spinal canal.

PEARLS

- *Screw entry points must describe a gentle curvature without sudden deviation—mark out their position before impaction.*
- *Visualize the vertebral end plates, spinal canal, PLL, posterior vertebral body, and rotation to assure accurate screw placement.*
- *Screws must be parallel to end plates.*
- *The screws should engage both cortices.*

PITFALLS

- *A deviantly placed screw will endanger the vessels and spinal canal, make rod placement difficult, and place unnecessary stresses on the anchors, at times leading to failure.*

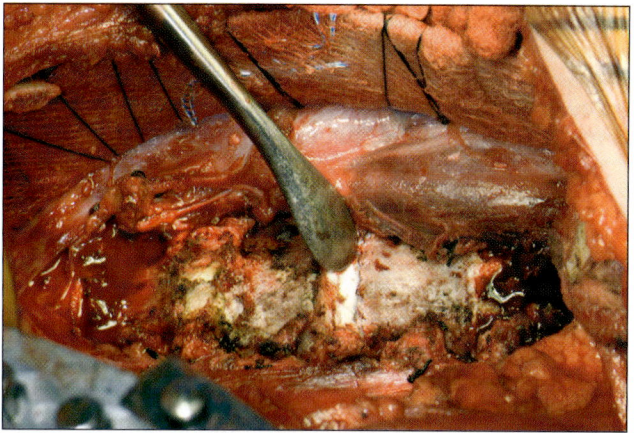

FIGURE 26

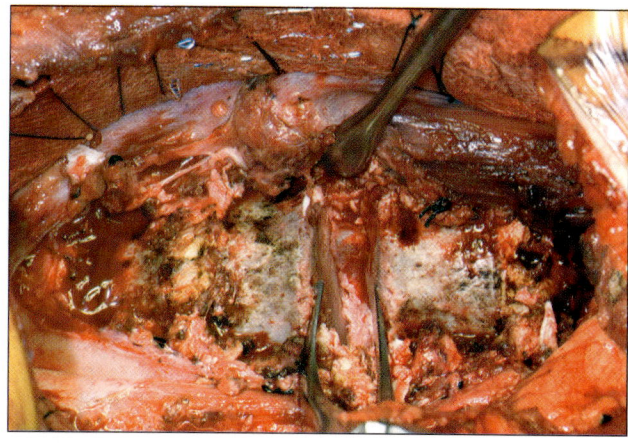

FIGURE 27

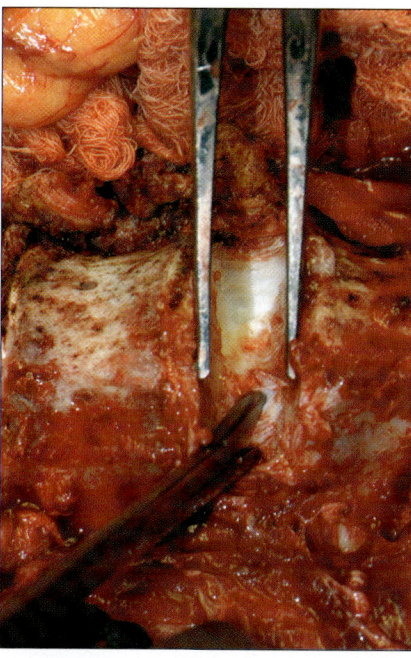

FIGURE 28

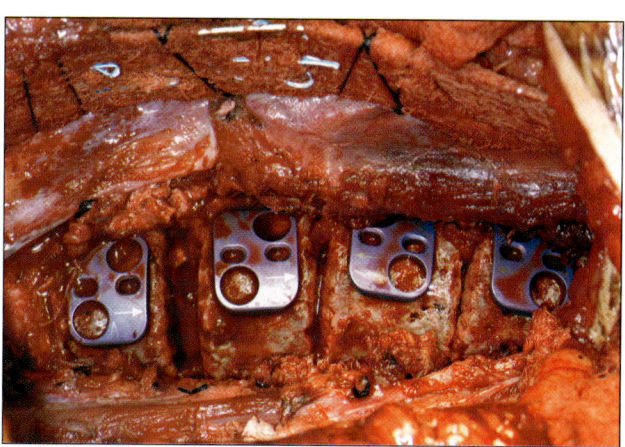

FIGURE 29

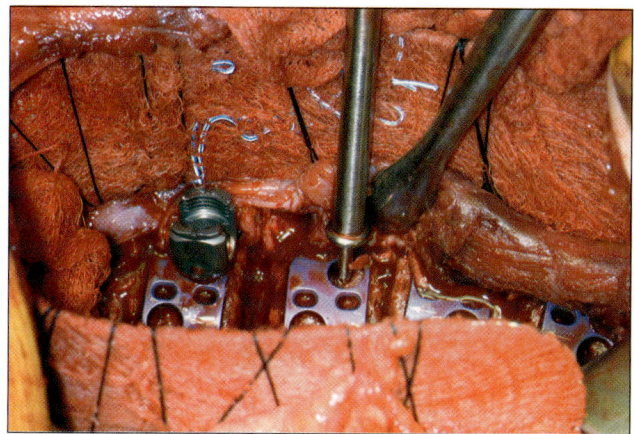

FIGURE 30

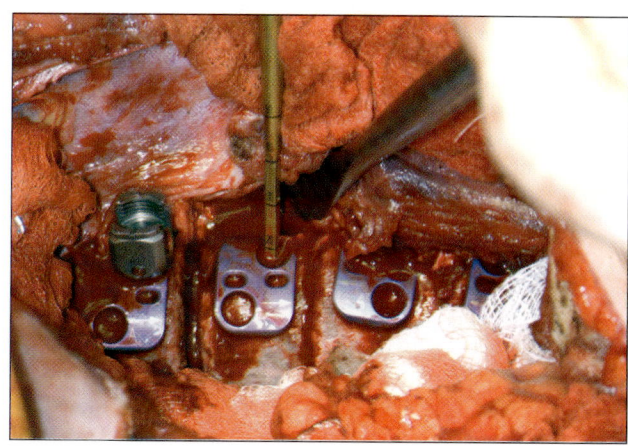

FIGURE 31

- In Figure 32, note that an obliquely placed screw is difficult to capture (Fig. 32A). Once engaged, further tightening is resisted by the deformity. If the curve rigidity is too great, the vertebral screw may plow (Fig. 32B). If the obliquely placed vertebral screw remains secure, full engagement of the rod will produce over- or undercorrection (Fig. 32C).
- The length of the screw to be used is measured by a caliper placed around the body or a depth guide placed through the screw hole to engage the far cortex (Fig. 33). The screw hole is now tapped with a tap 1–2 mm less than the diameter of the intended screw (Fig. 34) and the screw is placed (Fig. 35). The far cortex is engaged with one thread and the far side palpated to be sure the screw is not overly prominent.
- With a double-screw system, the staple will often have a guide to orient the screws. In addition to the orientation prerequisites as above, the screws must be divergent.
- The disk spaces may now be packed with morcelized bone graft. The spaces are opened with a laminar spreader and morcelized autologous rib graft is inserted. In general, the single removed rib is sufficient for two interspaces; supplemental allograft will be required for more.
- This may be a good time to verify screw placement with an image.

STEP 3: ROD INSERTION, DEFORMITY MANIPULATIVE CORRECTION, AND STRUCTURAL GRAFT PLACEMENT

- The rods are measured for length and cut, leaving an estimated 1 cm of length beyond the screw at each end.
- For single-rod system:
  - The rod is contoured. The scoliosis and rotation of the spine will describe a gentle arc and the rod is contoured to that shape. If the overcorrection method is used, the rod is bent with a bit more curvature so that, once rod rotation is performed, there will be a gentle arc in the sagittal plane and 10° overcorrection in the coronal plane.
  - The rod is placed and captured, but not bound, by loosely placing the set screws.
  - If a conventional table has been used, it is now adjusted to allow the spine to fall into correction. (With large curvatures, the surgeon may want to do this before rod contouring and placement.)

PEARLS

- *Allow the destabilization and table position to "help" with the correction. The instrumentation then holds the correction and the anchors avoid the stresses produced by manipulation. Eliminate the inertia of the spine.*

Controversies

- In the dual-rod technique, some prefer placing the anterior rod first.
- With the dual-rod technique, it is more difficult to overcorrect the deformity.

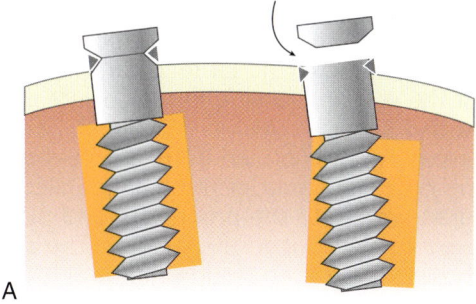

A

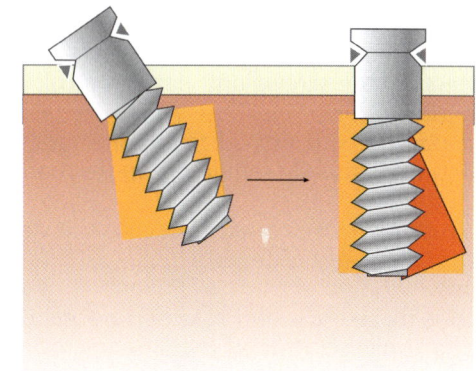

B

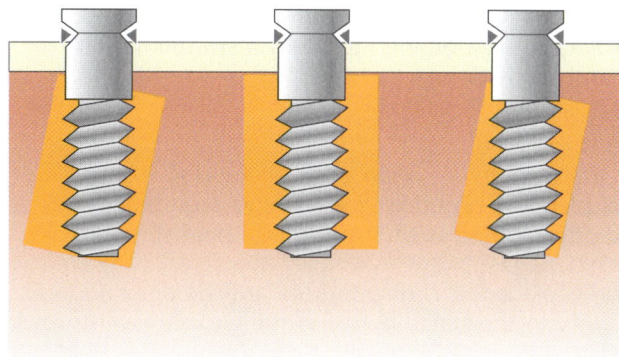

C   Over-correction   Under-correction

FIGURE 32

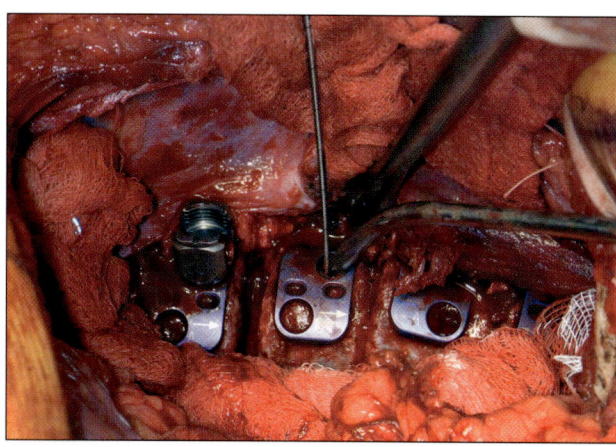

FIGURE 33

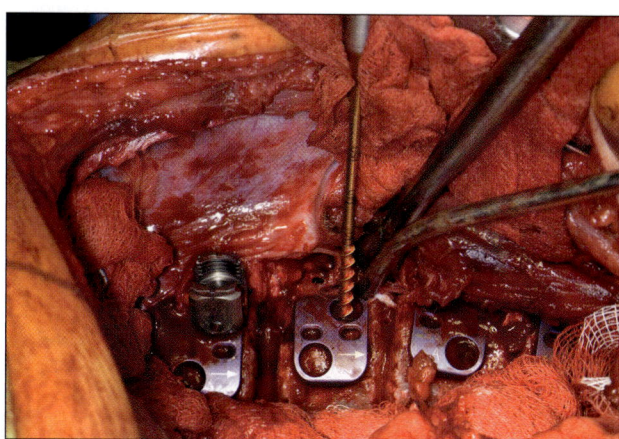

FIGURE 34

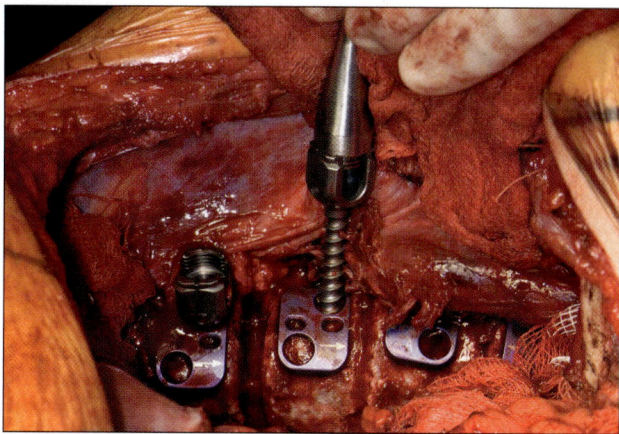

FIGURE 35

- The rod is rotated anteriorly, converting the scoliosis to lordosis. If overcorrection is planned, the rotation is continued, converting some of the lordotic curve to overcorrection of the scoliosis, dialing in the correct amount of each (Figs. 36 and 37).
- A structural interspace graft is placed in the single-rod technique. Either cortical allograft or mesh cages filled with cancellous autograft are cut to the proper size and placed in the anterior interspace to maintain the lordosis. The cortex is engaged. When using the overcorrection method, the structural graft is placed between the anterior and concave position to convert the concavity to convexity. To place the graft, the segment is first distracted. Ideally this can be performed with a laminar spreader placed in the interspace; alternatively, the adjacent screws may be distracted, although this will place stress on the screws and has some risk of causing them to plow.
- The disk space is packed with morcelized rib autograft; supplemental allograft is usually required if more than two interspaces are grafted.
- Each interspace is gently compressed to secure the structural graft and the set screws are tightened.

■ For dual-rod system:
- The posterior rod is placed first and rotated to obtain correction. Graft is applied and then the anterior rod is contoured and placed to maintain the lordosis. The anterior rod set screws are tightened. Finally, beginning at the apex and working in both directions, the posterior screws are sequentially compressed and the set screws tightened (Figs. 38–40).
- An AP radiograph is obtained to verify instrumentation position and correction.

STEP 4: CLOSURE

- ■ The wound is irrigated.
- ■ If possible, the periosteum is closed over the disk spaces.
- ■ The parietal pleura is closed with a running absorbable suture.
- ■ The diaphragm is closed with interrupted nonabsorbable sutures.
- ■ A chest tube is placed. It is directed toward the apex and exits the chest cavity in the space between the two subjacent ribs in the midaxillary region. A long subcutaneous tunnel is used and the tube is sutured in place.
- ■ The chest wall is closed by reapproximating the rib bed, avoiding the neurovascular bundle (pericostal sutures are rarely needed in the thoracolumbar area).
- ■ Anatomic closure of the split costal cartilage will align the abdominal musculature, which along with the chest wall musculature is now closed in layers.
- ■ The subcutaneous layer is closed and finally the skin; we use a running absorbable suture.

POSTOPERATIVE CARE AND EXPECTED OUTCOMES

- ■ The patient can be mobilized quickly as tolerated. Assuming stable fixation and satisfactory bone stock, postoperative immobilization is not required.
- ■ The chest tube is pulled pending the output—usually by 48 hours.

Complications

- • Though respiratory difficulties such as atelectasis or pneumonia should be anticipated, they are rarely problematic in the healthy population. Rare complications of the anterior approach also include pneumothorax, hemothorax, and chylothorax.
- • There will be a sympatheic affect on the side of the exposure. This does not seem to be long lived and has not been a problem. Retrograde ejaculation has been reported after lower lumbar approaches in males.
- • Pseudarthrosis and instrumentation failure are infrequent complications and infections are rare. Progression of the unoperated thoracic curvature when the selective technique is used have been discussed and can be avoided by proper patient selection.

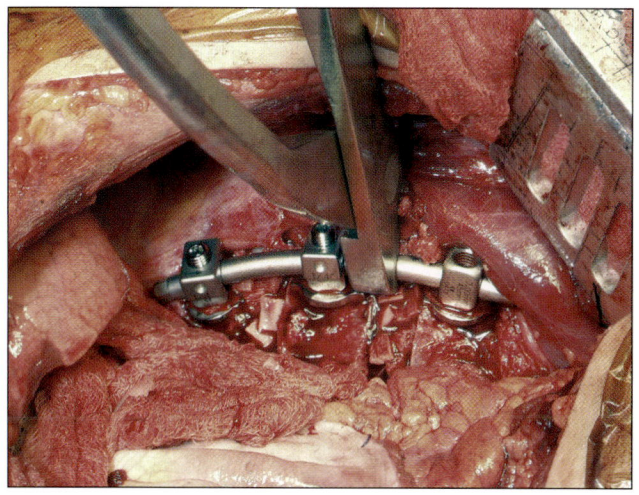

FIGURE 36

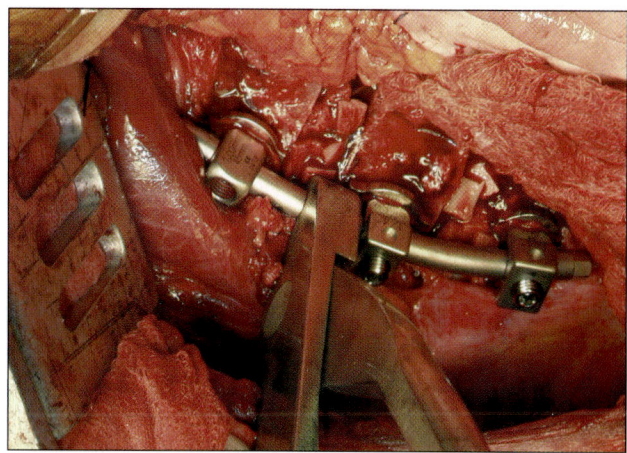

FIGURE 37

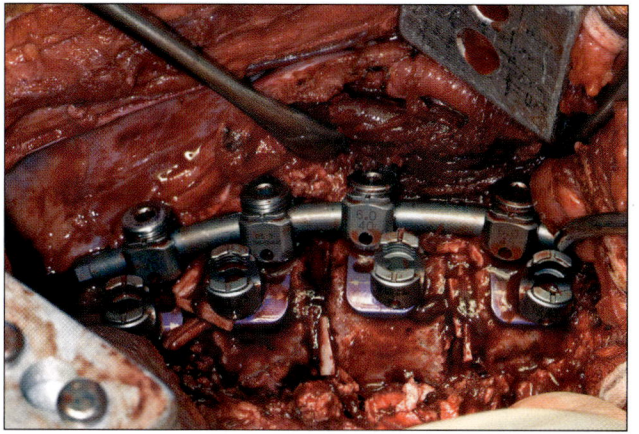

FIGURE 38

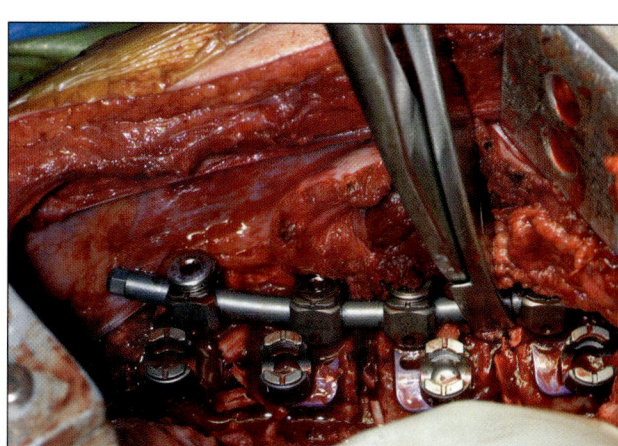

FIGURE 39

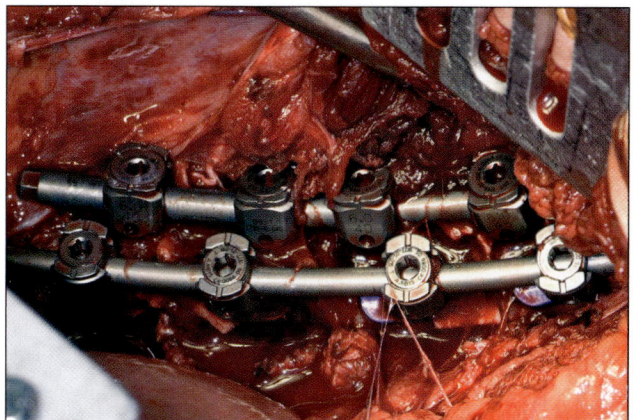

FIGURE 40

- A sedentary lifestyle is followed until fusion is noted; this usually extends to 6 months. At that time, gradual progression to noncontact activities is allowed.
- When done with an associated thoracic curvature, moderate spontaneous correction of that curve can be expected. The patients usually experience little if any perceived alteration in mobility.
- Long-term consequences of the fusion on the mobile subjacent segments is not known, but would seem to be no more of a problem than following posterior procedures.

EVIDENCE

Bernstein RM, Hall JE. Solid rod short segment anterior fusion in thoracolumbar scoliosis. J Pediatr Orthop. 1998;7:124–31.

Use of a solid rod without structural graft in the short-segment overcorrection technique for treatment of thoracolumbar scoliosis produced a 103% correction of the instrumented curvature at 2 years. Kyphosis of the instrumented segment increased 7°. (Level IV evidence)

Fricka KB, Mahar AT, Newton PO. Differences between single and dual rod systems with and without interbody structural support. Spine. 2002;27:702–6.

In bovine lumbar spines the addition of structural interbody graft in a single rod system increased the stiffness in flexion to a level comparable to that found in the dual rod construct.

Hall JE, Millis MB, Syder BD. Short segment anterior instrumentation for thoracolumbar scoliosis. In Bridwell KH, DeWald RL (eds). Textbook of Spinal Surgery, ed 2. Philadelphia: Lippincott-Raven, 1997:655–74.

The indications and selection techniques for the short-segment overcorrection method of thoracolumbar scoliosis correction is outlined.

Kaneda K, Shono Y, Satoh S, et al. New anterior instrumentation for the management of thoracolumbar and lumbar scoliosis: application of the Kaneda two-rod system. Spine. 1996;21:1250–61.

The two-rod technique produced excellent correction in the frontal plane and superior correction of the sagittal alignment. (Level IV evidence)

Sanders AE, Baumann R, Brown H, et al. Selective anterior fusion of thoracolumbar/ lumbar curves in adolescents—when can the associated thoracic curve be left unfused? Spine. 2003;28:706–14.

Successful results for a selective thoracolumbar/lumbar curve correction in the presence of a thoracic deformity were obtained when the TL/LT Cobb ratio was 1.25 or greater, and/ or the thoracic curvature corrected to 20° or less on supine side bending radiographs. (Level IV evidence)

Satake K, Lenke LG, Yongjung JK. Analysis of the lowest instrumented vertebra following anterior spinal fusion of thoracolumbar/lumbar adolescent idiopathic scoliosis: can we predict postoperative disc wedging? Spine. 2005;30:418–26.

Postoperative disc wedging below an instrumented anterior spinal fusion for thoracolumbar or lumbar adolescent idiopathic scoliosis occurred most often when the disc below the LIV is nearly parallel or when instrumentation is performed short of the LEV. (Level IV evidence)

Sweet FA, Lenke LG, Bridwell KH, et al. Maintaining lumbar lordosis with anterior single solid-rod instrumentation in thoracolumbar and lumbar adolescent idiopathic scoliosis. Spine. 1999;24:1655–62.

Lumbar lordosis was preserved with an anterior single solid-rod when a technique of a lordotically contoured rod and structural cages placed anteriorly in the disc spaces was used. (Level IV evidence)

Turi M, Johnston CE, Richards BS. Anterior correction of idiopathic scoliosis using TSRH instrumentation. Spine. 1993;18:417–22.

The technique of anterior instrumentation with a solid rod produced excellent frontal plane correction, but kyphosis of the instrumented segment increased 9 to 22° in 6 of 14 patients. (Level IV evidence)

Wang Y, Fei Q, Lee CI, et al. Anterior spinal fusion versus posterior spinal fusion for moderate lumbar/thoracolumbar adolescent scoliosis: a prospective study. Spine. 2008;33:2166–72.

In this prospective comparative study anterior spinal instrumentation and fusion using the Hall criteria produced correction and balance comparable to the posterior method while saving lumbar motion segments. (Level II evidence)

Posterior Instrumented Reduction and Fusion for Spondylolisthesis

Eric W. Tan and Paul D. Sponseller

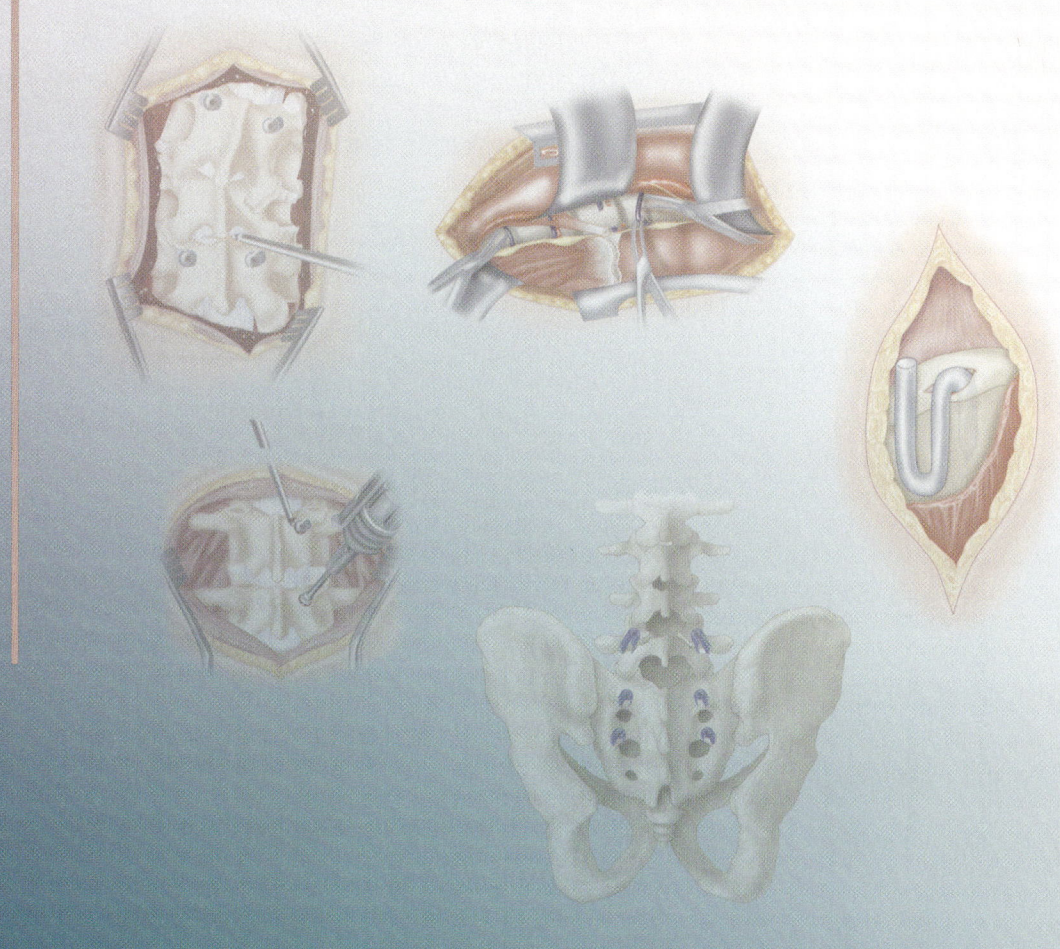

INDICATIONS

- Back pain not relieved by 6–12 months of conservative treatment: nonsteroidal anti-inflammatory drugs (NSAIDs), activity modification, back brace, physical/occupational therapy
- Radiculopathy of significant nature unrelieved by rest or analgesics
- Neurologic signs or symptoms (e.g., significant leg pain, bowel/bladder changes, claudication)
- Persistent postural/gait abnormalities
- Grade III spondylolisthesis or higher
- Pain or progression of spondylolisthesis of lower degree

Controversies

- Risk of neurologic injury and disk degeneration with surgical correction
- Risk of slip progression with posterior fusion secondary to shear forces on the fusion mass
- Risk of disk degeneration in adjacent segments
- Risk of pseudoarthrosis
- Need for reduction of spondylolisthesis. Alternatives to in situ fusion/fixation include open/closed reduction plus fusion, combined anterior-posterior approaches or posterior plus anterior interbody fusion, and fixation with pedicle screw constructs. In situ fusion without reduction is a time-honored procedure that works for many patients. It does require fusion to L4 in grade III and higher slips, and does leave the patient with some residual deformity. This can be done with posterior, anterior, or posterior interbody grafts. The Bohlman procedure is one that has a high rate of success with minimal incision.
- The patient may choose in situ fusion with a higher rate of pseudarthrosis and progression and residual deformity, but lower L5 nerve root risk; versus reduction and fusion of the slip with more correction of deformity, avoidance of fusion to L4, higher fusion rate, and higher risk of L5 nerve palsy.

Treatment Options

- No treatment in patients with nonprogressive and asymptomatic spondylolisthesis
- Activity modification with restriction of heavy lifting or excessive bending/hyperextension
- Physical therapy
- NSAIDS, analgesia
- Brace
- Surgical therapy (fixation, fusion, reduction, decompression)

EXAMINATION/IMAGING

- Anteroposterior (AP) and lateral plain film radiographs are obtained. Figure 1 depicts a preoperative lateral view of grade IV spondylolisthesis (L5-S1).
- Computed tomography (CT) scan of the lumbar spine is also obtained.
- Magnetic resonance imaging (MRI) of the lumbar spine is used to assess spinal cord/nerve integrity and ligamentous structures. Figure 2 depicts a preoperative sagittal MRI of grade II spondylolisthesis (L5-S1).

SURGICAL ANATOMY

- Palpable stepoff of spinous processes is one level above vertebral body stepoff.
- The posterior elements of the slipped vertebral body are hypermobile ("wobbly").
- L5 transverse processes are deeply recessed.
- Posterior elements of L5 and S1 may be bifid.

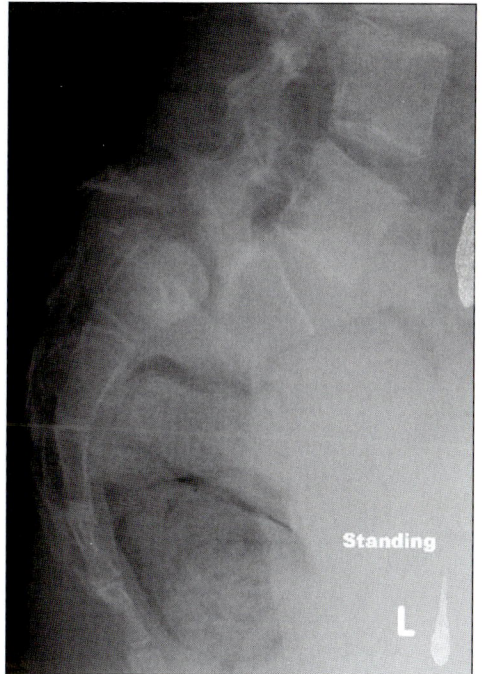

FIGURE 1

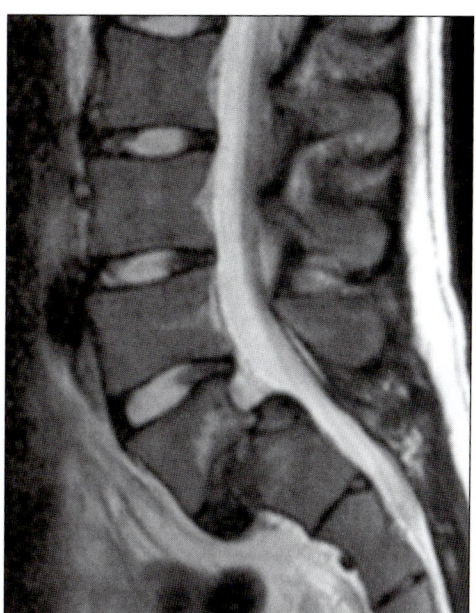

FIGURE 2

Equipment

- Radiolucent spine table

Instrumentation/ Implantation

- 6 mm or larger screws (preferred)
- Stimulate screws

Controversies

- Fixation of L4 may be employed if slip is severe or L5 pedicles are small (surgeon discretion).
- Insert screws in S1 pedicles. The authors also recommend inserting screws to the S2 ala.

POSITIONING

- The patient is placed prone on a radiolucent table. The table should produce no imaging artifact for PA and lateral projections of L4-S2.
- Spinal cord monitoring should include electromyography and nerve root monitoring and sphincter monitoring.

PORTALS/EXPOSURES

- A 4- to 6-cm midline posterior longitudinal exposure is made.
- Exposure continues to the transverse processes of L5.
- The ala of the sacrum is exposed.
- Posterior elements of L5 are excised below the pars defect after exposure is complete.

PROCEDURE

STEP 1

- The posterior elements from L5-S1 or S2 are exposed. This can be done through a midline or a Wiltse posterolateral fascial approach.

STEP 2

- The posterior elements of L5 are removed. The lamina and spinous process are removed down to the pars defect. Osteophytes and granulation tissue are removed from the pars region.
- Epidural bleeding should be minimized.
- The surgeon should visualize and decompress the L5 nerve root and obtain baseline stimulus threshold.
- Figure 3 depicts a preoperative sagittal MRI highlighting posterior elements to be removed (in rectangle).

STEP 3

- Pedicle starting points are localized on CT scans or MRI.
  - Figure 4 is a transverse CT scan demonstrating recommended pedicle starting points (indicated by *arrows*) and trajectories of the L5 (Fig. 4A), S1 (Fig. 4B), and S2 (Fig. 4C) screws.
  - The preoperative sagittal MRI in Figure 5 demonstrates the trajectories of the L5, S1, and S2 screws (*arrows*).
- Figure 6 illustrates AP (Fig. 6A) and lateral (Fig. 6B) views of screw placement prior to reduction.

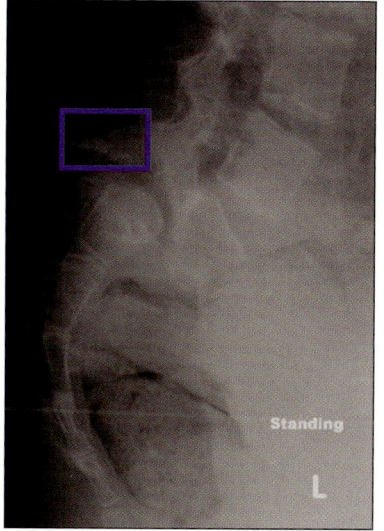

FIGURE 3

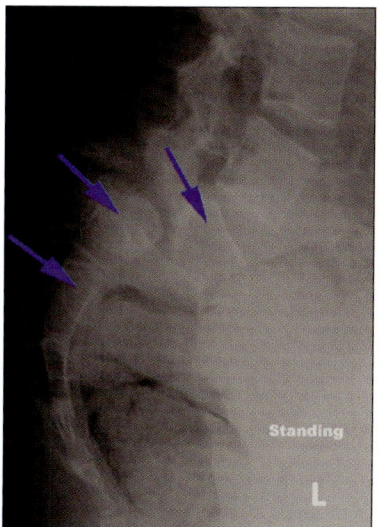

FIGURE 5

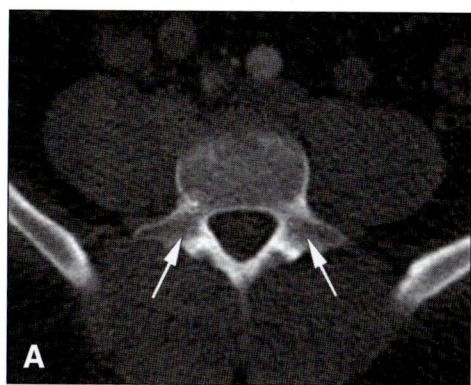

A

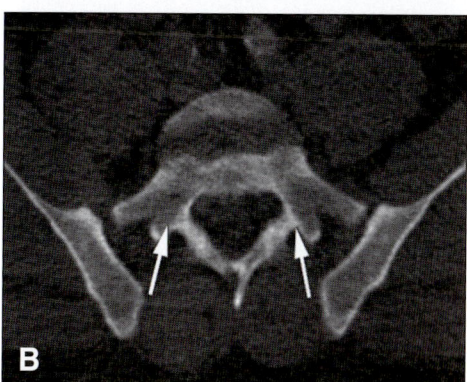

B

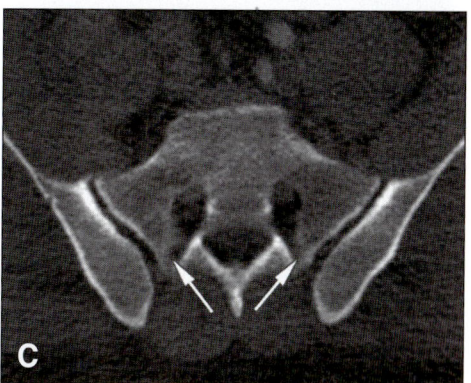

C

FIGURE 4

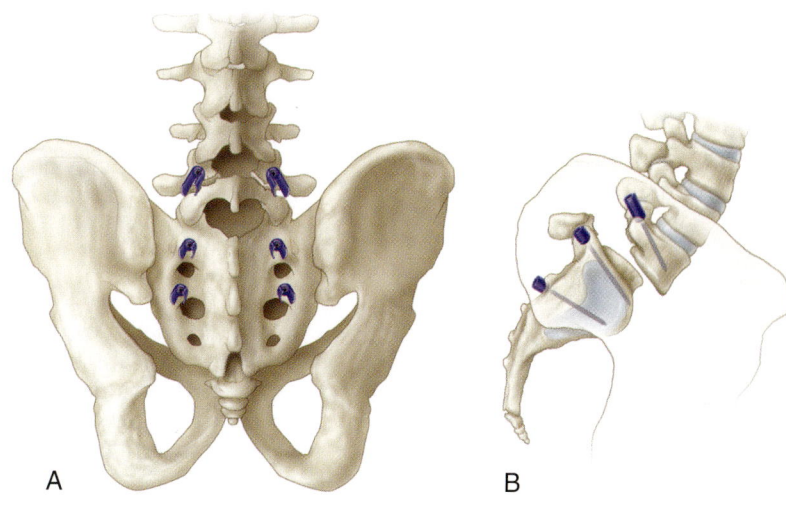

A

B

FIGURE 6

STEP 4

- Nerve roots are stimulated. The L5 nerve roots are decompressed; the ligamentum flavum and osteophytes around the defect are removed.
- The surgeon should visualize the L5 nerve roots and trace out past the transverse processes.
- Nerve roots are restimulated. The surgeon must be alert to spontaneous firing of nerve roots during reduction.

STEP 5

- Rods are inserted into L5-S2 and the S1 and S2 screws are locked down bilaterally.
- L5 is reduced on S1 slowly and bilaterally using reduction instruments or specially designed reduction screws.
- Iliac crest bone graft is harvested by dissecting laterally through the midline skin incision to the posterior iliac fascia. This should consist of cancellous strips and cortical strips that are at least 5 cm long.
- The L5-S1 interspace is gently distracted in preparation for interbody fusion.

STEP 6

- For transforaminal interbody graft/fusion, the thecal sac is retracted medially using a broad retractor and nerve root is visualized laterally. Epidural vessels are coagulated.
- The disk space is incised and the disk contents are resected in the midportion. The end plate cartilage of L5 and S1 is curetted down to bone. A structural interbody chisel and spacer are inserted, and then graft is inserted.
- Graft material may consist of bicortical autograft or allograft or a mixture of both. It may also consist of a structural cage. Structural graft may be either rectangular or slightly lordotic.
- The same process should be repeated on the right and the left sides.
- The L5-S1 screws are gently compressed to produce good bony contact between the vertebral bodies and the graft. Then the pedicle set-screws are locked to final tightness.
- Figure 7 shows an intraoperative fluoroscopy image of reduction and fixation of grade IV spondylolisthesis.
- The L5 nerve root is restimulated to make sure that the stimulus threshold has not gone up.

STEP 7

- The L5 transverse processes are gently decorticated.
- The sacral ala is decorticated and a trough is created in the ala just caudal to the L5 transverse processes.
- Cancellous strips are laid over the muscle between the L5 transverse process and the sacral ala.
- A 5-cm iliac cortical bone graft is placed into the alar trough and laid over the L5 transverse process on the right and the left sides.

STEP 8

- Any nonviable muscle is débrided and the fascia, subcutaneous tissue, and skin are closed in separate layers. A drain is palced at the surgeon's discretion.
- Local anesthesia may be infiltrated over the iliac crest and the paraspinous fascia.
- Figure 8 shows postoperative AP (Fig. 8A) and lateral (Fig. 8B) views of grade IV spondylolisthesis (L5-S1).

PEARLS

- *Perform a neurological examination of both ankles before leaving the operating suite. Check for ankle and toe dorsiflexion and plantar flexion.*

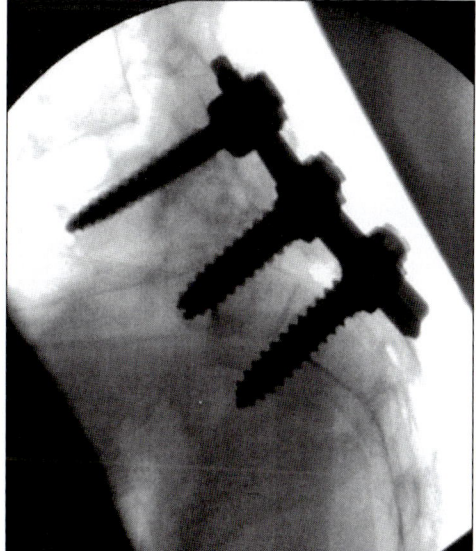

FIGURE 7

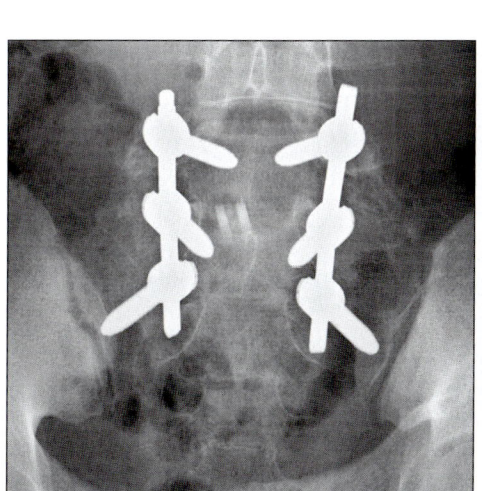

A
FIGURE 8

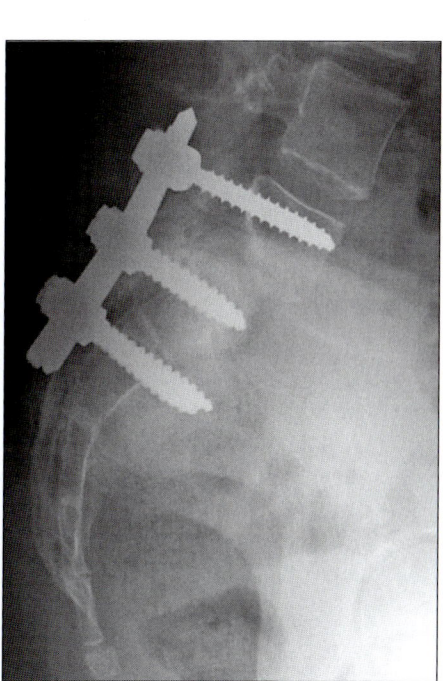

B

POSTOPERATIVE CARE AND EXPECTED OUTCOMES

- Patients are mobilized on postoperative day 1.
- The hospital stay is usually 2–4 days.
- The postoperative bracing regimen is variable; a soft brace may be used for comfort or no brace may be needed at all.
- Patients usually return to school or work in 3–6 weeks.
- Patients are restricted from contact sports for at least 6 months after surgery.

Controversies

- Reduction versus fusion in situ.
- Whether to add interbody fusion is controversial. It is more beneficial in older patients, those with foraminal narrowing, and those with small transverse processes.

PEARLS

- *Specify postoperative neurologic examinations every 2–4 hours for the first day.*
- *Patients may be more comfortable with the hips and knees flexed gently.*

PITFALLS

- *If a neurologic deficit is detected, obtain a CT scan to check for graft dislodgement or screw malposition. If none is detected, the surgeon may elect to treat severe motor weakness by returning to the operating room and decreasing the amount of reduction of the slip.*
- *After the reduction of a grade IV slip, a junctional kyphotic deformity may develop at L4-5. This is more likely to happen if L4 was exposed during the reduction procedure and especially if it was temporarily instrumented. The Wiltse approach may lessen this risk.*

EVIDENCE

Helenius I, Remes V, Poussa M. Uninstrumented in situ fusion for high-grade childhood and adolescent isthmic spondylolisthesis: long-term outcome. Surgical technique. J Bone Joint Surg [Am]. 2008;90(Suppl 2 Pt 1):145–52.

This retrospective comparative study suggested only slight improvement in long-term results with circumferential in situ fusion compared with posterolateral or anterior in situ fusion. (Level III evidence)

Lamberg T, Remes V, Helenius I, Poussa M. Uninstrumented in situ fusion for high-grade childhood and adolescent isthmic spondylolisthesis: long-term outcome. J Bone Joint Surg [Am]. 2007;89:512–8.

This retrospective comparative study suggested only slight improvement in long-term results with circumferential in situ fusion compared with posterolateral or anterior in situ fusion. (Level III evidence)

Ruf M, Koch H, Melcher R, Harms J. Anatomic reduction and monosegmental fusion in high-grade developmental spondylolisthesis. Spine. 2006;31:269–74.

The authors presented results indicating that reduction of L5-S1 with temporary instrumentation of L4 and monosegmental fusion of L5-S1 may be an effective alternative to fusion of L4-5 in the treatment of high-grade spondylolisthesis. (Level III evidence)

Schoenecker PL, Cole HO, Herring JA, Bradford DS. Cauda equina syndrome after in situ arthrodesis for severe spondylolisthesis at the lumbosacral junction. J Bone Joint Surg [Am]. 1990;72:369–77.

Decompression was recommended for patients with lumbosacral spondylolisthesis who either have preoperative nerve root dysfunction or acute cauda equina syndrome that follows arthrodesis. (Level III evidence)

Shufflebarger HL, Geck M. High-grade isthmic dysplastic spondylolisthesis: monosegmental surgical treatment. Spine. 2005;30(6 Suppl):S42–8.

The authors recommended anterior column structural support and posterior compressive instrumentation when treating high-grade spondylolisthesis to restore spinal balance and improve fusion. (Level IV evidence)

Smith MD, Bohlman HH. Spondylolisthesis treated by a single-stage operation combining decompression with in situ posterolateral and anterior fusion: an analysis of eleven patients who had long-term follow-up. J Bone Joint Surg [Am]. 1990;72:415–21.

This study found that single-stage operations involving posteriorlateral and anterior fusion with decompression provide solid fusion. (Level III evidence)

Thoracoscopic Release and Instrumentation for Scoliosis

John E. Tis and Peter O. Newton

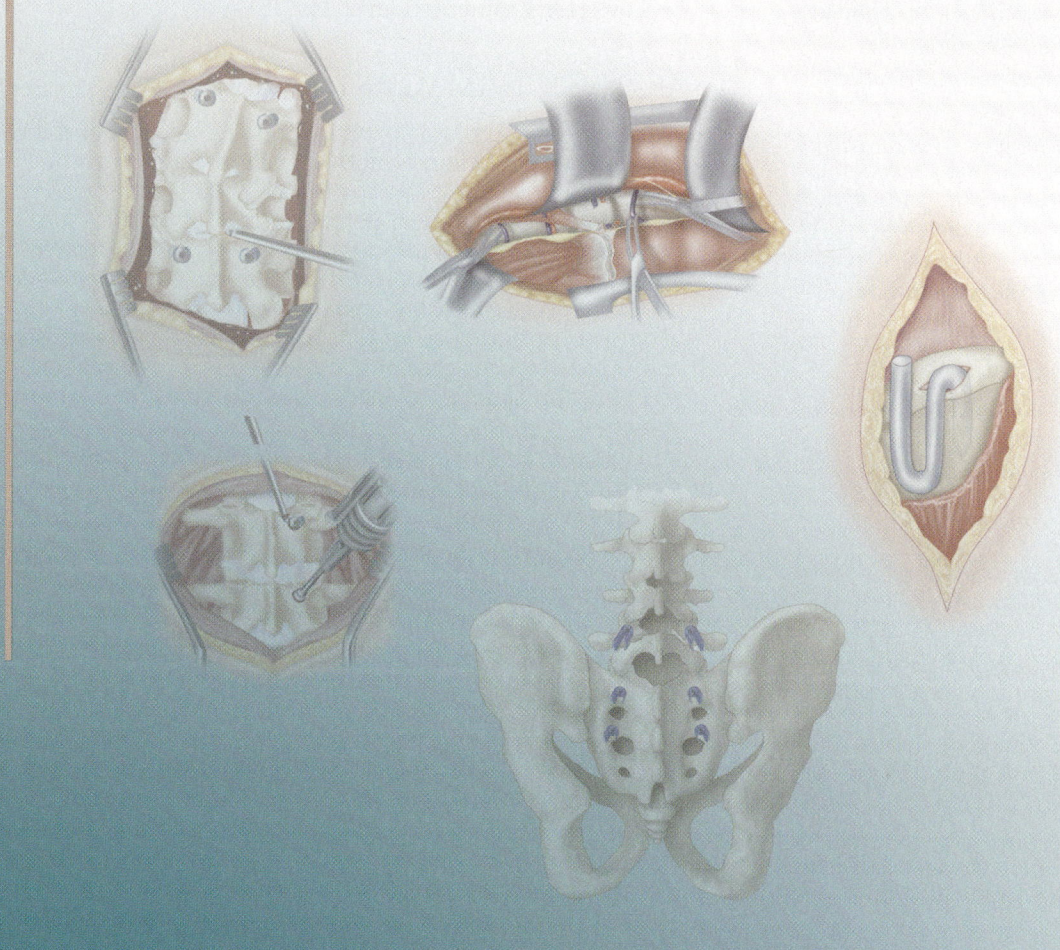

Controversies

- The upper limits for deformities requiring anterior release vary among surgeons. Thoracic pedicle screw use has reduced the indications for anterior release.

- Thoracoscopic anterior instrumentation remains a challenging operation with a substantial learning curve, limiting the adoption of the procedure.

Treatment Options

- Instrumented posterior spinal fusion

- Instrumented single-rod or dual-rod open anterior spinal fusion

INDICATIONS

- Thoracoscopic anterior release (diskectomy)
  - Rigid spinal deformity
  - Scoliosis greater than 70–80°
  - Thoracic lordosis greater than 10–20°
  - Thoracic hyperkyphosis greater than 90°
  - Pseudarthrosis risk
  - Juvenile patients at risk for crankshaft growth
- Thoracoscopic instrumentation for adolescent idiopathic scoliosis
  - Single structural thoracic curve (Lenke 1)
  - Cobb angle between 40° and 80°
  - Flexible main curve that bends to less than 35° (50% flexibility)
  - Normal or hypokyphotic sagittal contour
  - Lowest instrumented level T12 (L1)

EXAMINATION/IMAGING

- A complete neurologic examination of the trunk and lower extremities, including abdominal reflexes, needs to be performed.
- Assessment of rotational deformity is done using Adam's forward bend test, trunk shift, and pelvic and shoulder symmetry. Examination from the side must not be overlooked as well in order to assess sagittal contour.
- Standing posteroanterior (PA) and lateral scoliosis films should be obtained, with careful consideration of the Lenke curve type, coronal and sagittal balance, pelvic obliquity, and shoulder height.
  - Figure 1 shows standing PA (Fig. 1A) and lateral scoliosis (Fig. 1B) radiographs of a 15-year-old patient with Lenke 1A adolescent idiopathic scoliosis.
  - The instrumentation end vertebrae can also be planned using these radiographs.
- Left and right bending films are obtained to determine the flexibility of the compensatory upper thoracic and lumbar curves as well as the flexibility of the main thoracic curve. Figure 2 shows left (Fig. 2A) and right (Fig. 2B) bending films of the same patient as in Figure 1.

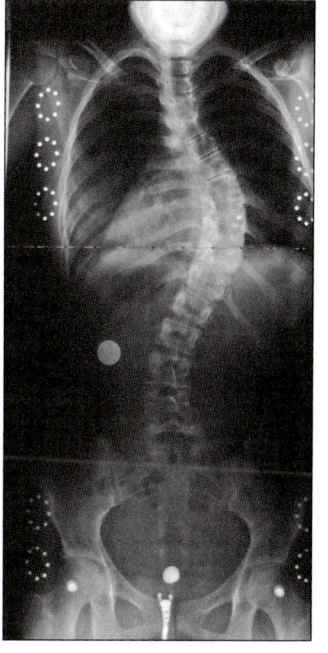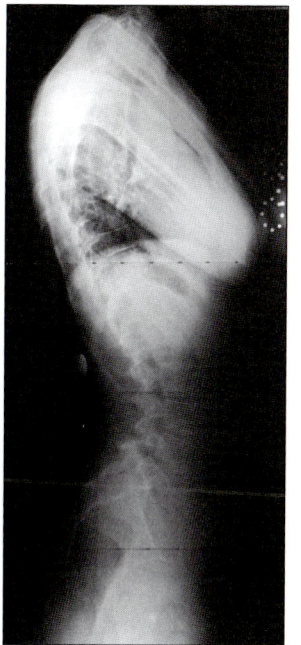

A   B

FIGURE 1

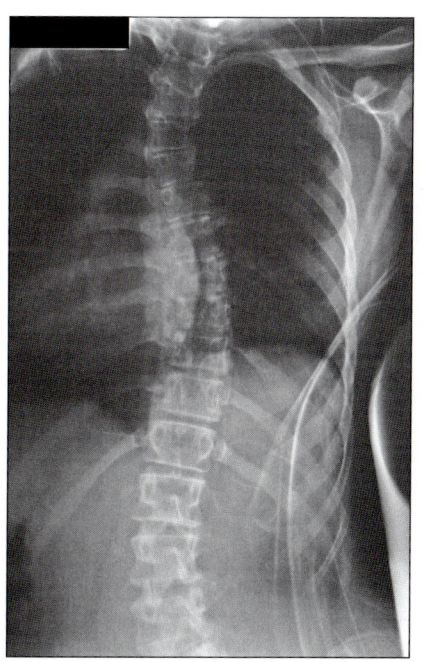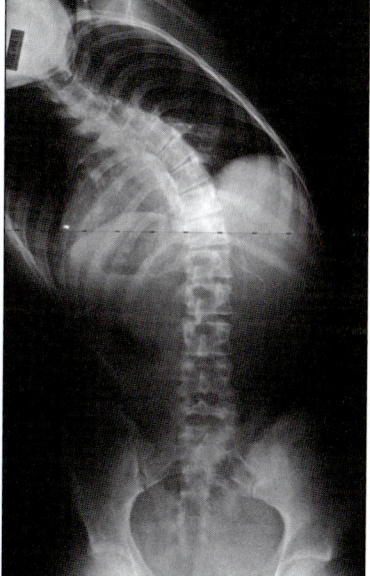

A   B

FIGURE 2

SURGICAL ANATOMY

- Figure 3 is an anatomic sketch of the right hemithorax demonstrating the major structures.
- The lung must be deflated prior to exposure and completely reinflated at the time of closure.
- Segmental vessels are at risk at two locations: during portal creation and during exposure of the vertebral body. Care must be taken when creating the portal to stay on the cephalad edge of the inferior rib. When exposing the vertebral body, segmental vessels must be carefully cauterized or clipped prior to division. Otherwise, bleeding may be difficult to control, requiring conversion to thoracotomy.
- The azygos vein is located anterior and slightly to the right of the vertebral bodies (Fig. 4). This large and friable vein is the most posterior longitudinal vessel in the right hemithorax. It receives intercostal vessels cepahalad to the T6 level (sometimes lower).
- The descending aorta is located on the left anterolateral spine from T4-8. The thoracic aorta crosses toward the midline at T9-12, and its location moves more anterior as the patient is moved from the supine to the prone position. The aortic arch is located cephalad to T4.
- The thoracic duct is on the left side of the vertebrae cephalad to T4, and it crosses to the right to follow the aorta in the right hemithorax between the azygos vein and aorta. Transection may produce a persistant chylothorax.
- The esophagus runs anterior to the vertebral column between the azygos vein and descending aorta.
- The sympathetic chain runs on both sides just anterior to the costovertebral joints.
- The splanchnic nerve branches out to form a network of fine fibers between the azygos vein and sympathetic chain. Transection of some of these fibers is unavoidable.
- The ribs of the thoracic spine articulate with the transverse process and bridge the disk space. The rib bridges the disk space at the same-number vertebra and the one cephalad (e.g., the fifth rib head lies at the T4-5 disk space).

POSITIONING

- The lateral decubitus position is described here because it facilitates retraction of the lung and great vessels and is the preferred position of the authors.
- The operating room table is placed in the center of the room parallel to its long axis. Monitors and other equipment are positioned as shown in Figure 5.
- Double-lumen endotracheal tube placement is performed in the supine position.
- For most situations, the patient is placed on the left side.
  - An axillary roll is placed under the left axilla and both shoulders and elbows are flexed 90°.
  - A pillow is placed between the elbows and one large "jelly" roll is placed behind the patient's shoulders and another in front to help hold the position.
  - Four-inch cloth or silk tape is placed over the right shoulder to maintain the lateral position.
- The hips and knees are slightly flexed in an offset position and two to three pillows are placed between the knees. Another strip of tape is placed over the hips and a safety strap over the legs.

PEARLS

- *Ensure that the patient is in the true lateral position. Obliquity may cause disorientation later during screw placement.*
- *The patient's shoulders must be distal to any pedestal or other blocks to fluoroscopic imaging.*
- *Ensure that the patient is well taped and padded prior to fluoroscopic marking.*
- *If iliac crest bone graft will be harvested, the posterior ilium must be kept exposed.*

PITFALLS

- *Inadequate padding of the greater trochanter and other bony prominences.*
- *Movement of the endotracheal tube during lateral positioning. This may prevent single lung ventilation and require repositioning.*
- *The upper arm is not flexed enough, blocking exposure to the upper spine.*

Controversies

- Some surgeons prefer the prone position, which allows simultaneous exposure of the posterior spine.

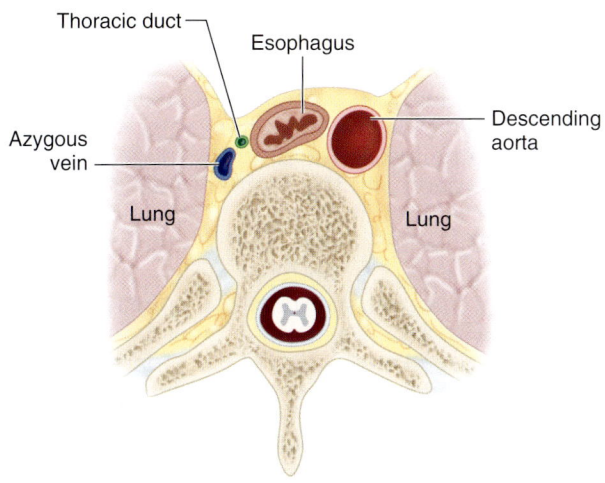

FIGURE 3

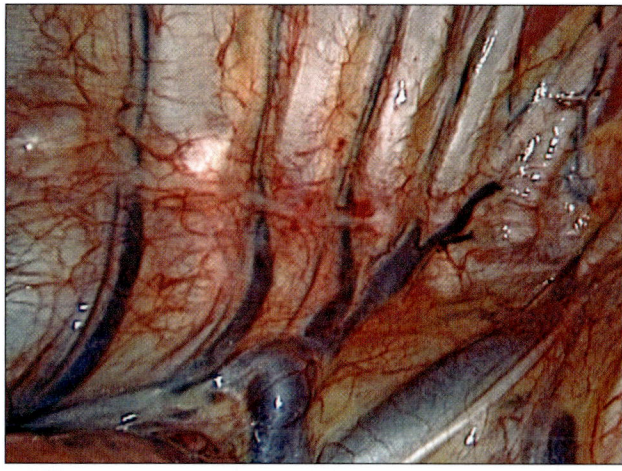

FIGURE 4

FIGURE 5

Instrumentation

• 11.5-mm disposable canula with blunt trocar

• 10-mm diameter 0° and 45° endoscopes

• Fan retractor (US Surgical)

• Harmonic scalpel laparoscopic coagulating shears (Ethicon)

PORTALS/EXPOSURES

■ Flouroscopic marking
   • The C-arm is brought in and placed into the lateral position (PA of the thorax). A line is drawn down the center of the spine over the levels to be fused. The C-arm is rotated to the anteroposterior (AP) position and the center of each vertebral body is marked with a straight line parallel to the end plate from the posterior to the anterior thorax. The intersection of these lines and the line along the posterior axillary line is the location of the posterior portals, which will be primarily used for screw placement (Fig. 6A).
   • The anterior portals are marked as follows: the proximal portal is in the "soft spot" distal to the latissimus in the anterior axillary line just distal to the axilla; the distal portal is in line with this and three interspaces distal (Fig. 6B). The anterior portals are used for exposure and diskectomy. If releases alone will be performed (no instrumentation), a third anterior portal is placed two to three interspaces distal to this; otherwise, the distal posterior portal is used as a distal portal (total three posterior and two anterior portals).

■ If autogenous bone graft is to be used, it is harvested now from the posterior ilium. The site is closed over a drain.

■ The right lung is deflated and the anterior cephalad portal is created first. A 3-cm longitudinal incision is made through the dermis. A curved Mayo scissors is used to bluntly dissect the external and internal oblique fibers. An 11.5-mm blunt disposable cannula is used to push through the deep fascia and pleura into the chest. The trocar is removed and a 45° endoscope placed.

■ The posterior caudad portal is then made using identical technique as for the cephalad portal. Figure 7A shows the creation of the caudal portal as seen through the midchest anterior portal. A disposable fan-shaped lung retractor is placed under direct visualization through this portal. The proximal lung is gently retracted with the fan retractor (Fig. 7B).

■ A third 11.5-mm portal is established in the anterior axillary line three interspaces distal to the anterior proximal portal. The harmonic scalpel (HS) is inserted through this portal. This will be the working portal (for now).

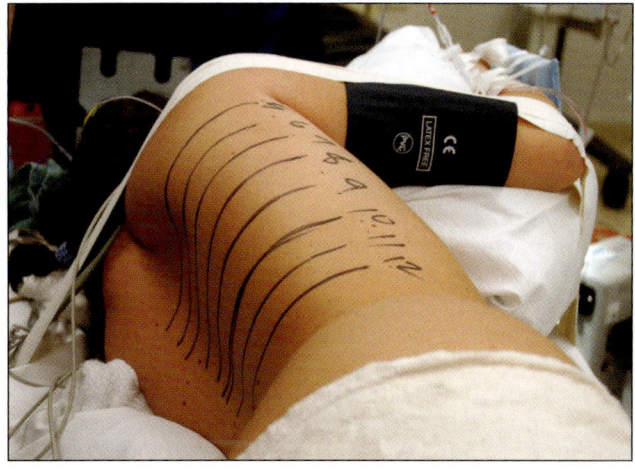

A

FIGURE 6

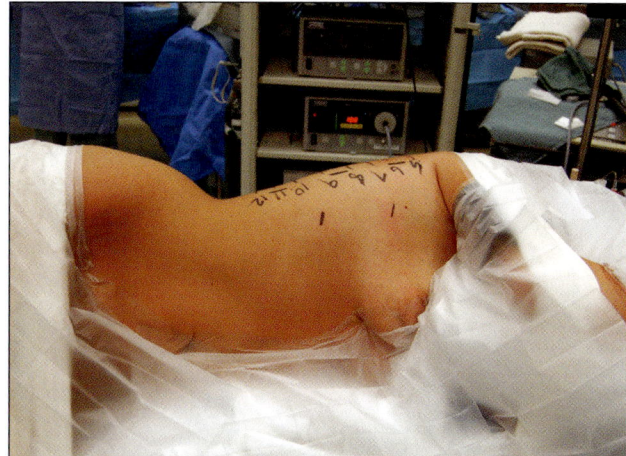

B

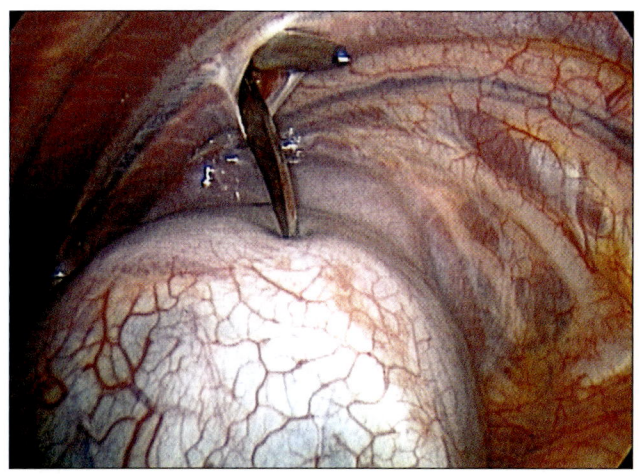

A

FIGURE 7

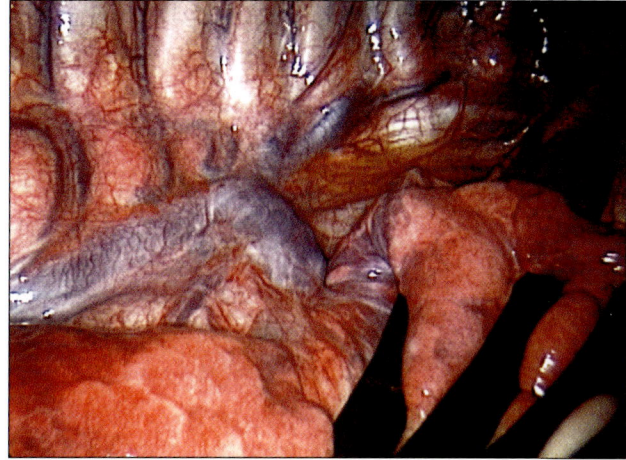

B

Instrumentation/ Implantation

- Scope holder (Koros Surgical)
- Suction-irrigator (Nezhat-Dorsey)
- Endo Peanut (US Surgical)

Controversies

- The need for autograft in adolescent idiopathic scoliosis fusion, and the harvest site, are controversial. Some surgeons harvest from the ilium, some take autograft rib, and others use banked allograft and/or demineralized bone matrix without autograft.

PEARLS

- *Prior to diskectomy, insert a 0.062-inch Kirschner wire (K-wire) into the most caudal disk and take a PA fluoroscopic image to confirm levels.*

- *Be sure to enter the disk parallel to the end plates. Do not violate the end plate bone (which causes bleeding) before the depths of the disk have been removed.*

PITFALLS

- *The disk must be completely excised. Incomplete diskectomy risks nonunion.*

PROCEDURE

STEP 1: EXPOSURE OF THE VERTEBRAE AND DISKS

- The blade of the HS is turned horizontal and the pleura incised from proximal to distal about 10 mm anterior to the rib heads. The segmental vessels are coagulated first and then slowly cut with the HS. Figure 8 shows the harmonic scalpel dissecting pleura from around the segmental vessel.
- After all the vessels are sectioned, the pleura is peeled anteriorly beyond the anterior longitudinal ligament (ALL). The passive arm of the HS is opened and used to retract the pleura anteriorly.
- Two to three Raytech sponges are packed in the far side gutter to protect the azygos vein, esophagus, and other anterior structures. In Figure 9, a fully dissected thoracic spine is seen with a sponge packed anterior to the spine.
- The HS is turned vertically with the passive arm closed and posterior and the posterior flap is peeled of pleura over the rib heads.

PEARLS

- *The key to good visualization is minimizing bleeding, which can be performed with patient technique utilizing the HS. Start on the far side of each segmental vessel and peel the pleura toward you with the scalpel off. Then incise the pleura with the scalpel on. Turn the HS vertical and run it up and down each side of the vessels until they are both coagulated. [Use the low setting (3) for all procedures except incising the disk; then use high (5)].*

- *When working on the distal (caudal) levels, move the fan retractor to the proximal portal and the HS to the middle, then distal portal.*

- *It is often possible to instrument L1 by taking down the attachments of the diaphragm at T12 with the HS. This must be repaired at the time of closure.*

- *Stop any bone bleeding with bone wax on the end of an Endo Peanut.*

STEP 2: DISKECTOMY

- Once the disks and vertebral bodies have been exposed, the HS is turned on high (5) and the center of the disk is incised from anterior to posterior (Fig. 10). An up-biting pituitary rongeur is used to remove the disk from anterior to posterior.
- The two end plates are exposed to define the boundries of the diskectomy. On the caudal two disks, the ALL is preserved to hold the structural graft in place. A PLIF shaver is inserted to scrape the end plates and flexibility is checked. Figure 11 shows a completed discectomy with cartilage removed from the end plates.
- A Surgicel sponge is inserted to aid hemostasis from the bleeding bony end plates.
- Repeat for all discs from proximal to distal.

Instrumentation/Implantation

- Thorascopic spine tools (Koros Surgical)
  - Pituitary rongeurs (4-mm straight, up-biting, right, and left; 6-mm straight and up-biting)
  - Curettes: straight, up
  - Small and large end plate shavers

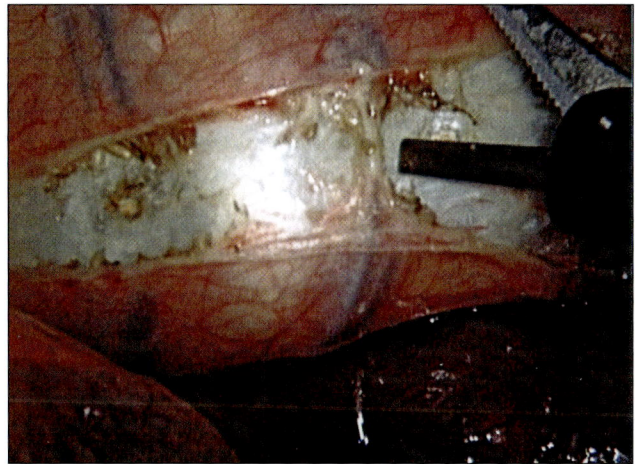

FIGURE 8

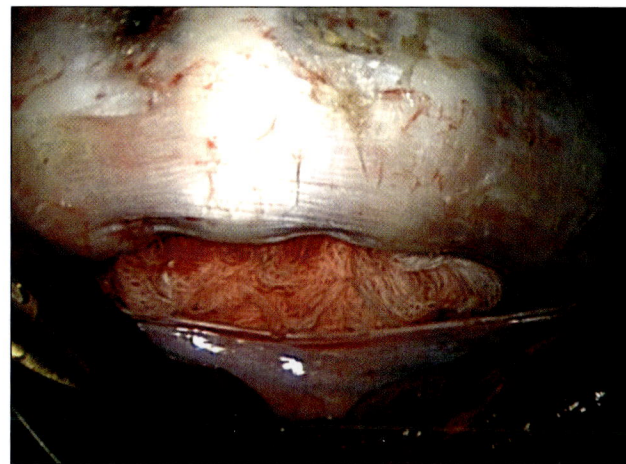

FIGURE 9

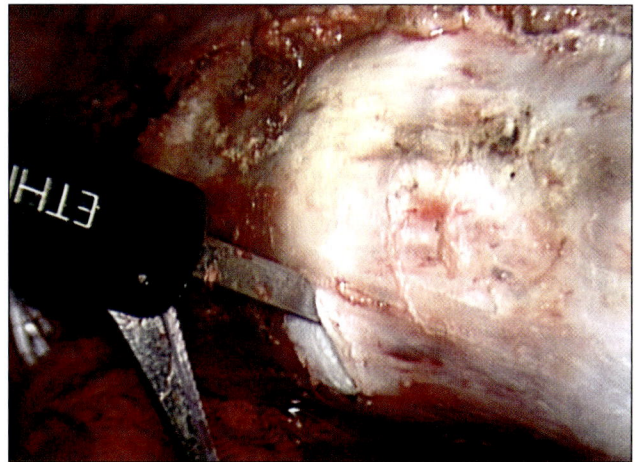

FIGURE 10

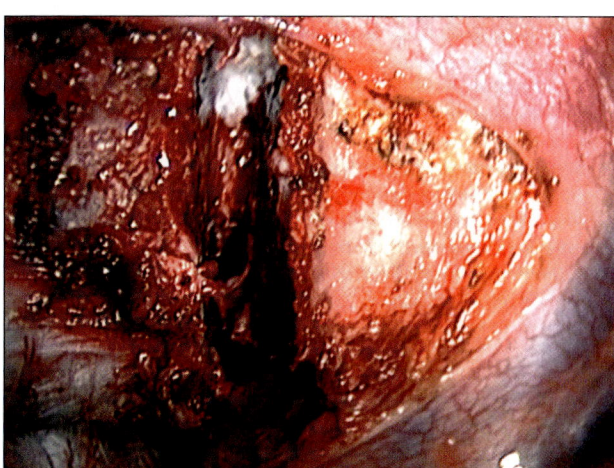

FIGURE 11

PEARLS

- *Often a nutrient foramen will be discovered about 1 cm anterior to the rib head and must be cauterized and packed with bone wax. This can be used to mark the insertion site of the screw.*

- *When checking the alignment and placement of the screws, it is often helpful to look directly through one of the portals at the K-wire or screw. A nasal speculum may be used to hold the portal open.*

PITFALLS

- *A starting point that is too anterior will tend to direct the screw posteriorly into the spinal canal.*

- *Screw pullout may occur (especially at the ends) if the screw is not in the center of the vertebral body. The most cephalad screw should be placed just caudal to the cephalad end plate to provide maximal purchase.*

- *Screws must be aligned in all planes. Be careful to place the second screw in line with the first screw and the proposed site of the most distal screw. Each screw must be the same height as the adjacent screw.*

- *When choosing a rod length, anticipate 1–1.5 cm of shortening due to compression.*

Instrumentation/ Implantation

- 15-mm disposable canula with blunt trocar
- Bone graft funnel and plunger
- Malleable rod or rod length gauge
- Rod reduction tool

Controversies

- Some surgeons prefer to use cannulated taps over a guidewire. This carries the additional danger of unintentional wire advancement into the contralateral chest if care is taken not to prevent this during tapping and screw insertion.

STEP 3: INSTRUMENTATION AND INSERTION OF STRUCTURAL GRAFT (FOR CASES WITH ANTERIOR INSTRUMENTATION)

- The Surgicel sponge is removed and a fibular ring allograft that has been trimmed to fit the interspaces distal to T11 is inserted (Fig. 12). Morselized autograft is inserted around the allograft with a special funnel.

- The posterior portals must be checked and established next for screw insertion from a perfectly lateral direction. Previously placed 11.5-mm cannulas will be exchanged for 15-mm cannulas (posterior portals only). All posterior portals lie roughly in the posterior axillary line.
  - A 0.062-inch K-wire is placed into the second most proximal vertebral body. It must be straight vertical in all planes. This is the center of the proximal portal and should be in about the center of an interspace so that the vertebrae proximal and distal can be placed through the same skin and fascial incision. The proximal portal will be used for the top three vertebrae, the middle for the middle two or three, and the distal for the bottom three.
  - The next K-wire should be placed into the center disk if an even number of vertebrae will be fused or the center vertebral body if an odd number will be fused. The final K-wire should be placed through the distal portal into the second most distal vertebral body.
  - The position of all K-wires is checked with an AP fluoroscopic view.

- The most proximal screw is placed first. The HS is used to trim any remaining pleura back to the rib head. All screws should be started about 8–10 mm anterior to the rib head and oriented straight across the anterior vertebral body parallel to the end plates.
  - An awl is inserted to create a starting hole. Next the calibrated tap is used to drill and tap the hole and get an idea of the required depth by feeling the second cortex. Depth is checked with the ball-tipped depth gauge and the screw is inserted.
  - A blunt-tipped screw should have one or two threads protruding from the far cortex. After placement of the first screw, the second screw is placed in an identical fashion. The portal must be re-established over the next most distal rib through the same skin incision.
  - After the first two screws are placed, an alignment guide may be placed to determine the starting position for the third and subsequent screws. After all the screws have been placed (Fig. 13), the C-arm is used to check screw placement on orthogonal views.

- Next, the malleable rod guide should be bent in a Z shape and inserted into the most distal portal. The length of the rod should be judged from this, keeping in mind that compression will be performed.
  - The rod guide is removed, and a rod is cut to length and contoured in slight kyphosis and a degree of scoliosis that is thought to be left after the correction. The rod is placed through the distal portal and locked into the most proximal screw using an end cap. The approximator is used, if needed, to lock the rod into the next screw with an end cap.
  - The first end cap is tightened to lock the rod rotation and torqued using the torque wrench and anti-torque device. The rod is inserted and locked into place in the subsequent screw, reducing the curve in a cantilever fashion.
  - In Figure 14A, a spinal rod is being cantilevered into the distal screws with an endoscopic approximator. A closure

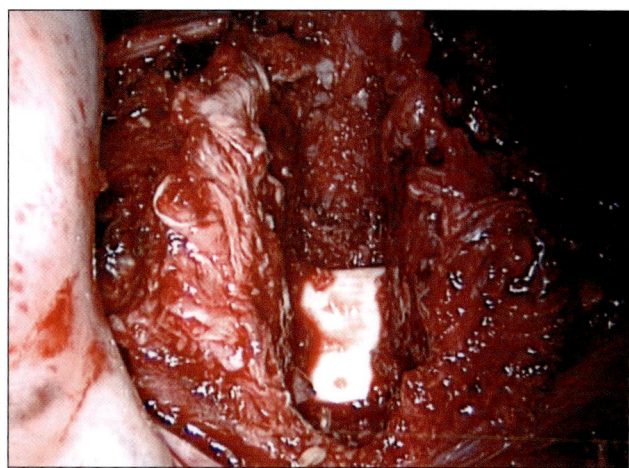

FIGURE 12

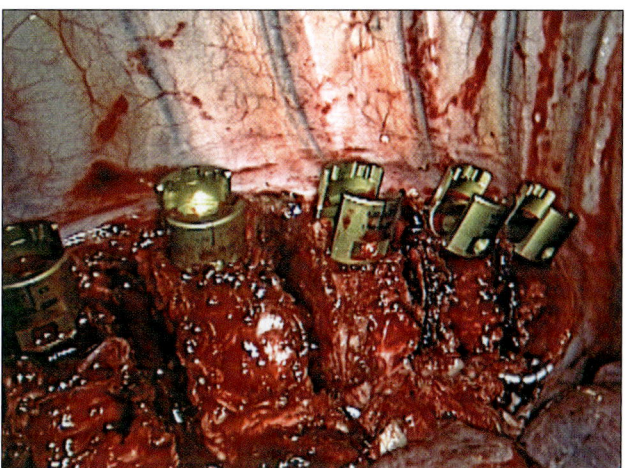

FIGURE 13

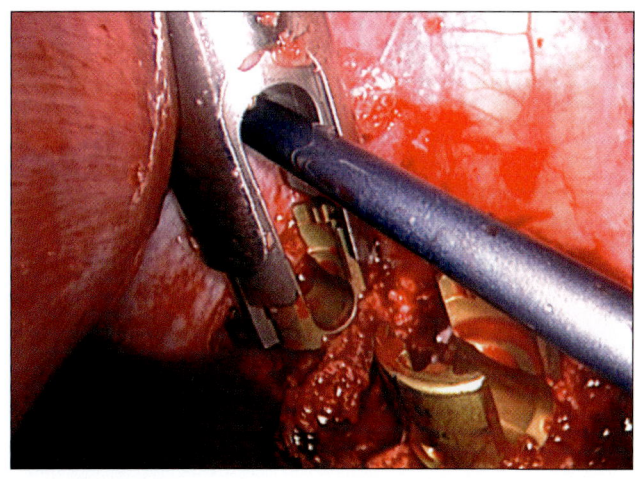

A

FIGURE 14

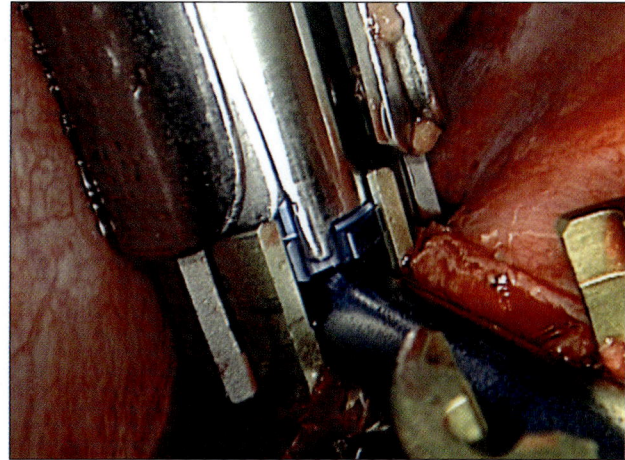

B

mechanism is used to lock the rod into the screw head (Fig. 14B).

- The Surgicel is removed from the most proximal disk space, and a mixture of cancellous autograft and demineralized bone matrix is inserted into the space using the special funnel. Compression is applied across the top two screws and the end caps are tightened. Bone graft is inserted into the adjacent disk space and then the next end cap is compressed and tightened.
- This sequence is continued for the remainder of the screws.

STEP 4: CLOSURE

- The pleura is closed with an Endostitch device from distal to proximal (Fig. 15).
- The chest cavity is irrigated and any remaining bits of disk are removed. A 20 Fr chest tube is inserted from the distal posterior portal and secured in place with a Monocryl suture.
- The fascia is closed with 2-0 Vicryl and the skin with 3-0 Monocryl.
- The chest tube is connected to 20 cm H_2O suction.

POSTOPERATIVE CARE AND EXPECTED OUTCOMES

- The patient is extubated and brought to the intensive care unit or floor.
- The chest tube is typically removed on postoperative day 2 or 3 when the drainage is serous and less than 75 ml per 8-hour period.
- The patient is typically discharged on postoperative day 5 and wears a custom-molded thoracolumbosacral orthosis for 3 months. The patient is restricted from running for 3 months and high-impact activity or gymnastics until solid fusion is obtained (~ 12 months).
- The patient can expect about 10–20% more correction than that observed on the preoperative bending radiographs and a slight increase in the thoracic kyphosis.
- Figure 16 shows postoperative standing PA (Fig. 16A) and lateral (Fig. 16B) radiographs of the Lenke 1A patient seen in Figures 1 and 2 at 1 year after thoracoscopic anterior spinal instrumentation and fusion from T6 to L1; the clinical photograph in Figure 17 was also taken 1 year after surgery.
- Figure 18 shows the appearance of the scars in this patient 2 months (Fig. 18A) and 2 years (Fig. 18B) after thoracoscopic surgery.

Instrumentation/ Implantation

- Endostitch Autosuture (US Surgical)

PEARLS

- *Maintain the chest tube until the drainage is less than 1 ml/kg of body weight per 12 hours.*
- *Limit activity with a brace to reduce the risk of implant loosening, rod failure, and pseudarthrosis.*

PITFALLS

- *Despite the small incisions, this remains major surgery and the patients must understand and comply with activity restrictions until a fusion is achieved.*

Complications

- Intraoperative complications include excessive bleeding and injury to the great vessels, lung, spinal cord, thoracic duct, and diaphragm.
- Postoperative complications include screw pullout, rod breakage, nonunion, and excessive kyphosis.

Controversies

- Some surgeons do not advocate the need for a brace postoperatively, and activity restrictions are variable.

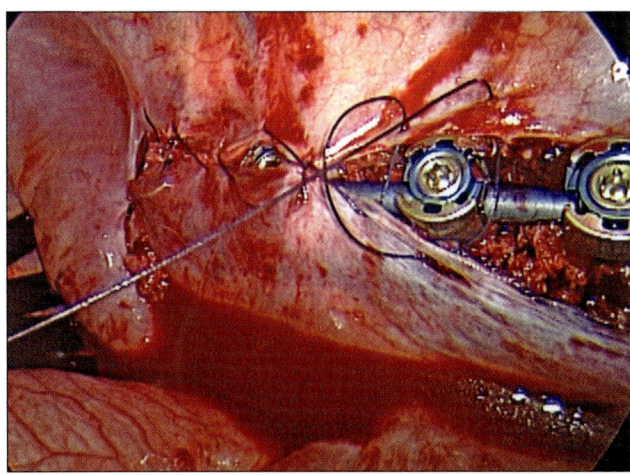
FIGURE 15

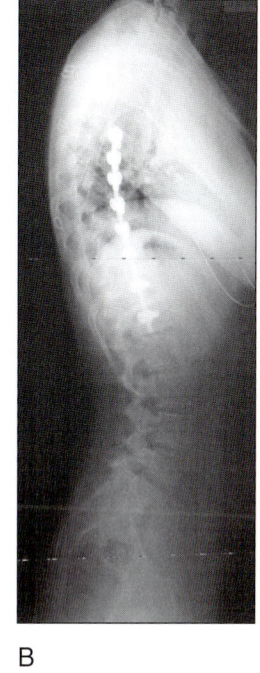

A
B
FIGURE 16

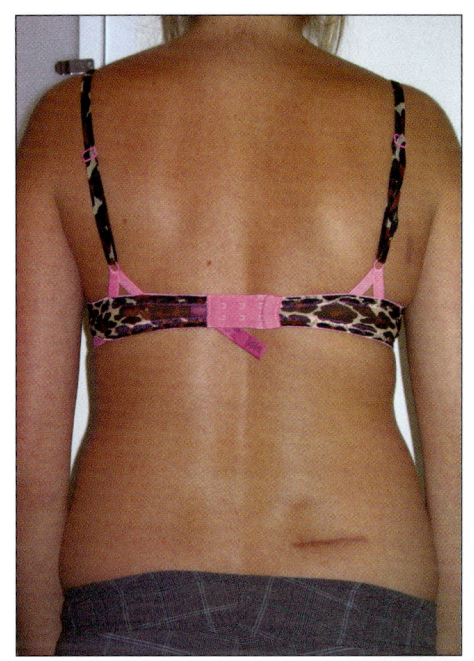
FIGURE 17

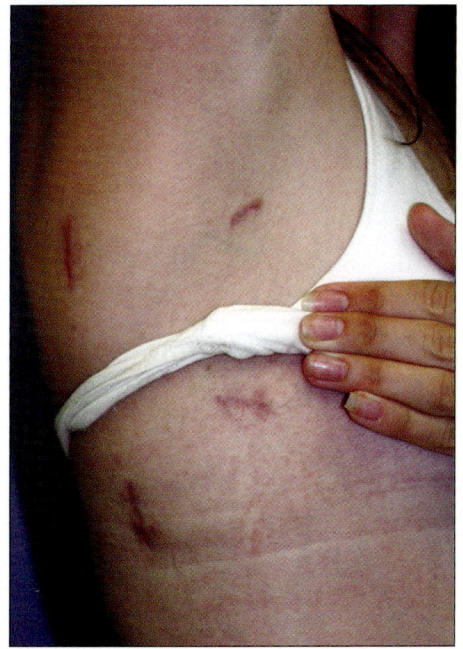
A

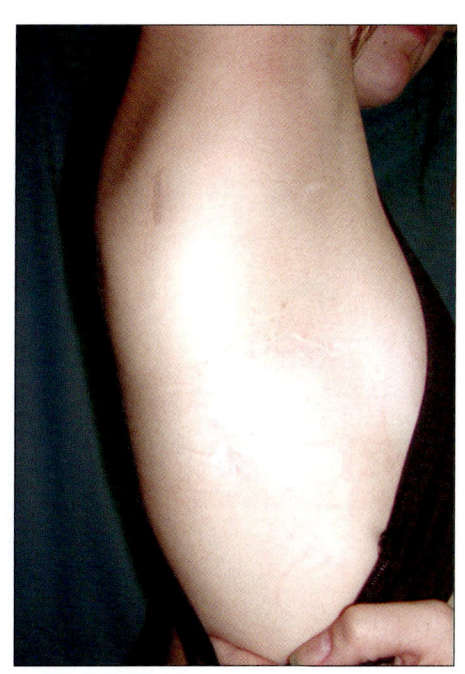
B

FIGURE 18

EVIDENCE

Early SD, Newton PO, White KK, Wenger DR, Mubarak SJ. The feasibility of anterior thoracoscopic spine surgery in children under 30 kilograms. Spine. 2002;27: 2368–73.

Thoracoscopic release and fusion (uninstrumented) was studied in patients under and over 30 kg. Smaller children had greater challenges, such as decreased working space within the chest and difficulties of selective intubation. Although the outcomes were similar in both groups, small children (under 20 kg) should remain a relative contraindication to thoracoscopic surgery, especially if surgeons are not extremely experienced with this procedure.

Huitema GC, Cornips EM, Castelijns MH, van Ooij A, van Santbrink H, van Rhijn LW. The position of the aorta relative to the spine: is it mobile or not? Spine. 2007; 32:1259–64.

This anatomic study utilized preoperative CT scans of patients in the supine and prone positions to document the position of the descending aorta relative to the spine. The aorta crosses toward the midline at T9-12, and its location moves more anterior (and the crossing point more proximal) as the patient is moved from the supine to the prone position.

Kishan S, Bastrom T, Betz RR, Lenke LG, Lowe TG, Clements D, D'Andrea L, Sucato DJ, Newton PO. Thoracoscopic scoliosis surgery affects pulmonary function less than thoracotomy at 2 years postsurgery. Spine. 2007;32:453–8.

This prospective study showed a substantial advantage to the thoracoscopic approach compared to open thoracotomy with regard to pulmonary function.

Lonner BS, Kondrachov D, Siddiqi F, Hayes V, Scharf C. Thoracoscopic spinal fusion compared with posterior spinal fusion for the treatment of thoracic adolescent idiopathic scoliosis. J Bone Joint Surg [Am]. 2006;88:1022–34.

This retrospective study of 28 patients who underwent thoracoscopic anterior spinal fusion compared to 23 patients who underwent posterior spinal fusion demonstrated better coronal and sagittal correction in the anterior group as well as an average savings of 3.5 levels of fusion. There was less blood loss and need for transfusion in the thoracoscopic group. The thoracoscopic operative time was nearly twice that of the posterior spinal fusion time.

Newton PO, Upasani VV, Lhamby J, Ugrinow VL, Pawelek JB, Bastrom TP. Surgical treatment of main thoracic scoliosis with thoracoscopic anterior instrumentation: a five-year follow-up study. J Bone Joint Surg [Am]. 2008;90:2077–89.

A cohort of 41 patients who underwent thoracoscopic anterior instrumentation was followed for a minimum of 5 years. There were no major intraoperative complications, and radiographic results were comparable to results reported for posterior spinal fusion and open anterior spinal fusion. There were three patients (7.3%) with rod failure and three patients who required revision to posterior spinal fusion.

Newton PO, White KK, Faro F, Gaynor T. The success of thoracoscopic anterior fusion in a consecutive series of 112 pediatric spinal deformity cases. Spine. 2005;30: 392–8.

The authors presented a retrospective review of 112 patients with a minimum of 2-year follow-up treated for scoliosis from a variety of etiologies. For this experienced surgeon, average operative time was 160 ± 41 minutes to excise and bone graft an average of 7 ± 2 discs, with an average blood loss of 285 ± 303 ml. Fourteen percent of the patients had perioperative respiratory complications that varied from atelectasis to chylothorax. There were no long-term complications associated with the anterior surgery. Evidence of a "solid" anterior arthrodesis (with > 50% filling of the disk space) was present radiographically in 75% of the disk spaces.

Reddi V, Clarke DV Jr, Arlet V. Anterior thoracoscopic instrumentation in adolescent idiopathic scoliosis: a systematic review. Spine. 2008;33:1986–94.

The authors presented a meta-analysis of thoracoscopic versus posterior spinal fusion. This study concluded that radiographic results are comparable, cosmesis is superior, operative and intensive care unit time is greater, and there are increased complications in the thoracoscopic group.

Sucato DJ, Kassab F, Dempsey M. Analysis of screw placement relative to the aorta and spinal canal following anterior instrumentation for thoracic idiopathic scoliosis. Spine. 2004;29:554–9; discussion 559.

Analysis of postoperative CT scans in 14 patients who underwent thoracoscopic instrumented fusion for right thoracic scoliosis demonstrated the proximity of screw tips to the aorta. The average distance from the posterior aspect of the screw to the spinal canal was 5.3 mm (range, 1.2–11.4 mm). Seventy-eight screws (73.6%) were distant from the aorta, 15 (14.2%) were adjacent to the aorta, and there were 13 screws (12.3%) that were thought to create a contour deformity of the aorta. There were no vascular complications at 2 years after surgery.

Yoon SH, Ugrinow VL, Upasani VV, Pawelek JB, Newton PO. Comparison between 4.0-mm stainless steel and 4.75-mm titanium alloy single-rod spinal instrumentation for anterior thoracoscopic scoliosis surgery. Spine. 2008;33:2173–8.

This paper is a single-surgeon retrospective clinical comparison of stainless steel and titanium rods. At a minimum of 2 years' follow-up, five patients (21%) in the stainless steel group had a pseudarthrosis, three (13%) experienced rod failure, and two (8%) required a revision posterior spinal fusion. In the titanium group, two patients (8%) had a pseudarthrosis, and no patient experienced rod failure or required a revision procedure. The authors concluded that titanium rods had fewer complications in this application.

INDEX

Note: Page numbers followed by f refer to figures; page numbers followed by b refer to boxes.